PERSPECTIVES IN PEDIATRIC CARDIOLOGY

Series Editor
Robert H. Anderson, M.D.

PERSPECTIVES IN PEDIATRIC CARDIOLOGY

Volume 3

Pediatric Cardiac Catheterization

Editors

William H. Neches, M.D.
Professor
University of Pittsburgh School of
Medicine
Children's Hospital of Pittsburgh
Cardiology Division
Pittsburgh, Pennsylvania

Sang C. Park, M.D.
Professor
University of Pittsburgh School of
Medicine
Children's Hospital of Pittsburgh
Cardiology Division
Pittsburgh, Pennsylvania

J. R. Zuberbuhler, M.D.
Professor
University of Pittsburgh School of
Medicine
Children's Hospital of Pittsburgh
Cardiology Division
Pittsburgh, Pennsylvania

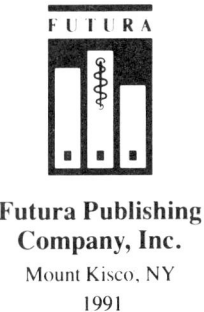

**Futura Publishing
Company, Inc.**
Mount Kisco, NY
1991

Dedication

This book is dedicated to our wives, Ellen, Sun and Jan, as well as the wives of all of our associates, who over the years have provided support and encouragement in all of our endeavors.

Contributors

Lee B. Beerman, M.D.
Associate Professor, University of Pittsburgh School of Medicine, Children's Hospital of Pittsburgh, Cardiology Division, Pittsburgh, Pennsylvania

José A. Ettedgui, M.D.
Associate Professor, University of Pittsburgh School of Medicine, Children's Hospital of Pittsburgh, Cardiology Division, Pittsburgh, Pennsylvania

Donald R. Fischer, M.D.
Associate Professor, University of Pittsburgh School of Medicine, Children's Hospital of Pittsburgh, Cardiology Division, Pittsburgh, Pennsylvania

F. Jay Fricker, M.D.
Associate Professor, University of Pittsburgh School of Medicine, Children's Hospital of Pittsburgh, Cardiology Division, Pittsburgh, Pennsylvania

Polly Grimminger, R.N.
Staff Nurse, Children's Hospital of Pittsburgh, Pittsburgh, Pennsylvania

Cora C. Lenox, M.D.
Professor Emeritus, University of Pittsburgh School of Medicine, Children's Hospital of Pittsburgh, Cardiology Division, Pittsburgh, Pennsylvania

Robert A. Mathews, M.D.
Senior Director, Regulatory Affairs, Merck, Sharp and Dohme Research Laboratories, West Point, Pennsylvania

William H. Neches, M.D.
Professor, University of Pittsburgh School of Medicine, Children's Hospital of Pittsburgh, Cardiology Division, Pittsburgh, Pennsylvania

Elfriede Pahl, M.D.
Associate Professor, University of Pittsburgh School of Medicine, Children's Hospital of Pittsburgh, Cardiology Division, Pittsburgh, Pennsylvania

Sang C. Park, M.D.
Professor, University of Pittsburgh School of Medicine, Children's Hospital of Pittsburgh, Cardiology Division, Pittsburgh, Pennsylvania

Richard A. Zoltun, R.Ph.
Director, Cardiac Catheterization Laboratory, Children's Hospital of Pittsburgh, Clinical Instructor, Pediatrics, University of Pittsburgh School of Medicine, Pittsburgh, Pennsylvania

J. R. Zuberbuhler, M.D.
Professor, University of Pittsburgh School of Medicine, Children's Hospital of Pittsburgh, Cardiology Division, Pittsburgh, Pennsylvania

Preface and Acknowledgments

The practice of pediatric cardiology has become increasingly complex over the last few decades. Recent technological advances have provided new insight into the function of the normal, as well as the abnormal, cardiovascular system, but these developments have made it difficult for the physician who has an interest in cardiovascular disease to remain knowledgeable in all areas. This is not only true of the family practitioner, internist, or pediatrician, but also of the pediatric and adult cardiologist and the cardiovascular surgeon as well.

Recent developments in the areas of cardiac catheterization, echocardiography, nuclear cardiology, and exercise physiology have enabled more precise anatomic diagnosis and functional assessment than has heretofore been possible. To these diagnostic advances must be added major therapeutic advances in cardiology and in cardiovascular surgery: interventional catheterization procedures, microsurgical techniques, new operative procedures, and the widespread use of profound hypothermia with circulatory arrest for the repair of cardiovascular anomalies in infants and young children. Last, but not least, are the advances in postoperative care, especially of the small patient.

At first glance, it would seem that advances in cardiac catheterization have not been as rapid as those in other areas. How-

ever, if one compares the catheterization laboratory of the late 1980s with that of 2 decades ago, great differences will be found. Improvements in image intensifiers, video monitors, and film quality have greatly enhanced resolution, permitting visualization of small structures and vessels while at the same time reducing radiation exposure to both the patient and physician. Radiographic equipment, with its more powerful, high-capacity generators and solid-state electronics, is faster and largely automatic, and yet is more compact. Biplane cineangiocardiographic units were not common even in the latter part of the 1960s, while in the 1980s it is rare for a pediatric laboratory to be without one. In fact, most pediatric cardiologists would agree that cardiac catheterization of infants and young children (and patients of any age with complex cardiac abnormalities) should not be performed in a single plane catheterization laboratory. In addition, with movable "C" or "U" arm, radiographic units, it is now possible to obtain angiograms in multiple complex angles of projection without the need to change the patient's position during the study.

Sensing and recording equipment have also been vastly improved over the last decade. Solid state recording equipment is more compact, is electrically isolated for greater safety and produces high-quality, hard-copy

ix

records immediately. Special catheters are available, even in small sizes, with sensors at the tip that record pressure, flow and sound directly within the patient's heart. Blood gases and oximetry are performed on automated solid state instruments that are accurate, reliable, and use very small volumes of blood. Computers are also well established in the catheterization laboratory and range from microcomputers that are helpful in the calculation of data or that measure cardiac output by indicator or thermal dilution methods, to large dedicated computers for digital subtraction angiography. Computers are available that record and analyze pressure, cardiac output and other signals directly from the recorder, and after other catheterization data are entered manually from a keyboard, a host of hemodynamic parameters are calculated, a hard-copy report printed and the data stored for future use.

It is no longer adequate to insert a catheter into the heart, measure a few pressures and a few oxygen saturations, perform a right or left ventricular angiogram, and consider the catheterization completed. Meticulous attention to detail is the rule rather than the exception. This is especially true in the patient with complex congenital heart disease, where anatomic variations that were once considered relatively unimportant in the overall picture may now have a significant effect on the outcome of cardiovascular surgical procedures. The pediatric cardiologist must thus determine the precise morphology and severity of outflow tract obstruction, valvar abnormalities, septal defects and vascular anomalies. New angiographic views have been developed and existing techniques further refined, all of which help to define cardiovascular anatomy more precisely.

Lastly, techniques have been developed that now make cardiac catheterization a therapeutic modality rather than a purely diagnostic tool. Balloon atrial septostomy, developed by Rashkind and Miller in 1964, has proven to be a relatively safe and effective method for enlargement of an interatrial communicationin in infants at the time of cardiac catheterization. Blade septostomy, developed by Park in the early 1970s, has enabled the enlargement of an interatrial communication even in older children in whom the atrial septum is too thick and stiff to be torn by a balloon catheter alone. The combination of blade septostomy with the transseptal technique has made possible the creation of an interatrial communication in a patient with an intact interatrial septum. Catheter closure of a patent ductus arteriosus has been accomplished using an Ivalon sponge technique, developed by Porstmann in East Germany, or by using a small mechanical "umbrella" device, developed by Rashkind in 1975. Atrial septal defects have also been closed together by catheter introduced mechanical devices developed over the last decade by King et al. and Rashkind. Although these techniques for ductal and atrial septal defect closure hold great promise, they are still experimental and their general clinical applicability has not yet been determined. Percutaneous transluminal angioplasty, developed by Gruentzig in Switzerland, has become widely and successfully used for dilation of stenosed coronary, renal, and ileofemoral arteries in adults. In the pediatric age group this technique has been used successfully to palliate valvar pulmonic and aortic stenoses, coarctation of the aorta and other vascular stenosis.

This proliferation of new equipment and techniques over the last decade has made it increasingly difficult for the cardiologist to acquire necessary information from a single source. Although there are a number of fine books on cardiac catheterization, most have little information about the specifics of cardiac catheterization in infants and young children, or are not recent enough to provide information about the newer techniques. The purpose of this book is to describe the current state of the art of pediatric cardiac catheterization. It is meant to complement and supplement those texts that are already available. *Pediatric Cardiac*

Catheterization consists of two parts. The first part provides specific information as to the principles, techniques, and methods that are used to perform this procedure on patients in the pediatric age group. The second part describes the approach to the catheterization of patients with specific lesions. It is hoped that these this text will serve as a handy reference source for the practicing pediatric cardiologist and as a "how-to" manual that describes many of the tricks of the trade for the pediatric cardiologist in training.

The preparation of a text such as this requires the combined effort of a number of individuals. We gratefully acknowledge the contribution of our associates at Children's Hospital of Pittsburgh for their time and effort in preparing their respective chapters. We would like to thank Beverly Davis for her hard work and long hours in the preparation of this book. We would also like to thank other members of the secretarial staff in the Cardiology Division, in particular Susan Powell, Carol Reder, Judy Doubt, and Joann Turk who assisted in the preparation of some of the manuscripts. Mr. Norman Rabinowitz of the Medical Photography Department, was of great help in preparing the illustrations.

In medicine, as in other aspects of life, knowledge is built by successive steps, but must first have a broad and secure foundation. It is impossible to begin to describe our gratitude to our teachers, friends, and colleagues who have helped provide this foundation. In particular, we thank Dan G. McNamara, M.D., Charles E. Mullins, M.D., Leonard Steinfeld, M.D., the late Richard D. Rowe, M.D., Francis C. Wood, M.D., and Richard S. Bauersfeld, M.D. who have not only been our mentors but have also provided us with the example and the desire to communicate and teach to others the knowledge that we have gained.

William H. Neches, M.D.
Sang C. Park, M.D.
J. R. Zuberbuhler, M.D.

Contents

Contributors   vii
Preface   ix

Part 1: Principles and Techniques

1   The Patient
    William H. Neches, M.D.   1
2   The Catheterization Laboratory
    Richard Zoltun, R.Ph. and Polly Grimminger, R.N.   9
3   Sequence of Procedure and Catheter Choice
    William H. Neches, M.D. 17
4   Catheter Introduction
    William H. Neches, M.D. 25
5   Catheter Manipulation and Guidewire Technique
    William H. Neches, M.D. 51
6   Shunt Detection
    Robert A. Mathews, M.D. 71
7   Pressure Measurement and Resistance Calculations
    Robert A. Mathews, M.D. 81
8   Measurement of Cardiac Output
    F. Jay Fricker, M.D. 93
9   Angiocardiography
    Sang C. Park, M.D. 101
10 Intracardiac Electrophysiology
    Lee B. Beerman, M.D. 121
11 Intracardiac Phonocardiography
    J. R. Zuberbuhler, M.D. 141
12 Atrial Septostomy
    Sang C. Park, M.D. 147
13 Balloon Angioplasty and Valvotomy
    José A. Ettedgui, M.D. 157
14 Special Procedures (Transseptal Puncture, Endomyocardial Biopsy,
    Pericardiocentesis, Foreign Body Retrieval)
    Sang C. Park, M.D. 171
15 Transcatheter Vascular Occlusion
    William H. Neches, M.D. 185

16   Complications Associated with Cardiac Catheterization
       William H. Neches, M.D. 203

Part 2: Approach to Specific Lesions

17   Atrial Septal Defect
       Sang C. Park, M.D. 217
18   Ventricular Septal Defect
       Sang C. Park, M.D. 227
19   Atrioventricular Septal Defect
       Sang C. Park, M.D. 241
20   Patent Ductus Arteriosus
       Donald R. Fischer, M.D. 251
21   Aortopulmonary Window
       Donald R. Fischer, M.D. 257
22   Common Arterial Trunk
       William H. Neches, M.D. 261
23   Pulmonary Stenosis with Intact Ventricular Septum
       William H. Neches, M.D. 267
24   Pulmonary Atresia with Intact Ventricular Septum
       William H. Neches, M.D. 277
25   Tetralogy with Pulmonary Stenosis and/or Atresia
       William H. Neches, M.D. 285
26   Double Outlet Right Ventricle
       Elfriede Pahl, M.D. 301
27   Transposition of the Great Arteries
       Lee B. Beerman, M.D. 309
28   Corrected Transposition
       Lee B. Beerman, M.D. 327
29   Ebsteins' Anomaly of the Tricuspid Valve
       J. R. Zuberbuhler, M.D. 337
30   Atrioventricular Valve Atresia
       Robert A. Mathews, M.D. 345
31   Double Inlet Ventricle
       J. R. Zuberbuhler, M.D. 357
32   Left Heart Inflow Obstruction
       José Ettedgui, M.D. 365
33   Aortic Stenosis and Atresia
       F. Jay Fricker, M.D. 375
34   Interrupted Arch and Coarctation
       F. Jay Fricker, M.D. 389
35   Anomalous Pulmonary Venous Connection
       Cora C. Lenox, M.D. 399
36   Systemic Venous Anomalies
       J. R. Zuberbuhler, M.D. 411
37   Vascular Ring and Pulmonary Sling
       Sang C. Park, M.D. 419

Index 437

Part I
Principles and Techniques

The Patient

William H. Neches, M.D.

In the early years after its introduction as a clinical tool, cardiac catheterization was considered a rather dangerous undertaking, especially in infants and young children. Even in the early 1960s cardiac catheterization was performed with some trepidation in newborns, and patients were sometimes sent to surgery without invasive study. It was thought, with some justification, that catheterization might reduce their chance of surviving surgical intervention. Today, cardiac catheterization and angiocardiography have become indispensable to the pediatric cardiologist. Although primarily a diagnostic procedure, cardiac catheterization may also include therapeutic maneuvers, especially in infants with inadequate mixing at atrial level (e.g., transposition of the great arteries), with obstruction to flow across an atrial septal defect (e.g., in mitral or tricuspid atresia), or with valvar obstruction (e.g., pulmonary or aortic valve stenosis). It is also important to remember that physical examination, noninvasive studies, and cardiac catheterization are complimentary and each provides valuable diagnostic information. A careful evaluation prior to cardiac catheterization provides information that facilitates the cardiac catheterization and makes it a safer, shorter, and more complete procedure.

Today, cardiac catheterization is a relatively safe procedure even in a sick newborn infant when it is performed by a skilled pediatric cardiologist and an experienced team. In general, the cardiac center where this procedure is to be performed should be part of a major pediatric care facility, so that once an accurate anatomic and hemodynamic assessment of an infant's abnormality has been made, the necessary pediatric and surgical care will be readily available.

Indications for Cardiac Catheterization

Cardiac catheterization and angiocardiography are basically diagnostic procedures, enabling rather precise anatomic diagnosis as well as an estimation of the nature and degree of hemodynamic abnormalities. In the older child, cardiac catheterization is usually performed electively as a prelude to cardiac surgery. In some cases, the need for cardiac surgery may be in doubt, even after complete noninvasive evaluation, and catheterization is undertaken to acquire data that are currently unobtainable in any other way. This is particularly true when the differential diagnosis includes a serious congenital abnormality for which cardiac surgery is indicated. As an example, an infant or young child with cardiomegaly and congestive heart failure may seem to have myocarditis or a cardiomyopathy, but cardiac catheterization may be indicated to rule out anomalous origin of a coronary artery, a potentially correctable anomaly.

In the past, the presence of cyanosis and congestive heart failure were strong indications for cardiac catheterization in any age child, while in the newborn, the indication was most pressing, and the study was often done on an emergency basis. The techniques of cross-sectional and Doppler echocardiography have greatly enhanced the ability to make an accurate anatomic diagnosis noninvasively. The combination of this accurate anatomic diagnosis and the use of prostaglandin E_1 to maintain patency of the ductus arteriosus enable deferring cardiac catheterization until an infant has been stabilized and, in some cases, may even eliminate the need for this procedure. It must be remembered, however, that in the hands of a skilled pediatric cardiologist experienced in the care of critically ill newborns, no infant is too sick to undergo cardiac catheterization and subsequent surgery. Although the morbidity and mortality of cardiac catheterization in an extremely sick infant may be considerable, the likelihood of death from the natural progression of the patient's cardiovascular malformation is usually greater.

Lastly, cardiac catheterization is often indicated for the postoperative hemodynamic and anatomic assessment of patients with complex cardiac abnormalities, whether the operative procedure has been reparative or palliative, such as banding of the pulmonary artery or a systemic-to-pulmonary artery anastomosis. In either circumstance, the determination of the anatomic and physiologic effects of the surgical procedure provides important information as to prognosis in the individual patient and is also critical in the general evaluation of the surgical procedure in that institution.

Psychological Concerns

The psychological effects of congenital heart disease on the patient and his family are important concerns of all pediatric cardiologists. Despite the greater risk, "invasiveness," and cost of cardiac surgery, it is surprising to find that many patients and their families find cardiac catheterization to be the more frightening procedure. In view of this, more attention should be paid to the psychological needs of the child undergoing cardiac catheterization and those of his family. These psychological needs can be approached in several ways. Precatheterization parent groups have been in existence for almost two decades at Children's Hospital of Pittsburgh. These groups are held twice monthly, and parents whose children are about to undergo cardiac catheterization are invited to attend. A social worker or a clinical nurse specialist spends the first portion of the group session describing the upcoming hospitalization as well as the cardiac catheterization procedure itself. The parents are shown the catheters used, view a cineangiogram, and are given a tour of the catheterization laboratory. For the remainder of the group session, which generally lasts about 2 hours, the parents interrelate with each other and with the social worker. There is an extensive discussion about ways to approach hospitalization and how much and what kind of information to tell their child about the cardiac catheterization procedure itself. If there are parents in the group whose children have had prior cardiac catheterizations, they can often provide helpful ideas and insights. Many parents have remarked that meeting with the other parents whose children were about to undergo cardiac catheterization was a valuable experience for them. As an outgrowth of the response to the precatheterization group sessions, we have subsequently formed parent groups in a number of the surrounding communities to enable families to experience these interrelationships at times other than the stressful period of cardiac catheterization.

It is also important to focus on the psychological needs of the patients themselves. In children over 2 years of age, some comprehension of the forthcoming event is possible. Obviously the extent of preparation will depend upon many factors, including the age of the child, his or her ability to understand, and the level of sophistication of the parents. A variety of tools are available for patient preparation.

Puppet Therapy or Other Forms of Hospital Play

These are effective means of preparation, especially in the young child. The availability of skilled professional personnel and the distance of the patient's home from the hospital may limit the applicability of this tool. In the young child, play therapy is usually most practical and useful on the day prior to the catheterization procedure.

Booklets or Other Literature

Some literature is available from the American Heart Association and many pediatric cardiology centers have their own descriptive materials and pamphlets. Such literature is generally written for parents and is thus of use mainly for the older child, adolescent, or young adult. Some centers, including our own, have prepared special materials that are directed toward patients in the younger age group. At Children's Hospital of Pittsburgh, a coloring book entitled "So You're Having a Heart Cath" has been developed in conjunction with our parent support group "Heart-to-Heart" and the Western Pennsylvania Heart Association. This book was adapted from a narrative written by a 12-year-old patient describing his experiences surrounding cardiac catheterization. It was illustrated by one of our Heart-to-Heart parents and uses line drawings and cartoon figures to depict the experiences that a child has from the time of admission until discharge. It gives visual representation of the hospital environment and thus enables the younger child to have a mental image of the experiences he will encounter. Having "seen" these things before makes the experience a little less frightening. Such booklets can be given to the child at the time of an outpatient visit or mailed to the family in advance of the child's hospital admission.

Audiovisual Materials

A number of pediatric cardiology centers have prepared film strips or videotapes as a means of preparing the young child and his family for cardiac catheterization. In general, a friendly individual—an animal, clown, or some other figure—is used to take a child through the experience from admission to discharge. Films and tapes are useful, but in general are limited to the time of an office visit, a preadmission group session, or the hospital stay.

Adolescent Materials

Adolescents have specific needs that unfortunately are not readily met by the usual available materials. Adolescents are too sophisticated for the "childish" materials available for younger children and are not sophisticated enough for materials available for adults. They probably need more attention before, during, and after the procedure than any other age group. In general, their fears are not verbalized since they do not wish to behave like small children. Yet the adolescent usually has all of the fears of a young child added to the fears of disfigurement, disability, and death that are found in the adult patient. We have found that it is best to introduce an adolescent to one of the social workers of the cardiology division prior to the time of hospital admission. This often can be done at the time of the outpatient visit when the decision is made to perform a cardiac catheterization. After a brief interview, additional contacts can be initiated either by the patient or by the social worker, depending on the patient's needs. We have prepared instructional materials that are specifically directed toward the adolescent. These are given to the patient at the time of this first interview. At the time the adolescent is admitted for cardiac catheterization, he or she is given a tour of the catheterization facility and an explanation of the procedures that will follow the next day. The adolescent will usually identify this social worker or nurse as a friend and will often gain considerable comfort from the presence of that individual. When indicated, the social worker or nurse accompanies the adolescent to the catheterization laboratory and remains during the procedure.

Parent's Role

Lastly, the importance of the continued presence and support of the parents during any hospitalization is well recognized in most pediatric centers. Although a hospital may not have provisions for a parent to sleep in the same room as the child, any pediatric care facility should provide for round-the-clock parent visitation and should make it as easy as possible for the parents to stay in the hospital area if they so desire.

Premedication

In general, prior to the cardiac catheterization, food or drink is not given after midnight. In the case of infants, it is preferable for the last feeding to be at least 4 hours prior to the procedure. If a procedure is planned for the afternoon, the older patient is usually allowed a liquid breakfast prior to 8 AM.

The goal of premedication is to provide some degree of analgesia and amnesia for the procedure, and there are several acceptable combinations of premedications and dosages. The most important consideration is that the physician be familiar with the effects, complications, and contraindications of the particular medication being used.

At Children's Hospital of Pittsburgh, the following scheme is generally used, although there is some variation with individual cardiologists. Infants under 6 months of age generally require no sedation since a pacifier is usually sufficient to quiet the patient. If desired by the individual cardiologist, morphine sulfate, 0.1 mg/kg intramuscularly, may be used in children from 1 to 6 months of age; others use this drug intramuscularly or intravenously once

the catheter has been inserted, but only on a PRN basis. For patients from 6 months to 1 year of age, morphine sulfate in the same dosage is used intramuscularly as premedication 1 hour prior to the procedure.

After 1 year of age, meperidine, promethazine, and chlorpromazine are given intramuscularly in the following dosages:

1. Meperidine hydrochloride (Demerol)—2 mg/kg
2. Promethazine hydrochloride (Phenergan)—0.5 mg/kg
3. Chlorpromazine (Thorazine)—0.5 mg/kg

These drugs are mixed together in the same syringe. In our laboratory, the maximum dose is 50 mg of meperidine, 12.5 mg of promethazine, and 12.5 mg of chlorpromazine. In larger, very apprehensive patients, the maximum dosage of promethazine and chlorpromazine can be increased to 25 mg of each. In our experience, this combination of intramuscular premedication works quite effectively. In some circumstances, however, it provides too much sedation, especially if patient cooperation is needed in performing a stress exercise study during the cardiac catheterization. In this situation, 5–10 mg of diazepam (Valium) intramuscularly or orally may suffice.

It is sometimes necessary to supplement the premedication during the cardiac catheterization procedure. In the small child, morphine sulfate can be given intravenously in a dose of 0.1 mg/kg. *An important word of caution!* Morphine sulfate comes in a standard vial containing 15 mg/mL, and a dose of 0.5 mg for a 5 kg infant is a volume of only 0.03 mL. For infants and small children, morphine sulfate must *always* be diluted prior to administration.

In older children, either meperidine hydrochloride (1 mg/kg) or diazepam (0.1 mg/kg) can be given intravenously. With special procedures such as transseptal catheterization, small doses of ketamine hydrochloride (1 mg/kg intravenously) can be used.

Because ketamine may cause laryngeal spasm and airway compromise, atropine sulfate (0.01 mg/kg intravenously) is usually given 5–10 minutes before to prevent or minimize this side effect. Ketamine is a potentially hazardous drug and should only be administered by individuals familiar with its use. In the laboratory where this medication is not regularly administered, it may be preferable to have an anesthesiologist come to the catheterization laboratory for the brief period of time that the ketamine is to be utilized.

Immobilization

It is important to properly immobilize the patient on the catheterization table. This is generally accomplished by restraining ankles and wrists with additional restraint across the lower extremities. The small infant is easily restrained by taping the legs to two sandbags (Fig. 1, Top). After the electrocardiographic electrodes have been placed on the legs, a small piece of paper tape is applied over the connector to prevent it from becoming dislodged. Paper tape is then used to secure the child's lower extremities to the sandbags. The tape is applied at mid thigh and lower calf levels. The lower extremities are fixed in slight abduction and with some external rotation. To give some additional stability, a loose tie of gauze is wrapped about each ankle and wrist and each tie is then attached to the table. After electrocardiographic electrodes have been placed on the upper extremities, strips of gauze are applied around the wrists and are tied to the sides of the table (Fig. 1, Bottom). In older infants and children, restraints are placed about the ankles and wrists and secured to the sides of the table (Fig. 2, Top). These restraints are made of cloth and are washable. The inner surface is covered with soft fleece-like material and the band has a Velcro fastener that enables a secure attachment but is adjustable for different sized patients. The lower extremities are then secured using crossing strips of 2-inch adhesive tape (Fig. 2, Bottom). Pieces of 4 x 4 gauze are placed on the patient's legs over the area to be crossed by the adhesive tape, facilitating removal at the completion of the catheterization. In our laboratory, we use an additional retraining device, an 8-inch-wide strip of cloth that is positioned across the lower extremities just above the knee. One end of the cloth has a loop that is secured to one side of the table with a rod. The other end of the cloth strip is attached to a roller device that enables easy adjustment of the tension on the cloth and thus of the pressure on the patient's legs. This device limits the amount of motion of the lower extremities and minimizes the amount of tension on the restraints about the ankles.

The Newborn

Cardiac catheterization is often performed as an urgent or emergency procedure on many newborn infants with cyanosis and/or congestive heart failure. The condition of a cyanotic newborn may be unstable, and once such an infant has been referred to a cardiac center, an accurate anatomic and physiologic assessment should be performed as soon as possible. Prostaglandin E_1 (0.1 μg/kg/min intravenously) is usually started as soon as the diagnosis is suspected. The necessary noninvasive diagnostic procedures should be performed expeditiously, and the infant's temperature, metabolic state, and acid-base balance should be addressed. If the infant's condition cannot be stabilized within a few hours after arriving at a cardiac center, it is likely that treatment of the underlying hemodynamic abnormality is urgently necessary.

In addition to the usual electrocardiographic monitoring in the cardiac catheterization laboratory, it is essential to maintain a neutral thermal environment for the newborn infant. An electronic thermistor rectal

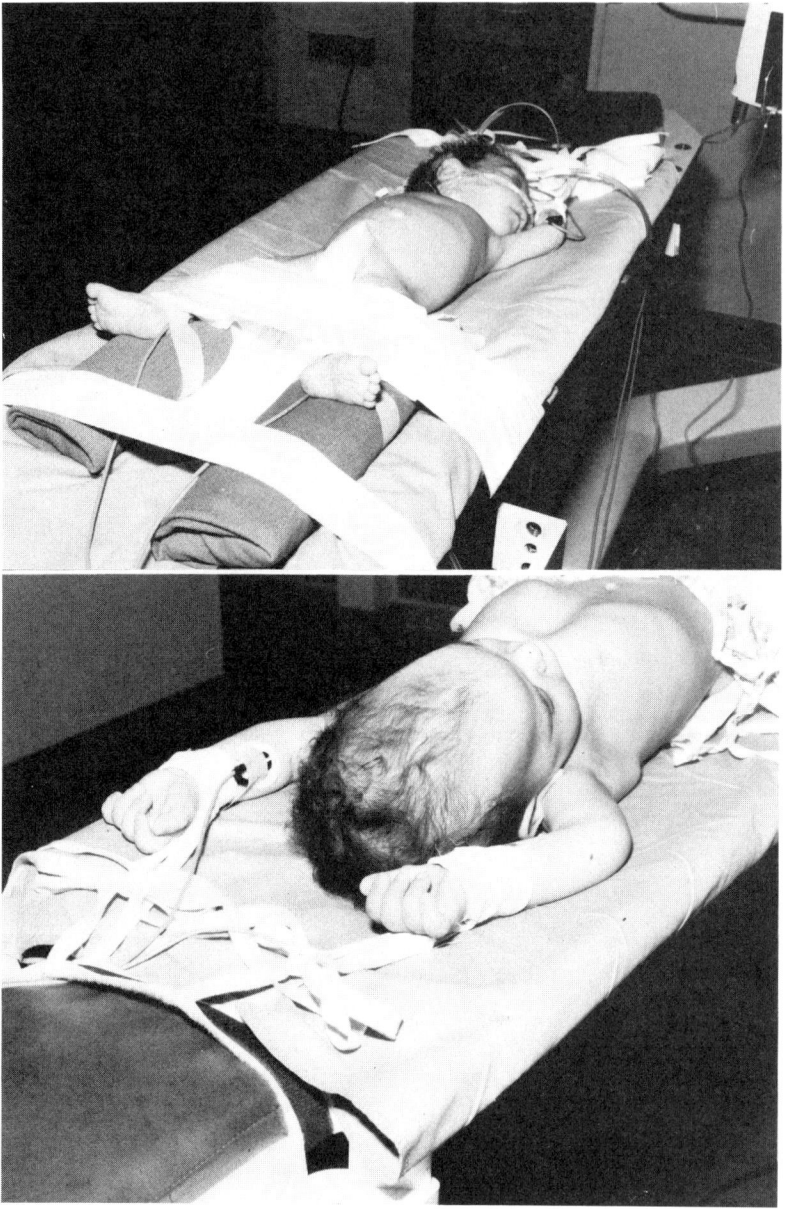

Figure 1. Infant restrained with sandbags.

probe that provides a direct read out is used to monitor temperature during the entire catheterization procedure. Hypothermia is avoided by the use of a warming mattress placed under the patient prior to the beginning of the procedure (Fig. 3) or with a radiant heating device that is affixed to the overhead image-intensifier housing.

Metabolic abnormalities may also adversely effect the newborn infant whose cardiovascular system has already been compromised by hypoxemia or congestive heart failure. Hypocalcemia or hypoglycemia are frequent problems in the newborn and should be corrected prior to cardiac catheterization. In addition, significant abnor-

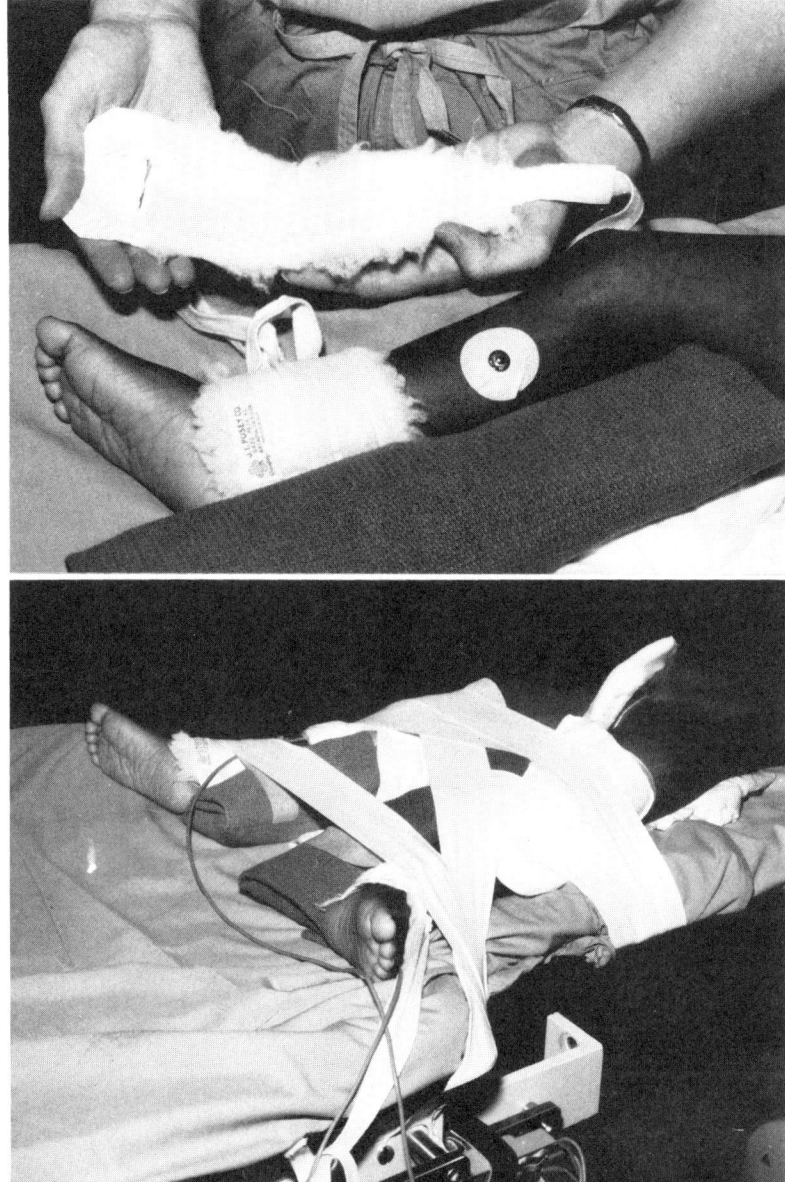

Figure 2. Older child restrained on the table prior to catheterization. Top: Lower extremities—a restraint lined with a soft, fleece-like material is applied to the patient's ankle. Bottom: Cross-taping of the legs using 2-inch adhesive tape.

malities of acid-base equilibrium frequently accompany hypoxemia or congestive heart failure in the newborn and small infant. Thus, blood gas analysis equipment should be available in the catheterization laboratory to enable blood gas and acid-base determinations as often as necessary.

Humidified oxygen is administered to patients with cyanosis and a PO_2 of less than 35 torr. As was indicated previously, prostaglandin E_1 is used to dilate the ductus arteriosus in those patients with severe cyanosis and a congenital cardiac lesion in whom patency of the ductus arteriosus is

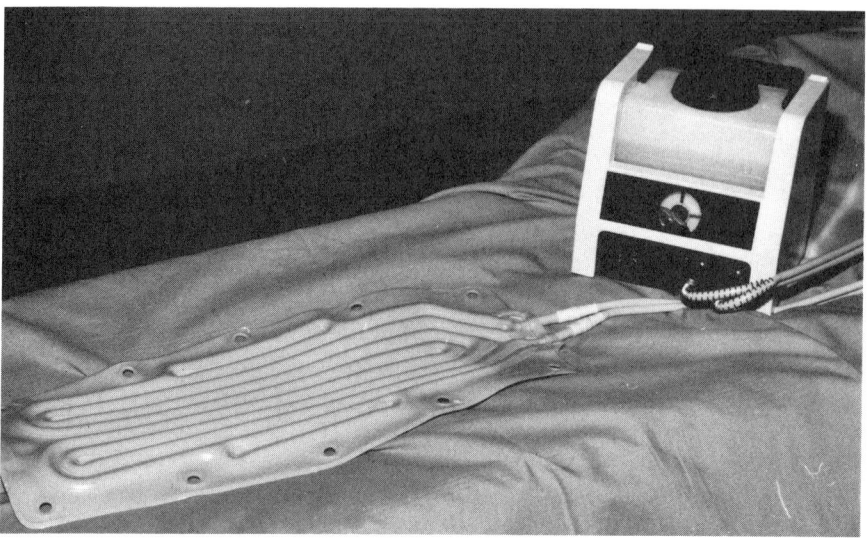

Figure 3. A warming mattress with a thermostatically controlled water heater used to maintain normothermia in neonates.

essential (e.g., pulmonary atresia). This drug should only be utilized with careful monitoring of the patient because hypotension, apnea, and bradycardia may occur during its administration.

Although cardiac catheterization is basically a diagnostic procedure, it may also include therapeutic maneuvers, especially for infants with inadequate mixing at atrial level (transposition of the great arteries), obstruction to flow across an atrial septal defect (mitral atresia or tricuspid atresia), or valvar obstruction (pulmonary or aortic valve stenosis). Balloon atrial septostomy is an effective procedure for enlarging an intra-atrial communication in the newborn and a blade atrial septostomy combined with balloon atrial septostomy has been used in older infants and children. Balloon valvotomy has been used to treat valvar obstruction. These therapeutic procedures are described in detail in Chapters 12 and 13.

2

The Catheterization Laboratory

Richard A. Zoltun, R.Ph. and Polly Grimminger, R.N.

The catheterization laboratory should be efficient and provide a safe environment for both the patient and the laboratory personnel. Ideally, the laboratory should be a dedicated pediatric care facility with no space limitations or budgetary constraints. Unfortunately, this is usually not possible, but this chapter will deal with generalizations about the ideal situation. It will include discussions of appropriate physical layout, the equipment in the laboratory, the materials needed for percutaneous or cutdown cardiac catheterizations, and the duties and responsibilities of the nursing and technical personnel.

Room Design and Layout

If one has the opportunity of designing a catheterization laboratory in a new facility, several factors should be considered in its location.

1. The laboratory should be near an elevator or close to patient access corridors. The access route to the laboratory should avoid patient waiting areas or corridors with high traffic flow.
2. The area immediately adjoining the cardiac catheterization laboratory should be available for support facilities, including a) a clean supply and work room, b) a dark room, and c) a computer room (in automated catheterization laboratories).

Other support areas that add to the convenience and effectiveness of the catheterization laboratory include dressing areas for physicians and technical personnel, film viewing areas with adjacent film storage facilities, and storage areas for linen and laboratory supplies.

The ideal cardiac catheterization laboratory includes a procedure area, a control room, and a separate area for the generator and power modules. A floor space of at least 600 square feet is required, with the procedure area itself needing approximately 500 square feet. The procedure area contains radiographic equipment, the catheterization table, monitors, movable equipment such as the angiographic injector, a defibrillator, exercise equipment, and blood gas analysis units. Storage cabinets, counter space, and work table surfaces are also required. The control room houses recording equipment, radiographic controls, a computer console, and videotape recorders. This area should be accessible both from the catheterization laboratory and from outside the procedure area. Protective, leaded glass windows should be large enough to make all portions of the procedure area visible from the control room. To facilitate communication between the control room and procedure area, either the wall separating the control room from the procedure area should be open at the top, or a microphone or intercom device should be mounted near the table. In the control room area, the x-ray controls should be flush mounted on vertical panels to conserve space. Various counter tops and work areas should also be provided.

Important additional considerations in the design and construction of the cardiac catheterization laboratory are the appropriate shielding of the walls, ceiling, and floor. A minimum ceiling height of 10 feet should be provided and the ceiling should be capable of supporting radiographic equipment, table, monitors, and surgical lights, thus removing as much equipment from the floor area as possible.

The concept of free and easy accessibility to the patient must be of primary concern in placement of equipment in the procedure area. This will influence the location of the patient junction interface to which will be connected cables from the electrocardiographic leads, transducers, and other measuring devices. This will, in turn, determine placement and location of conduits in the floor and ceiling for connecting cabling between the patient junction, recording devices, and monitors. It is also important to pay special attention to the grounding (earthing) system in the room. An equal-potential grounding system, consisting of permanent hard wiring of the equipment table and all electrical equipment outlets to a large grounding buss, is strongly recommended.

Lastly, the type, style, and number of storage cabinets (Fig. 1) and the location of counter and table surfaces and a scrub area for physicians are important considerations during the design of the catheterization laboratory. It is also important to decide on the type, location, and environmental controls of air conditioning and humidity systems.

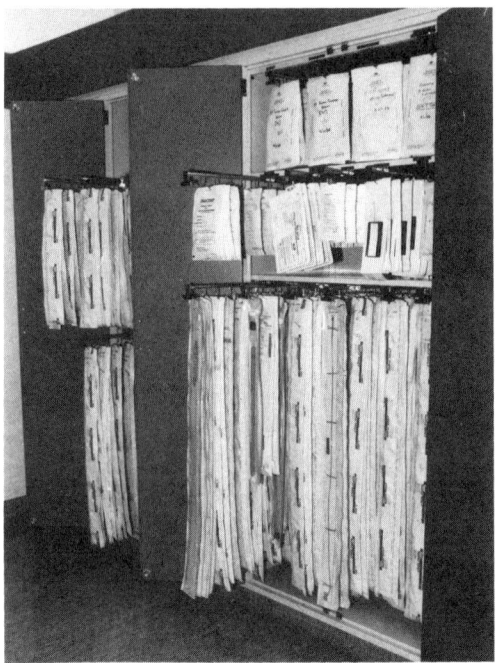

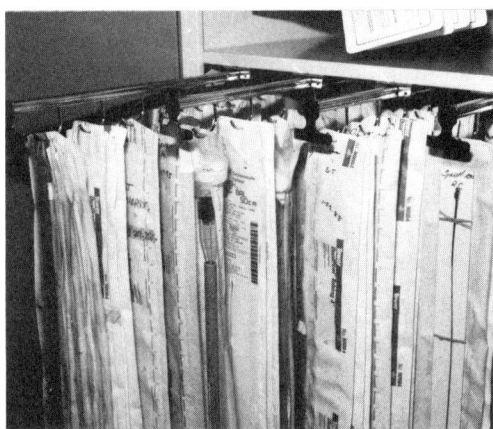

Figure 1. Storage racks for easy access to cardiac catheters. Note that the catheters do not have to be coiled in small packages and can be extended to their full length with this storage system.

Equipment

Radiographic Units

Radiographic equipment is very expensive and makes up the bulk of the cost of a new laboratory. There are a number of man-

ufacturers of high-quality radiographic equipment for the catheterization laboratory. Although initial cost is a major factor, other considerations are very important. A considerable saving in the purchase price is of no value if the catheterization laboratory is frequently "down" because of equipment malfunction. Radiographic equipment is complex and requires expert service and maintenance. In selecting a supplier, it is highly desirable to select a company with an established local office and a reputation for prompt expert service. The physician should plan to visit a few centers where this equipment has been previously installed to see the physical layout of the equipment and to consult with physicians who are using the equipment on a daily basis. If possible, one should visit a center where this manufacturer's equipment has been used for a number of years. This may provide useful information as to long-term reliability and potential for equipment update as design changes are made.

An exhaustive description of radiographic equipment and the technical aspects of its use is beyond the scope of this book. A few important points, however, will be mentioned. An important consideration at the outset is whether the laboratory will be a shared facility or dedicated to pediatric usage. Because the requirements for catheterization of pediatric patients are considerably different than those for adults, some compromises may have to be made if the same laboratory is to be used for both groups of patients. Most pediatric cardiologists would agree that biplane angiographic equipment is mandatory for a pediatric cardiac catheterization laboratory that will care for newborns, small infants, and patients with complex congenital heart disease. Biplane, 35-mm cineangiography is used in most laboratories, but biplane cut film equipment is also available and will be discussed further in the chapter on angiocardiography. "C-arm" or other varieties of movable-arm radiographic equipment enable the physician to obtain oblique- and compound-angle radiographic views without moving the patient, and having this capability in at least one plane is highly desirable. This equipment requires more floor space than standard, fixed-position, anteroposterior and lateral radiographic tubes and it is also more expensive.

The resolving power of the radiographic equipment is another important consideration. It is usually described as the number of line pairs per mm that can be visualized on the photographic image of a calibrated reference grid. Current image intensifiers incorporate rare-earth element output phosphors and are interfaced with high-resolution television tubes. It is important for the pediatric catheterization laboratory to have at least dual-mode capability, usually 6- or 7-inch and 9- or 10-inch modes. The smaller mode provides a magnified image for the smaller patient and the larger permits large-field visualization in older children or adults.

Patient Table

The laboratory table is another important and expensive piece of equipment. Again, compromises may have to be made if the catheterization laboratory is to be used for adults as well as pediatric patients. If coronary artery studies are to be performed, then a tilting, cradle-type table is mandatory, unless a C-arm is available. If the laboratory is only for pediatric use, a flat, floating-top catheterization table is quite satisfactory. Unless C-arms are available, it is helpful to have a table that tilts in its long axis, because this facilitates the obtaining of special angled views. The table-locking mechanism should have both operator- and remote-switch operation. The operator switches may be table mounted or on the floor. We prefer the latter and use a model with three pedal switches: one for fluoroscopy in each plane and one for the table lock. An additional switch is mounted on the housing for angiography.

Multichannel Recorder

There are a number of high-quality, multichannel recording devices available on the market today. Cost, reliability, repair service, and the potential for future updates are important considerations in choosing the best device. It is preferable to purchase a multichannel recording device with the option of adding additional channels as necessary. The additional cost for the capability of adding channels in the future is small compared to the cost of the equipment itself and is good insurance for future needs. A physiologic catheterization laboratory recorder should have at least six input channels and several DC input channels. This combination permits the recording of pressures, indicator dilution curves, intracardiac sound, and high-fidelity pressures using micromanometer-tipped catheters and simple electrophysiologic studies such as His-bundle recordings with simultaneous surface electrocardiograms. As was discussed earlier, current equipment is solid-state and electrically isolated from the patient for safety. The ideal recorder is an optical photographic device that provides immediately available, high-fidelity recordings, at paper speeds up to 200 mm/sec.

Oximeter and Gas Analyzer

The determination of oxygen saturation by oximetry is standard in all cardiac catheterization laboratories. In the pediatric laboratory the device should provide accurate reproducible data from a small volume of blood. Current devices provide a digital readout of hemoglobin and oxygen saturation within 15 to 60 seconds. In addition to oximetry, it is essential that the pediatric cardiac catheterization laboratory have the capability of blood gas analysis as well. Again, current equipment is solid-state and provides rapid digital readout of pH, PCO_2, and PO_2 from a sample of less than 0.5 mL of blood.

Emergency Equipment

Emergency equipment must be readily available in the catheterization laboratory and should be checked daily. A synchronized cardioverter/defibrillator should be no more than one or two steps away from the catheterization table and should be switched on and ready to use during the procedure. Infant-size, as well as adult-size, paddles should be available on the machine, and the appropriate size paddles should be plugged into the device prior to the beginning of the catheterization procedure. Oxygen and suction should be available at the head end of the table and ready for use. A full supply of emergency equipment, such as laryngoscopes, endotracheal tubes, ambubags, suction catheters, etc., should be available a few steps from the table and, again, ready for use at any time. The same also applies to a full line of emergency medication.

Catheterization Laboratory Personnel

Ideally, the catheterization laboratory is staffed with at least three individuals: a nurse, a cardiovascular technician, and a cardiovascular aide. Although the laboratory can be run adequately by two individuals, the third provides a comfort margin for routine simple procedures and an important additional pair of hands when dealing with critically ill patients or performing special studies such as exercise testing. In addition, the third individual provides valuable backup when others are on vacation or are ill. Although each member of a catheterization laboratory technical and nursing team has a specific job description, it is desirable that each person be skilled in all areas. This is particularly important if only one technician or nurse is on call, because he or she must be able to perform all technical functions for an emergency cardiac catheterization during off hours.

Each member of the cardiac catheterization laboratory team has responsibility to the patient and to his or her primary function. In addition, each is responsible for cross-training. Each individual thus functions as both teacher and student: teaching others the elements of his or her primary function and, in turn, learning the functions of all other individuals in the laboratory.

Cardiac Catheterization Laboratory Nurse

This position requires an individual with both nursing and technical skills. The primary responsibility of the nurse is to the patient and this begins when the patient enters the cardiac catheterization laboratory. Because many new and potentially frightening things are happening to the patient from the moment that he or she enters the laboratory, the nurse must serve as a calming and settling influence. In effect, the nurse serves as the mediator between the patient and the catheterization "environment." In addition to introducing the patient to other laboratory personnel, the nurse should explain the various preparatory procedures to

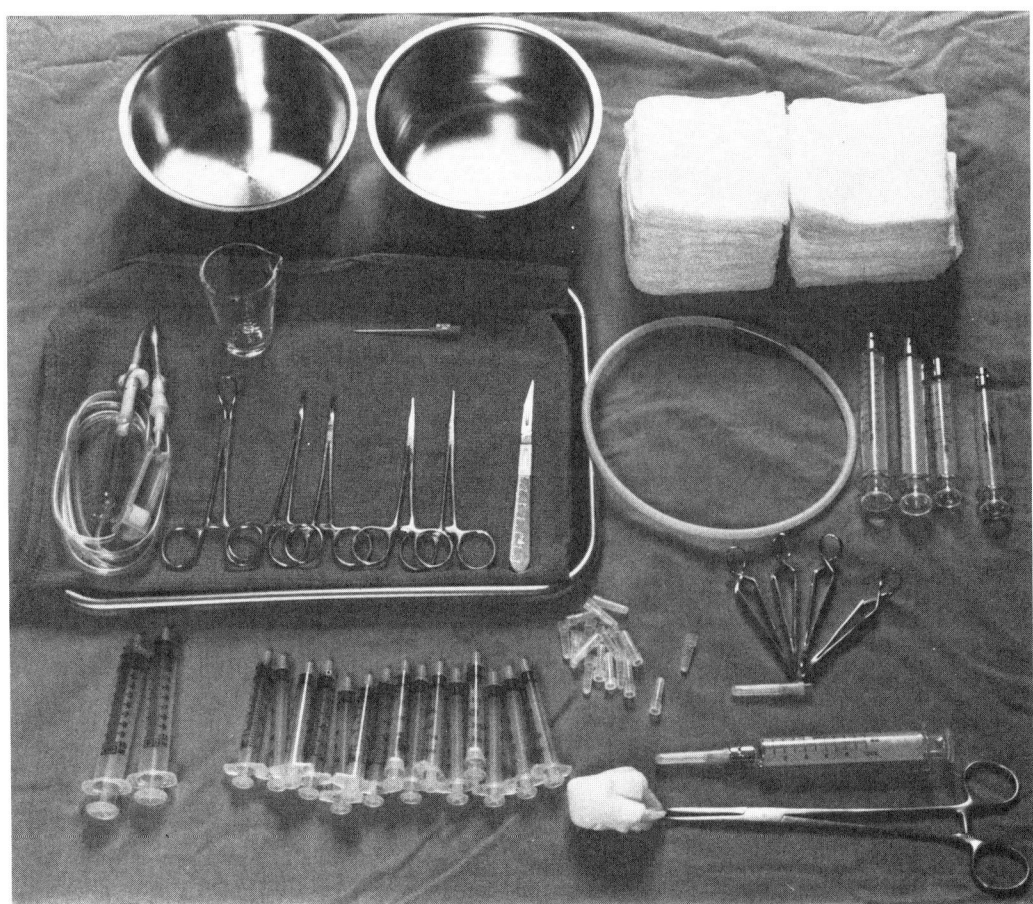

Figure 2. Percutaneous instrument tray. Two 6-inch round stainless-steel solution bowls; 1 sponge stick; 2 straight mosquito hemostats; 2 curved mosquito hemostats; 5 small cross-action Jones towel clamps; 1 5-inch towel clamp; 1 1-oz medicine glass; 1 knife handle; 1 #11 knife blade; 2 percutaneous needles (19-gauge, 1 1/2-inch, short-bevel, thin-wall); 2 20-gauge, 1–inch disposable needle; 1 25-gauge, 1 1/2-inch disposable needles; 15 3-cc disposable syringes; 2 10-cc disposable syringes; 3 10-cc glass syringes; 2 5-cc glass syringes; 1 IV tubing; 1 plasticized linen wrap; 40 4 x 4-inch gauze sponges.

the patient just before they are carried out. At other times during the catheterization, the nurse should be available to relate to the patient as much as possible, to allay anxiety, and to provide reassurance. The nurse also monitors the patient during the procedure and prepares and administers any medication required during the catheterization.

The nurse is responsible for prepara-tion of the sterile catheterization table, the instruments, and the intravenous flushing solutions (Figs. 2 and 3 and Tables 1 and 2). She should be skilled in sterile technique and in the use of all cardiac catheterization instruments. Because she supervises all sterile equipment used, she should have in-timate knowledge of cleaning, packing, ster-ilization, and storage of such equipment. In

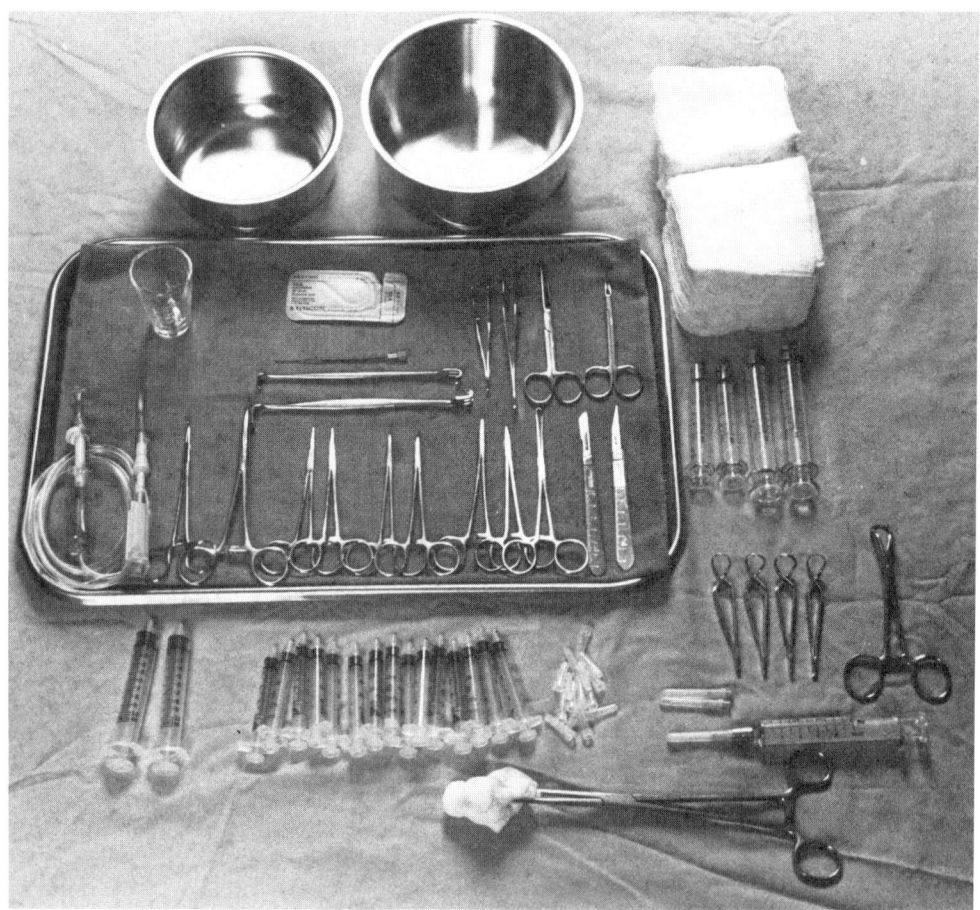

Figure 3. Cutdown instrument tray. Two 6-inch stainless steel solution bowls; 1 sponge stick; 1 Allis forceps; 2 needle holders; 4 curved mosquito hemostats; 3 straight mosquito hemostats; 1 suture scissors; 1 curved iris scissors; 1 right-angle clamp; 5 Jones cross-action towel clamps (small); 1 5-inch towel clamp; 1 Miller-Senn retractor; 1 mouse-tooth (Adson) forceps; 1 iris forceps; 1 1-oz medicine cup; 2 knife handles; 1 #10 knife blade; 1 #11 knife blade; 1 vessel dilator; 1 package vessel loops (silicone vessel holders); 1 package 4–0 silk suture strands; 1 4–0 (or 5–0) silk on skin needle; 2 20-gauge disposable needles; 1 26-gauge, 1/2-inch dis-posable needle; 15 3–cc plastic disposable syringes; 2 10-cc plastic disposable syringes; 3 10-cc glass syringes; 2 5-cc glass syringes; 1 IV tubing; 1 plasticized linen wrap; 40 4 x 4-inch gauze sponges.

Table 1

Items To Be Added to Percutaneous or Cutdown Tray

1	Linen pack*
1	Camera cover (linen or plastic)
1 (or 2)	Pressure transducer(s)
1	Paley stopcock bank (single or double, depending upon number of transducers used)*
1	Injector pack for pressure injector*
2	Plastic steridrapes
1	1,000-cc (or (500-cc) heparinized 5% D/W
1	Surgical lampholder (if cutdown)

* See detail in Table 2.

our laboratory, the nurse is responsible for maintaining the sterile inventory and for ordering new supplies and equipment as consumables are depleted.

Ideally, the nurse should be experi-

Table 2

Detailed Listing of "Packs"

Linen pack:
  8 Hand towels
  1 Rolled sheet (72″ × 72″)
  1 Small sheet (36″ × 36″)
  1 Small fenestrated sheet
Gown Pack:
  1 Hand towel
  1 Surgical scrub gown
Paley stopcock bank:
  1 Modified USCI Paley Manifold—single bank
  1 3-way stopcock with male Luer-Lok rotating tip
  1 3-way female-female to male Luer-Lok tip (left-side) stopcock
  1 1-way stopcock male-female
  2 Knurled nuts
  1 Anesthesia extension tubing—31″ length (Travenol—2C0050)
Transducer Pack:
  1 Statham-Gould p-23 series—ID pressure transducer with reusable plastic dome with Linden fittings

enced in critical care nursing in order to be better able to assist the physician in emergency situations. She should at least be capable of initiating resuscitation, assembling the necessary resuscitation equipment, and preparing and administering emergency medications. Lastly, as was mentioned previously, it is essential that the nurse be able to function as a cardiovascular technician if she is to take night and weekend call.

Cardiovascular Technician

This individual should have intimate knowledge of all the equipment in the cardiac catheterization laboratory. In addition to being able to operate all this equipment, the individual should be capable of teaching the operation to other laboratory personnel. In our laboratory, the cardiovascular technician is responsible for oximetry and blood gas analysis during the initial phase of the catheterization procedure and for operation of the radiographic equipment during angiography. He is also responsible for preparing and calibrating the equipment prior to the procedure and for cleaning and maintenance following catheterization. This individual is also expected to observe the patient during the catheterization procedure and be able to assist if any emergency or therapeutic procedures become necessary.

Cardiovascular Aide

This third support individual in the catheterization laboratory operates the recording equipment, enters data into the cardiac catheterization computer, and maintains the written log or record of the cardiac catheterization procedure. Once a new aide has become sufficiently skilled in the operation of the recording equipment, this individual should then be trained by the other catheterization laboratory personnel in the performance of duties in other areas.

3

Sequence of Procedure and Catheter Choice

William H. Neches, M.D.

To perform a cardiac catheterization that will provide maximum information at minimum risk to the patient, one does not just insert a catheter and subsequently "hope for the best." The physician should carefully plan an approach to the cardiac catheterization in light of the information available from the history, physical examination, and noninvasive studies. In general, after the catheter has been introduced, baseline, resting hemodynamic measurements are made (Table 1), including pressure and oxygen saturation in each cardiac chamber and great artery and determination of cardiac output. Any special studies that are required are then performed, followed by angiocardiography and indicated therapeutic procedures. (These therapeutic maneuvers are described in detail in subsequent chapters.) It is also important to remember that the above sequence of procedures can, and should, be changed under certain circumstances. For instance, it is generally better to record hemodynamic data before performing angiocardiography, because contrast medium affects hemodynamics. However, if one is catheterizing a patient with severe pulmonary stenosis or pulmonary atresia and a previous subclavian-to-pulmonary artery anastomosis, and if the catheter is manipulated into the anastomosis early during the procedure, it is worthwhile to perform selective angiocardiography at that site. It may subsequently be difficult to reenter the anastomosis, and in addition, the

information obtained may be helpful in planning the remainder of the catheterization (e.g., discontinuity between the right and left pulmonary arteries).

Hemodynamic Measurements

The various hemodynamic parameters that are measured during the catheterization are described in Chapters 6 through 8. An end-hole catheter is usually preferable during the initial phase of the cardiac catheterization. Such a catheter is necessary for the measurement of pulmonary artery wedge pressure and in obtaining wedge blood for oximetry. An end-hole catheter is also safer for exploring the interior of the heart and in making difficult passes, because the pressure wave will become damped if the catheter tip is against the wall or trapped between trabeculae. In addition, a guidewire can be used if difficulty is encountered in entering the pulmonary artery. (This technique is described in detail in Chapter 5.) Lastly, an end-hole catheter enables more precise determination of the site of a gradient within the heart or a great artery.

A number of end-hole catheters are available, including the Lehman, the Cournand, and the Swan-Ganz type, flow-directed balloon catheters (Fig. 1). The Goodale-Lubin catheter has an end hole and two distal side holes. Because the side holes are very close to the tip, they are occluded when

Table 1

Catheterization Outline

A. Resting hemodynamics
   1. Shunt determination
   2. Pressure determinations
   3. Resistance calculations
   4. Cardiac output measurement
B. Special studies
   1. Intracardiac electrocardiography
   2. Intracardiac phonocardiography
   3. Exercise studies
   4. Miscellaneous—flow studies, drug
      studies, research protocols, etc.
C. Angiocardiography
D. Therapeutic procedures

the catheter is in the wedge position, and accurate wedge pressure and oxygen saturation can be obtained. Some physicians prefer the Goodale-Lubin catheter for routine hemodynamic measurements at the beginning of the catheterization, because it can be used for wedge pressure measurement like the end-hole catheter but pressures are not dampened and it is still possible to withdraw blood for oximetry when the tip of the catheter is against the myocardial wall. There are a number of disadvantages, however, in using this catheter. The lack of damping of the pressure contour when the catheter is against the myocardial wall removes a safety factor during catheter manipulation. Also, the side holes of this catheter make it somewhat less precise in identifying the site of a gradient.

Most pediatric cardiac catheterizations are now performed using a femoral approach. The pulmonary artery is the most difficult area to enter from this route. It is therefore preferable to attempt this catheter pass at the beginning of the catheterization procedure, because a catheter becomes softer and more difficult to maneuver with time. After the main pulmonary artery has been entered, the catheter is maneuvered into one of the branch pulmonary arteries and then advanced as distally as possible. Once the catheter has been "wedged" into a pe-

ripheral pulmonary artery branch, the catheter will no longer transmit pulmonary artery pressure, but rather the pressure from a pulmonary vein and the left atrium.

Once a catheter has been inserted into the pulmonary artery wedge position a blood sample is obtained. Only gentle traction should be applied to the syringe barrel because vigorous traction pulls the arterial wall against the tip of the catheter. It is sometimes easier to obtain a wedge sample with a glass rather than a plastic syringe, because there is less resistance with the glass variety. A saturation of over 95% confirms a wedge position. After the wedge blood sample is obtained, the catheter is gently flushed and pressure is recorded.

Once the pulmonary artery wedge pressure and saturation have been obtained, the catheter is withdrawn to the branch pulmonary artery and the pressure and saturation sequence is again repeated. The contralateral pulmonary artery is then entered, and a blood sample obtained. The catheter is then withdrawn successively to the main pulmonary artery, right ventricle, and right atrium, sampling at each site.

At this point, the evaluation of left-sided hemodynamics is undertaken. If an interatrial communication is present, entry to the left-sided chambers can be accomplished with the venous catheter. An angiographic catheter is used, because an end-hole catheter is not needed for the left-sided study and angiography will probably be performed after the catheter is inserted into the left ventricle.

It must be remembered that the above outline is a guide for the catheterization of individuals with normally connected atria, ventricles, and great arteries. If there is severe stenosis or atresia of a valve or subvalvular area, or if there is complex congenital heart disease, this approach must often be modified. For example, in a patient with tetralogy of Fallot with severe pulmonary stenosis, it may be difficult to traverse the stenosis with a catheter. In this situation, it may be better and safer to proceed to

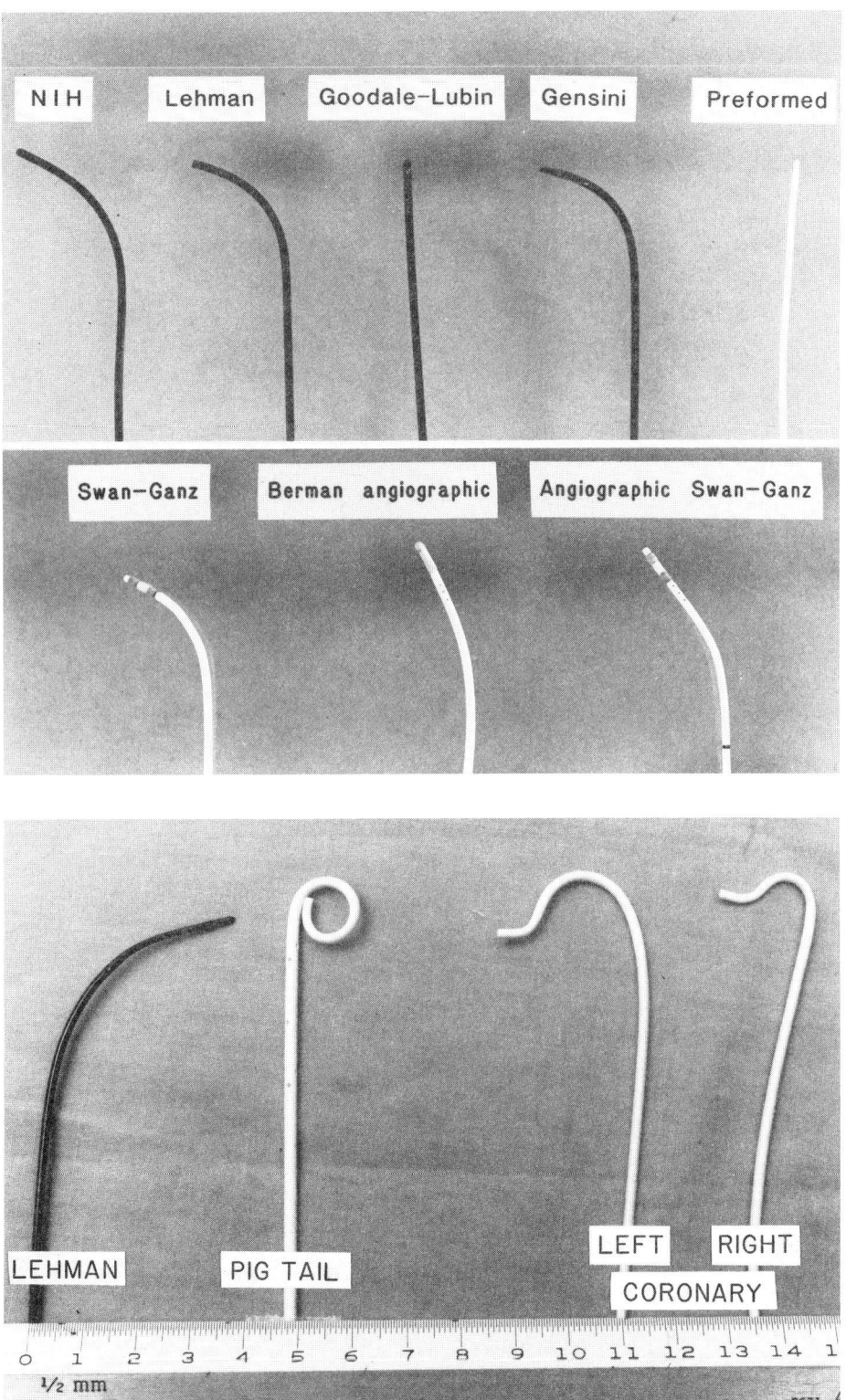

Figure 1. Top: Various types of cardiac catheters. Middle: Flow-directed cardiac catheters. Bottom: Other angiographic catheters.

other measurements and defer entry into the pulmonary circulation until later during the procedure. After the other hemodynamics have been measured, a small, selective hand injection of contrast media just below the region of stenosis may delineate it adequately. If passage of the catheter into the pulmonary artery is necessary and it appears that it may be possible to traverse the obstruction, the physician may then proceed with a guidewire or a flow-directed catheter, aided by the knowledge of the anatomy gained from the angiogram. As another example, in a patient with severe, isolated, valvar pulmonary stenosis with systemic or suprasystemic pressure in the right ventricle, traversing the area of pulmonary stenosis with the catheter for an extended period of time may significantly increase obstruction and thereby decrease forward flow. The resulting reduction of cardiac output may initially result in tachycardia, which then may progress to bradycardia and hypotension. In such cases, it is preferable to complete other hemodynamic measurements prior to attempting to enter the pulmonary artery.

In most pediatric catheterization laboratories, fluid-filled catheters are utilized for routine hemodynamic measurements. When stenotic lesions are present, however, the spike artifacts so commonly seen with fluid-filled catheters (see Chapter 7) interfere with the accurate assessment of the pressure gradient. If management of the patient (i.e., surgery or balloon valvotomy) depends upon the magnitude of the gradient, high-fidelity, micromanometer-tipped catheters should be utilized for the hemodynamic assessment. The most accurate way of determining a pressure gradient is by simultaneous measurement of proximal and distal pressures with equally sensitive systems. In some circumstances, this may not be technically feasible and one must rely on withdrawal of the catheter across the stenotic area with continuous pressure monitoring. This "pullback" tracing gives a close approximation of the gradient as long as hemodynamics are stable during the recording. Measurement of the proximal and distal pressures across a stenotic area at two different times during the catheterization is of less value because of variations in the steady state of the patient.

Angiocardiography

The selection of a catheter with an appropriate diameter is influenced by the size of the patient. In addition to the obvious relationship between the caliber of the vessel into which the catheter is to be introduced and the patient's size, the volume of contrast material to be utilized is generally determined on the basis of the patient's body weight. As a general rule, with children under 35 kilograms, 1 mL/kg of contrast material is delivered in 1 to 1.5 seconds for standard biplane cineangiography. If digital subtraction techniques are to be used, then substantially less contrast can be injected at a much lower delivery rate. The delivery of a given volume of contrast media in a given period of time depends upon a number of factors: the pressure used, the viscosity of the contrast media, and the resistance to flow in the catheter. The last factor is in turn dependent upon the internal diameter and length of the catheter. A catheter must be chosen for angiography that will have the capacity to deliver the desired volume of contrast material in a specified period of time.

In each laboratory that performs cardiac angiography, a pressure volume chart (Table 2) should be constructed for the various types and sizes of catheters and type of contrast material used in that laboratory. The physician can then select the proper catheter for delivery of a given volume and flow rate of contrast material (Table 3).

In general, with standard biplane cineangiocardiography, contrast material that is not injected within 2 seconds does little to enhance the quality of the angiogram and is therefore wasted. This, to a degree, depends upon the heart rate. With more rapid

Table 2

Pressure–Volume Table

NIH catheter size*	Volume ml/sec							
	4	8	12	16	20	25	30	35
5F–50	300	700	—	—	—	—	—	—
6F–50	100	300	400	600	700	—	—	—
5F–80	500	900	—	—	—	—	—	—
6F–80	200	400	600	800	—	—	—	—
7F–80	<100	200	300	400	500	700	900	—
6F–100	300	400	700	—	—	—	—	—
7F–100	<100	<100	<100	200	300	400	500	600
8F–100	<100	<100	<100	200	300	400	500	600

Renografin–76 (room temperature); pressure in pounds/square inch—PSI.

* Catheter size expressed as diameter (French)–length (cm).

heart rates, the injected contrast clears more rapidly and thus the contrast should be delivered more rapidly. Also, the largest catheter that can be used safely should be selected because it allows for a rapid delivery of a given volume of contrast material at less pressure and thus permits better quality angiograms. In addition, there is less catheter recoil during delivery of contrast and thus less risk of an intramyocardial injection.

There are many different types of catheters available for angiography (Fig. 1). Many have a closed tip and multiple side holes. Although open end straight catheters can be utilized for small hand injections of

Table 3

NIH (Woven Dacron) Catheter Selection for Angiography

Body wt. (kg)	NIH catheter size*	Maximum flow rate at 700 PSI (ml/sec)
<8	5F–50	8
8–25	6F–80	15
26–50	7F–100	25
>50	8F–100	40

* Catheter size expressed as diameter (French)–length (cm); PSI, pounds/square inch.

contrast material, they are not suitable for pressure angiography because of catheter recoil and the potential hazard of endomyocardial injury by a jet stream from the end hole. In our laboratory, either the NIH catheter, which has a closed end and six side holes, or the pigtail catheter is used. The NIH catheter is relatively stiff and maneuverable. Intraluminal guidewires can be utilized for difficult catheter passes (Chapter 5).

The Lehman ventriculography catheter is occasionally used in our laboratory, especially when it is difficult to maneuver a catheter across the aortic valve. This catheter also has a closed end and side holes, but has a tapered flexible tip that facilitates passage across a stenotic aortic valve. Also, because the side holes are somewhat proximal to this "rat-tail" tip, the tip of the catheter can be against the myocardial wall or even in a trabeculated area during pressure angiocardiography. Unfortunately, arrhythmia is more common with this type catheter.

The pigtail catheter is also in common use for ventricular angiography. As its name implies, the tip of this catheter is curled and it has an end hole and a number of side holes. The main advantage of this catheter is the low risk of an intramyocardial injection. Because it has an end hole, it can be used for angiography in those laboratories where percutaneous catheterization is utilized without a sheath introducer. With this technique, the guidewire is advanced into the aorta and the pigtail is straightened and advanced over the guidewire. When the guidewire is removed, the catheter again forms the pigtail and can be advanced across the aortic valve and into the left ventricle. It may be difficult to pass the pigtail catheter directly across the aortic valve, especially in a patient with aortic stenosis. In that case, the guidewire may be extended beyond the tip and passed across the aortic valve and into the left ventricle. The catheter is advanced over the guidewire and, after the wire is withdrawn, again assumes its pigtail configuration. These catheters are now available in a variety of sizes beginning with #4 French.

Balloon-tipped, flow-directed catheters (see below) can also be used for angiography (Fig. 1). In fact, in some centers they are the catheters of choice. Balloon angiographic catheters are particularly useful when an injection must be made in an area that is difficult to enter; for example, an antegrade pass into the aorta from the left ventricle, especially in the small infant. Unfortunately, the angiographic holes are proximal to the balloon and in a small infant it may be difficult to position the catheter so that the side holes are within the chamber or artery to be opacified.

Flow-Directed Catheters

Flow-directed catheters were first developed by Swan and Ganz in the 1960s and were originally used for monitoring in the intensive care unit. These catheters are currently marketed by several companies but all have the same basic design. There are a minimum of two lumens, one of which opens into a balloon near the distal end of the catheter. The second lumen may open at the distal tip of the catheter, enabling its use for wedge pressure as originally described by

Swan and Ganz. Subsequent modifications of the original balloon catheter include angiographic catheters with a closed end and multiple side holes, electrode catheters for atrial pacing or electrophysiologic studies, and thermal-dilution, cardiac-output catheters with a sensor at the tip and a proximal side hole for injecting cold fluid.

Since balloon-tipped catheters are flow-directed, they are soft and lightweight and are usually constructed of thin polyethylene. Unfortunately, this construction limits the ability of the physician to maneuver the catheter in a direction other than the blood flow. This may make it difficult to pass the catheter into an area of low flow when there is an alternate area of high flow. Examples include a pass into the pulmonary artery in a patient with tetralogy of Fallot and a large right-to-left shunt at ventricular level, or into the aorta from the left ventricle in an infant with a large ventricular septal defect and very large pulmonary blood flow. In each case, the balloon catheter tends to follow the direction of greatest flow.

The balloon of a flow-directed catheter can be inflated either with a gas or with liquid. Air may be used for inflation when the catheter is used only in the right side of the circulation. Although there is always a small risk of balloon rupture and escape of a small volume of air into the circulation, there is no problem if the air enters only the pulmonary artery. There is considerably greater risk, however, if air is used as the inflation material in patients with an actual or potential right-to-left shunt. Therefore, if gas is to be used for inflating the balloon of a flow-directed catheter in patients with congenital heart disease, carbon dioxide is recommended. It is so soluble in blood that rupture of the balloon carries little or no risk of air embolism. The use of carbon dioxide is somewhat cumbersome, however, because it requires a tank of carbon dioxide with sterile connecting fittings. Also, the gas slowly leaks from the balloon and must be replaced if the balloon is to be kept inflated for any length of time. In our laboratory, dilute contrast media (0.5 mL contrast in 2 mL of catheter flushing solution) is used to inflate the balloon of some flow-directed catheters, eliminating the risk of air embolism and the inconvenience of carbon dioxide. This technique can be used only with flow-directed catheters that have a large enough lumen to permit easy withdrawal of the fluid and rapid balloon deflation. (The physician should test the balloon catheters of a given manufacturer *prior* to introduction into the patient.) One would expect a fluid-filled balloon to be less "flow-directed" than a gas-filled balloon, but in practice there is little difference between the two.

Ideally, the external diameter of the balloon should be the same as that of the body of the catheter, allowing introduction of the balloon through a percutaneous sheath without subsequent back-bleeding. Unfortunately, the deflated balloon diameter is greater than the diameter of the shaft in many catheters, necessitating a larger sheath for balloon introduction. Also, considerable back-bleeding occurs during manipulation of the catheter unless a special type of sheath is used to prevent this (see Chapter 4). In some commercially available catheters, balloon and shaft diameters are equal but the lumen leading to the balloon is very small and carbon dioxide must be used for inflation. The ideal flow-directed catheter should be soft enough to float easily and yet be stiff enough to permit some manipulation. As mentioned above, the balloon should be easy to deflate, especially if fluid is used as the inflation medium. Since no catheter is ideal in every respect, in our laboratory we have a number of different brands of catheters available. If external diameter is the most crucial factor (i.e., a very small patient with small vessels), then the smallest catheter is used and carbon dioxide is used for inflation. If size is not crucial, a catheter is utilized that will permit inflation of the balloon with fluid.

Special Catheters

There are a wide variety of special catheters available for use in the catheterization laboratory.

Micromanometer-Tipped

These catheters provide high-fidelity pressure and sound recordings from a sensor at the tip of the catheter. They are available in a variety of sizes with single or double sensors, and with and without a lumen.

Balloon Atrial Septostomy

Balloon atrial septostomy was developed by Rashkind and Miller in 1964. The procedure has become indispensable in the management of the newborn with transposition of the great arteries and is also useful in other anomalies in which a large interatrial communication is desirable (e.g., tricuspid atresia, total anomalous pulmonary venous connection, and pulmonary atresia with intact ventricular septum). There are currently two types of catheters available for balloon septostomy; the Rashkind catheter, manufactured by USCI, and the Fogarty balloon septostomy catheter, manufactured by Edwards Laboratories. The Rashkind catheter has a recessed balloon and can be used with a #6 French sheath (the same diameter as the catheter shaft), whereas the Fogarty catheter requires a #7 French sheath. Despite this disadvantage of requiring a larger sheath size, the Fogarty balloon septostomy catheter is superior to the USCI Rashkind catheter in a number of ways and is preferred for use in our laboratory (see Chapter 12).

Blade Atrial Septostomy

This procedure involves the use of a special catheter containing a tiny surgical blade within the tip. The blade can be protruded from the catheter when it is in position in the patient's heart and has been used successfully to create or enlarge interatrial communications. This catheter is commercially available (Cook Incorporated) and further description of this catheter and its use is provided in Chapter 12.

Transseptal Puncture

The transseptal procedure has been used for many years for the introduction of a catheter into the left atrium by puncture of the atrial septum. A transseptal sheath technique developed by Dr. Charles E. Mullins of Houston, Texas, has greatly facilitated the use of this procedure in small children. In addition, the biplane radiographic equipment available in most pediatric catheterization laboratories makes this procedure less hazardous. The transseptal technique is discussed further in Chapter 14.

Electrode Catheters

These catheters are used for intracardiac pacing and recording. They have from one to six platinum electrodes in various arrangements at the distal end of the catheter. A further description of these catheters and their use is found in Chapter 10.

Thermal-Dilution Catheters

Thermal-dilution catheters are available in sizes from #4 French upward and in both regular and flow-directed varieties. These catheters are used for measuring cardiac output in the cardiac catheterization laboratory, the intensive care unit, and the surgical recovery area (Chapter 8).

Flow-Velocity Catheter

The electromagnetic flow-velocity catheter was first introduced by Mills in Eng-

land in 1966. In our laboratory, a square wave electromagnetic flow meter catheters (Carolina Medical Electronics) and flow probe catheters (Millar Instrument Company, Houston, Texas) are used. Electromagnetic flow and micromanometer pressure sensors are located on the same #6 French catheter, allowing for accurate and simultaneous measurement of pressure and flow velocity at the same point in the circulatory system. The catheter is small enough to use in infants and children. Volume of flow can be calculated by multiplying instantaneous flow velocity by the cross-sectional area of the vessel at the site of the flow sensor. Although the clinical usefulness of this catheter is limited at the present time, it is a valuable research tool and is currently the only accurate means of measuring intravascular pressure and instantaneous flow simultaneously outside the operating room.

Fiberoptic Oximetry

The fiberoptic catheter is connected to an instrument that provides direct readout of oxygen saturation. This enables continuous monitoring of oxygen saturation during manipulation of the catheter and eliminates the necessity for withdrawal of blood samples. Fiberoptic oximetry has not attained wide use because of the considerable cost of the system and the fact that newer oximetric devices require only a small volume of blood.

Balloon Angioplasty/Valvotomy

This procedure was first described by Gruentzig in Switzerland in 1977. It has been used for dilatation of stenosed coronary, renal, and ileofemoral arteries. This technique has been used in relieving vascular or valvar stenosis in the pediatric age group and it is currently in use in many pediatric cardiology laboratories. (see Chapter 13)

4

Catheter Introduction

William H. Neches, M.D.

General Considerations

For many years, cardiac catheterization was performed only by the cutdown method, inserting the catheter directly into a blood vessel after it had been surgically exposed. In 1953, Seldinger described a technique for percutaneous insertion of catheters into the femoral vessels by the use of guidewires. This technique was subsequently modified by Desilets and Hoffman in 1965 to permit the introduction of a sheath into the vessel, with the catheter then being inserted through the sheath. Either the standard percutaneous Seldinger technique or the percutaneous sheath method are preferred in most centers for the catheterization of patients in the pediatric age group. These techniques are generally utilized for vessels in the inguinal region, although they also can be used in the brachial area. In most centers the cutdown technique is now used only as an alternative method in newborns or small infants if the percutaneous technique is not successful. If arm vessel catheterization is required in infants and small children, a cutdown is usually performed in the axilla, because the brachial vessels are almost always too small to admit a useful size catheter in such patients. In older children or adults, the brachial vessels are often utilized, using either the percutaneous or cutdown technique. On some occasions, jugular veins can be utilized for venous catheterization if the femoral, axillary, or brachial vessels are not accessible, or for repeated endomyocardial biopsies in patients who have undergone heart transplantation. In the newborn infant, the umbilical vessels provide easy access to both the arterial and venous circulations and often can be used for the complete cardiac catheterization, especially if the infant is less than 48 hours old.

In the past, there was much discussion regarding the relative advantages and disadvantages of the percutaneous and cutdown techniques. Although the percutaneous technique is now the preferred method in almost all pediatric centers, a discussion of the merits and drawbacks of each seems appropriate. The percutaneous technique is relatively easy to learn and greatly facilitates changing catheters during the procedure. Another advantage of this technique is that a particular vein or artery can usually be used again at a subsequent catheterization. Also, the percutaneous method is faster than a cutdown in most circumstances, especially when the physician performing the catheterization is relatively inexperienced in the cutdown method. However, occasionally even the experienced operator has difficulty passing the guidewire through the needle into the vessel, often for no apparent reason. At some point in such frustrating cases, the judgment of the physician will dictate a resort to the cutdown method.

In our laboratory, although percutaneous entry is usually successful even in a newborn or small infant, we do not hesitate to resort to the cutdown technique if percutaneous entry is unsuccessful within about 30 minutes. The cutdown method is often utilized more in some patients, especially if the infant is sick and speed is important. If percutaneous entry is not initially successful, it may be quicker to cutdown on the saphenous vein than to continue to try to enter the femoral vein percutaneously. In addition, if the percutaneous method is unsuccessful, hematoma formation obscures landmarks and makes a subsequent cutdown more difficult and time consuming. However, except in the very small infant, percutaneous entry is almost always possible.

Although the preparation of the catheterization site is the same for both the cutdown and percutaneous procedures, the postcatheterization care is easier and complications are fewer with the percutaneous method. The site of percutaneous entry is small and is essentially sealed within 24 hours. There are no sutures that may serve as a route of entry of infection through the skin and that must be removed a week following the procedure. (We know of no single infection of a percutaneous catheterization site in our laboratory). The percutaneous technique does require closer observation immediately following the catheterization, because bleeding may occur. It has been our experience that proper application of a pressure bandage minimizes the risk of bleeding. With the percutaneous technique, some bleeding into the tissues surrounding the catheterization site does occur, both during and following the procedure. Although this is not harmful to the patient, it may result in a fairly large ecchymosis around the catheterization site a few days later. This is especially true if an arterial puncture has been performed. It is important that the patient and the parents be informed about the possibility of a sizable "bruise" appearing after a percutaneous catheterization.

Percutaneous Technique

The percutaneous technique used in our laboratory was described by Neches et al. in 1972 and is a modification of the tech-

niques described by Seldinger (1953), Lurie et al. (1963), and Desilets and Hoffman (1965). The use of a sheath facilitates substitution of one catheter for another and permits the use of a wide variety of catheters including electrode- or micromanometer-tipped catheters, closed-end catheters for angiocardiography, and balloon catheters. Bleeding can be controlled easily during catheter changes, thus minimizing blood loss. A sheath of any internal diameter can be changed to a larger one by a series of simple maneuvers, described later, which permit the use of a variety of catheter sizes. Lastly, trauma to the vessel wall and surrounding tissues from prolonged catheter manipulation or repeated catheter changes is less common with the sheath technique.

Site Preparation

Although the percutaneous technique can be used for either the femoral or brachial vessels, the femoral vessels are preferred for almost all cardiac catheterizations in the pediatric age group. The larger size of the femoral vessels permits the use of much larger catheters and the femoral approach provides a greater chance of entering the left heart with a prograde venous catheter via a patent foramen ovale. Most major arterial branches and surgically created aorta-to-pulmonary artery shunts can be entered with a retrograde femoral arterial catheter. If the brachial vessels are being utilized, usually only that site is prepared. However, if the femoral vessels are to be used, we prefer to prepare both the right and left groins for possible catheterization. If the patient is a newborn, the right groin and the umbilical area are usually included in the sterile field.

The skin of the selected site is prepared with an antiseptic solution povidone-iodine (Betadine), which is then washed off with 70% isopropyl alcohol. The site is then dried thoroughly and covered with sterile drapes. Some of us prefer to cover the catheterization site with sterile plastic aperture drapes (Steri-Drape, no. 1020, 3M Company) that have an adhesive backing on the underside. Two of these drapes are utilized, one for each groin area. They are then covered by sterile drapes, as is the rest of the table, allowing for enough of an opening for easy access to the catheterization site. Others in our group prefer to do this in the reverse, with sterile drapes being initially placed around the site. An adhesive plastic drape (Steri-Drape, no. 1040, 3M Company) is then placed over the opening, with a portion of the adhesive contacting the patient's skin and the rest firmly applied to the surface of the sterile drapes. Either way, the end result is a large, sterile operative field with adequate room to work, good exposure of the catheterization site, and readily palpable landmarks.

Local anesthesia of the catheterization site is achieved with 1% lidocaine hydrochloride (Xylocaine) *without* added epinephrine. In contrast to the small amount of local anesthesia that is utilized in preparing the skin surface for a cutdown procedure, preparation for percutaneous catheterization requires anesthetizing not only the surface but also the deeper tissues. In our laboratory, a 1 ½-inch, 25-gauge needle is used to inject 1–5 mL of local anesthetic at the site to be utilized (depending on the size of the child). Some of us also inject a small amount of local anesthetic in the opposite groin with the idea that anesthetizing the surface tissues may later make deep local anesthesia easier for the patient should it become necessary to utilize that side. It is a good idea to make the needle entry point for the local anesthesia at approximately the point that one chooses to insert the needle for the attempt at percutaneous catheterization. This has the advantage of marking that site in case some of the landmarks are obscured by the volume of local anesthesia used or by a transient decrease in the femoral artery pulse as a result of the anesthetic injection. If local anesthetic is injected *slowly* and *intermittently,* the pain associ-

ated with the administration is minimal. Allowing a short time interval after each portion of the injection enables the anesthetic to take effect before the needle is advanced deeper toward the vascular sheath. Rapid injection is quite painful and should always be avoided.

Methods

Femoral Vein and Artery

Prior to percutaneous catheterization, it is essential to ascertain the location of the various landmarks in the femoral triangle (Fig. 1). The superior margin of this triangle is formed by the inguinal ligament, which runs between the antero-superior iliac spine and the lateral superior margin of the pubis. The femoral artery can easily be palpated within the triangle, and its course is approximately perpendicular to the inguinal ligament. The femoral vein lies just medial and slightly superficial to the femoral artery and runs parallel to it. It is important for the physician to ascertain the course of the femoral artery and femoral vein by palpating the arterial pulse and determining its relationship to the inguinal ligament. The position of these vessels is an important consideration during the early stages of the procedure, since entry into the vessels is best accomplished when the needle is following the course taken by the vessel. A variety of needles can be used for percutaneous catheter introduction. Disposable percutaneous needles are available and consist of a plastic hub with side flanges and a stylet that is contained in the needle during entry. These needles are expensive and we have found them to be cumbersome to use, especially in infants and small children. We prefer a standard 1 ½-inch, 19-gauge, thin-walled, short-bevel needle. It is much less expensive and can be obtained from a number of suppliers. In some cases, a wire-introduction adapter may be necessary if the needle does not have a sufficiently tapered hub. We have

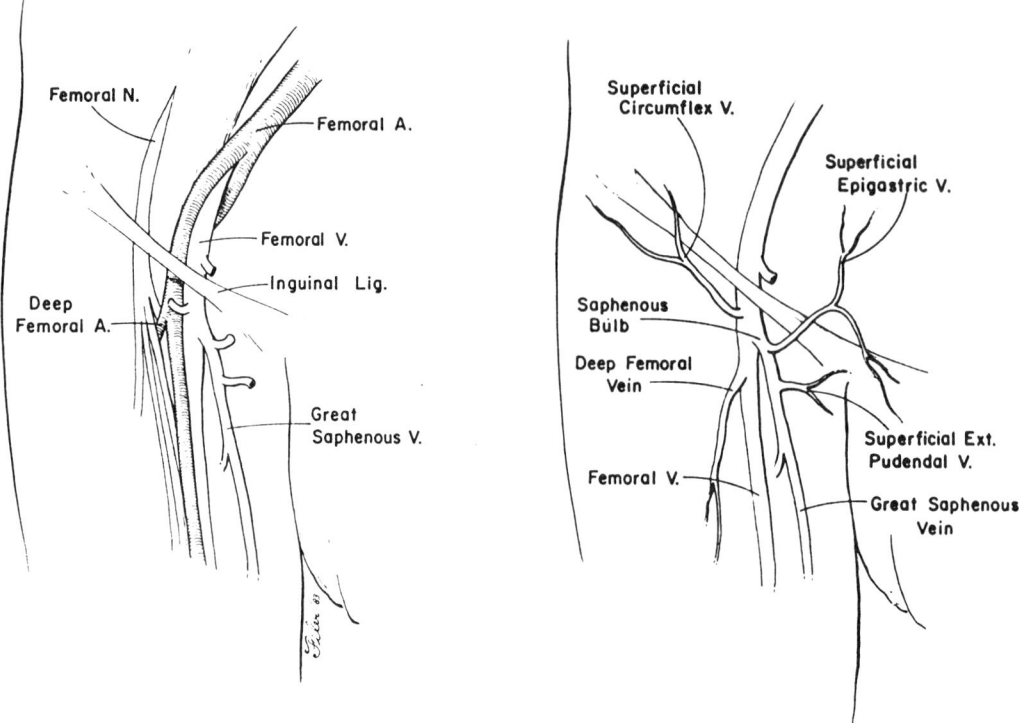

Figure 1. Anatomy of the femoral triangle (the right femoral artery and right femoral vein run perpendicular to the inguinal ligament at the point where they cross).

been able to use this type of needle for percutaneous catheterization of patients weighing from 2.5 to over 80 kg. In infants we sometimes prefer to use a 21-gauge, thin-walled needle or even the 21–gauge, thin-walled needle of a scalp vein infusion set to initiate the percutaneous procedure.

The technique for percutaneous sheath cardiac catheterization is outlined in Figures 2 and 3. The letters in the paragraphs below correspond to the illustrations in the figures.

A. The position and angulation of the needle as it is inserted through the skin and into the vessel lumen determines the ease with which the rest of the percutaneous catheter insertion is accomplished. After the position of the femoral artery has been ascertained, the needle is inserted over the femoral artery for arterial puncture and medial to that position for venous catheterization. In either case, the needle should be parallel to the long axis of the vessel being

entered. Some physicians prefer to enter the vessel close to the level of the inguinal ligament, and here the needle should maintain an angle of 45° to 75° with the surface of the skin. Others prefer to enter the skin from 1 to 3 cm below the level of the inguinal ligament, depending upon the size of the patient. In this situation, the course of the needle will be at a smaller angle to the surface of the skin. Once the needle has been inserted through the skin and advanced in an appropriate direction, free flow of blood should occur when the vessel is entered: an even flow of dark blood from the femoral vein and a pulsatile flow of bright red blood from the femoral artery. The use of a needle without a stylet is preferred since entry of the needle into the vessels is then accomplished "on the way in." Ideally, the needle will puncture only the anterior wall of the vessel, avoiding trauma to the posterior wall and surrounding tissues.

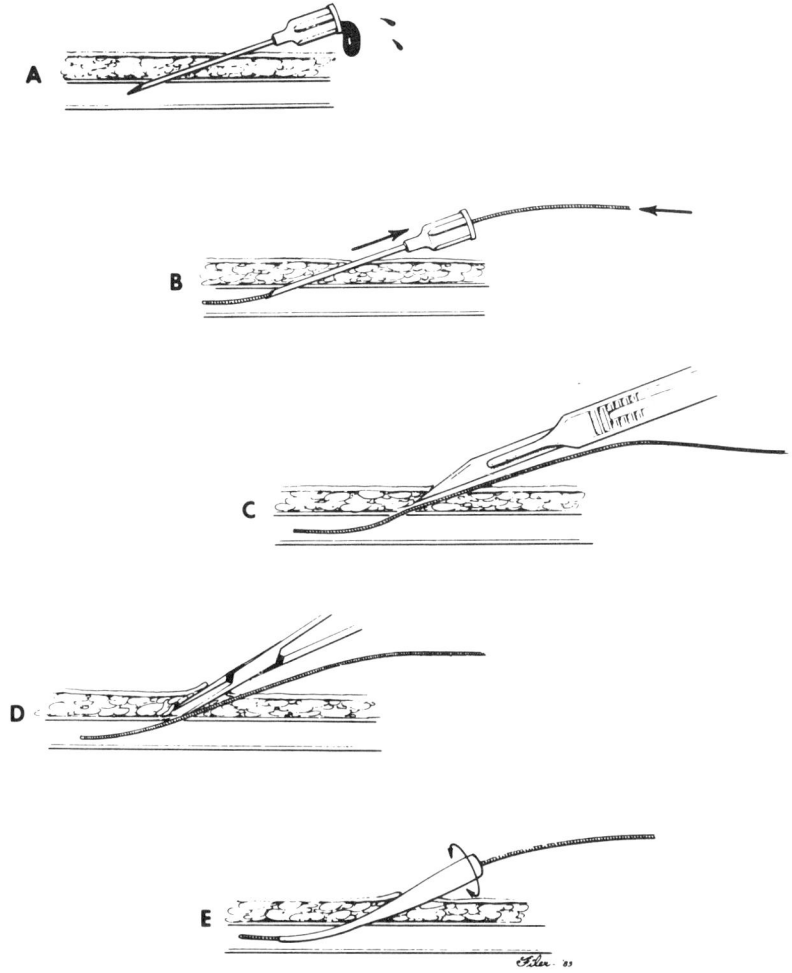

Figure 2. Percutaneous catheter insertion. See text for the description of this figure. The letters in the figure correspond to the letter headings of the paragraphs in the section on Methods: Femoral Vein and Artery. A: Insertion of needle into the vessel. B: Insertion of wire into the needle. C: Lancing the skin with a scalpel blade. D: Dilation of the soft tissue with a hemostat. E: Dilation of the soft tissue with a plastic cannula.

B. After the needle has been inserted and a free flow of blood obtained, the soft flexible end of the guidewire is passed through the needle and into the vessel lumen. (A 19-gauge, thin-walled needle accepts a guidewire of 0.025-inch maximum diameter. With a 21-gauge, thin-walled needle the maximum guidewire diameter is 0.021 inches.) The guidewire should pass through the needle and into the vessel lumen smoothly and without resistance. *Force should not be used* in attempting to advance the guidewire if it does not pass easily through the needle. If the patient experiences discomfort or if the wire does not advance without resistance, the needle tip may not lie completely within the lumen of the vessel and the wire tip may be outside the wall of the vessel or within the wall. In either case, attempting to force the wire through the needle can result in significant trauma to the vessel or surrounding tissues. In this situation, the bevel of the needle should be repositioned after the wire has been with-

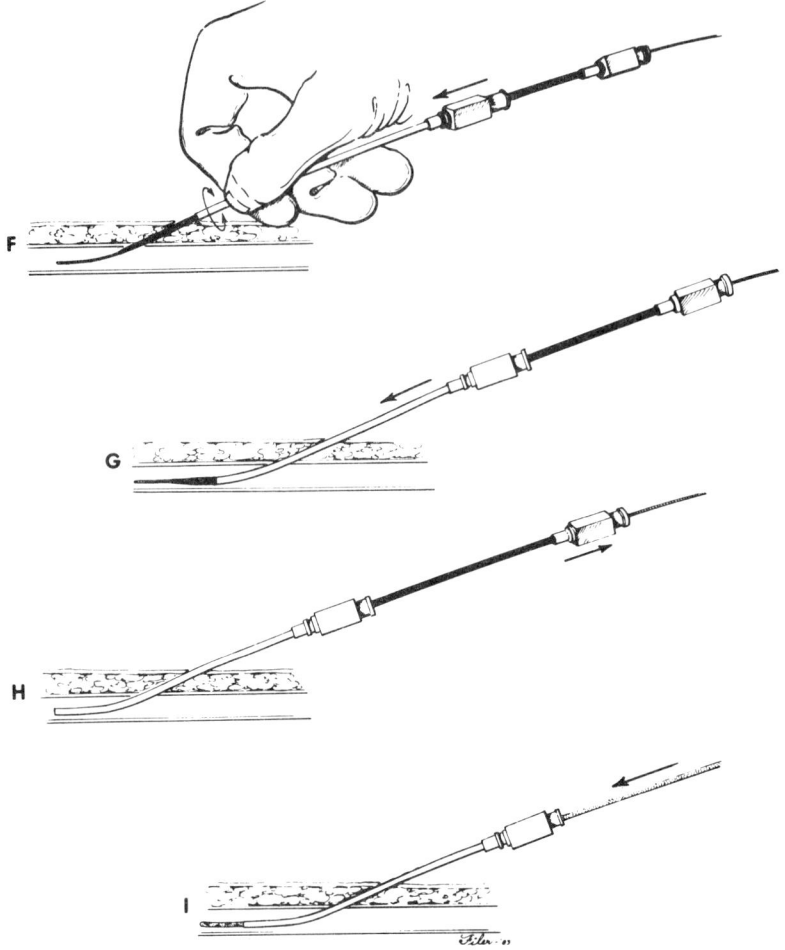

Figure 3. F: Insertion of the introducing unit. See text for the description of this figure. The letters in the figure correspond to the letter headings of the paragraphs in the section on Methods: Femoral Vein and Artery. G: Introducing unit is advanced into the vessel. H: Removal of the guidewire and dilator leaving the sheath alone in the vessel. I: Catheter introduced through sheath into vessel.

drawn either into the needle or completely out of it. Occasionally, rotating the hub on its axis may eliminate the problem. In some cases, the angle between the needle and vessel lumen is too great and repositioning the needle so it is more parallel to the surface of the skin may be helpful. In other cases, the needle may not have been parallel to the vessel and has therefore entered it at an angle. Movement of the needle in the horizontal plane, first to one side and then the other, may position the needle within the vessel lumen. It is also possible that the needle either may not have been advanced far enough or may have been advanced too far so that the bevel does not lie entirely within the vessel lumen. Here, either slightly advancing or withdrawing the needle may position it properly. After one of these maneuvers (rotation of the needle or movement in any direction), the guidewire may be advanced when there is free flow of blood. (If there is no free flow of blood, either the needle is not in the vessel lumen or a clot has formed within the needle.) Also, if the guidewire still does not pass through the needle, the needle should be withdrawn and pressure applied for adequate hemostasis. Another word of caution: Under no circumstances should the needle be advanced over the guidewire. Also, if resistance to withdrawal of the guidewire from the needle is encountered, no attempt should be made to forcibly pull the guidewire back through the needle. Rather, the needle and guidewire should be withdrawn together. In either of the above situations, there is a risk of the needle severing the guidewire tip while the wire is still in the patient.

Once the guidewire has been passed through the needle, it is advanced under fluoroscopic control up the inferior vena cava to the right atrium or, in the case of an arterial procedure, into the aorta to the level of the diaphragm. There are two advantages to this maneuver. First, the physician is able to ascertain that the wire is definitely within the vessel lumen and has not passed into the retroperitoneal space. (The wire can sometimes be advanced a considerable distance despite the fact that is not within a vessel lumen.) Second, the passage of the wire to the level of the diaphragm enables the physician to determine whether the wire has been passed into the arterial or venous system. Extraluminal or intra-arterial, rather than intravenous, positioning of the wire are errors that may not be recognized if the wire is advanced only a short distance, especially if fluoroscopic guidance is not utilized. In either situation, subsequent introduction of a percutaneous sheath, especially a larger one, may be harmful to the patient.

After passage of the guidewire through the needle, resistance may be met within the vein itself because of entry into a tributary or into a tortuous portion of the vessel. In some cases, simple manipulation of the guidewire under fluoroscopic control may be sufficient to position the wire in the main channel. If this is not possible, the guidewire should not be removed if the physician feels that it is located within the vessel lumen.

Instead, the metal needle should be withdrawn slowly while a gentle forward pressure on the guidewire is maintained to keep it in position. Once the metal needle has been withdrawn, a plastic cannula (e.g., Medicut, Long-dwell, etc.) can be introduced over the wire into the vessel. The wire can now be maneuvered or withdrawn without the risk of damage to the wire by the metal needle. It is often helpful at this point to gently advance the guidewire against the resistance, under fluoroscopic control. If only a small portion of the flexible tip is lodged in a tributary, it may be possible to buckle the soft end of the wire into a rounded J shape. This should be done with caution and only with gentle pressure, especially if the physician is not experienced in this maneuver. This maneuver should only be utilized in a venous channel, because in an artery the guidewire is almost always advanced in a straight course into the iliac arterial system. If the guidewire cannot easily be advanced, it should now be removed from the plastic cannula. If there is free flow of blood, the plastic cannula must lie within the vessel lumen. At this point, a small amount of contrast material should be injected through the plastic cannula to define the vascular anatomy. After the site of the difficulty has been determined, the guidewire can again be inserted through the plastic cannula. Manipulation under fluoroscopic control should be sufficient to bypass the problem area. It is also helpful, before reintroducing the guidewire, to curve slightly the flexible tip of the wire by pulling it gently over the end of the hemostat. The curved tip permits some control of the direction of the guidewire advance and also facilitates the buckling of the tip into a J position as described above. If these maneuvers are not successful and the contrast injection has demonstrated that the vessel is patent, a smaller guidewire can be tried. Sometimes a 0.021-inch or even a 0.018-inch guidewire can be maneuvered through a tortuous area that cannot be traversed with a stiffer guidewire.

Once the guidewire has been advanced to the level of the diaphragm, the needle is removed, leaving the guidewire in the vessel. To prevent bleeding, pressure should be applied with the left hand to the site of the guidewire entry, especially during arterial procedures. At the same time, the guidewire is grasped between the left thumb and forefinger. Using the right hand, a gauze sponge saturated with heparinized flushing solution is used to wipe the wire and remove any blood clots from its surface. The wire must be held firmly to prevent accidental withdrawal as the gauze is drawn over it. At this point, either of two maneuvers can be used to enlarge the opening along the guidewire and facilitate entry of the sheath assembly.

C and D. With one method, a 2- to 3-mm skin incision is made with a #11 scalpel blade at the site of needle entry. A small, straight hemostat is inserted into the tract along the guidewire as far as possible. The needle tract is widened by slowly opening and closing the jaws of the hemostat once or twice. The hemostat is then closed and removed, leaving a much wider opening along the wire tract.

E. With an alternative technique, a tapered plastic cannula (e.g., Medicut) is threaded over the guidewire and advanced with a twisting motion as far as possible through the skin. This enlarges the needle tract and facilitates sheath introduction. In many cases, especially in small patients and those who do not have a scar from a previous procedure, this method is quite sufficient. When a thick, heavy scar is present, especially if it is related to a previous surgical procedure for femoral artery cannulation at the time of open heart surgery, a sufficiently large tract may be more easily achieved using the hemostat. In cases with considerable scarring, it may even be necessary to use the hemostat followed by dilation with the plastic cannula. Occasionally, successive introduction of progressively larger sheaths is required until the appropriate diameter sheath can be successfully introduced.

F. The introducing unit consists of a sheath of a specified internal diameter and a dilator with a tip tapered to an opening just large enough to admit a specific size guidewire (Fig. 3). The Teflon dilator fits snugly within the sheath. The sheath and dilator unit has a gradual taper from the wire diameter up to the external diameter of the sheath. This permits gradual dilation of the wire tract and facilitates entry of the percutaneous sheath unit. The dilator is passed through the skin first and with a rotary motion is advanced into the vessel. In some cases, the dilator passes into the vessel lumen with only minimal resistance. Most often, however, some degree of resistance is met. It is important to press firmly over the skin proximal to the entry site as the dilator is rotated becasue an attempt simply to force the dilator over the wire and into the vessel lumen may result in buckling and kinking of the dilator and/or wire. When there is considerable resistance and the dilator cannot easily be advanced, rotary motion first in one direction and then in the other, with constant forward pressure, will usually be successful. If the dilator still cannot be advanced into the lumen there are a number of alternative courses of action. After withdrawing the dilator and sheath together, making sure that the wire remains in the vessel lumen, an attempt may again be made to enlarge the wire tract using either a hemostat or plastic cannula (as in step E). If this still is not sufficient, a smaller diameter sheath and dilator may be used to dilate the opening enough to permit introduction of the desired diameter unit. Lastly, it is possible that the angle of entry into the vessel lumen is too acute, making it difficult for the dilator to enter the vessel lumen. If this seems to be the case, the substitution of a larger diameter wire may help. First, the sheath and dilator unit is removed from the standard guidewire and a plastic cannula is advanced over the wire. (The plastic cannula should be tested first to make sure that it is large enough to permit introduction of a larger guidewire). In some cases another sheath also may have to be selected to fit the larger guidewire). After the plastic cannula has been advanced over the wire, the standard guidewire is removed and a larger guidewire substituted. The increased stiffness of this larger guidewire will tend to straighten out the course from the skin surface into the vessel lumen and facilitate entry of the dilator and subsequently the sheath.

G. The sheath is advanced over the dilator and into the vessel. There are a number of different types of sheaths available. All of those that are relatively rigid can be advanced by the rotation method, similar to that described above for the dilator. However, if a thin-walled polyethylene sheath is used for percutaneous catheterization on the arterial side, especially if there is a "tight fit," rotation may wrinkle the sheath. For the proper introduction of a thin-walled sheath in this situation after the dilator has been introduced, the sheath is grasped tightly between the thumb and index finger and the sheath and dilator are advanced together over the guidewire with only a slight twisting motion. Occasionally, it may be possible to introduce an appropriate size dilator into the vessel and yet not be able to pass the sheath. In this case, it may be helpful to use a smaller diameter sheath and dilator unit first, to provide gradual dilation of the entry site.

H. The dilator and guidewire are removed, leaving the sheath in the vessel for the duration of the catheterization. To avoid excessive bleeding (or, in the case of a venous sheath, the possibility of air aspiration), the physician should always occlude the orifice of the sheath with the index finger or thumb after the dilator has been removed or at the time of any catheter change. A sheath can be changed to one of a larger diameter by reversal of steps H through F. Briefly, the dilator and guidewire are reinserted and the wire passed up to the level of the diaphragm. The dilator is removed and the desired size dilator and sheath are introduced.

I. Any appropriate diameter catheter can now be inserted through the sheath into the vessel. The external diameter of most catheters is matched to the internal diameter of the sheath and little bleeding occurs during the procedure. Some balloon catheters have a larger external diameter at the tip (i.e, the balloon) than at the shaft, and there is considerable space around the catheter once the balloon portion has been advanced into the vessel. This may result in either blood loss or thrombus formation within the sheath. To solve the problem of catheter diameter–sheath size mismatch, a special sheath with a side port for continuous fluid infusion should be used (Hemaquet, USCI Corp.) (Fig. 4). This type of sheath, manufactured by a number of companies, has a seal about the hub opening that prevents back-bleeding.

Internal Jugular Vein

Premedication and local anesthesia are the same as that used with the percutaneous femoral approach. Some children who have undergone multiple internal jugular vein procedures for endomyocardial biopsy following heart transplantation have preferred to forego premedication and have tolerated the procedure well with only local anesthesia.

The patients are positioned with a pillow beneath the shoulder and with their arms at their sides. The patient's head is turned toward the left and the entire right anterior neck is therefore exposed in the sterile field. Landmarks for identifying the anterior triangle of the neck are shown in Figure 5. The anterior triangle of the neck is bordered by the medial and lateral heads of the sternocleidomastoid muscle and by the clavicle. The internal jugular vein courses through this triangle in an orientation from the apex of the triangle toward the patient's right nipple. Local anesthesia is administered with a 25-gauge needle, puncturing the skin at the apex of the triangle and infiltrat-

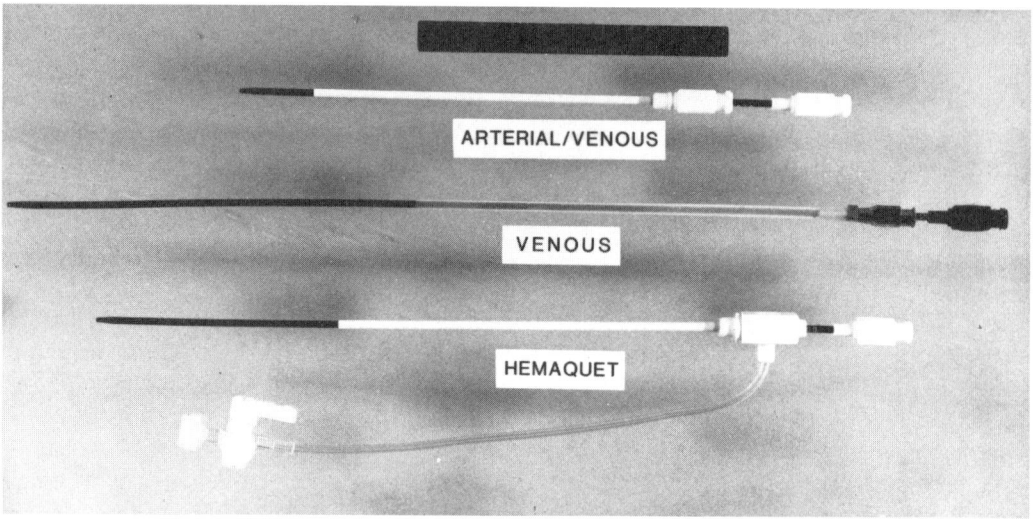

Figure 4. Sheath and dilator units. A: Thin-walled polyethylene introducer (arterial or venous). B: Teflon percutaneous catheter introducer (venous only). C: Side-arm flushing sheath (Hemaquet, USCI Corp).

ing along the expected course of the internal jugular vein. Some centers have described a "low approach" to the vein, puncturing the skin at the base of the triangle near the clavicle. However, in our institution, the approach has been from the apex of the triangle.

There are two similar methods, either of which may be used to enter the internal jugular vein. A 21-gauge needle is attached to a 3-mL syringe filled with heparinized flush solution and this is used to locate the vein. The needle enters the skin at the apex of the triangle and is advanced in the direction of the course of the internal jugular vein (toward the patient's right nipple) while maintaining an angle of 45° with the skin. Constant negative pressure is applied to the syringe until a free flow of blood is obtained. Once the vein has been entered, the needle is fixed in place with one hand while the syringe is removed with the other. A 0.021-inch or smaller guidewire is advanced through the needle and into the vein. Bleeding or air aspiration have not been a problem due to the small caliber of the needle. On the other hand, the use of this small caliber 0.021-

gauge needle necessitates the use of a small guidewire with a maximum diameter of 0.021 inches. This may make sheath insertion difficult in some cases with scared subcutaneous tissues. In an alternative method, the same technique is used to locate the vein. However, once the vein has been entered, the syringe is removed and the needle left in place as a guide to the location of the vein and to the angle of insertion of a larger needle. A 19-gauge, 1 ½-inch, thin-walled, short-bevel needle with an attached syringe is then used to puncture the skin immediately behind the guide needle. When the vein is entered by the larger needle, as evidenced by free flow of blood, the syringe is removed and a larger guidewire can be advanced into the right atrium under fluoroscopic control. The two needles can then be removed and a venous sheath and dilator advanced over the guidewire. Regardless of which initial technique is used, once the guidewire has been introduced through the needle and advanced to the right atrium, the needle is withdrawn leaving the guidewire in place.

The subcutaneous tissues are dilated with a Medicut plastic needle (Argyle), or a

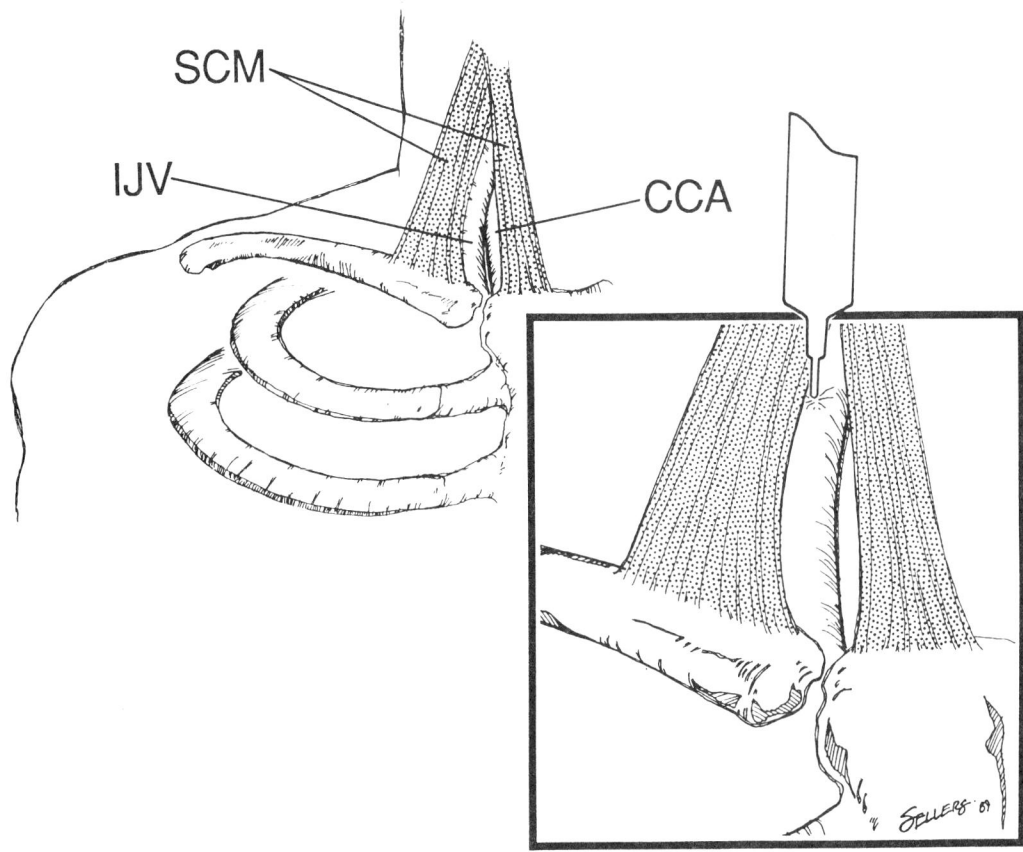

Figure 5. Anatomy of the anterior triangle of the neck (see text). CCA = common carotid artery; IJV = internal jugular vein; SCM sternocleidomastoid muscle.

hemostat, as was described in the technique for percutaneous femoral insertion. When the small needle and guidewire are used, or in some cases where multiple prior procedures have resulted in scar tissue, a scalpel blade is used to nick the skin adjacent to the wire before dilation with either the plastic needle or hemostat.

Because this route of access is generally used for right heart catheterization and endomyocardial biopsy in patients who have undergone cardiac transplantation, side-port sheaths are usually used to accommodate a variety of catheter sizes, to enable frequent irrigation of the sheath to prevent clot formation and to avoid inadvertent air embolization during catheter exchange. A variety of catheter types are then used including flow-directed thermodilution catheters, woven Dacron catheters, and endomyocardial bioptomes.

Right heart catheterization is carried out in the usual manner. Balloon-tipped catheters are not required to enter the pulmonary arteries because this catheter pass is even easier from the internal jugular route as compared to the femoral venous route. When biplane cineangiography is performed, it is necessary to reposition the patient's arms above the head. After completion of the procedures, the catheters are removed and hemostasis is achieved with firm hand pressure, followed by a light dressing. Children are returned to their rooms and receive routine postcatheterization care. Observation in an intensive care setting is not necessary from this route either. A particular advantage of internal jugular catheterization is that ambulation is possible once the patient is fully awake. Unusual or excessive bleeding, or hematoma formation, have not been encountered.

Heparinization—Yes or No?

The loss or diminution of a peripheral arterial pulse is a common complication of retrograde arterial cardiac catheterization, regardless of the technique utilized. Causes include spasm and/or thrombosis of the artery and the differential diagnosis is difficult immediately following the procedure. Simple spasm resolves in a few hours but the persistence of pulse abnormalities more than 24 hours after the procedure suggests thrombosis. Fortunately, thrombosis occurs in less than 5% of patients undergoing percutaneous catheterization and the actual number of patients who require surgical thrombectomy is quite small. A description of vascular problems following cardiac catheterization and their management is found in Chapter 16.

The argument regarding the use of systemic heparinization at the time of cardiac catheterization has yet to be resolved. Some centers recommend administration of a bolus of 100 units of heparin/kg of body weight at the time of insertion of the retrograde arterial catheter. In other centers, heparinization is recommended at the beginning of the catheterization procedure whether or not a retrograde catheterization is to be done. In our laboratory, systemic heparinization is used routinely by some physicians for retrograde arterial procedures, while others do not use heparin routinely except for patients with low cardiac output or those with cyanosis and a hematocrit >65%. The incidence of vascular complications in our patients when heparin is not used is similar to that in centers that use

heparin. This suggests that the use of an arterial sheath that reduces trauma to the vessel wall and surrounding tissues, combined with careful attention to technique at the beginning of the catheterization, minimizes local tissue injury and is more important than the use of heparin in avoiding arterial thrombosis.

Postcatheterization Care

Once the procedure is completed, the catheters are removed and hemostasis obtained with pressure on the catheterization site. (It is generally a good idea to withdraw the catheter from the sheath first to allow any clots that may have formed on the side or end of the catheter to be flushed through the sheath by the intravascular pressure.) Generally, after a period of about 10 minutes, active bleeding has stopped and a pressure bandage is applied to the catheterization site. The patient is then returned to the room and is usually kept in bed for 6 hours following a venous procedure and for 8 hours if an artery was also used. Smaller children may be allowed out of bed to be held by their parents, but walking is not allowed for at least these minimum periods. If the patient is unstable, closer observation in a recovery room or intensive care setting may be warranted.

Cutdown Technique

Direct surgical exposure of the vessels by cutdown technique can be utilized in the inguinal area as well as in the axilla or antecubital fossa. In the newborn or small infant, the leg vessels are preferred for catheter introduction for reasons described earlier in this chapter. In general, an arm cutdown for a venous catheterization is done only if the femoral route is not possible, usually because of iliac or inferior vena cava thrombosis from a previous catheterization. At one time, an arm approach was preferred if absence of the intrahepatic portion of the inferior vena cava was suspected, because of the 180° turn required at the junction of the azygos vein and the superior vena cava. Now, with flow-directed catheters, an inguinal approach is usually successful.

If an arterial catheterization is necessary and if the femoral artery cannot be entered percutaneously, we prefer an arm cutdown to an inguinal one. Repair of a femoral artery is more difficult than repair of a brachial or axillary artery, largely because of a more difficult exposure. In addition, there is more likely to be functional disability if the femoral artery is lost. In an older child weighing over 15 kg, an antecubital cutdown is preferred, since exposure and repair of the brachial artery is easier than that of the axillary artery. In an infant or small child, an axillary approach is advisable since the brachial artery is likely to be too small.

Another indication for an arm approach to an arterial catheterization is in the occasional child with coarctation of the aorta in whom the coarcted segment cannot be traversed from below.

Femoral Vessels

The femoral triangle contains the femoral artery, vein, and nerve, Its apex points caudally and the base is formed by the inguinal ligament (Fig. 6). The vessels run perpendicular to the inguinal ligament and are relatively superficial as they pass below it. The femoral artery is usually located near the mid point of the inguinal ligament, with the femoral vein located just medial, and slightly more superficial than, the artery. Both vessels are enclosed by the femoral sheath. The femoral nerve is located just lateral to the femoral artery and runs parallel to it through the femoral triangle. The mnemonic NAVE describes the relationships of the structures in the femoral triangle from lateral to medial: Nerve, Artery, Vein, Empty space. Although either the right or left groin can be used for catheterization of the fem-

oral vessels, the right groin is preferred because it allows a straighter catheter pass into the inferior vena cava and makes manipulation of the catheter inside the heart easier. If for some reason the right groin cannot be used, a left groin approach is quite satisfactory.

The area of cutdown is cleaned with antiseptic solution, dried, and draped in the same manner as that described for percutaneous catheterization. Local anesthesia is accomplished using 1% lidocaine, injected subcutaneously over the femoral artery and medially over the femoral vein for a distance of 1 to 2 cm. Most of the local anesthetic should be injected rather superficially; there is no need for deep infiltration unless more than usual dissection is required. The site of the skin incision for cardiac catheterization in the newborn or young infant differs from that in older infants and children. In the latter group, the saphenous bulb lies 1 to 3 cm caudal to the inguinal crease, whereas in newborn infants, the saphenous bulb and sapheno-femoral junction lie just below the inguinal crease. If the saphenous vein of a newborn is not large enough to admit even a #5 French catheter, the saphenous bulb or femoral vein must be used. This is especially common if a cutdown is required for balloon atrial septostomy. The skin incision for cardiac catheterization in a newborn is made parallel to, and just below, the level of the inguinal crease. In older infants the incision is made about 1 cm below the inguinal ligament, and in older children from 2 to 3 cm below this structure. The skin incision is started over the femoral artery and carried medially 1 to 2 cm.

After the skin incision has been made, a small curved hemostat is used to gently dissect the underlying tissue. At this point, it is important to stress the necessity for the physician to be very careful and gentle in dissecting and handling the vessels, especially in small infants. The small branches tend to be fragile and spasm of even the major vessels is a common consequence of rough handling.

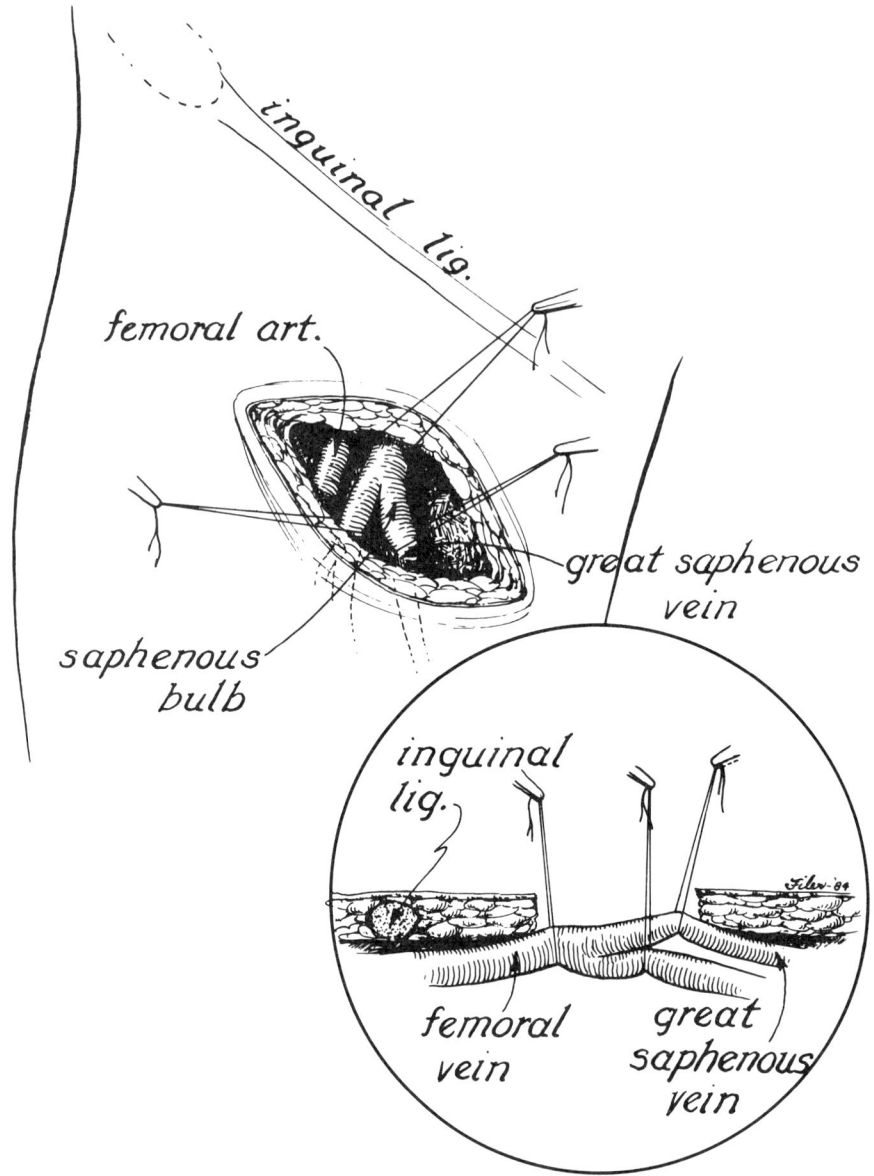

Figure 6. Anatomy of the femoral venous system.

As the dissection proceeds, one first encounters either the long saphenous vein or one of the many branches that drain into the sapheno-femoral junction (Fig. 6). Once a vessel has been identified, blunt dissection is carried down along its course toward the femoral vein. At this point, a decision is made as to which vessel is to be used for the introduction of the catheter. If balloon septostomy is not contemplated and the long saphenous vein is of adequate size for the desired catheter, further dissection is unnecessary once this vessel has been exposed. Black silk threads (size 4–0) are then placed proximal and distal to the proposed site of catheter introduction. The distal thread is tied and held with a hemostat. Once the area has been adequately exposed and provisions have been made to control bleeding, venotomy and catheter insertion are performed in the manner described later in this section.

If circumstances necessitate the use of the saphenous bulb, the sapheno-femoral junction, or the femoral vein itself, careful dissection and adequate exposure of the saphenous bulb, all of its tributaries, and both the proximal and distal femoral vein should be a standard procedure. Although this additional dissection is time consuming, it is time well spent if problems are encountered. In contrast to the usual saphenous vein cutdown, where bleeding is easily controlled by traction of the vessel, insertion of a catheter into the femoral vein or sapheno-femoral junction can be accompanied by considerable bleeding. In addition, should a vessel accidently be torn, it is much easier to control the bleeding and identify the proximal and distal ends of the vessel if adequate dissection has been carried out beforehand. Needless to say, it is very difficult to adequately dissect the main vessels while blood is pouring from the ends of a torn vessel and obscuring the operative field.

If the saphenous bulb is to be used, ties should be placed around the femoral vein proximal and distal to entry of the saphenous vein, around the saphenous vein between the bulb and the femoral vein, and around each vein entering the bulb (Fig. 6). It is important to note that there is usually a deep perforating vein that enters the dorsal aspect of the saphenous bulb. It will be missed unless searched for and will cause considerable bleeding when the bulb is subsequently opened. If possible, the saphenous bulb should be repaired, and if this repair is contemplated the long saphenous vein and any other large feeder vein should not be permanently ligated. A single knot will usually occlude the vein and can be easily removed after repair. (If bleeding occurs with a single knot, a double knot can be used and

the tie can subsequently be cut. Smaller feeder veins should be ligated.

If the femoral vein is used for the catheterization, the catheter should be inserted into the femoral vein just caudal to the sapheno-femoral junction. The femoral vein is fairly large at this point and is usually of adequate size to accommodate even a balloon catheter. If this area of the vein is utilized, it is wise to leave the saphenous bulb and its tributaries undisturbed. Even if the femoral vein is ligated after the procedure, the long saphenous vein and its branches will allow blood flow to bypass this obstruction. Whenever possible, the femoral vein should be repaired after removal of the catheters. A further description of venotomy, catheter insertion, and vessel repair is found later in this chapter.

Axilla

The axillary region is usually used only in infants or young children in whom the inguinal approach is not practical, although some physicians prefer to utilize the axillary artery for retrograde arterial catheterization in a newborn or small infant. It is important to remember that some patients have an anomalous retroesphageal right subclavian artery that arises from the descending aorta rather than from the brachiocephalic artery. If this abnormality is present, a catheter that is introduced into the right axillary artery will pass directly into the descending aorta and cannot be maneuvered into the ascending aorta and left ventricle. It is thus important to determine whether or not the right subclavian artery arises normally prior to commencing an axillary or brachial artery cutdown, especially if this procedure is contemplated prior to the start of the catheterization. This is accomplished by careful examination of a "four-view" cardiac series with barium esophagram. If the posterior indentation of the esophagus characteristic of an anomalous right subclavian artery is seen, another artery should be used.

After the axillary region is cleaned and draped, local anesthesia is obtained using 1% lidocaine. The anesthetic is injected relatively superficially in the area just distal to the axillary fold and over the axillary arterial pulsation. As in the inguinal region, only superficial injection of the local anesthetic is used because deep dissection is usually unnecessary. The skin incision is made perpendicular to the course of the axillary artery 1 to 2 cm distal to the axillary crease. In this area, as in the femoral triangle, initial injection of the anesthetic agent should be over the axillary artery so that the needle mark in the skin serves as a guide to where to begin the incision.

The skin incision is initiated over the axillary artery (Fig. 7). Dissection is then carried down to the level of the axillary sheath, which encloses the axillary artery,

vein, and the brachial plexus nerves. The axillary vein is medial and slightly superficial to the axillary artery and often overlaps it partially. The medial cord of the brachial plexus and its branches are usually found between these two vessels but somewhat deep to them in the axilla. During the dissection, it is always important to ascertain the location of these brachial plexus nerve branches. If deeper dissection is necessary, additional injection of lidocaine can be done under direct vision to avoid injection into the nerves. It is important to distinguish between the axillary artery and nerve before opening this "artery." The nerve is "shiny," has longitudinal striations, and does not pulsate. Traction on the artery, both proximally and distally, should eliminate the pulsation and definitely identify it. If there is any doubt, a 25-gauge needle should be inserted

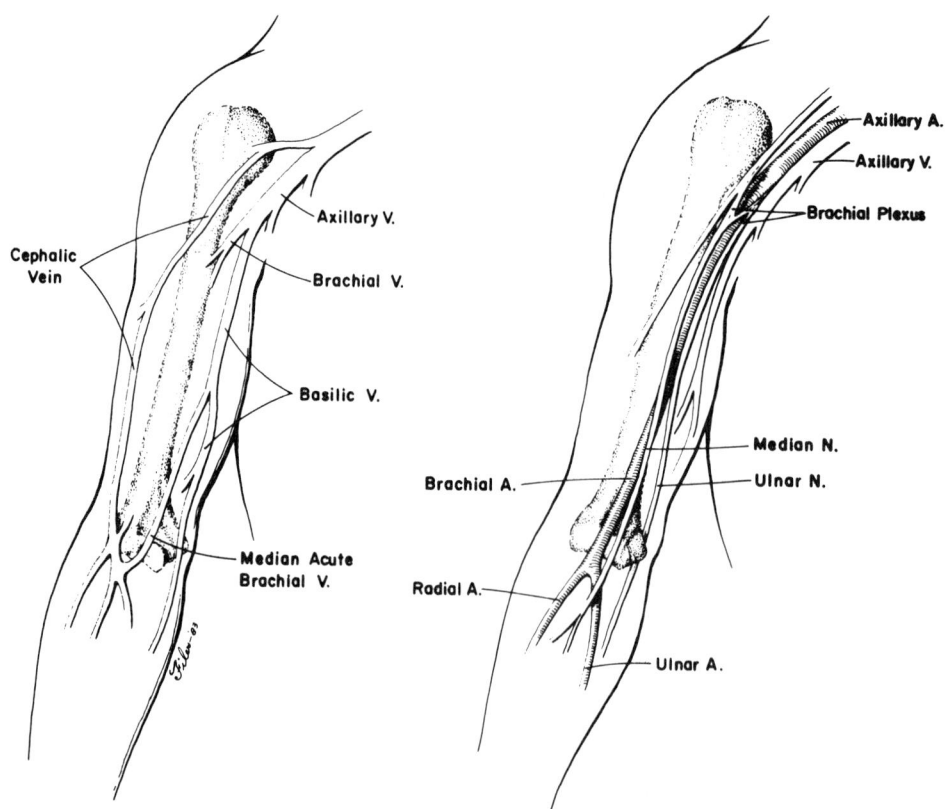

Figure 7. Vascular anatomy of the upper extremity.

to verify that the structure is an artery. After the vessels have been adequately identified and isolated and adequate control of potential bleeding obtained, catheterization of the vessels is accomplished as described in the sections on venotomy, arteriotomy, and catheter introduction.

Antecubital Fossa

The brachial vessels are generally used only in older children because they are too small to accept an adequate size catheter in infants. As with axillary vein catheterization, the most common indication for an antecubital venous cutdown is thrombosis of the femoral and/or iliac vein from a previous procedure. Less common indications are absence of the intrahepatic portion of the inferior vena cava (relative) and a previous superior vena cava-to-right pulmonary artery (Glenn) anastomosis (absolute, if the right pulmonary artery is to be entered). Indications for brachial artery cutdown are the same as for the axillary approach, except in a larger child. For a venous catheterization, the right arm is preferred to the left. If the left arm is used and a left superior vena cava is present and drains to the coronary sinus, a complete right heart catheterization is difficult because the catheter enters the heart via the coronary sinus. The caution is again made that, if catheterization by the brachial artery route is considered, the physician must first exclude the presence of an anomalous retroesophageal right subclavian artery.

Local anesthetic is infiltrated in an area just over and medial to the brachial artery pulsation about 1 cm above the skin crease. The skin incision is centered over the brachial artery pulsation. The median cubital vein traverses the antecubital fossa as it courses medially and superiorly to join the basilic vein (Fig. 7) and is ideal for catheterization. If it is unavailable, the cephalic vein can be used. It is of similar size to the median cubital vein but is more lateral. Un-

fortunately, it joins the subclavian vein in the shoulder at very sharp angle and it may be difficult to pass a catheter around this bend.

If both venous and retrograde arterial catheterizations are to be performed, it is generally worthwhile to dissect out the brachial artery prior to beginning the venous catheterization. The brachial artery follows a course parallel but deep to the median cubital and basilic veins. In the mid portion of the antecubital fossa, at about the level of the skin crease, the aponeurosis of the biceps muscle lies between the brachial artery and the more superficial median cubital vein. If the incision has been made in the position described above, the brachial artery will be found in a more superficial position and will not be covered by this thick layer of fascia. It is important to make certain that it is the artery and not the nerve that has been selected for cannulation. Only after the vessels have been identified, isolated, and controlled for bleeding should one proceed with catheter introduction.

Umbilical Vessels

During the first 48 to 72 hours after birth, and rarely even up to 1 week of age, it is often possible to perform a cardiac catheterization using the umbilical artery and vein. Although the superficial portion of these vessels may be cannulated after the third day of life, the catheters generally cannot be passed from the umbilical into the central vessels. Infection is a major concern with an umbilical approach and considerable care must be given to adequate cleansing of the umbilical region prior to catheter introduction and appropriate care of the area following the study. Cannulation of the umbilical vessels is easiest if the obstetrician has left a long umbilical stump and if there have been no previous attempts at cannulation of the umbilical vessels. Prior to cleansing the area, the cord is cut with sterile scissors or a scalpel blade, as close to the stump as possible. (The cord clamp cannot be sterilized adequately and should be removed before the area is prepared.)

With today's aggressive neonatal care, it is common for a patient to arrive in the catheterization laboratory with an umbilical artery line already in place. This makes isolation of the other cord vessels more difficult and often means that the umbilical cord has also been cut off very close to the skin. In addition, if there has been extensive manipulation of the cord in an attempt to introduce the umbilical artery line or if the line has been sutured to the umbilical stump, the remaining area may be so macerated as to preclude location of the other vessels. If the umbilical artery line is positioned in the descending aorta, it is not adequate for angiographic evaluation of the thoracic aorta. If aortography is necessary, the line should be replaced.

After the umbilical cord clamp has been removed, the umbilical region and the right inguinal area are cleaned using antiseptic solution. The area is draped with sterile towels and eye-hole drapes so that both the umbilicus and right inguinal catheterization sites are included in the sterile field. If an umbilical artery line is in place it is moved laterally and taped to the infant's left flank. Five or 6 cm of the line closest to the umbilicus are cleaned at the same time as the skin surface and this portion of the arterial line is included in the sterile field. If the arterial line is not to be removed, the transducer and the nonsterile portion of the line can be connected with plastic tubing. If the line is to be removed, a #5 French polyvinyl feeding tube with a closed end and multiple side holes is filled with heparinized flushing solution, the old arterial line is removed, and the new line inserted in its place and advanced until it is in the thoracic aorta at the level of the ductus arteriosus. If an end-hole arterial line is in place in the umbilical artery, it may be possible to introduce a larger diameter, end-hole, soft, flexible catheter using a guidewire as an exchange wire.

The umbilical cord contains a single vein and two arteries and is surrounded by a thick tubular sheath. The cord is filled with Wharton's jelly, a gelatinous substance. Because the cord vessels readily contract upon contact with air, it is rare for bleeding to occur when the cord clamp is removed after the patient is more than a few hours old. Although the umbilical vein enters the abdominal wall cephalad to the umbilical arteries, which lie side by side, there is a variable degree of spiral rotation of the vein around the cord. It is therefore not possible to rely on the position of the vessels in the umbilical cord to determine whether they are arteries or veins. Usually, the vein can be identified as a larger, thin-walled structure that often courses obliquely around the side of the cord. The arteries are paired, smaller, and thicker walled structures and are usually more centrally located in the cord. There may be only a single umbilical artery. Once a vessel has been identified, a small, curved iris forceps is introduced a short distance into the vessel lumen and gently opened and closed a few times to dilate the opening. The umbilical cord stump is then held with a toothed forceps and a #5 French polyvinyl feeding tube is advanced a short distance into the vessel. The position of the catheter should now be observed fluoroscopically to be certain whether it is positioned either in the arterial or venous system. If the catheter has been introduced into the umbilical vein, it will advance in a cephalad direction toward the liver. If in the artery, it will advance caudally into the pelvis and then turn cephalad into the abdominal aorta. Ideally, the umbilical arterial catheter should be introduced first and advanced into the aorta to obtain a systemic oxygen saturation and blood gases and to monitor pressure.

The umbilical arteries arise as branches of the internal iliac arteries, subtending a rather sharp angle at their point of origin. If difficulty is encountered in maneuvering the umbilical arterial catheter past this junction, the catheter should be moved in and out with a short motion or advanced with gentle forward pressure and some twisting. Occasionally, it may be helpful to gently aspirate the catheter and slowly withdraw it from the umbilical artery. The catheter may have a small clot at its distal end, which can then be removed with flushing solution. The catheter is then reintroduced into the umbilical artery.

If these maneuvers are not successful, it may be possible to advance the catheter into the appropriate position by inserting the soft, flexible end of a 0.018-inch or 0.021-inch coil-spring guidewire into the catheter to increase its stiffness. The flexible tip will allow the catheter to bend around the sharp angle while the stiffer more proximal part of the guidewire will increase the maneuverability of the catheter. As a last resort, the stiff end of an 0.018-inch guidewire can be gently curved at the tip by pulling this end over the rounded edge of a hemostat. This curved portion of the wire can then be introduced into the catheter and carefully and slowly advanced under fluoroscopic control until it is at the catheter tip. (It is mandatory for the physician to make certain that the wire tip is always within the lumen of the catheter or laceration of the intima of the arterial wall may occur.) Once the guidewire is positioned at the tip of the catheter, the curved end may sufficiently bend the catheter to permit passage around the arterial junction into the iliac artery and then into the aorta. The wire is then removed and 1 mL of blood is aspirated from the catheter and discarded, removing any air bubbles and clots that may be present. The catheter is then rinsed with flushing solution and advanced into the thoracic aorta to the level of the ductus arteriosus.

The umbilical venous catheter is usually easily advanced in a straight pass into the liver. We have developed a method in our laboratory to facilitate multiple catheter changes when the umbilical vein is used. A #5 French polyvinyl feeding tube is passed through a #5 French thin-walled sheath and then advanced into the umbilical vein. Once the catheter has been advanced into the um-

bilical vein for a few centimeters, all further manipulation should be done under fluoroscopic control. It is usually preferable to start out with a soft, flexible catheter to avoid any trauma to the liver. If the feeding tube enters the ductus venosus in what appears to be the low to mid portion of the liver on the fluoroscope screen, the catheter will course posteriorly and slightly to the patient's left. After another centimeter or so, the catheter will then course superiorly and enter the suprahepatic portion of the inferior vena cava and the right atrium. Once the catheter is in the right atrium, the sheath is advanced over the catheter until it is also in the right atrium. The feeding tube catheter can be then withdrawn and exchanged with any other type of catheter, which is then readily introduced through the sheath into the right atrium. Because this sheath provides a short, direct route into the heart, it is advisable to use a side-port sheath with a back-bleed prevention device to avoid inadvertent introduction of air into the heart and/or excessive blood loss during catheter exchange. The sheath is then withdrawn back onto the catheter and is only advanced again if another catheter change has to occur.

If resistance is encountered while the feeding tube catheter is initially being advanced, especially if the catheter has not followed the course described above, it should be withdrawn slightly and advanced again. Because this feeding tube catheter is quite soft and flexible, the physician will have little control over the direction of the catheter tip. If the catheter has not passed across the ductus venosus after a few attempts, it should be withdrawn to the low border of the liver and a small amount of contrast material injected to determine whether or not the ductus venosus is patent. If the ductus venosus is already closed, the feeding tube can be withdrawn about half way and left in place during the procedure. If it is completely withdrawn at this point, bleeding from the umbilical vein may occur and delay the catheterization.

If the ductus venosus is patent but small, the physician must decide the appropriate course of action. A critically ill infant, particularly one who requires a balloon septostomy, is not a suitable candidate for prolonged manipulation in the hope of traversing the ductus venosus, and the catheter should be inserted into an inguinal vessel either percutaneously or by cutdown. If a continued effort to use the umbilical route seems warranted, a standard woven Dacron catheter or a flow-directed balloon catheter may be tried. In both cases the sheath technique described above can be used to facilitate subsequent catheter changes if entry into the heart is successful. Although it is easier to maneuver a Dacron catheter because of its increased stiffness, it also increases the danger of trauma to the liver. A flow-directed balloon catheter may be a better choice in this situation because it is relatively soft and flexible like the feeding tube yet has more maneuverability. It should not be inflated in the ductus venosus or liver because the vessels are small and easily damaged. Once the flow-directed balloon catheter enters the heart it can be passed across the atrial septum and the balloon can be used to enter the ventricles from their respective atria. In addition, the balloon catheter can be floated out into the pulmonary artery, a catheter pass that is difficult to achieve from the umbilical route using a woven Dacron catheter.

After completion of the cardiac catheterization, the umbilical catheters are usually removed. If the patient is going to cardiac surgery within a short time following the catheterization, the umbilical artery line may be withdrawn to the descending aorta and left in place to monitor systemic pressure and blood gases. Following removal of the catheters, bleeding must be controlled. If the umbilical cord is of adequate length, it may be sufficient to tie a suture ligature around the base of the cord. Usually, the cord has been cut short and it is necessary to put sutures through the cord and tie them. In some circumstances it may be necessary

to include some umbilical skin to prevent the suture from tearing out of a macerated cord stump.

Arteriotomy and Catheter Introduction

After the artery to be used has been exposed surgically, controlling ties of umbilical tape or soft, flexible silicone material (Vesseloops, Medgeneral, Minneapolis, MN) are placed proximal and distal to the proposed site of cannulation (Fig. 8A). Whenever possible, a 1.5- to 2-cm segment of vessel should be exposed. It is again important to stress the necessity for gentle and careful introduction. Rough handling may result in spasm of vessels, making catheterization difficult or impossible.

If a long segment of artery can be exposed, a pair of miniature bulldog vascular clamps are applied at the proximal and distal ends of the vessel as far as possible from the proposed site of arteriotomy. This method puts no tension on the arteriotomy site. If only a short segment of vessel is exposed, usually in an infant, the proximal and distal umbilical tapes or silicone threads can be used to elevate the artery and control bleeding. Alternatively, a forceps or a small hemostat can be placed under the vessel and then opened slightly, bringing the vessel further into the field and making arteriotomy easier. If this is not sufficient to control bleeding, gentle traction on the umbilical tapes usually suffices. In each of the above techniques, a transverse arteriotomy is then made perpendicular to the long axis of the blood vessel. The incision can be made with a pair of iris scissors or with a #11 scalpel blade (Fig. 8B). The incision must be carried through the full thickness of the arterial wall and into the lumen. Too large an incision results in back-bleeding around the catheter and also weakens the arterial wall, risking disruption of the artery during manipulation. On the other hand, too small an opening may

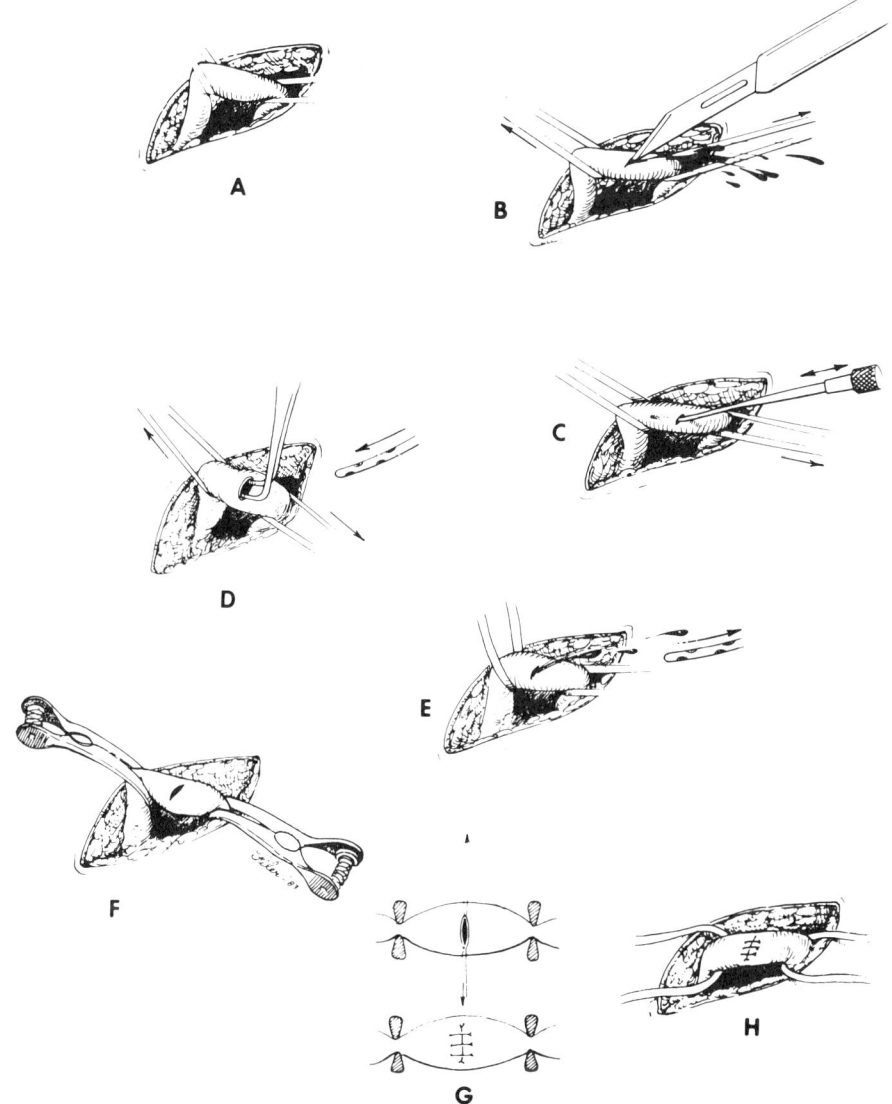

Figure 8. Arteriotomy and repair (see text). A: Vessels exposed, loops on artery. B: Arteriotomy using a knife blade. C: Use of the vessel dilator. D: Iris forceps are inserted into the lumen of the vessel and the catheter will then pass between the jaws of the forceps. E: Catheters have just been removed from the vessel and free back flow of blood is spurting from the open end. F: Bulldog clamp is applied to the proximal and distal segments of the vessel. G: Suturing of the vessel—mattress sutures or interrupted sutures. H: Suturing of vessel is completed.

result in dissection or tearing of the vessel wall at the time of catheter introduction or manipulation. Needless to say, if an error is made, it is better to be on the side of too small an opening than one that is too large. Although it is not ideal, it is possible sub-

sequently to enlarge an opening that is inadequate. After the arteriotomy has been made, a dilute heparin solution (100 units/mL) is injected into the distal segment through a small plastic cannula. Two milliliters of this solution are used for infants and

5 mL for older children and adults. The cannula is then removed and traction is reapplied to prevent back-bleeding. A vessel dilator is inserted into the proximal segment and advanced to its maximum diameter (Fig. 8C). The dilator has a soft, rounded tip and a gradual taper from the tip to the mid point of the instrument, permitting gentle enlargement of the opening without tearing. An alternative method of arteriotomy consists of making a small stab wound in the artery with a #11 blade, then inserting first one and then both blades of an iris forceps into the wound. A vessel dilator is then used to enlarge the opening to the desired size. With this method there is much less risk of creating an arteriotomy that is too large.

There are several methods for introduction of the catheter into the vessel lumen. In one, the lateral portion of the arteriotomy incision is picked up with a fine iris forceps and elevated, giving the arteriotomy site a fish-mouthed appearance. The catheter is then inserted into the arteriotomy site and gently advanced into the vessel lumen, often with a small degree of rotation in one direction or the other. In another technique, the ends of a small pair of curved iris forceps are inserted into the arteriotomy site and advanced a few millimeters into the lumen (Fig. 8D). The anterior wall of the vessel is elevated slightly by the forceps while the instrument is tilted cephalad and the jaws are allowed to open, separating the edges of the incision. The catheter is then inserted into the arteriotomy site and gradually advanced as the forceps are withdrawn. If the vessels are small this is a difficult and delicate maneuver. The catheter must be advanced just far enough so that the tip is within the lip of the arteriotomy site before the forceps are completely withdrawn. Otherwise, the tip of the catheter may catch on the edge of the incision and it may not be possible to advance it into the lumen. In a third technique, only one blade of the iris forceps is inserted into the arteriotomy, the anterior wall of the artery is grasped with the forceps and is elevated, permitting introduction of the catheter.

There are a number of techniques for controlling bleeding and getting adequate exposure during introduction of the catheter. One that we have found to be quite effective will be described. A single loop of umbilical tape, silk, or any other suitable material is placed proximal to the arteriotomy and another distal. A hemostat is placed on each about 2 cm from the skin. The hemostat on the proximal loop is placed on the drapes cephalad to the cutdown site and is held in place with the fifth finger of the left hand with enough tension to prevent bleeding. The iris forceps is grasped by the thumb and forefinger of the left hand. The heel of the right hand is used to anchor the hemostat on the distal loop, exerting enough tension to prevent bleeding. The catheter is then grasped by the thumb and forefinger of the right hand and is inserted. This technique has the advantage of requiring no "extra hands" and with a little practice can be accomplished by a single operator.

Once the catheter has been inserted into the vessel lumen and reaches the site of the proximal loop or clamp, this proximal control is released and the catheter is advanced into the central circulation. At this point, the umbilical tapes or other ties encircling the artery are allowed to lie loosely with the ends clamped in a hemostat. Should it be necessary to occlude the vessel during the catheterization to control bleeding, tension can be applied to the artery by pulling the hemostat and tightening the loop around the vessel. Should troublesome bleeding around the catheter persist, it may be helpful to loop the tape or suture material a second time around the artery. Traction on the hemostat securing the loop is then more effective.

After the catheterization is completed and the catheter has been withdrawn, it is essential to make certain that there is adequate flow from the proximal and distal segments of the artery. As the catheter is being withdrawn, good blood flow from the proximal segment washes out any clots that may have formed in the vessel or that may have been stripped off the end of the catheter (Fig. 8E). Bleeding is then controlled by tension of the proximal encircling tape while the same maneuver is performed with the distal segment. If free flow of blood is not obtained from either direction, then the previously used vessel dilator can be inserted into the lumen and advanced a few centimeters. This may dislodge a small clot and allow it to be flushed out with the pressure of blood behind it. If adequate blood flow is still not obtained, a small plastic cannula can be inserted. Suction is maintained with a syringe as the cannula is inserted and advanced into the vessel. If blood does not flow freely into the syringe after the tubing has been advanced for a distance of 4 to 5 cm, the tubing is withdrawn while maintaining constant suction with the syringe. Often a clot will either be withdrawn or a portion of it may be sucked into the tubing. If free flow of blood is still not obtained by this maneuver, the tubing can be filled with flushing solution and the segment irrigated. If, after all of the maneuvers, blood flow is still not adequate from the proximal or distal segment, it may be necessary to insert a small Fogarty embolectomy catheter into the vessel past the presumed site of obstruction. The balloon of the Fogarty catheter is then inflated and the catheter is withdrawn through the arteriotomy incision, pulling any clot in front of it.

Once adequate blood flow is obtained from both segments of the artery, a small plastic cannula is inserted into the distal segment and a few milliliters of dilute heparin solution are again infused. The cannula is withdrawn and a small bulldog clamp is applied to the distal segment. The same maneuver is repeated for the proximal segment and the bulldog is then applied to this area as well. The encircling tapes are loosened so that they now lie only under the posterior surface of the artery. The bulldog clamps control bleeding from the artery while allowing approximation of the edges of the incision for suturing (Fig. 8F)

There are several methods for suturing the arteriotomy incision. Regardless of which technique is used, careful approximation of the intimal surfaces must occur to prevent subsequent complications. Simple interrupted sutures are usually preferred using silk or synthetic suture material (6–0, 7–0) and an atraumatic needle. Two "corner" sutures should be placed first, near the ends of the incision (Fig. 8G). These should be tied and can then be used for traction to better expose the rest of the arteriotomy. Two or more additional interrupted sutures, depending on the size of the vessel, are then placed (Fig. 8H). It is better to delay tying these sutures until all are in place (as each suture is inserted, the ends are clamped in a small hemostat). This will permit adequate visualization of the intima and will insure proper placement of each suture.

Regardless of the technique used, the sutures must be placed through the full thickness of the arterial wall without injuring the intima of the opposite surface. In adults, an alternate technique consists of placing interrupted sutures at each end of the arteriotomy incision and continuous sutures between the two ends. This technique may be adequate for the repair of larger arteries but its use in infants and small children may result in inadequate approximation of the intima due to poor visualization. Other techniques such as longitudinal arteriotomy or arteriotomy with purse string sutures should not be used in children, because there is a considerable risk of arterial stenosis.

After the arteriotomy has been closed and adequate hemostasis obtained, the physician must be certain that there is adequate flow past the arteriotomy site. If there is evidence of inadequate flow and the distal artery is collapsed, the site may be gently massaged with iris forceps. If this is not effective in restoring flow, the vessel should be reopened.

Venotomy and Catheter Introduction

The techniques of placing catheters in the venous system are similar to those that have just been described in the previous section. The vein to be cannulated is adequately dissected and sutures are placed at appropriate sites on the vessel to control bleeding. In contrast to the umbilical tape used for bleeding control during arteriotomy, 3–0 or 4–0 silk is used for venous control. Again, as in the case of arteriotomy, gentleness is necessary to avoid spasm and to avoid tearing the rather fragile vessels of infants and children.

As a result of the lower pressure in the venous system, bleeding from the venotomy is easily controlled by gentle traction on the sutures surrounding the venotomy site. The venotomy is made in an identical manner to an arteriotomy, using a #11 scalpel blade or sharp iris scissors. The incision into the vein should be transverse. A longitudinal incision is more likely to tear and repair of a transverse incision is less likely to cause stenosis. A vessel dilator is used to size and/or enlarge the venotomy and the catheter is inserted with the assistance of forceps as described in the arteriotomy section above. Neither local nor systemic heparinization is used in our laboratory for venous catheterization.

In contrast to arterial catheterization, the vein caudal to the venotomy site is ligated unless the vein is to be repaired. With the exception of the femoral vein, saphenous bulb, or axillary vein, the cephalad portion of the vein is also ligated following removal of the catheter. We prefer to try to repair these large veins, and this is accomplished with continuous or interrupted sutures as was described for arterial repair. During the repair, bleeding is controlled by proximal and distal ties. If the vein is deep, exposure may be facilitated by gentle traction on these proximal and distal ties. After repair, the proximal and distal controlling sutures

should be removed. If they have been loosely tied with a single knot, the knot can usually be easily undone with the iris forceps. If this suture must be cut off it is prudent to have another temporary suture around the vessel, in case the vessel is nicked during cutting the suture or in case bleeding is brisk from the repaired venotomy site. There is commonly some oozing, which is easily controlled with pressure.

Skin Closure

After the catheters have been removed, the vessels sutured or ligated, and adequate hemostasis obtained, all loose sutures are removed. The incision should be meticulously irrigated with clean flushing solution to remove all blood and clots. The skin is then closed. Interrupted sutures or interrupted mattress sutures of 4–0 or 5–0 silk or synthetic material are commonly used. These sutures are removed 5 to 7 days following the catheterization, assuming that no infection has occurred. Another good technique for skin closure uses 5–0 polyglycolic acid material, a synthetic absorbable suture (Dexon, Davis and Geck Company). This suture is used subcutaneously with final skin approximation by sterile paper adhesive strips (Steri-strips). The advantage of this technique is that there are no sutures through the skin following the procedure. This eliminates a potential route of infection, especially in the inguinal region.

References and Suggested Reading

Desilets DT, and Hoffman R. A new method of percutaneous catheterization. Radiology 1965; 85:147–148.

Lurie PR, Armer RM, Klatte EC. Percutaneous guide wire catheterization: Diagnosis and therapy. Am J Dis Child 1963; 106:189–196.

Neches WH, Mullins CE, Williams RL, Vargo TA, and McNamara DG. Percutaneous sheath cardiac catheterization. Am J Cardiol 1972; 30:378–384.

Prince SR, Sullivan RL, Hackel A. Percutaneous catheterization of the internal jugular vein in infants and children. Anesthesiology 1976; 44:170–174.

Seldinger SI. Catheter replacement of the needle in percutaneous arteriography, a new technique. Acta Radiol 1953; 39:368–376.

5

Catheter Manipulation and Guidewire Technique

William H. Neches, M.D.

When a physician initially learns to maneuver a cardiac catheter, considerable thought is necessary to determine the connection between movement and rotation of the catheter outside the patient and motion and rotation of the catheter tip within the vascular system. Eventually, these thought processes become subconscious and similar to other acquired motor skills such as riding a bicycle or driving a car. Although this motor skill is readily learned and may become highly polished with time and experience, some difficult catheter maneuvers are learned only by long experience or from the experiences of others. This chapter will describe the various techniques of catheter manipulation, particularly those procedures that are useful in advancing the catheter into positions that are usually difficult to attain.

It should be emphasized that the physician may need to try a variety of catheters for a difficult pass. For example, if a pulmonary arteriogram is required, a side-hole catheter such as an NIH, is ideal. However, if such a catheter cannot be maneuvered into the pulmonary artery, another less ideal catheter, such as one with an end hole, may be advanced there with the use of a guidewire. Although with this latter catheter contrast must be injected much more slowly, it may still provide useful information.

Guidewire Uses

The use of guidewires for difficult catheter manipulation has become much more common with the widespread use of percutaneous catheterization techniques. Guidewires help to avoid the trauma to the patient's myocardium that may occur with prolonged catheter manipulation. On the other hand, when a guidewire is used, the physician must use meticulous technique to avoid embolic complications related to thrombus formation. Heparinized flushing solution should be infused into the catheter prior to the introduction of a guidewire to clear the lumen of any accumulated blood. Once the guidewire has been inserted into the lumen, maneuvers should be accomplished expeditiously since blood flows back into the catheter along the guidewire and a thrombus may form. Once the catheter has been manipulated into the desired position, the guidewire is removed. A few milliliters of blood should *immediately* be withdrawn from the catheter and discarded to remove any thrombi that may have formed within the catheter lumen. Heparinized flushing solution should then be infused into the catheter and the catheter reconnected to the pressure monitoring system. The guidewire should be wiped clean with a gauze pad saturated with heparinized flushing solution and then coiled and placed in a basin of heparinized flushing solution. This serves to remove residual dried blood or fibrinous material from the spaces between the coils of the guidewire.

Guidewires can be introduced into the catheter lumen for a number of different purposes:

1. A straight guidewire can be used to stiffen the catheter and facilitate its manipulation.

2. The soft flexible end of a guidewire can be introduced into an end-hole catheter and then carefully advanced through the catheter tip and into a desired location (Fig. 1A). The catheter is then advanced over the wire and into the proper position (Fig. 1B, 1C). Entering a pulmonary artery wedge position is an example of this application.

3. Either a closed-end or an end-hole catheter may be maneuvered around a bend or sharp curve with the use of a guidewire. The stiff end of the guidewire is curved using the technique shown in Figure 2. The curved end of the guidewire is then introduced into the catheter lumen and advanced to the tip of the catheter, taking care to keep the tip of the wire within the lumen if an end-hole catheter is being used. The J-shaped curve on the stiff end of the wire will help to pass a straight or slightly curved catheter around a relatively sharp bend. This is particularly useful in advancing a catheter from left atrium to left ventricle or in passing a retrograde femoral artery catheter around the aortic arch.

4. Complex curves can be added to a guidewire for certain passes. For example, an S-shaped curve may facilitate passage of a cath-

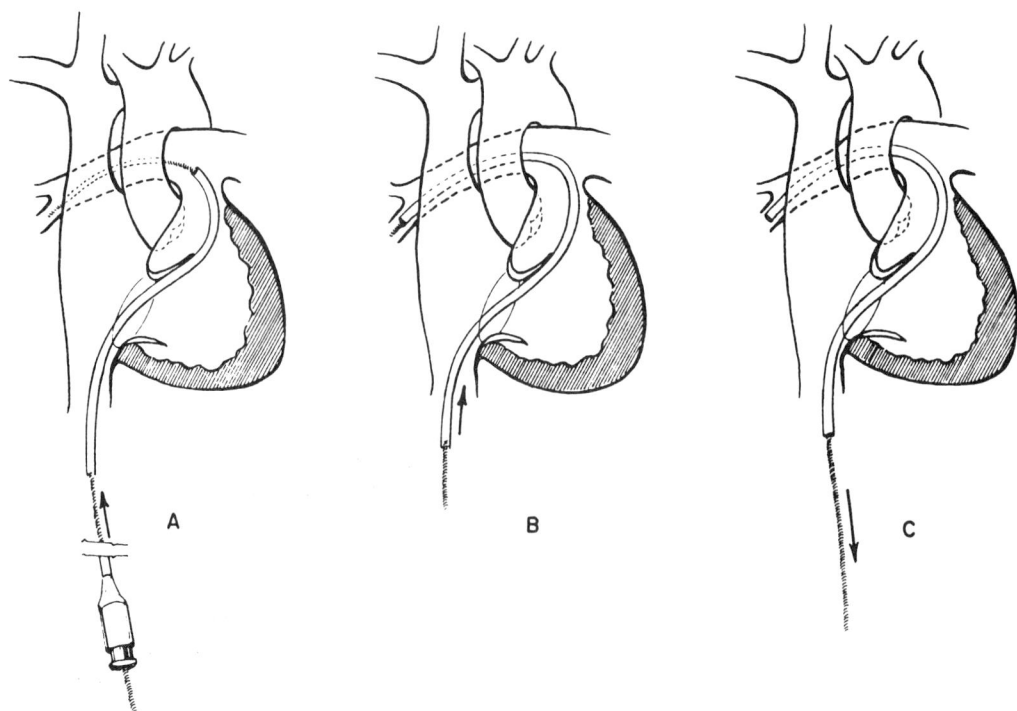

Figure 1. (A) A catheter is placed in the main pulmonary artery from the femoral vein and a wire is advanced through the catheter into the right pulmonary artery. (B) The catheter is advanced over the wire to the right pulmonary artery position. (C) The wire is removed, leaving the catheter in place.

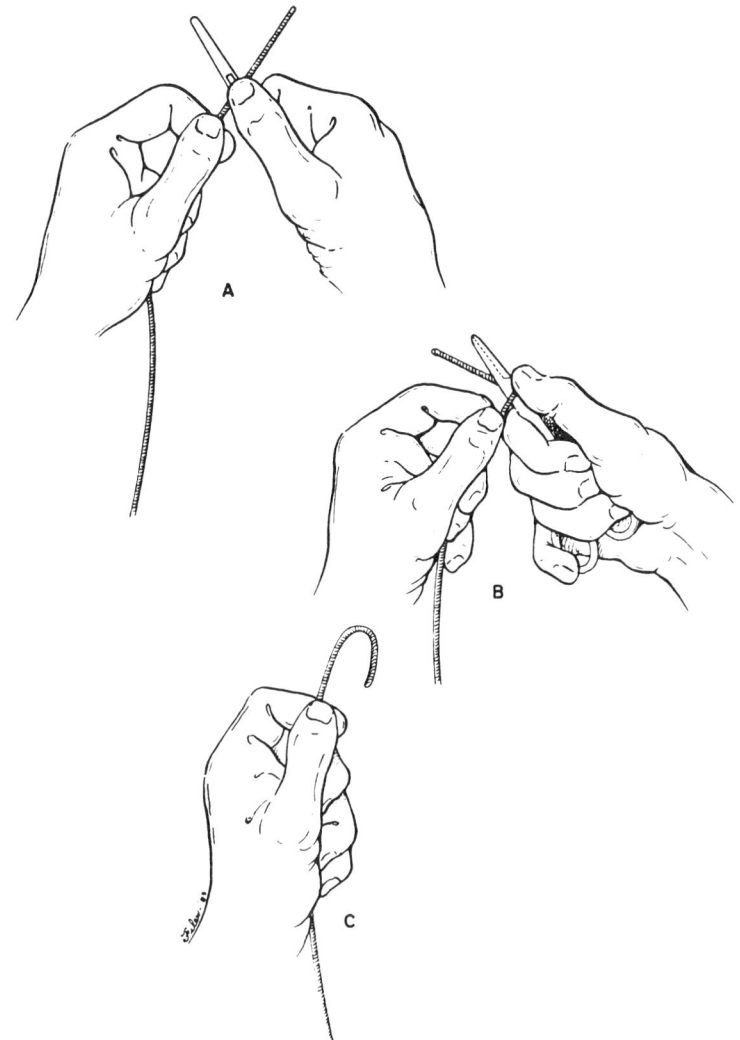

Figure 2. Bending the stiff end of a guidewire into a J shape. (A) The stiff end of a guidewire is placed over a straight hemostat 2–3 cm from the tip of the wire. (B) The guidewire is withdrawn over the curved side of the hemostat while gently pressing the wire between the thumb and the instrument, as if one were attempting to coil the end of a fancy ribbon on a present. (C) A guidewire with 180° curve in the stiff end after this maneuver.

eter from the right ventricle through a ventricular septal defect and into the aorta. The catheter is positioned in the right ventricular outflow tract as if it were to be maneuvered into the pulmonary artery (Fig. 3A). The stiff end of the wire is bent into an S shape (Fig. 3E) and is advanced to the catheter tip. (As a result of the double curve, it may be difficult to advance the wire and it may kink at the catheter hub if it is not advanced slowly). As the wire is being advanced into the distal portion of the catheter, the reverse curve on the wire will tend to withdraw the catheter from the

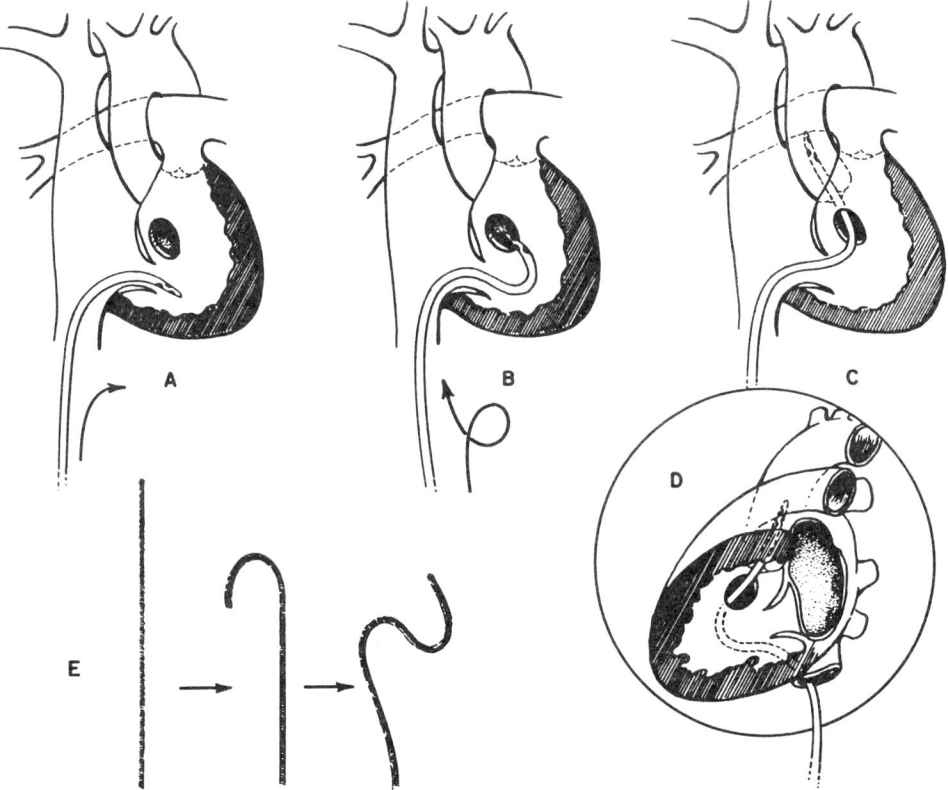

Figure 3. Bending the stiff end of a guidewire into a S shape to facilitate passage from the right ventricle into the aorta. (A) Position of the catheter in the right ventricle. (B) The wire is advanced into the catheter that is still positioned in the region of the right ventricular outflow tract. (C) The catheter is rotated clockwise and the tip flips up into the aorta. (D) Lateral view corresponding to Figure 3C. (E) A reverse 180° bend is placed on the wire forming it into an S shape. The maneuver used is similar to that described in Figure 2 for initial forming of the J.

right ventricular outflow tract. It is therefore advisable to advance the wire under fluoroscopic control and to advance the catheter slightly as it begins to withdraw from the desired position. Once the wire has reached the catheter tip, which should be in the mid right ventricular outflow tract (Fig. 3B), the catheter is rotated clockwise. This causes the catheter tip to flip cephalad. In many cases, the S shape causes the catheter to advance through the ventricular septal defect and out into the aorta (Figs. 3C and 3D). Once this has occurred it is usually not possible to advance the catheter further into the ascending aorta until the guidewire has been removed from the catheter. To prevent the catheter from flipping back into the ventricle during withdrawal of the guidewire, gentle forward pressure should be maintained on the catheter with one hand as the guidewire is slowly removed with the other hand. As the guidewire is withdrawn from the distal portion of the catheter, the gentle forward pressure tends to advance the tip further into the ascending aorta. If necessary, passage of the catheter around the aortic arch and into the descending aorta can then be accomplished using a guidewire with a simple curve at the stiff end. The catheter should be advanced well into the ascending aorta or even into one of the proximal brachiocephalic arteries to prevent the catheter from flipping back into the ventricle as the stiff J wire is advanced.

The variety of other maneuvers using guidewires is limited only by the ingenuity and skill of the individual performing the catheterization. For example, it may be difficult to pass a slightly curved catheter across a tight coarctation or across a stenotic or even a normal aortic valve. An end-hole catheter can be used and the soft end of a guidewire advanced through the catheter and across the stenotic area. The catheter is then advanced over the guidewire and into the desired position. If a closed-end angiographic catheter is preferred, the stiff end of a guidewire can be used to straighten the catheter, sometimes facilitating its passage across the coarctation or the aortic valve.

Catheter Manipulation

Manipulation in the Venous System

It is not unusual to encounter difficulties in advancing the catheter into the heart from either the femoral or antecubital venous route. In most cases, a catheter with the standard gentle curve at the tip can be maneuvered, with a little patience, into the inferior vena cava and subsequently into the right atrium. If this proves to be impossible, the catheter may be changed for one with a more suitable curve or a guidewire may be used.

A guidewire is especially useful in the patient with an absent intrahepatic inferior vena cava and an azygos continuation to the superior vena cava. Although a flow-directed, balloon-tipped catheter can be used to secure right heart pressures and oxygen saturations, it may be necessary to maneuver an angiographic catheter around the 180° angle at the azygos–superior vena cava junction. This is facilitated by inserting the tightly curved stiff end of a guidewire after the catheter has been positioned high in the azygos vein, near its junction with the superior vena cava. Once the catheter has been advanced around the tight bend, the guidewire is removed, the catheter is aspirated, and the aspirate is discarded. The physician is now left with a slightly curved catheter that can then be advanced into the right ventricle. Since the pass from the right ventricle into the pulmonary artery is difficult with this anomaly, the stiff end of the J-shaped wire can be used again. A larger (and therefore stiffer) guidewire (0.035-inch) can be tried if the thinner wire does not give the desired result.

It may be difficult from the arm approach to advance a catheter from the right subclavian vein into the right superior vena cava. This may be a fairly acute bend, especially if the cephalic vein has been used, and a catheter with a gentle curve at the tip may pass into the innominate vein rather than caudally into the superior vena cava. If the child is old enough to cooperate, taking a deep breath while the catheter is advanced may result in the desired catheter pass. Alternatively, raising the patient's arm cephalad and/or externally, compressing the axillary area, may align the subclavian vein with the superior vena cava. If these maneuvers are not successful, a J-shaped guidewire can be used to increase the curve at the tip.

Another means of bypassing side channels and manipulating a catheter into the inferior vena cava from the leg, or into the superior vena cava from the arm, is by buckling the catheter in a branch vessel and

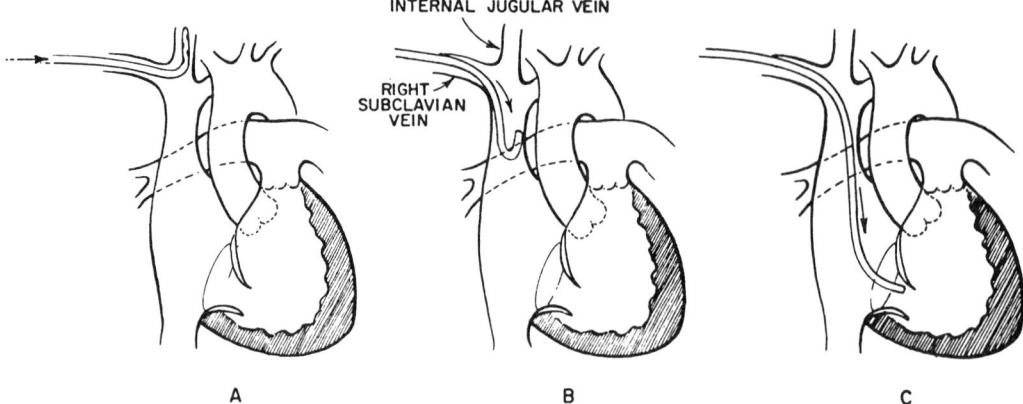

Figure 4. A catheter looped in the jugular vein and advanced into the right atrium.

forming a loop at its distal end (Fig. 4A). As the loop forms, it will gradually advance into the main channel (Fig. 4B). The catheter is then advanced, using this loop as the leading edge. (This maneuver must be performed carefully and gently to avoid trauma to the wall of the vein and can be done only in larger vessels.) Usually, after the loop forms at the distal catheter end, the tip will pop free and the whole U-shaped end of the catheter can be advanced, loop end first, into the heart (Fig. 4C). Once the leading edge of the loop has been advanced into the right atrium, the catheter is rotated and the loop is removed by slow withdrawal of the catheter. *A word of caution:* This looping of the catheter tip should only be done with fluoroscopic control so as to avoid forming too tight a curve at the very distal end of the catheter near the side holes. If the physician observes formation of a sharp angle, rather than a gentle curve, the catheter should be removed and inspected for a cracked wall. If a crack in the wall occurs and it is not recognized, subsequent manipulation of the catheter can result in embolization of the catheter tip.

Right Atrium to Superior Vena Cava

The catheter pass from the right atrium to the superior vena cava can be a difficult one unless done properly. The catheter should be rotated clockwise until the tip points toward the patient's right. The catheter is then slowly advanced, keeping the tip pointed in the same direction and the catheter as straight as possible. If the catheter bends even slightly during this maneuver, the tip is caught in a trabeculation and must be freed before the pass can be completed. This is accomplished by withdrawing the catheter slightly and changing the clockwise torque to alter the tip position. The catheter tip is again advanced. This maneuver can be thought of as sliding the catheter tip up the lateral wall, allowing the wall to guide the tip into the superior vena cava rather than into the right atrial appendage. It is quite effective and is safe, much safer than simply probing the superior aspect of the right atrium, hoping to enter the superior vena cava "sooner or later." With the latter random manipulation technique, the right atrial appendage will be entered more often than the superior vena cava. (The appendage is a thin-walled structure that can be easily perforated.)

Atrium to Right Ventricle

Passage of the catheter from right atrium to the right ventricle is generally an easy maneuver, particularly if the catheter has a gentle curve at the distal end. The catheter tip is positioned in the low right atrium with the tip pointing superiorly and to the left (and also anteriorly if viewed with the lateral fluoroscopy unit). The catheter is then advanced, either into the right ventricle or up along the atrial septum if the catheter curve is too gentle or if the right atrium is large. If, after several tries, the right ventricle cannot be entered, the catheter should be looped in the right atrium by advancing it with the tip pointed toward the right wall of the heart (Fig. 5A). The tip usually catches on a trabeculation and a loop will form as the catheter is advanced. The catheter is withdrawn slightly until the tip is free and it is then rotated counterclockwise so that the tip end of the loop is oriented toward the left. The tip may then flip directly into the right ventricle. If it does not, the catheter should be alternatively withdrawn and advanced slightly until it does. Occasionally it may be necessary to form a fairly large, almost 180° loop on the end of the catheter in order to enter the right ventricle. This may be difficult if the catheter only catches at the high lateral wall of the right atrium. When this occurs, the catheter can be "walked" down the lateral wall of the atrium by making a gentle loop, withdrawing the catheter until the tip is free and rapidly repositioning the tip in a slightly more caudal position. This is repeated a few times until the desired loop is obtained. Once the desired catheter loop has been formed, the catheter is withdrawn from the lateral wall of the right atrium and the tip turned around and flipped into the right ventricle (Fig. 5B, C). On occasion, especially in a patient with a large right atrium, it may not be possible to catch the catheter tip on the lateral wall of the right atrium. If this occurs, the initial curve on the catheter tip may be obtained by positioning the tip in a hepatic or renal vein in the abdomen or in the innominate vein in the chest.

As an alternative to building a loop within the right atrium to facilitate the pass into the right ventricle, the curved stiff end of a guidewire can be used to give the catheter a sharper curve.

On occasion, entering the right ventricle is more difficult, especially if the tricuspid valve is small or abnormally positioned. For instance, in patients with corrected transposition, the right-sided atrioventricular valve orifice is obliquely rather than vertically oriented. The atrial aspect of the plane of this valve faces superiorly and to

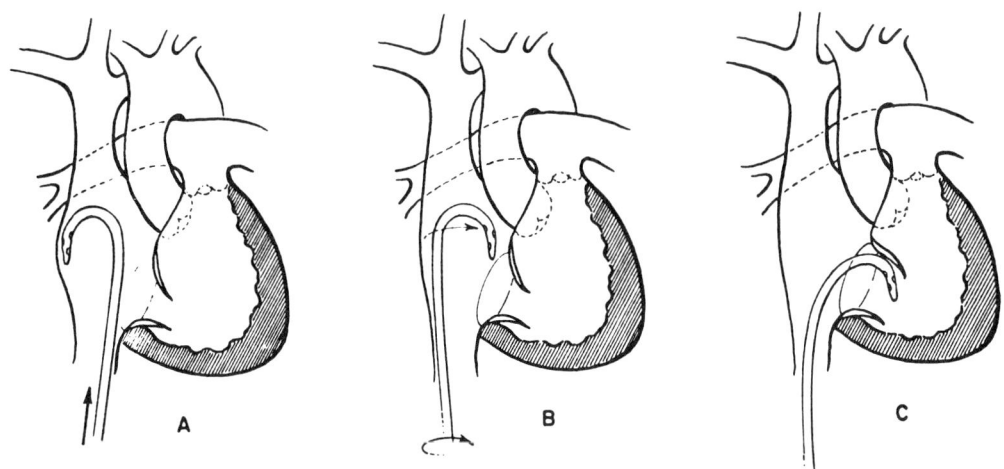

Figure 5. Manipulation of a catheter from right atrium to right ventricle (see text).

the right, and it is from that direction that the valve must be approached. This means that, from the femoral approach, the catheter must be looped within the atrium so that the tip points caudally. This position simulates the catheter pass from the superior vena cava. The catheter is then rotated until the tip lies anterior and to the left of the more proximal limb of the loop. The catheter is then alternately advanced and withdrawn—taking care to retain the loop—until the tip enters the ventricle. It is important to note that the atrioventricular valve orifice is more cephalad than normal in corrected transposition, and therefore the catheter tip will enter the right-sided ventricle from a position rather high in the right atrium.

Right Ventricle to Pulmonary Artery

In general, when there is normal right ventricular anatomy, passage of the catheter from right ventricle to the pulmonary artery is not particularly difficult. A catheter with a gentle curve is passed across the tricuspid valve and positioned in the body of the right ventricle just below the right ventricular outflow tract (Fig. 6A). The catheter is then rotated clockwise and as the catheter tip flips up and points toward the pulmonary artery the catheter is advanced forward and across the pulmonary valve. It should be remembered that the right ventricular outflow tract is usually located medial to the lateral heart border as seen fluoroscopically. If the catheter tip is too lateral it tends to lodge in an intertrabecular space. Even if the catheter tip seems properly positioned it may not readily turn superiorly during clockwise rotation of the catheter. If so, the tip is probably caught in a septal trabeculation. The catheter should be slightly withdrawn and clockwise rotation again attempted. If the catheter tip is caught and the catheter is not withdrawn as more and more rotational torque is placed on the catheter, when the tip eventually springs free it often ends up medial to the desired position.

When infundibular pulmonary stenosis is present, it may be difficult or even impossible to pass a catheter across the stenotic area. In patients with tetralogy of Fallot, the right ventricular outflow tract is positioned more laterally (leftward) than usual and this also may make the catheter pass even more difficult. Since the right ventricular outflow tract is relatively thin, forceful manipulation of the catheter in this area should be avoided. Lateral plane fluoroscopy is often helpful when attempting to traverse the right ventricular outflow area. When passage of the catheter across a stenotic area has not been accomplished despite repeated attempts, it is often valuable to visualize this area angiographically with a small hand injection of contrast material. The catheter should be placed proximal to the stenotic area and a few milliliters of contrast material injected slowly, recording the injection on the video recorder. If the outflow region is found to be atretic or so severely stenotic that catheter passage seems impossible, another hand injection of contrast material can be recorded cineangiographically for a permanent record.

The presence of corrected transposition should also be considered if the pulmonary artery cannot be entered despite repeated efforts. In this anomaly, the pulmonary artery arises medially and slightly posteriorly, making the pass from the abnormally positioned right-sided atrioventricular valve uncommonly difficult. This congenital abnormality may be recognized only after the exploratory injection of contrast media.

If the pass into the pulmonary artery can still not be made even after the right ventricular outflow tract anatomy has been adequately delineated, it can sometimes be accomplished with the help of a guidewire (Fig. 6B). An end-hole catheter must be used for this maneuver since it involves passage of the soft end of a guidewire through the catheter tip, past the stenotic area, and out into the pulmonary artery. This is best accomplished with a thin guidewire (e.g.,

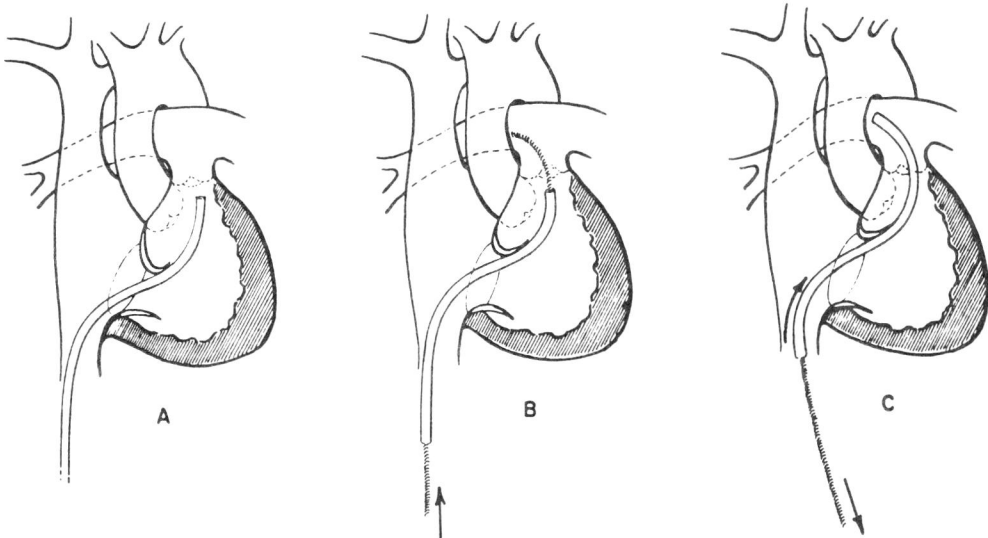

Figure 6. Manipulation of a catheter from right ventricle to pulmonary artery.

0.025-inch or less) since a smaller wire has a more flexible tip. However, the guidewire cannot bend readily until the tip protrudes a centimeter or more from the catheter. This maneuver must therefore be performed carefully so that the tip of the guidewire does not perforate the right ventricular outflow tract. Putting a slight curve on this soft end of the guidewire facilitates manipulation through the stenotic area. Once the wire is passed through the stenotic area and into the pulmonary artery, it should be advanced distally into a pulmonary artery branch. The catheter is then slowly advanced over the wire, while the end of the wire outside the patient is maintained in a fixed position. This prevents the tip of the wire from advancing further as the catheter is being maneuvered into the pulmonary artery. Once the catheter has been advanced into the desired position, the wire is removed, the catheter is aspirated and the aspirated blood discarded, and the catheter is flushed (Fig. 6C).

Pulmonary Artery Branches

Once the catheter enters the main pulmonary artery, it should be rotated clock-wise and advanced to enter the right pulmonary artery, or rotated counterclockwise and advanced to enter the left pulmonary artery. Either of these passes may be easy or difficult, depending on the curve of the catheter and the individual patient's anatomy. If a patent ductus arteriosus is present, passage into the right and/or left pulmonary arteries may be especially difficult since the catheter may preferentially traverse the ductus into the descending aorta. Whether or not a ductus is present, passage into the distal pulmonary arterial tree may be facilitated by substituting a catheter with a more sharply curved tip or by using the stiff end of a guidewire with a J curve. If an end-hole catheter is being used, the soft end of a guidewire, preferably with a rather sharp curve, can be advanced through the catheter into the right or left pulmonary artery and the catheter then advanced over the wire. If the guidewire makes a relatively sharp bend entering one or the other pulmonary arteries, it may be very difficult to advance the catheter over the wire. Slowly withdrawing the wire while advancing the catheter usually facilitates the maneuver.

The pulmonary artery "wedge" position can usually be attained by simply advancing the catheter far distally into the right or left pulmonary artery. Occasionally, the catheter "hangs up" too proximally, despite repeated probing with clockwise and counterclockwise torque on the catheter. In such cases, the soft end of a guidewire can usually be advanced distally and the catheter then advanced over the wire into the desired "wedge" position.

Right Atrium to Left Atrium

The ease of passing a catheter from the right to left atrium across an interatrial communication is one of the advantages of catheterization from the leg. In patients with an interatrial septal defect, this is a very simple catheter pass, but it may be equally easy in a patient who has just a patent foramen ovale. (Therefore, the ease with which a catheter passes from right to left atrium is not an indication of the presence of an actual interatrial septal defect or of its size.) To traverse the atrial septum, a catheter with a gently curved tip is used. It is advanced from the inferior vena cava into the right atrium and is directed toward the left shoulder. If the catheter passes freely beyond the left border of the vertebral column, the left atrium may have been entered. This can be confirmed by a change to a left atrial pressure contour, by aspiration of highly oxygenated blood from the catheter, by passage of the catheter beyond the left border of the heart into a pulmonary vein, or by demonstrating the posterior location of the catheter tip by lateral fluoroscopy. If the catheter has passed into the right ventricle, instead, a ventricular pressure contour will be seen. In addition, premature ventricular contractions often result when the catheter touches the right ventricular wall. If entry into the right ventricle has occurred, the catheter tip was directed too anteriorly during the maneuver. The catheter should be slowly withdrawn from the right ventricle until the pressure curve changes from a ventricular to an atrial pressure, and then rotated slightly clockwise to point more posteriorly but still to the left. The catheter is again advanced and should traverse the atrial septum.

The catheter sometimes enters the coronary sinus during an attempt to cross the atrial septum. This is particularly likely if there is a persistent left superior vena cava draining to the coronary sinus, since the coronary sinus is unusually large in this anomaly. If the catheter has been passed into what appears to be a left atrial position and there is still a right atrial pressure curve and dark venous blood is obtained upon aspiration, the catheter tip is probably in the coronary sinus. If a persistent left superior vena cava is present, it can be entered by clockwise rotation of the catheter tip as it is advanced. Once the left superior vena cava has been entered, a small amount of contrast material should be hand injected and the angiogram recorded on film. This serves to document the size and location of the left superior vena cava and its entry into the coronary sinus. It will also demonstrate the rare occurrence when a left superior vena cava enters the left atrium directly. The pass into it via an atrial septal defect or patent foramen ovale may then resemble the pass into the much more common coronary sinus drainage site. The cineangiogram also demonstrates the presence or absence of a left innominate vein, important information if open heart surgery is contemplated. If an innominate communication is present, the surgeon can snare and temporarily occlude the left superior vena cava during operation without fear of increasing venous pressure in the left side of the cerebral circulation. We routinely attempt to enter the left innominate vein and demonstrate its presence whenever the catheter is first passed into the right superior vena cava. Inability to enter the left innominate vein from the right superior vena cava should suggest the possibility of a persistent left superior vena cava draining to the coronary sinus.

The right atrial appendage can also be

entered during attempts to pass the catheter across the atrial septum. This catheter position is similar to, and only slightly more cephalad than, the catheter position that is actually desired and is also anteriorly positioned on lateral fluoroscopy. When the right atrial appendage is inadvertently entered with the catheter, it may appear that the catheter is advancing in an appropriate direction and the physician may be tempted to continue advancing the catheter despite some resistance. *CAUTION*: The right atrial appendage is a very thin walled structure and perforation is quite possible. Motion of the catheter tip is an important clue as to the actual catheter location. If the tip has traversed the interatrial septum or the tricuspid valve, it moves only slightly or not at all as the heart beats. In contrast, the right atrial appendage moves vigorously during atrial systole and imparts a brisk rocking motion to a catheter tip positioned there. If there is any doubt about the catheter location, a small hand injection of contrast material will establish the true position of the catheter tip. In patients with mitral atresia or mitral stenosis, the interatrial septum tends to bulge toward the right atrium. An interatrial communication is more superiorly and posteriorly located in these patients. The catheter pass across this communication is often difficult and will be located more cephalad than usual.

On occasion, it may be necessary to introduce a relatively stiff catheter into the left atrium (e.g., an electrode catheter or special sensor). If the catheter does not have an appropriate curve, this pass may be difficult and is potentially dangerous. A long percutaneous sheath or a Mullins transseptal sheath (USCI) facilitates this maneuver. The sheath can easily be passed across the atrial septum with a standard catheter or with its own introducer. After the catheter or introducer is withdrawn, the sheath remains in the left atrium and the special catheter or instrument can then be passed through it. The sheath can be withdrawn if it is nec-essary to expose the distal "working" portion of the catheter.

Left Atrium to Pulmonary Veins

The pulmonary veins enter the posterior wall of the left atrium, near the left border of the vertebral column as visualized fluoroscopically. The left pulmonary veins are generally easier to enter since the catheter tip is directed toward their orifices as it crosses the atrial septum. The right pulmonary veins are more difficult to enter and require a posterior and fairly sharp rightward angulation of the catheter after it crosses the atrial septum. This catheter pass is accomplished by advancing the catheter across the atrial septum and then rotating it clockwise. With a gently curved catheter, the right, upper lobe pulmonary vein is more easily entered than the lower lobe vein. The latter requires a more sharply curved catheter tip, which sometimes can be obtained by buckling the catheter. If this is not successful, substitution of a catheter with a more sharply curved tip, or the use of a guidewire with a sharply curved tip as described earlier, should be considered. It is important to remember that a catheter with a guidewire within its lumen is a much more rigid instrument than the catheter alone and must be manipulated with caution.

Since the left atrial appendage is located at the upper left heart border, a catheter pass that appears to be entering the left upper pulmonary vein may instead be entering the left atrial appendage. If the catheter is in a pulmonary vein, the tip will advance readily beyond the left heart border and there will be almost no motion of the catheter in a cephalo-caudal direction. In contrast, if a catheter has been inadvertently introduced into the left atrial appendage, it will not advance beyond the left heart border and the catheter tip will move rather briskly. If there is any doubt, the catheter position should be documented with a cautious, slow hand injection of contrast medium, since the left atrial appendage, like the right, may be relatively easily perforated.

Left Atrium to Left Ventricle

The ease with which a catheter can be passed from the left atrium to the left ventricle is determined by the curve on the catheter and the angle of the plane of the mitral valve. In general, a catheter with a curve that is ideal for passage across the atrial septum is too straight to pass easily across the mitral valve. A more sharply curved catheter may easily traverse the mitral valve but be more difficult to get across the atrial septum. It is generally preferable to use a catheter with a gentle curve to cross the atrial septum and then use one of a number of maneuvers to pass this catheter across the mitral valve. On some occasions, simply advancing the catheter may suffice. More often, the catheter preferentially enters a left pulmonary vein or the left atrial appendage. It is also possible to curve the catheter by gently buckling it against the posterior or lateral wall of the left atrium. The catheter can then be withdrawn, rotated in a counterclockwise manner, and advanced across the mitral valve.

In an alternative technique of traversing the mitral valve, the catheter tip is first positioned in a right pulmonary vein. The catheter is then cautiously advanced until it begins to buckle. It is then rotated counterclockwise and advanced further. The tip usually "pops" out of the pulmonary vein and as it does, the counterclockwise torque causes it to sweep posteriorly, to the left, and then inferiorly. The tip then is usually quite near the mitral orifice, and either slightly advancing or withdrawing the catheter will cause the tip to cross the mitral valve and enter the left ventricle. (This maneuver is most easily accomplished with a relatively soft catheter and must not be used if the catheter is stiff. It requires a certain amount of "touch" and should be used only by an experienced operator.)

Another, more usual method for advancing the catheter from the left atrium to left ventricle involves the use of the stiff end of a guidewire. The catheter is passed across the atrial septum and positioned in the mid portion of the left atrium. When using a #6 French catheter, the stiff end of a 0.025-inch guidewire is formed into a J shape. If a larger catheter is used, it is preferable to use a 0.035-inch guidewire. The J-curved stiff end of a guidewire is then introduced into the catheter hub. If this is done slowly, the straight catheter lumen will gently unbend the J tip of the guidewire. If it is difficult to insert the curved wire into the catheter, the soft end of the wire should be introduced into the sharp end of a percutaneous needle (or into the tip of a sheath dilator). The needle (or dilator) is then advanced over the wire to the stiff end, thus straightening the J curve. The tip of the needle (or dilator) is inserted into the hub of the catheter and the wire advanced 5 to 10 cm. The needle or dilator can then be removed while holding the guidewire in position. The guidewire is advanced slowly under fluoroscopic control until it reaches the catheter tip. (It is important to be certain that the catheter has not been inadvertently advanced too far to the left so that it lies in a pulmonary vein or in the left atrial appendage). If the catheter tip is lying freely within the left atrium, the catheter will curve easily as the curved guidewire reaches the catheter tip. The catheter is then rotated counterclockwise and advanced across the mitral valve into the left ventricle. (This maneuver is even easier if lateral plane fluoroscopy is available and the physician can be certain that the catheter tip has been rotated anteriorly and is properly positioned before it is advanced.) If the catheter does not rotate freely or meets resistance when it is being advanced toward the left ventricle, the physician should again make certain that the catheter tip is not in a pulmonary vein or in the left atrial appendage. To check this without removing the guidewire, the catheter is withdrawn slightly and rotated counterclockwise. If the catheter is in a pulmonary vein or in the left atrial appendage, the tip often pops free as the catheter tip is being withdrawn. Once this occurs, the catheter can then be advanced across the mitral valve as described above.

Once the left ventricle has been entered, removal of the guidewire should be monitored fluoroscopically. The catheter should be held firmly and the guidewire withdrawn slowly with the other hand. As this withdrawal takes place, the catheter often loses much of the curve induced by the guidewire and may hit against the left ventricular wall and cause arrhythmia. If this occurs, the catheter should be repositioned slightly.

If a catheter is too straight after the guidewire has been removed, proper positioning of the catheter in the left ventricle may be impossible. A more sharply curved catheter can be used or a curve can be "custom made" prior to catheter insertion. This is accomplished by having a boiling sterile waterbath available in the catheterization laboratory. (This may be a small instrument sterilizer or even a hot plate with a sterile, covered metal container filled with sterile water.) A 10-mL syringe is filled with heparinized flushing solution and attached to the catheter without filling the catheter with the fluid. The catheter tip is dipped for a few seconds into the sterile boiling water, then removed from the water, and bent into the desired curve. The room temperature solution is then infused through the catheter, fixing the curve in this position. Although the catheter loses some of this bend after it is inserted into the patient, the tendency to reform this curve will be retained and will facilitate positioning of the catheter in the left ventricle. This technique is also useful for forming a catheter tip into complex shapes for entry into peripheral arterial branches or for selective coronary angiography.

Aorta to Left Ventricle

Passage of a catheter from the aorta into the left ventricle may be easy or maddeningly difficult. Surprisingly, there is poor correlation between the difficulty of the pass and the degree of abnormality of the aortic valve. It may be very difficult in a patient with a normal valve or easy in a patient with rather severe aortic stenosis. In adult cardiology, a "pigtail" catheter is widely used and is probably the easiest to get across the aortic valve. It is less used in small children because of the size of the leading loop and because of the difficulty in introducing it through a percutaneous sheath. It is also not possible to localize a left ventricular outflow gradient using the pigtail catheter.

A standard catheter can be maneuvered across the aortic valve in a number of different ways. The catheter may simply be advanced across the aortic valve without meeting any resistance. It is often necessary to advance and withdraw the catheter repetitively while simultaneously turning it in one direction or another to change the orientation of the catheter tip. (In this maneuver, once the catheter meets resistance, the tip lies in one of the sinuses of Valsalva and further advancing will never be successful. Since repeated vigorous probing of a sinus may cause perforation, the catheter should be advanced only until it *begins* to buckle, then withdrawn and advanced again.) If this maneuvering is still not successful, it is usually possible to form a 180° loop at the tip of the catheter by continuing to advance the catheter slowly and carefully after the tip has lodged in a sinus of Valsalva. Care must be taken to stop advancing the catheter if it enters one of the coronary arteries.

If it is difficult to form a loop in the aortic root, the catheter may be withdrawn and the tip positioned in the innominate artery. Advancing this catheter may then cause it to buckle as the tip "hangs up" within the artery. Further advancing then usually causes the loop to pop into the ascending aorta. Once the 180° loop is formed at the distal end of the catheter, this loop may sometimes be easily advanced across the aortic valve into the left ventricle. As soon as the loop passes across the aortic valve and into the left ventricle, the catheter tip will spring against the left ventricle wall and considerable arrhythmia may result. The catheter should be withdrawn until the loop is removed, then advanced until the tip is in a stable position without arrhythmia.

Unfortunately, it may not be possible to successfully back a loop of catheter across the aortic orifice. In this situation, a relatively straight catheter may be substituted. A curved guidewire is usually needed to manipulate the catheter around the aortic arch. Alternatively, the stiff end of a 0.025- or 0.035–inch guidewire may be used to straighten whatever catheter is already in place. An advantage of this method lies in the fact that as the stiff end of the guidewire approaches the end of the catheter, the curve on the distal end is *gradually* straightened. In general, it is preferable to insert the guidewire all the way to the catheter tip and attempt passage across the aortic valve with the nearly straight catheter. If this is not initially successful, the guidewire can be withdrawn in successive steps, each time probing the aortic valve with a slightly different curve on the catheter, rotating it as it is repeatedly advanced and withdrawn. One of the combinations of catheter shapes and angles of approach to the aortic valve may be the proper one to allow the catheter to traverse the valve.

If the above approaches fail, a Lehman ventriculography catheter may be tried. This catheter has multiple side holes and a closed end and can therefore be used for angiocardiography. It has, however, a distal "rattail" tapered tip. This tip is much more flexible than the rest of the catheter and it is easy to loop in the aortic root. The loop is small, facilitating passage across the aortic valve. With this catheter, the more proximal location of the side holes lessens the possibility of an intramyocardial injection, but the long "rat tail" seems to increase arrhythmia.

If all of the above maneuvers fail, it may be possible to pass a catheter into the left

ventricle with the use of a guidewire. The soft end of the guidewire is passed through the distal tip of an end-hole catheter. Attempts are then made to cross the aortic valve with the guidewire, either directly or by forming a small loop on the flexible tip. If this is successful, the catheter can then be advanced over the guidewire and into the ventricle. If a Lehman catheter has been used for this maneuver, it is possible to measure and localize an aortic gradient, but high-quality angiocardiography is not possible. A "pigtail" catheter will enable fine angiography, but will not permit localization of the gradient. It is also possible to use a Gensini catheter, whose multiple side holes facilitate angiocardiography. Because of the end hole on this catheter, however, recoil may be a problem, and the injection rate must be slower than with either a closed-end or a pigtail catheter.

If passage of a guidewire across the aortic valve was not too difficult, a long sheath may be used to pass a closed-end catheter across the aortic valve. To do this, the standard percutaneous sheath is replaced by a long sheath that is then advanced around the aortic arch. The end-hole catheter is advanced through the sheath and the guidewire advanced through the catheter tip. Once the wire has passed across the aortic valve and the catheter is advanced over it, the sheath is advanced over the catheter into the left ventricle. The catheter and wire are then removed, the sheath aspirated and flushed, and the desired closed-end or micromanometer catheter advanced through the sheath into the left ventricle.

Retrograde Passage Across an Atrioventricular Valve

In certain circumstances, a catheter may be passed retrogradely across an atrioventricular valve when an approach via the interatrial septum is not feasible. Examples include patients with a Mustard or Senning repair of complete transposition of the great arteries and patients with concordantly connected great arteries who have an intact interatrial septum and in whom a transseptal approach is not possible (e.g., thrombosed iliofemoral vein, azygos continuation of the inferior vena cava). In such situations, the atrium can usually be entered retrogradely from the left ventricle (or from the right ventricle in a patient with complete transposition of the great arteries). In our experience, the pass into the pulmonary venous atrium can best be accomplished by looping the catheter in the aortic root, with the tip of the J loop pointing to the patient's right. The loop is then backed across the aortic valve into the ventricle. The catheter tip then usually points toward the mitral valve (tricuspid valve in a patient with complete transposition of the great arteries) and can be advanced across it by repeated gentle probing.

If this technique is not successful using an NIH or other closed-end catheter, it may be tried using an end-hole catheter. Once the catheter is positioned near the atrioventricular valve, the soft flexible end of a guidewire is passed through the catheter. This soft tip may pass through the valve directly or it may buckle and form a loop that can then be passed across the valve. The catheter is then advanced over the wire into the pulmonary venous atrium.

Removal of a Catheter Loop

During attempts to pass a catheter from the aorta to the left ventricle across the aortic valve or retrograde across an atrioventricular valve, a loop may form that is inappropriate for the desired maneuver. If the loop is in the left ventricle, it can generally be removed by withdrawing the catheter across the aortic valve, the tip usually catching somewhere within the left ventricle and releasing the loop as the catheter is gently withdrawn. If the undesired catheter loop is in the ascending aorta (Fig. 7A), the catheter

can be withdrawn until the tip catches in one of the brachiocephalic branches (Fig. 7B). (The catheter can be advanced and withdrawn repetitively with clockwise and/or counterclockwise torque to accomplish this.) If the catheter tip does not lodge in one of the brachiocephalic branches, it may then be necessary to withdraw the catheter further into the abdominal area and attempt to have the catheter tip catch in either a renal artery or one of the other abdominal aortic branches (Fig. 7C). If this is not successful, the catheter may be withdrawn into the lower abdominal aorta to the aortic bifurcation, where the tip will usually catch in the contralateral internal iliac artery (Fig. 7D). A word of caution: If this latter maneuver is attempted in a small child, it must be remembered that the abdominal aorta is a narrow vessel, and as the catheter is withdrawn closer and closer to the aortic bifurcation, the catheter loop will become tighter and tighter until a 180° angulation of the catheter occurs. This may cause fracture of the catheter wall, making it even more difficult to straighten the catheter, or even result in the tip breaking off.

If manipulation of the catheter tip into a brachiocephalic vessel or abdominal aortic branch has not been successful in removing the loop, the catheter should be readvanced to the level of the aortic arch. The stiff end of 0.35-inch guidewire (a 0.45-inch wire can be used for a #7 or #8 French catheter) should then be advanced into the catheter to the beginning of the catheter loop. Considerable resistance to advancing the wire will probably be met once this area is reached. The catheter is now slowly withdrawn as the guidewire is advanced, tending to straighten out the proximal end of the catheter loop and facilitating the entry of the catheter tip into one of the brachiocephalic or abdominal aorta branches. In our experience, the combination of a stiff guidewire and catching the catheter tip in an aortic branch has not failed to uncoil a catheter loop.

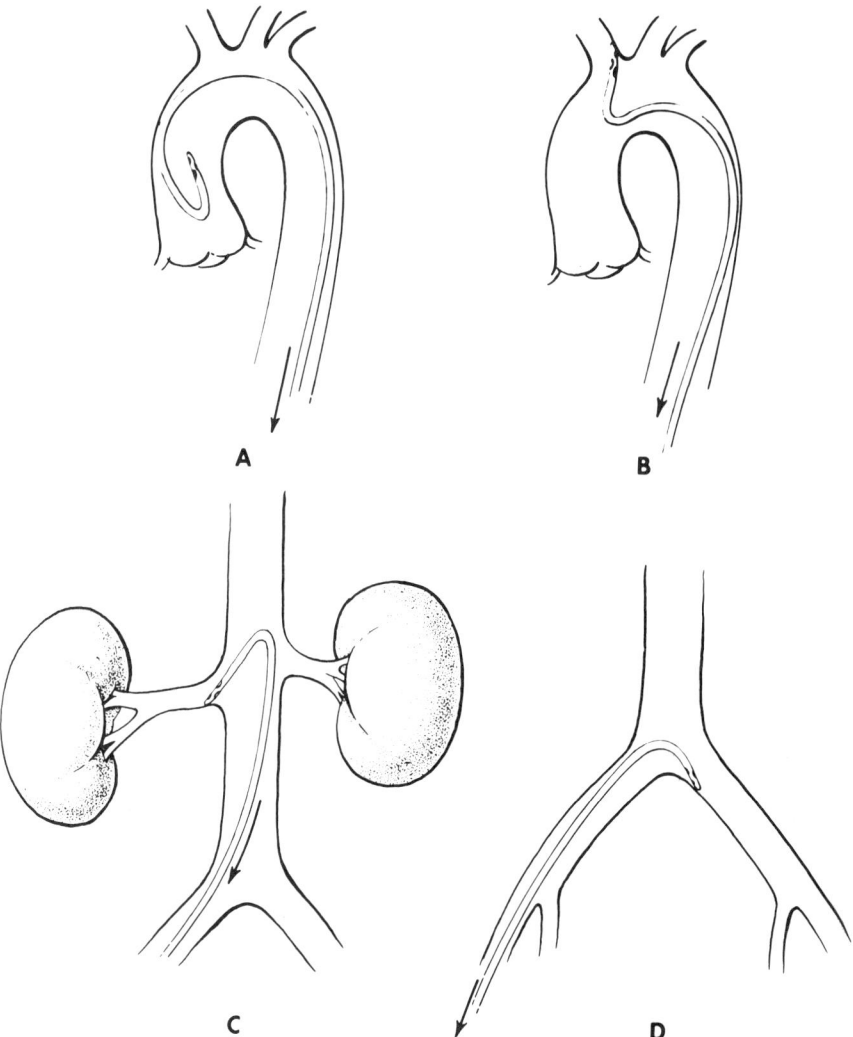

Figure 7. Removal of a catheter loop. (A) Catheter loop in the ascending aorta. (B) The catheter withdrawn to a brachiocephalic vessel for uncoiling. (C) Catheter withdrawal to the renal artery for uncoiling. (D) Catheter withdrawal to the aortic iliac bifurcation for uncoiling.

Manipulation of Flow-Directed Balloon Catheters

Some difficult catheter passes have become relatively simple with flow-directed balloon catheters. In general, any area in which there is blood flow is accessible to a flow-directed balloon catheter. The most notable exception to this rule is in passage of a balloon catheter across a very stenotic area, especially when there is an alternative route for the blood to travel. For instance, in a patient with tetralogy of Fallot with very severe, right ventricular outflow obstruction, a flow-directed balloon catheter almost always passes into the aorta from the right ventricle rather than into the pulmonary artery. The same situation exists in complete transposition of the great arteries with ventricular septal defect and pulmonary stenosis or in double inlet ventricle. Difficulty may also be encountered when there is no stenotic area but the predominant blood flow is away from the region the physician is attempting to enter with the catheter. For example, in a patient with a large ventricular septal defect and very large pulmonary blood flow, it may not be possible to enter the aorta prograssiely from the left ventricle, since a flow-directed catheter follows the predominant flow of blood and passes from the left ventricle through the ventricular septal defect into the pulmonary artery. In spite of these limitations, flow-directed balloon catheters are often useful in catheterizing infants and young children.

There are several types of flow-directed balloon catheters currently available. The two most commonly used in the pediatric cardiac catheterization laboratory are the standard distal end-hole catheter (Swan-Ganz) and the angiographic balloon catheter with multiple side holes proximal to the balloon (Berman or Schwartz). As was noted in Chapter 3, we prefer to use a catheter with a large enough lumen to the balloon so that it can be inflated with fluid rather than gas. (Carbon dioxide, rather than air, must be used in most pediatric patients because of the potential of right-to-left shunting, and the balloon must be refilled frequently when this gas is used.) In our experience, inflation of the balloon with fluid is adequate for catheter manipulation and is more convenient.

Although the movement of a balloon catheter is basically controlled by the blood flow, there are certain techniques that improve physician control. Unfortunately, most balloon catheters have straight rather than curved distal ends when they come packaged and sterilized from the manufacturer and this makes certain passes more difficult. For example, it may be very difficult to pass a straight catheter across the atrial septum. It may also be very difficult to make an appropriate loop in a ventricle with a perfectly straight catheter tip. In our laboratory, therefore, we precurve these catheters just as standard catheters are precurved. A thin, curved, stainless steel wire is inserted into the lumen through the distal end hole of a Swan-Ganz catheter, or a piece of curved, plastic tubing is used for an angiographic balloon catheter (Fig. 8). The catheters are then resterilized using standard gas sterili-

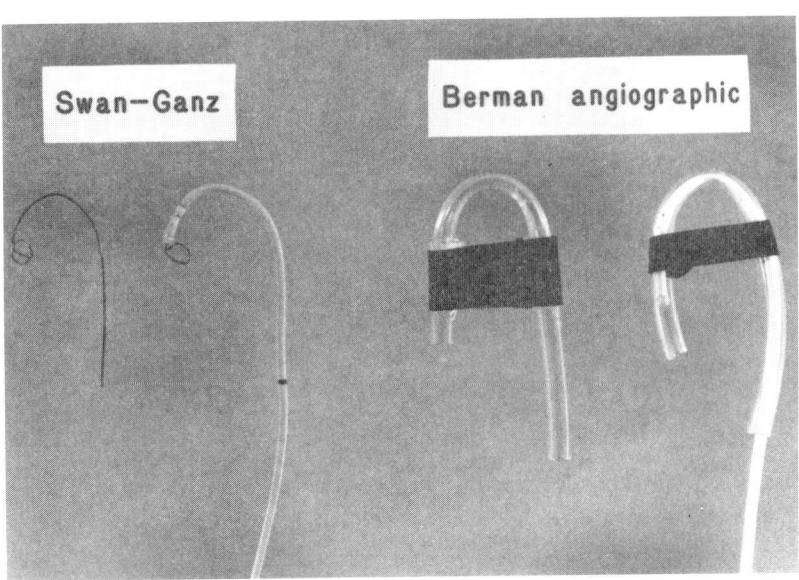

Figure 8. Balloon catheters with either end hole or angiographic balloon that have been prepared with a curve at the tip and placed for resterilization.

zation technique. These procedures serve to fix a gentle curve at the distal end of the catheter, and this curve facilitates passage of the balloon catheter across the atrial septum. In addition, especially in small infants, the curved tip makes it easier to loop the catheter in either ventricle without the catheter tip lodging in the apex of the ventricle. In some circumstances, a more sharply looped catheter tip is helpful, and we keep a supply of sterile, sharply curved balloon catheters on hand. They are especially useful for entering the aorta progradely from the left ventricle. Using these catheters, it is almost always possible to enter the pulmonary artery in a patient with complete transposition of the great arteries, even a newborn or premature infant.

Flow-directed balloon catheters are much more flexible than standard catheters, and usually it is easy to form a loop in a balloon catheter in either an atrium or a ventricle. A loop formed in the atrium can often be backed across the atrioventricular valve and into the ventricle, the tip then advancing into a great vessel (Fig. 9). These maneuvers

can be performed with the balloon deflated or partially or fully inflated. There are many variations, such as starting out with the balloon deflated and then inflating it once the loop of the catheter has been passed into the desired area. Sometimes it is helpful to inflate and deflate the balloon gradually while attempts are made to float it into the desired position. When floatation of a balloon catheter is being attempted, it must be remembered that occasionally a fully inflated balloon will lodge within a chamber. This problem may be overcome by partially deflating the balloon or simply by withdrawing the catheter slightly without changing the balloon size. In this latter case, the balloon will often dislodge. As soon as it comes free, it will move in the direction of blood flow and float out into the desired area. This latter technique of withdrawal of the catheter is sometimes quite helpful in passing the catheter from the left ventricle to the pulmonary artery in an infant with complete transposition of the great arteries. *A word of caution:* The balloon catheter must be inflated carefully when the catheter tip is in a

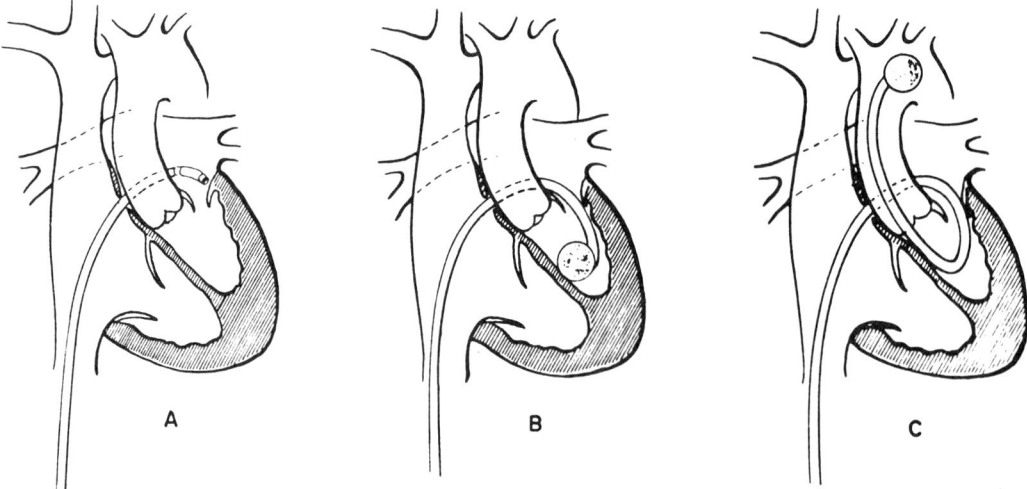

Figure 9. Passage of a balloon catheter from left atrium to left ventricle and out into the aorta. (A) A loop is formed in the left atrium at the lateral border (or by passage of the catheter into the right upper pulmonary vein). (B and C) As the loop advances across the mitral valve the balloon catheter is inflated and the balloon will then be directed toward the aorta.

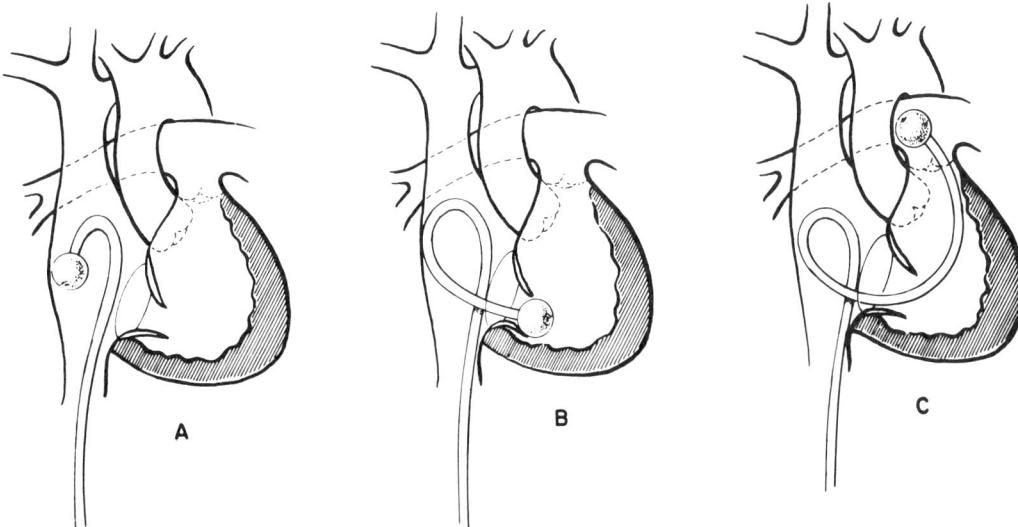

Figure 10. Passage of the catheter from right atrium to right ventricle and pulmonary artery. (A) A loop is made in the lateral wall of the right atrium. (B) The balloon is inflated and it will be carried in the direction of flow into the right ventricle. (C) The balloon catheter is carried by the balloon out into the right pulmonary artery.

ventricle. The balloon tip may be caught within the delicate chordal structures of the atrioventricular valve. If the catheter does not appear to move freely as the balloon is inflated, *DO NOT* forcefully pull the catheter. Instead, deflate the balloon, slightly withdraw the catheter, and start again.

In a patient with normally connected great arteries, catheterization of the pulmonary artery may be facilitated by forming a loop in the right atrium with the balloon deflated. Then, as the balloon is inflated, it advances across the tricuspid valve (Fig. 10). This reversed atrial loop simulates a superior vena cava approach.

It is also possible to change the shape of the tip of the balloon catheter by the use of guidewire techniques that have been described previously in this chapter. With a #5 French end-hole or angiographic balloon catheter, it is usually possible to pass an 0.0l8-inch guidewire. The stiff end of the guidewire is shaped with the desired curve and the wire is then passed into the sampling lumen of the catheter. While this is being done, the catheter should be held as straight as possible on the table so that the wire does not make unnecessary bends. Since these catheters are quite soft, it is very easy to tear the lumen, especially if one attempts to force the stiff end of a guidewire around a sharp bend in the catheter. It is also possible to use a wire to stiffen the balloon catheter and make it more maneuverable. The soft flexible end of the guidewire can be used for this purpose and considerably lessens the possibility of tearing the catheter wall with the wire. Since the catheter lumen is so small, the catheter should be adequately flushed prior to introduction of the wire. The wire should not be left in the catheter longer than necessary, since the combination of a small lumen and a wire predisposes to thrombus formation. Aside from the risk involved, it is distressing to manipulate a catheter into a difficult area and then find the catheter has clotted.

6

Shunt Detection

Robert A. Mathews, M.D.

Shunt detection, localization, and quantification are important components of the hemodynamic assessment of the patient with congenital heart disease. Many patients with congenital heart disease have some type of intracardiac shunting, and several methods to determine the site and amount of shunting have been developed. This chapter will explore the methods currently used to define intracardiac shunts in pediatric patients. This chapter and the next two chapters are meant to be brief overviews rather than exhaustive treatises in their respective areas.

Oximetry

Oximetry is perhaps the most commonly used and easiest method of determining the presence of an intracardiac shunt. This technique utilizes blood sampling from each cardiac chamber and great vessel and analysis of this blood for oxygen saturation and/or content. Originally, this required relatively large amounts of blood and was done by the complex, time-consuming Van Slyke oxygen analysis method (Van Slyke and McNeill 1924) according to the following formula:

$$\% \text{ Oxygen saturation} = \frac{\text{Oxygen content}}{\text{Oxygen capacity}}$$

Now analysis is done by absorption spectrophotometry and requires only small amounts of blood (0.5 mL). This technique measures the absorption by blood of light in the red wave length portion of the spectrum (540 nanometers), absorption being directly proportional to the oxygen saturation.

Although this method is generally reproducible, simple, and requires only small volumes of blood for sampling, it has a number of limitations. The relationship between light absorption and oxygen saturation is nonlinear at the extremes of the normal physiologic range (i.e., $< 60\%$ and $> 95\%$). In addition, the reliability of this method depends upon *rapid* sequential sampling from cardiac chambers and great arteries, which may be difficult or impossible in some cases. Even with rapid sampling, the patient may not be in a steady state during all sampling. Streaming of blood introduces another problem. For example, it is especially difficult at times to obtain consistently similar oxygen saturations from the venae cavae or right atrium. In the superior cava, the stream of blood from the subclavian vein and from the jugular system are quite dissimilar in oxygen saturations, jugular venous blood being consistently less fully saturated. Similarly, highly saturated, renal venous blood and much less saturated blood from the hepatic venous system produce inconsistent oxygen saturations from repeated inferior vena cava sampling. Streaming of the inferior and superior caval return, plus the influx of highly unsaturated coronary sinus blood, may produce variable atrial saturations, even in patients with no interatrial shunting. A variation of oxygen content up to 1.9 vol% (saturation, 10%) within the right atrium, 0.9 vol% (saturation, 5%) between the right atrium and the right ventricle, and 0.5 vol% (saturation, 3%) between the right ventricle and the pulmonary artery may be normal because of streaming of blood flow in the right heart. A left-to-right shunt is thus suggested if measured oxygen content or saturation exceed these ranges of normal variation from one area to the next. In any good laboratory, however, shunt detection and quantitation can be carried out by more than one method, and an oxygen saturation or content step-up of more than the above values should lead to a further search for a left-to-right shunt.

It has been suggested that, since inferior vena cava flow is roughly twice superior vena cava flow, mixed venous saturation be estimated by the following equation (Dalen and Grossman 1980):

$$\text{Mixed venous oxygen saturation} = \frac{2\ (\text{IVC saturation})\ +\ \text{SVC saturation}}{3}$$

In our own laboratory, however, we have found that the oxygen saturation in the low superior vena cava, just above the junction with the right atrium, correlates best with the pulmonary artery (or true mixed systemic venous saturation) in patients who do not have a left-to-right shunt. We use this value as the mixed systemic venous saturation in all calculations except when there is a shunt into the superior vena cava such as in anomalous pulmonary venous return or cerebral arteriovenous fistulae.

Abbreviations

MV = mixed venous   PV = pulmonary vein

PA = pulmonary artery   SA = systemic artery.

Estimation of shunt flow by oximetry and the Fick principle (Fick 1870) used the following equations:

$$\text{Flow (Q) (L/m)} = \frac{O_2 \text{ consumption (ml/min)}}{\text{Arteriovenous difference (ml of oxygen/L of blood)}}$$

Thus, for pulmonary flow (Qp):

$$\text{Qp (L/min)} = \frac{O_2 \text{ consumption (ml/min)}}{\text{PVO}_2 \text{ content (ml O}_2\text{/L)} - \text{PA O}_2 \text{ content (ml O}_2\text{/L)}}$$

and for systemic flow (Qs):

$$\text{Qs (L/min)} = \frac{O_2 \text{ consumption (ml/min)}}{\text{SAO}_2 \text{ content (ml O}_2\text{/L)} - \text{MVO}_2 \text{ content (ml O}_2\text{/L)}}.$$

Effective pulmonary blood flow (Qep) is another commonly used term and refers to the volume of systemic venous return being oxygenated in the lungs. It is determined by the following formula:

$$Qep \text{ (L/min)} = \frac{O_2 \text{ consumption (ml/min)}}{PVO_2 \text{ content (ml } O_2/L) - MVO_2 \text{ (ml } O_2/L)}.$$

Obviously, if there is no shunt, all three flows (Qp, Qs, Qep) are equal. If there is a right-to-left but not a left-to-right shunt, pulmonary flow and effective pulmonary flow are equal.

In each of the above equations, oxygen contents are used in the calculations. Since oxygen contents are no longer measured in most laboratories, it is necessary to calculate oxygen content from oxygen saturation data. Since 1 gm of hemoglobin can combine with 1.34 mL of oxygen:

$$Oxygen \text{ content (ml/L)} = oxygen \text{ saturation } (\%) \times Hgb \text{ (gm/dl)} \times 1.34 \times 10.$$

(The figure "10" in the right hand member of the equation is necessary since hemoglobin is expressed in gm/dL rather than gm/L.

The dissolved oxygen in the plasma must be added to this number to give the true oxygen content. Since it is a negligible portion of the total content with a patient breathing room air (0.3 mL oxygen/100 mL blood/100 torr PO_2) and requires determination of the partial pressure of oxygen (PO_2), it is usually disregarded. However, if shunt calculations are performed with the patient breathing oxygen (see below), the dissolved oxygen *must* be calculated and considered in the total oxygen content.

Right-to-Left Shunt

Arterial unsaturation may, or may not, be due to actual right-to-left shunting within the heart or great arteries. Other causes include pulmonary disease with impaired diffusion, ventilation/perfusion imbalance, or hypoventilation, either induced by sedation or caused by airway obstruction. The latter can be due to hypertrophied tonsils and adenoids or, in a child with Down's Syndrome, to a small oropharynx and relatively large tongue.

The volume of a right-to-left shunt can be calculated using the following formula:

Qs (L/min)

= Qep (L/min) + R → L shunt (L/min),

thus:

R → L shunt (L/min)

= Qs (L/min) − Qep (L/min).

Left-to-Right Shunt

The net left-to-right shunt can be calculated by the equation:

Qp (L/min)

= Qep (L/min) + L → R shunt (L/min),

thus:

L → R shunt (L/min)

= Qp (L/min) − Qep (L/min).

This is more commonly described as a percentage of the total pulmonary blood flow:

% shunt (L → R)

$$= \frac{Qp \ (L/min) - Qep \ (L/min)}{Qp \ (L/min)} \times 100.$$

Flow Ratios

Another means of expressing flow in patients with left-to-right, right-to-left, or bidirectional shunts is by a pulmonary-to-systemic flow ratio (Qp/Qs). If oxygen consumption has been measured and oxygen contents calculated, then Qp and Qs are determined separately, and determining the ratio between them simply involves division of Qp by Qs. However, the pulmonary-to-systemic flow ratio can be calculated without measuring or assuming O_2 consumption and from oxygen saturation values rather than from oxygen content since:

$$Qp \ (L/min) = \frac{O_2 \ consumption \ (L/min)}{PVO_2 - PAO_2}$$

$$Qs \ (L/min) = \frac{O_2 \ consumption \ (L/min)}{SAO_2 - MVO_2},$$

then:

$$\frac{QP}{QS} \ (L/min) = \frac{\dfrac{O_2 \ consumption \ (L/min)}{PVO_2 - PAO_2}}{\dfrac{O_2 \ consumption \ (L/min)}{SAO_2 - MVO_2}},$$

and cancelling out, we have:

$$Qp/Qs = \frac{SAO_2 - MVO_2}{PVO_2 - PAO_2}$$

Since content is proportional to saturation, saturation can be substituted for content, leaving:

$$Qp/Qs = \frac{SAO_2 \ Sat - MVO_2 \ Sat}{PVO_2 \ Sat - PAO_2 \ Sat}.$$

Although calculation of Qp/Qs ratio is a simple matter, Qp/Qs should not be equated with pulmonary flow. Thus, if a patient has a pulmonary flow of 6 L/min, the Qp/Qs will be 1.5 if the systemic flow is 4 L/min. But if systemic flow is only 2 L/min, the calculated Qp/Qs will be 3.0. As will be described further in the next chapter, these two sets of numbers give very different impressions of the status of the pulmonary vascular bed. However, for any given pulmonary artery pressure, both would have the same calculated level of pulmonary vascular resistance.

Shunt Determination with Oxygen Administration

If there is a left-to-right shunt and pulmonary hypertension, the shunt and resistance ratios are usually determined with the patient breathing room air and during inhalation of 100% oxygen (Fishman 1961). Since tolazoline (Priscoline) (Grover et al. 1961) and oxygen are potent pulmonary vasodilators in normal individuals, an assessment of the reactivity of the pulmonary arterioles to either agent is necessary in patients with elevated pulmonary artery pressures. As mentioned previously, in room air, the amount of oxygen dissolved in the plasma can be disregarded since it is small (0.3 mL O_2/dL blood/100 torr PO_2). However, when breathing 100% oxygen, the amount of dissolved oxygen increases and a flow ratio based only on saturation will be spuriously high. In this situation, it is mandatory to determine blood gases (including PO_2) in samples taken from the pulmonary vein, systemic and pulmonary arteries, and the superior vena cava and to use content rather than saturation in calculating Qp/Qs.

For example, in a patient breathing 100% oxygen and with a hemoglobin of 14.9 gm/dL:

O_2 capacity $= 14.9 \times 1.34 =$

20.0 ml O_2/dl blood.

If we assume the following data:

	Oxygen Saturation (%)	PO_2 (torr)
SVC	75	45
MPA	94	90
PV	100	500
AO	100	400

using oxygen saturations alone (or calculated oxygen contents without consideration of dissolved oxygen):

$$Qp/Qs = \frac{Ao - SVC}{PV - PA} = \frac{100 - 75}{100 - 94} = \frac{4.2}{1}$$

However, if O_2 content, including dissolved oxygen, is used and:

O_2 content = [O_2 capacity

    × saturation (%) + dissolved oxygen]

then:

SVC O_2 content

    = 20 × 75% + (0.3 × .45)

    = 15 + .14 = 15.14 ml O_2/dl blood

MPA O_2 content

    = 20 × 94% + (0.3 × 0.9)

    = 18.8 + 0.27 = 19.07 ml O_2/dl blood

PV O_2 content

    = 20 × 100% + (0.3 × 5.0)

    = 20.0 + 1.5 = 21.5 ml O_2/dl blood

Ao O_2 content

    = 20 × 100% + (0.3 × 4.0)

    = 20.0 + 1.2 = 21.2 ml O_2/dl blood

and:

$$\frac{Qp}{Qs} = \frac{Ao - SVC}{PV - PA}$$

$$= \frac{21.2 - 15.4}{21.5 - 19.07} = \frac{6.06}{2.43} = \frac{2.5}{1}$$

Obviously, this considerable difference in Qp/Qs will result in an error in the estima-

tion of pulmonary vascular resistance if dissolved oxygen is ignored (Chapter 7).

Indicator Dilution Method

Indicator dilution techniques can also be used to identify, localize, and quantify intracardiac shunts and to measure cardiac output (Bloomfield 1974, Wood 1962, Yang 1988) (See Chapter 8). However, it requires a complex recording device and a skilled technician to operate the system. The indicator dilution curve depends on the principle that an indicator injected into the blood stream can be identified and its concentration measured when blood is sampled from another site in the circulation. Figure 1A depicts a normal, indicator time-concentration curve obtained when indocyanine green is injected into the pulmonary artery and sampled from a systemic artery. When the cardiac output is low, the curve is usually broader and has a delayed and much lower peak (Fig. 1B). The concentration of the dye in the sampled blood is proportional to the height of the curve at any given point. The appearance time (AT) is the interval between injection and the first appearance of dye at the sampling site. In this curve, the first hump represents the first pass of the dye through the circulation. Recirculation, or reappearance, of the injected dye in its second passage past the measuring site, is evidenced by the second and lower hump. The area under the curve can be used to calculate cardiac output (see Chapter 8).

Indocyanine green is a commonly used indicator substance. It is nontoxic and rapidly cleared from the circulation by excretion through the liver. Other substances that have been used include radioactive material (radioactive albumin, labeled red cells, etc.) and cold fluid (with a thermodilution analyzer). Ascorbic acid and/or hydrogen gas are detected with a platinum-tipped electrode and can be used for qualitative shunt determination (Clark and Bargeron 1959, Carter et al. 1960). The use of hydrogen as an indicator has an advantage in that only

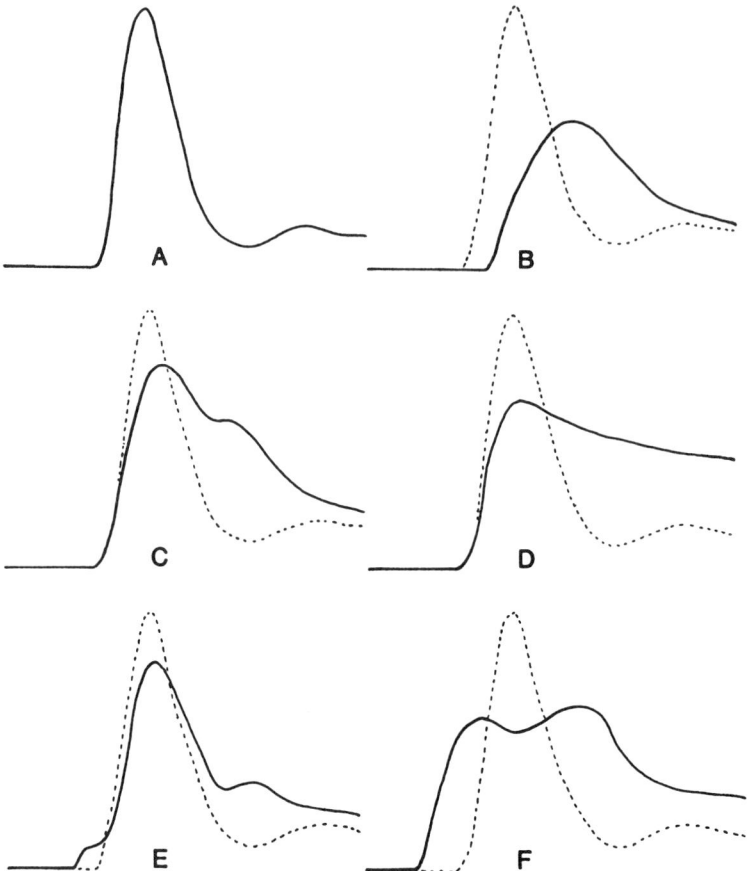

Figure 1. Indicator dilution curves (broken line indicates normal curve). (A) Normal indicator dilution curve (no shunt). (B) Low cardiac output. (C) Mild-to-moderate left-to-right shunt. (D) Marked left-to-right shunt. (E) Mild right-to-left shunt. (F) Marked right-to-left shunt.

a single catheter is necessary to detect a shunt. In this technique, hydrogen is administered by face mask. Dissolved hydrogen gas causes a change in the electrical conductivity of the blood, which can be detected by an electrode catheter. An electrode positioned distal to a left-to-right shunt will register this change in conductivity when hydrogen is breathed. Although this is an extremely sensitive way to detect a left-to-right shunt, it is not widely used because of the need for storage and handling of this highly explosive gas.

The shape of an indicator dilution curve, regardless of the indicator used, is helpful in determining the presence and magnitude of shunting. Figures 1C and 1D depict typical left-to-right shunt curves from patients with a ventricular septal defect. Injection of dye is into the pulmonary artery and sampling is from the aorta. The upstroke is normal. The maximal height of the curve is reduced since the left-to-right shunt contains no dye and reduces the maximal concentration of dye at the sampling site. The distortion of the downstroke results from dye in the left-to-right shunt reentering the pulmonary circulation and again passing the sampling site.

Figures 1E and 1F show right-to-left indicator dilution curves from patients with tetralogy of Fallot. Injection is into the right ventricle and sampling is from the aorta. The right-to-left shunt results in a shortened appearance time and a deflection before the main portion of the curve.

The site of an intracardiac shunt may be demonstrated by indicator dilution curves. If there is a right-to-left shunt, it can be localized by injection into several sites in the right heart; a site that fails to show an early appearance time must be distal to the shunt. Left-to-right shunts are localized by injection into different sites in the left heart and sampling from the pulmonary artery. If the curve shows no distortion of the down slope, the injection site must have been distal to the shunt.

Two venous catheters can be used to localize a left-to-right shunt. One is used for sampling and the other for injection. The injection catheter is placed in the distal right or left pulmonary artery and the sampling catheter's position is varied. If the sampling catheter is proximal to the shunt (e.g., right atrium with a ventricular septal defect), a single low-amplitude deflection with a long appearance is then observed. If the sample site is at, or distal to, the shunt, an early, relatively sharp deflection will precede the main curve.

Quantitation of Intracardiac Shunts

A number of different methods have been utilized to quantitate the amount of intracardiac shunt. In patients with left-to-right shunts, early recirculation will alter the down slope of the curve (Fig. 1C). In some patients, the left-to-right shunt causes a distinct second peak, especially following injection of the dye in the pulmonary artery. This type of curve is more likely if withdrawal is from the central aorta rather than from a peripheral artery. The ratio of the height of the second peak to the first (P2/P1) provides an estimate of the left-to-right shunt expressed as a percentage of the pulmonary blood flow.

More often there is no well-defined second peak (Fig. 1D). Carter et al. (1960) described two empiric equations for calculating left-to-right shunts based upon the rate of disappearance of an indicator at specific intervals following the time of peak concentration (Fig. 2). The magnitude of left-to-right shunt, expressed as a percentage of pulmonary blood flow, is derived from the following equations:

$$L \rightarrow R \text{ shunt } (\% \text{ } Qp_1) = 141 \frac{PC_2}{PC_1} - 42$$

$$L \rightarrow R \text{ shunt } (\% \text{ } Qp_2) = 135 \frac{PC_3}{PC_1} - 14$$

Example based on Fig. 2A:

$$Qp_1 = 141 \times \frac{41}{55} - 42 = 63\%$$

$$Qp_2 = 135 \times \frac{33}{55} - 14 = 67\%$$

$$\text{Average } \frac{Qp_1 + Qp_2}{2} = 65\%$$

In these calculations, PC_1 refers to the initial peak concentration of the curve and PC_2 and PC_3 refer to the maximum concentrations on the curve at two and three times the initial build-up time, respectively. The values obtained from the two equations are averaged to give an approximation of the left-to-right shunt. This method may be inaccurate, especially if the shunt is less than 40% of the total pulmonary blood flow (i.e., Qp/Qs <1.7:1). However, the information may be useful particularly when there is a disparity between the magnitude of the shunt as calculated from oximetry data and the angiographic appearance.

The magnitude of a right-to-left shunt, expressed as a percentage of the total systemic flow, can be calculated from the dye dilution curve. The right-to-left shunt is quantitated from the area of the first portion of the curve, and the total systemic flow is estimated by the sum of the area of the first

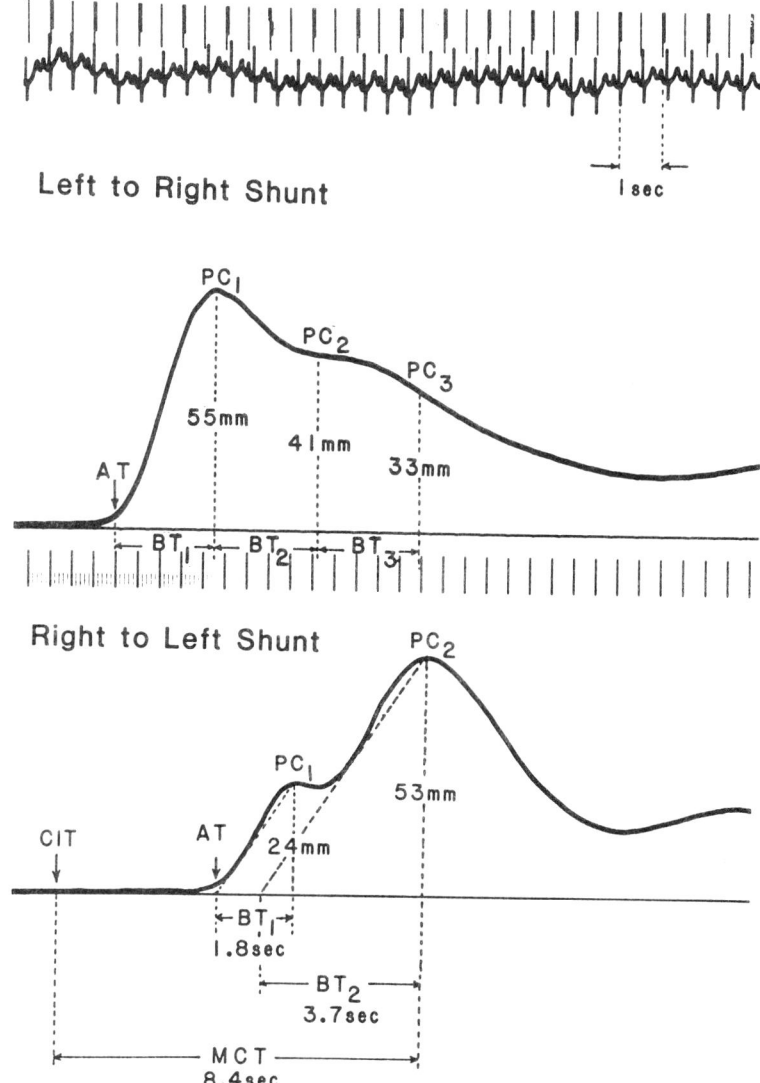

Figure 2. Calculation of shunt from indicator dilution curves. Top: Left-to-right shunt (see text). AT = appearance time; BT = build-up time (to peak concentration); PC = peak concentration. Bottom: Right-to-left shunt (see text). AT = appearance time; BT = build-up time; CIT = corrected injection time; MCT = maximum concentration time; PC = peak concentration.

portion of the curve plus the area determined from the major portion of the curve by extrapolation of the upslope back to the baseline (Fig. 2). The right-to-left shunt is then expressed as a percentage of the total systemic flow using the following formula:

$R \rightarrow L$ shunt (%Qs)

$$= \frac{(PC_1 \times BT_1)}{(PC_1 \times BT_1) + (PC_2 \times BT_2)}$$

In this formula, PC_1 refers to the height of

the first peak, BT_1 to the build-up time to this peak. PC_2 and BT_2 refer to the height and build-up time of the second peak. BT_2 is calculated from the following formula:

$$BT_2 = MCT$$

$$\times\ 0.44\ (\text{empirical correction factor})$$

where MCT is the maximum concentration time.

Example based on Figure 2:

$R \rightarrow L$ shunt (%Qs)

$$= \frac{(24 \times 1.8)}{(24 \times 1.8) + (53 \times 3.7)} = 18\%$$

Radioactive materials can also be used as indicators to detect and quantitate shunt flow (Long et al. 1960). For radioactive gas methods, a gamma camera is necessary to measure venous, arterial, and background activity. With computer assistance, a left-to-right or right-to-left shunt can be identified, localized, and quantitated, and regional blood flows to each lung can be obtained.

References and Suggested Reading

Bloomfield, DA (ed). Dye Curves. Baltimore, MD, University Park Press. 1974.

Carter SA, Bajec DF, Yannicelli E, Wood EH. Estimation of left-to-right shunt from arterial dilution curves. J Lab Clin Med 1960; 55:77–88.

Clark LC, Jr, Bargeron LM, Jr. Left-to-right shunt detection by an intravascular electrode with hydrogen as an indicator. Science 1959; 130:709–710.

Dalen JE, Grossman W. Chapter 12 in Grossman W (ed), Cardiac Catheterization and Angiography. 2nd ed. Philadelphia, PA, Lea & Febiger. 1980.

Fick A. Uber die Messung Des Blutquantums in den Herzventrikeln. Sitz der Physik—Med Ges Wurtzberg. 1870.

Fishman AP. Respiratory gases in the regulation of the pulmonary circulation. Physiol Rev 1961; 41:214–280.

Grover, RF, Reeves JT, Blount SG, Jr. Tolazoline hydrochloride (Priscoline): An effective pulmonary vasodilator. Am Heart J 1961; 61:5–15.

Long RTL, Braunwald E, Morrow AG. Intracardiac injection of radioactive Krypton: Clinical applications of new methods for characterization of circulatory shunts. Circulation 1960; 21:1126–1133.

Van Slyke DD, Neill JM. The determination of gases in blood and other solutions by vacuum extraction and manometric measurements. J Biol Chem 1924; 61:523–573.

Wood EH. Diagnostic application of indicator-dilution technics in congenital heart disease. Circ Res 1962; 10:531–568.

Yang SS, et al. (eds). From Cardiac Catheterization Data to Hemodynamic Parameters. 3rd ed. Philadelphia, PA, FA Davis Co. 1988.

7

Pressure Measurement and Resistance Calculations

Robert A. Mathews, M.D.

Direct measurement of pressure in all intracardiac chambers that can be entered is a vital part of cardiac catheterization in infants and children with congenital heart disease. Since reentering a chamber or great artery may be difficult, pressure measurements and blood samples for oxygen determination should be obtained when a chamber or artery is first entered. This chapter will be concerned with a description of the measuring devices and the calibration technique commonly used in most laboratories. Pressure contours commonly seen in the pediatric cardiac patient will be illustrated.

Instrumentation

A fluid-filled catheter system is most commonly used to measure intracardiac pressure, with the catheter connected directly, or by plastic tubing, to a stopcock and then to a pressure transducer. Interposition of plastic tubing between the catheter and stopcock bank alters damping of the system, but the pressure contours are usually acceptable.

A strain gauge transducer is used in most laboratories. The metal diaphragm of the transducer is part of a Whetstone bridge, an electrical circuit that measures resistance. When the pressure changes within the transducer, the diaphragm is deformed and this changes the resistance in the Whetstone bridge. The change in resistance is directly proportional to the degree of deformation of the diaphragm and to the amplitude of the input pressure. This resistance change alters the voltage of a calibrated electrical signal that has a linear relationship to the pressure being measured. Gould-Statham P-23-ID transducers are used in our laboratory and have the advantage of being isolated, preventing inadvertent electrical shock. The electrical isolation also protects the transducer during electrical current surges and need not be disconnected if a defibrillator is used. Air bubbles can easily be expelled from the clear plastic dome of these transducers.

Pressure measurement transducers should be accurate and yet have an adequate range. Most strain gauge transducers in use today can accurately measure pressure up to 400 mm Hg. Another important characteristic of the pressure transducer is its frequency response. This describes the transducer's ability to follow rapid alterations of an input signal with a linear output signal and without alterations of the amplitude or phase characteristics of the harmonic components of the pressure wave form. Any physiologic wave form can be separated into its harmonic components by Fourier analysis, giving a series of sine waves, each of which is a multiple of the fundamental frequency of the patient's heart rate (e.g., 2 Hz for a heart rate of 120 beats/min.) The pressure wave form can be reconstructed as the sum of these various sine waves. For most pressure wave forms there are no significant harmonics greater than the 10th harmonic of the fundamental frequency. If the transducer is not flat (i.e., linear) within this range, the amplitude of the sine waves at higher harmonics will not be reproduced as faithfully as those of the lower harmonics. This will result in distortion of the summated wave form and the output signal will not be quite accurate. A transducer that is flat to about 40 Hz is capable of reproducing most pressure signals up to a heart rate of 240 beats/min (i.e., 4 Hz x 10 harmonics = 40 Hz). Most strain gauge transducers are flat to a frequency range far above this level and distortion of the actual recorded signal is largely related to the dynamics of a fluid-filled catheter system. The frequency response of a fluid-filled catheter and a plastic connecting tube interposed between the catheter and transducer may be 20 Hz or less. Although this may introduce inaccuracies in pressure measurement, from a practical point of view they are usually unimportant.

If extreme accuracy in pressure measurement is desirable (e.g., in determining transvalvular gradient or the rate of rise of ventricular pressure [dp/dt]), micromanometer-tipped catheters should be used. These commercially available catheters have miniature transducers at the tip and can be used to measure intracardiac pressure directly. They have excellent frequency-response characteristics and are generally flat into the kilohertz range. They have the additional advantage of having no time delay. With the use of appropriate filters, an intracardiac phonocardiogram can also be recorded with these catheters. Micromanometer-tipped catheters are available in #5 French and can thus be used in infants and small children. Disadvantages include relatively high cost ($500 or more) and stiffness. Many other forms of larger size micromanometer-tipped catheters (>#7 French) are currently available and include those with multiple pressure sensors, a lumen for blood sampling, or pressure and

flow velocity sensors. Figure 1 compares pressure waves recorded simultaneously from the same site with fluid-filled and micromanometer systems.

The recording system is another important consideration in accurate pressure measurement and at minimum should have frequency-response characteristics that enable it to linearly record to at least the highest frequency of the transducer output.

Measurement of Pressure

A number of practical points should be stressed, which are necessary to obtain accurate and reproducible pressure curves. Prior to the start of a cardiac catheterization, it is important to have the pressure transducer connected to its recording device to allow for proper warm-up of the components. The transducer should be flushed with heparinized solution and be free of all air bubbles. It should be positioned on the side of the catheterization table at mid chest level (the level where the venae cavae enter the right atrium). When open to air at this level, the transducer output is taken as the zero, or reference point, for all pressure measurements. Prior to and following *all* pressure recordings, the transducer should be calibrated to its zero and maximum points to insure standardization. The shortest and largest diameter catheter that is practical to use in a given patient will provide the most accurate tracings. Although stopcocks and connecting tubing can reduce the system's resonant frequency, as was stated previously, their disadvantages must be weighed against the benefits of their use. The cardiac catheters must be kept free of clotted blood by flushing periodically with a heparinized solution.

In the infant, it is important to use only small amounts of fluid for flushing the catheter system. The volume given tends to accumulate rapidly and in an infant can result in serious volume overload. Air should be kept out of catheters, stopcocks, and pres-

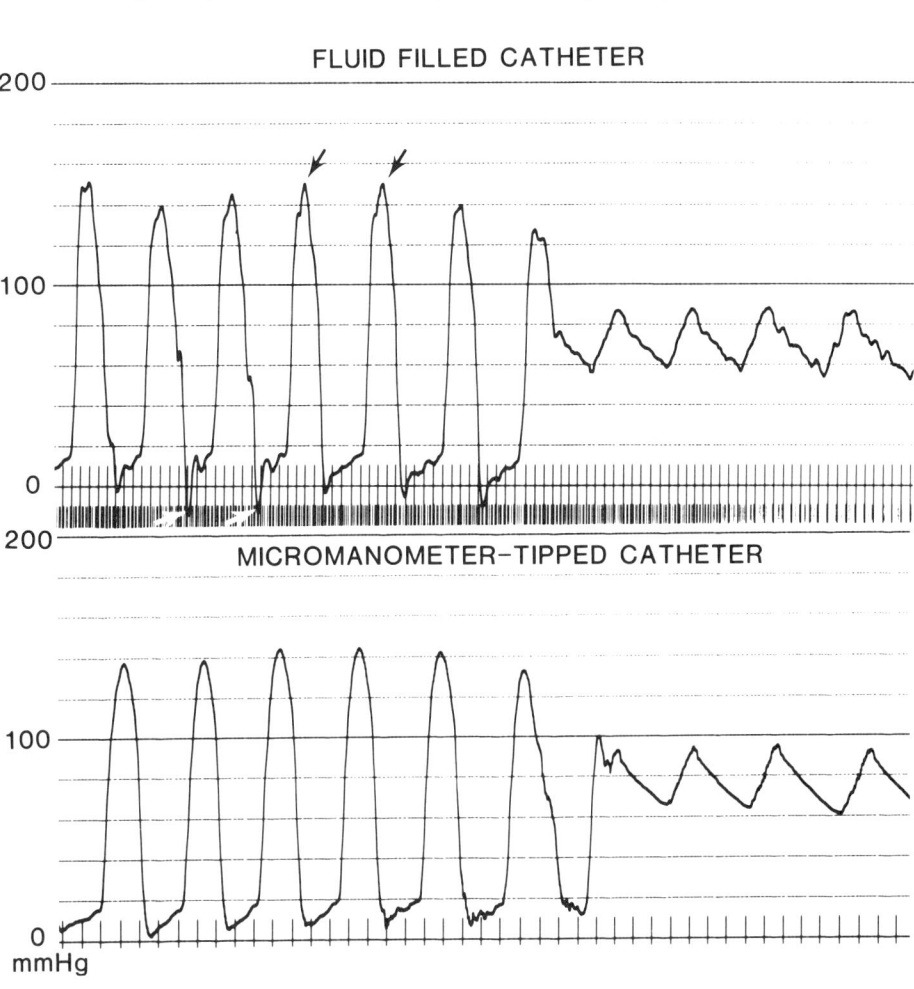

Figure 1. Micromanometer versus fluid-filled pressure curves.

sure transducers, since it damps the pressure tracing and may cause damage or even death if it is inadvertently flushed into the patient. A continuous pressure tracing should be obtained for at least 10 cardiac cycles because of respiratory variation in pressure measurements. In order to standardize pressure measurements and minimize the effects of marked respiratory variation, pressure curves should be measured consistently in all chambers at end-expiration. Pressures should be measured routinely in all catheter positions, and whenever possible, pullback (or withdrawal) pressure recordings should be obtained when a catheter is initially passed across a valve or septum. Bilateral pulmonary artery wedge pressures should also be measured routinely in all pediatric cardiac patients, especially when pulmonary hypertension is present. This can be done with either an end-hole catheter or a Swan-Ganz balloon catheter. If possible, the wedge position of the catheter should be verified by obtaining a blood sample, which will be fully saturated if the catheter is truly wedged.

Figure 2 shows pressure tracings that are underdamped, overdamped, and properly damped. Clots or air bubbles within the catheter system or transducer can cause overdamping, and in some cases simply the presence of blood rather than flushing solution may be responsible for overdamping. The reverse of this, a seriously underdamped pressure tracing, may also occur, especially in the pulmonary artery or in a ventricle. When this occurs, withdrawal of blood into the catheter will provide proper damping.

The normal contours of right and left atrial pressures are shown in Figure 3A. As a general rule, right atrial pressure is higher during atrial systole (A wave > V wave), while in the left atrium the reverse is true (V wave > A wave). Atrial pressures are usually recorded with phasic and mean contours at either 25 or 50 mm/sec and 10 mm/sec paper speeds, respectively. Mean pressures are usually recorded in atrial chambers and in great vessels but not in the ventricles. Figures 3B and 3C demonstrate simultaneous recordings of normal right and left ventricular pressures with corresponding atrial pressures. Peak systolic pressure is measured in each ventricular chamber at

a paper speed of 50 mm/sec. Diastolic pressures are measured at a paper speed of 100 mm/sec, and end diastole is considered to occur 0.04 sec after the Q wave of the electrocardiogram. Simultaneous recording of normal pulmonary artery and ventricular pressure is also shown in Figure 3D. A gradient between two cardiac chambers or a cardiac chamber and a great artery can be most accurately estimated from simultaneous pressure recordings from the two areas. In practice, however, especially in infants and small children, pullback pressures are more easily obtained and usually suffice.

When mitral stenosis or some other left atrial obstructive lesion is suspected, either simultaneous left atrial or pulmonary artery wedge and left ventricular end-diastolic pressures should be obtained (Fig. 4). Although pulmonary artery wedge pressure is an indirect measure of left atrial pressure, it is usually accurate and is much easier to obtain if the interatrial septum is intact, since direct measure of left atrial pressure requires either a transseptal puncture or a retrograde approach from the left ventricle.

Typical pressure curves from several common congenital cardiac defects are shown in Figures 5 and 6. The contour of the

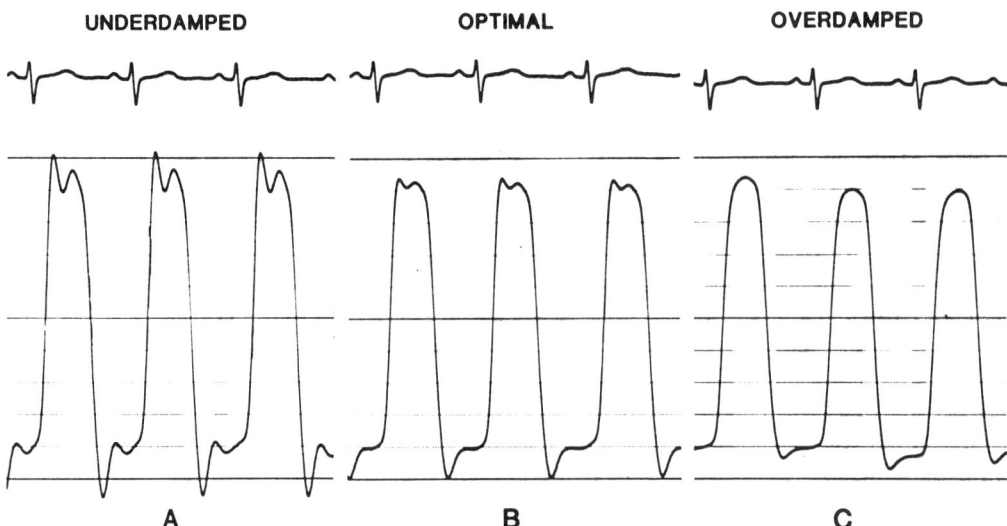

Figure 2. Underdamped, overdamped, and properly damped pressure tracing.

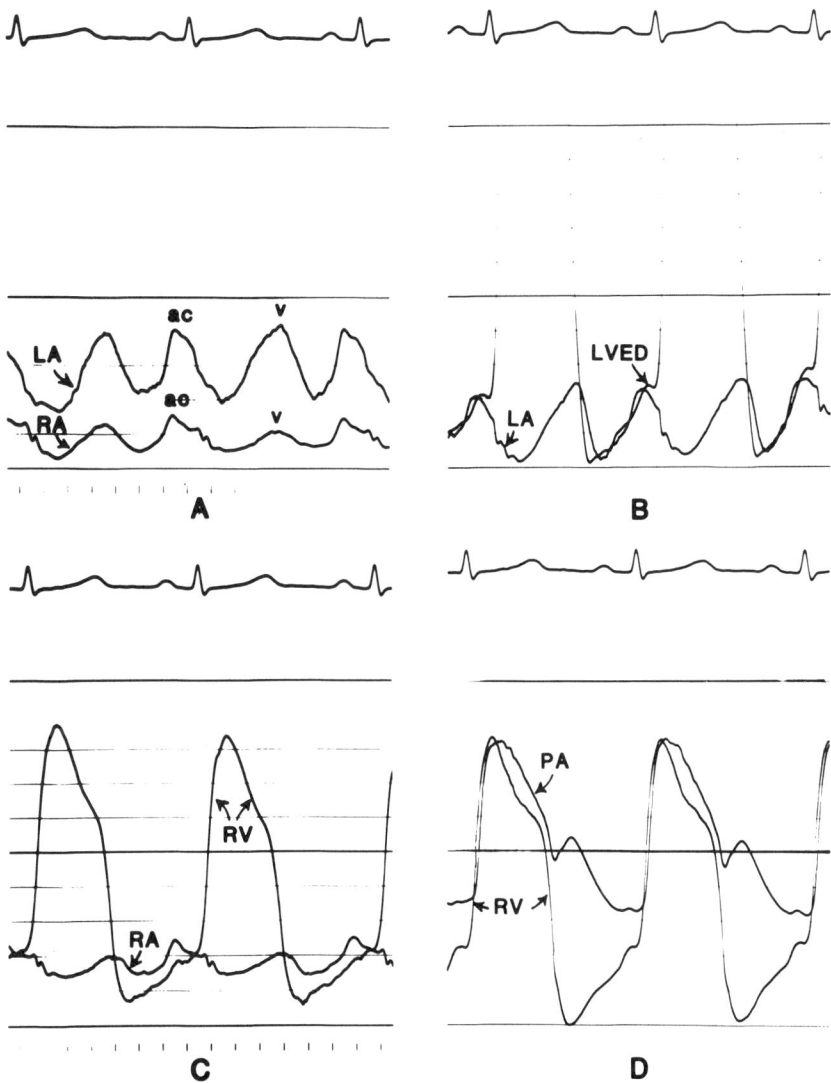

Figure 3. Intracardiac pressure tracings. A: Simultaneous normal right (RA) and left (LA) atrial pressures. B: Simultaneous tracing of the left ventricular end-diastolic (LVED) and left atrial pressures. C: Simultaneous tracing of the right ventricular (RV) and right atrial pressures. D: Simultaneous tracing of the right ventricular and pulmonary artery (PA) pressures.

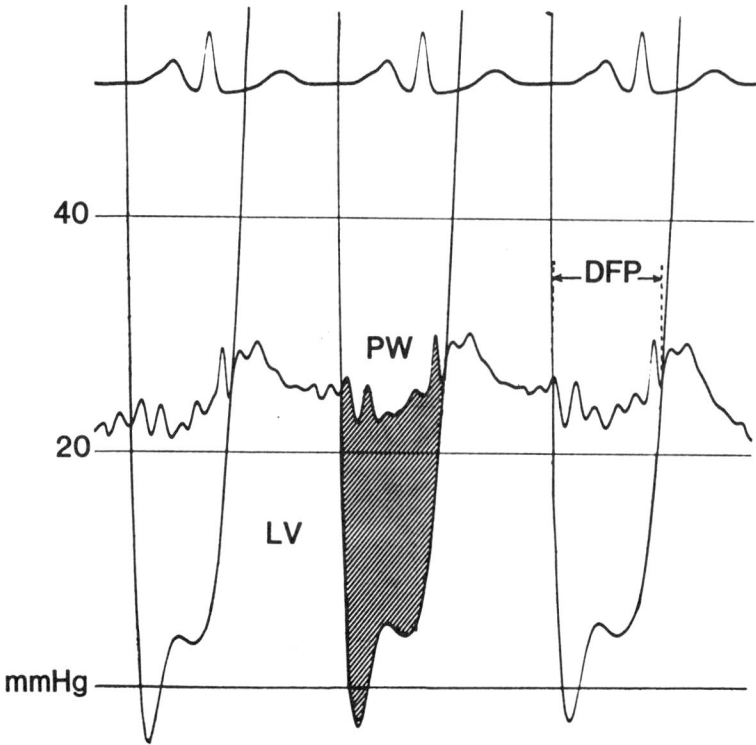

Figure 4. Simultaneous left ventricular end-diastolic and pulmonary artery wedge (PW) pressures in a patient with mitral stenosis. Shaded area indicates the pressure gradient. DFP = diastolic filling period.

pressure tracing will usually clearly localize obstruction to the supravalvar, valvar, or subvalvar level if it is remembered that an arterial pressure is present on either side of a supravalvar stenosis and a ventricular pressure is found on either side of a subvalvar stenosis (Fig. 5). With pulmonary artery stenosis, very low diastolic pressure can occur in the main pulmonary artery and the contour will resemble right ventricular pressure (Fig. 6C). On occasion, a negative pressure may be seen just distal to the site of obstruction, the so-called Venturi effect. In the patient with severe semilunar valve stenosis, the upstroke of the pressure curves is slow, the anacrotic notch often obliterated, and the pulse pressure small.

Characteristic wave forms occur in patients with cardiac tamponade. In this situation, right atrial, right ventricular end-diastolic, pulmonary artery wedge, and left ventricular end-diastolic pressures are similar. (These revert to their normal contour after pericardiocentesis.)

With atrioventricular dissociation or with complete heart block, "cannon" waves occur when atrial contraction occurs against a closed tricuspid valve (Fig. 7). The height of the cannon wave is variable and depends upon the phase of systole in relationship to atrial contractions.

Resistance Calculations

The resistance to flow in a vascular bed is described by the following equation:

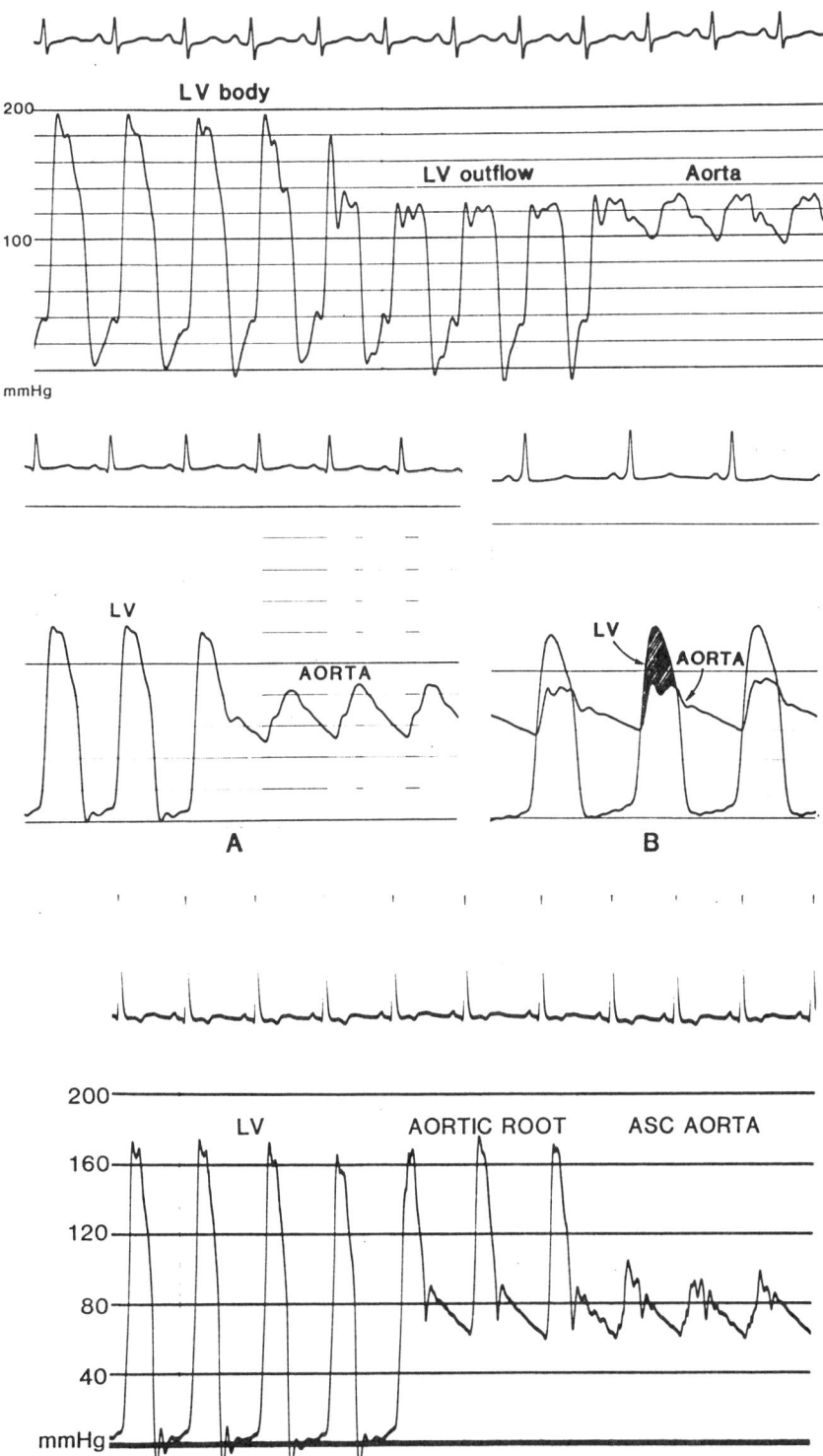

Figure 5. Various levels of aortic outflow obstruction Top: subvalvar. Middle: valvar; (A) withdrawal tracing; (B) simultaneous tracing. Bottom: supravalvar level.

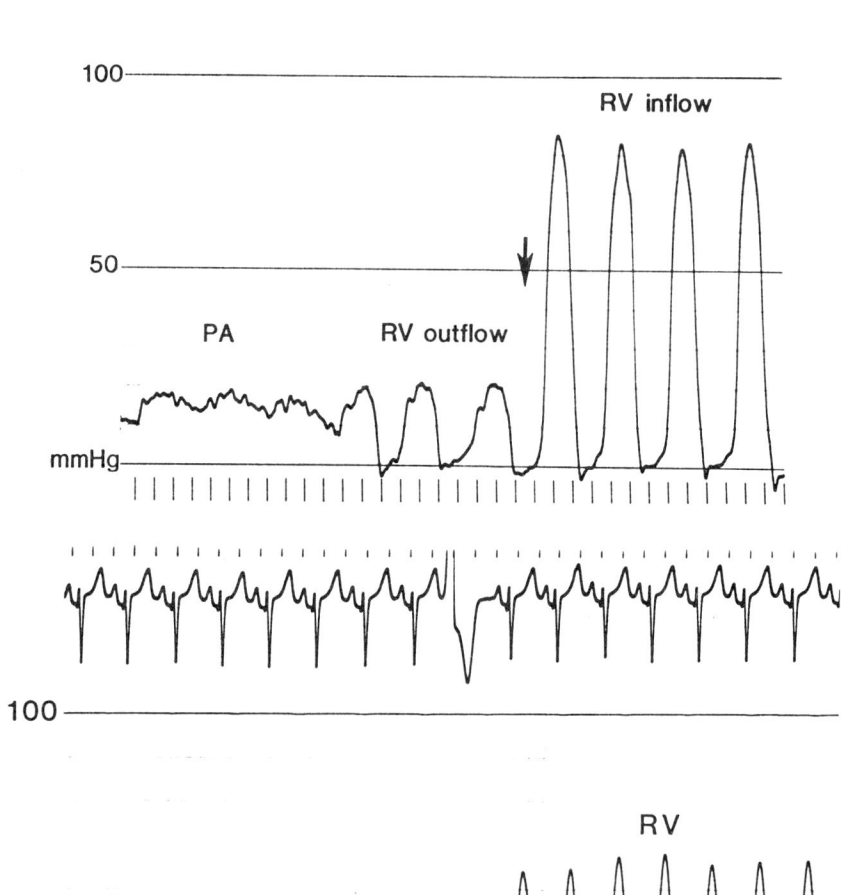

Figure 6. Various levels of right ventricular outflow obstruction. (A) Top: subvalvar; B: valvar. (B) Bottom: valvar; (C) *continued next page.*

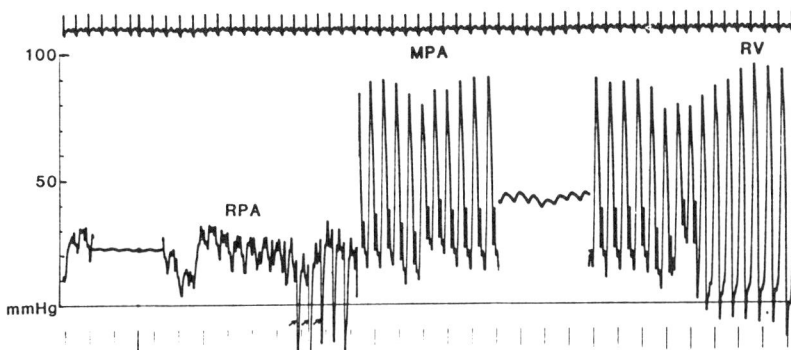

Figure 6. (*Continued*) C: supravalvar level or pulmonary artery branch (arrows indicate Venturi effect).

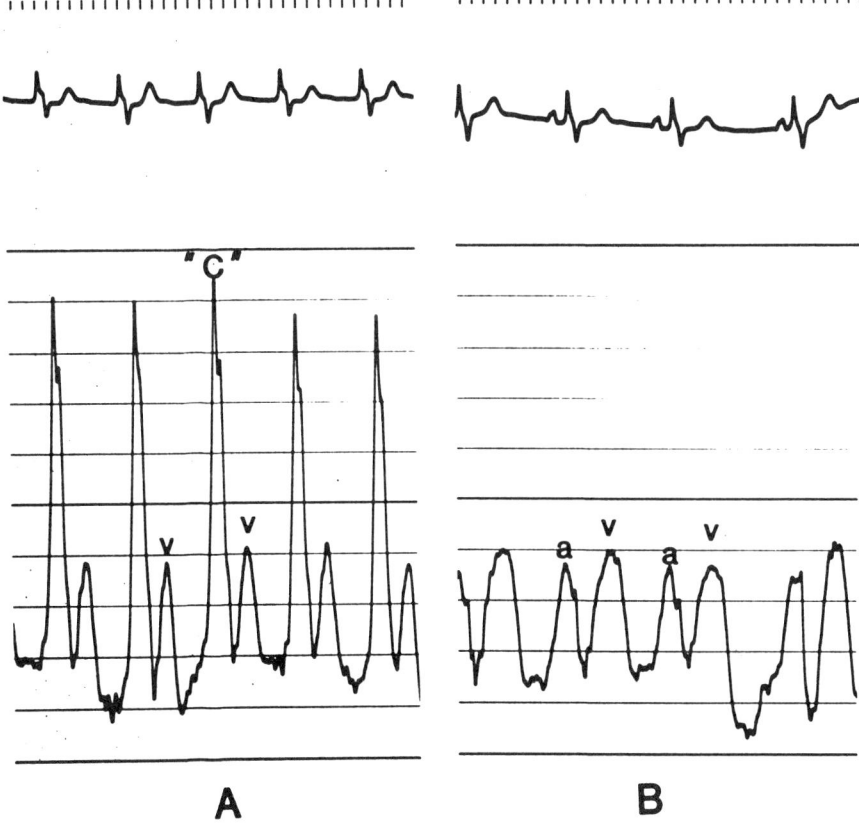

Figure 7. Atrial pressure tracings. A: Complete heart block with giant A waves. C = cannon waves. B: During sinus rhythm. Normal A and V waves.

$$\text{Resistance (mmHg/liter/min)} = \frac{\text{mean pressure drop (mmHg)}}{\text{mean blood flow (liters/minute)}}$$

Thus for systemic vascular resistance (Rs)

$$Rs = \frac{\substack{\text{Systemic arterial (aortic)} \\ \text{pressure (mmHg)}} - \text{right atrial pressure (mmHg)}}{\text{Systemic blood flow (Qs) (L/min)}}$$

and for pulmonary vascular resistance (Rp)

$$Rp = \frac{\substack{\text{Pulmonary arterial} \\ \text{pressure (mmHg)}} - \substack{\text{Pulmonary arterial wedge or} \\ \text{left atrial pressure (mmHg)}}}{\text{Pulmonary blood flow (Qp) (L/min)}}$$

A flow index ($L/min/m^2$) rather than actual flow (L/min) is usually used in calculating resistance and reduces the effect of variation of body size. For example, an infant with an appropriate cardiac output for its size would have a high calculated pulmonic and systemic resistance, but normal vascular resistance indices. The normal pulmonary vascular resistance is 1–2 mm $Hg/L/min/m^2$, while the normal systemic vascular resistance is 15–20 mm $Hg/L/min/m^2$.

The calculation of pulmonic and systemic resistances requires measurement of pulmonary and systemic blood flows as well as pressures. For many years, it was impossible to accurately measure the oxygen consumption (and therefore the blood flows) in infants and children. Thus, pediatric cardiologists have instead tended to use the ratio between pulmonary and systemic resistances. As was discussed in Chapter 6, this eliminates the need to measure actual blood flow, a flow ratio obtainable from oxygen saturation data sufficing.

$$Rp/Rs = \frac{\dfrac{PA - LA\,(PW)}{QP}}{\dfrac{SA - RA}{Qs}}$$

where PA = pulmonary artery pressure; PW = pulmonary artery wedge pressure; LA = left atrial pressure; SA = systemic artery pressure; RA = right atrial pressure.

(Note: All pressures are mean pressures) Thus

$$\frac{Rp}{Rs} = \frac{PA - LA}{Qp} \times \frac{Qs}{SA - RA}$$
$$= \frac{PA - LA}{SA - RA} \times \frac{Qs}{Qp}$$

The normal pulmonary-to-systemic resistance ratio is approximately 0.1 to 0.2.

Since the resistance ratio eliminates the need to measure pulmonary or systemic flow, it is a very practical means of estimating pulmonary vascular resistance in infants and small children if oxygen consumption cannot be measured. However, Qp/Qs depends on both pulmonary and systemic flows. In the example given in Chapter 6, two patients, each with a Qp of 6.0 $L/min/m^2$, had a different QP/Qs since their Qs was different. The patient with a Qs of 4.0 $L/min/m^2$ had a Qp/Qs of 1.5, while the other, with a Qs of 2.0 $L/min/m^2$, had a Qp/Qs of 3.0. If we assume equal pulmonary and systemic arterial pressures (Pp/Ps = 1), then one patient (Qs of 4.0 $L/min/m^2$) has an Rp/Rs of 0.67, while the other (Qs of 2.0 $L/min/m^2$) has a Rp/Rs of 0.33, in spite of *both* patients having the same pulmonary vascular resistance index. Thus, the resistance ratio is most useful if there is relatively normal systemic flow.

The response of the pulmonary arteriolar resistance to vasodilator agents (e.g., tolazoline, oxygen inhalation) is a measure of the lability or reactivity of the pulmonary vascular bed. In general, most laboratories near sea level have not seen a significant response of the pulmonary vascular bed to tolazoline. On the other hand, there is usually an increase in Qp/Qs and a decrease in Rp/Rs with oxygen administration (see Chapter 6). Unfortunately, the correlation between the Rp/Rs ratio, its response to oxygen inhalation, and the actual histology of the pulmonary vascular bed (or the patient's postoperative hemodynamics) is often not a particularly good one. However, it is still the best (and only) guide we presently have.

8

Measurement of Cardiac Output

F. Jay Fricker, M.D.

Cardiac output measurement in the catheterization laboratory is an integral part of the hemodynamic evaluation of heart disease in children, and it is essential that reliable and reproducible methods be used. Although blood flow is pulsatile and undergoes phasic variations with respiration and the cardiac cycle, methods for measuring cardiac output ignore these variations and measure mean flow over time. The direct Fick and indicator dilution methods are the standard techniques used in most laboratories. In the absence of an intracardiac shunt, both the direct Fick and indicator dilution methods measure pulmonary blood flow, which is the same as systemic blood flow with a small error introduced by the bronchial circulation. The principle for both methods is the same. Flow through a vascular bed (e.g., the lungs) can be determined if the amount of a substance entering the blood stream during a given period of time is divided by the difference in concentration of that substance between the inflow and outflow of that vascular bed.

$$\text{Flow (Q)} = \frac{\text{Amount of indicator introduced or absorbed}}{\text{Mean concentration difference (outflow } - \text{ inflow)}}$$

These methods assume that the indicator substance is completely mixed with the blood at each sampling point and that there is no indicator lost during the transit through the vascular bed in which flow is being measured. The normal range for cardiac index is 3.5 ± 0.7 L/min/m^2 of body surface area (Yang et al. 1988).

Direct Fick

It was not until the mid 1940s, when cardiac catheterization came into use, that the direct Fick method began to be used clinically for the measurement of cardiac output (Cournand et al. 1945). Oxygen is the "indicator" substance used in this method. In the lungs, a volume of oxygen (O_2 consumption or $V \cdot O_2$) is added to the oxygen content of mixed venous blood (MVO_2 in mL O_2/100 mL of blood). End capillary blood oxygen content (pulmonary venous) is designated as PVO_2 (in mL O_2/100 mL of blood). Therefore, each 100 mL (dL) of blood takes up $PVO_2 - MVO_2$ mL of oxygen as it passes through the lungs. If the amount of oxygen taken up by the lungs (oxygen consumption or $V \cdot O_2$) is known, pulmonary blood flow (Qp) can be calculated:

$Qp(L/min/m^2)$

$$= \frac{V \cdot O_2 \text{ (ml/min)}}{PVO_2 - MVO_2 \text{ (ml } O_2/100 \text{ ml blood)}}$$

$$\times 10.$$

The number "10" in the right hand part of the equation converts O_2 content from mL/

100 mL of blood to mL/L of blood. Thus, flow will be expressed in liters of blood/min.

The determination of cardiac output by the direct Fick method requires the measurement or estimation of oxygen consumption and the determination of the oxygen content of mixed venous and arterial blood (SAO_2 = systemic arterial O_2 content). Thus, systemic blood flow (Qs) is

$$Qs(L/min/m^2)$$

$$= \frac{V\cdot O_2 \text{ (ml/min)}}{SAO_2 - MVO_2 \text{ (ml/}O_2\text{/100 ml blood)}}$$

$$\times 10.$$

The oxygen content of arterial blood is easily determined, but the measurement of oxygen consumption and mixed venous (pulmonary artery) oxygen content deserves further comment. The direct measurement of oxygen consumption can be difficult and fraught with errors, particularly in young children. The Douglas bag, commonly used in adult laboratories for collecting expired gas, is not practical in infants and children. We use a flow-through oxygen consumption computer (e.g., Waters Instrument Co. MRM-2). Various sizes of clear plastic hoods are available to cover the patient's head. In this device, a polarographic cell determines the decrease in concentration of oxygen when expired air is mixed with a known volume of room air being withdrawn through the hood.

In general, VO_2 determined by this method has correlated with expected and assumed oxygen consumption both for patient size and type of disease. Accurate estimation of VO_2 is essential if reliable blood flow and resistance calculations are to be obtained. When VO_2 is not measured, estimation of oxygen consumption can be made by multiplying body surface area (m^2) × 150 mL/min. Values in normal children have also been reported by La Farge (La Farge and Mienttinen 1970) and others, based on sex, age, BSA, and heart rate.

The reliability of the Fick method also depends on the accurate measurement of the arteriovenous oxygen content difference ($SAO_2 - MVO_2$). Ideally, the mixed venous oxygen content should be measured in the pulmonary artery, requiring pulmonary artery catheterization. Sampling from more proximal sites gives only an estimation of true mixed venous oxygen content since there is considerable streaming of flow from different vascular beds in the SVC and IVC (Wood et al. 1955). In our laboratory, however, samples taken from the low superior vena cava have proven to be very similar to those from the pulmonary artery in patients who do not have a left-to-right shunt and, therefore, are the best approximation of mixed venous blood in patients with a left-to-right shunt. Arterial oxygen content can be obtained from any peripheral artery. Although there is variation in end capillary partial pressure of oxygen (pO_2) from moment to moment, such variation does not substantially influence arterial oxygen content. Under ordinary circumstances, arterial oxygen saturation is on the plateau portion of the oxyhemoglobin dissociation curve, and a modest change in pO_2 will not affect oxygen content. However, in patients with lung disease who have a reduced end capillary pO_2 and systemic arterial hypoxemia, small changes in pO_2 have a more profound effect on the arterial oxygen content, since the pO_2 falls on the steep portion of the oxyhemoglobin dissociation curve.

Another obvious source of error is in the measurement of O_2 content. In most laboratories, O_2 content is calculated from O_2 saturation measured by a photometric method and dissolved oxygen is not included. At normal alveolar pO_2, the error is small since the amount of oxygen dissolved in blood is only 0.3 mL/100 mL of blood/100 torr pO_2. If blood flow is determined with the patient breathing 100% oxygen, the amount of dissolved oxygen increases arterial oxygen content by approximately 1.8 mL/100 mL of blood. If dissolved oxygen is not considered in this circumstance, cardiac output is substantially overestimated (Visscher and Johnson 1953).

Indicator Dilution Method

This method was first suggested by Stewart in 1897, but most of the research in establishing it as a useful clinical tool was done by W. F. Hamilton from 1928 to 1948 (Stewart 1897; Hamilton et al. 1932). If a known quantity of an indicator substance (I) is injected as a bolus into the circulation, flow (Q) can be determined by sampling the concentration of that substance over time down stream. [C (mg/L) × t (min) = mean concentration of indicator.] This method assumes complete mixing and no loss of the indicator substance. Thus

$$Q(L/min) = \frac{I\ (mg)}{C\ (mg/L) \times t\ (min)} .$$

Indocyanine Green

Indocyanine green (Cardiogreen) is the indicator currently used and it has a number of advantages over Evans blue, a substance used in the past. Both dyes are nontoxic and, since they combine with proteins, they leak from the circulation slowly. Cardiogreen has the advantage of not discoloring the patient's skin. The point of maximal light absorption on the spectrum is also more favorable for indocyanine green, and small quantities of dye can be detected in the circulation without interference from hemoglobin. Solutions of either 2.5 mg/mL or 5 mg/mL are prepared by dissolving 25- or 50-mg vials of indocyanine green in 10 mL of diluent. A standard volume (1 mL) is injected into a selected site and sampled from the aorta or from a peripheral artery. A more proximal site of injection in the venous system and/or a low cardiac output flattens the indicator dilution curve and may hinder recognition of the beginning of recirculation. Injection of dye into the pulmonary artery or a pul-

monary artery wedge position is therefore advisable. Blood is sampled from the arterial line by a constant flow pump (e.g., Sage Instruments) at a rate of 25 mL/min. The blood is aspirated into a sterile syringe through sterile tubing positioned across a densitometer. Since the blood does not leave the sterile system, it can be reinfused into the patient after the dye curve has been obtained. The curves are recorded on the physiologic data recorder and the signal can also be fed into a computer (Fig. 1, Left top). Standard calibration dilutions are made by diluting 20 lambda (0.020 mL) of the Cardiogreen solution with 10 mL of blood.

Methods for calculation of cardiac output from indicator dilution curves utilize either the standard Stewart-Hamilton logarithmic extrapolation method or the "Fore 'n Aft Triangle" method of Bradley and Barr (Bradley and Barr 1969). The accurate determination of cardiac output depends upon measuring the mean concentration under the first pass curve. Unfortunately, recirculation occurs before complete inscription of the primary curve and the terminal part of the curve must be estimated. It has been demonstrated that the disappearance phase of the primary curve is logarithmic. Therefore, if the logarithm of the concentration of dye is plotted against time, the downslope and the intercept of the curve on the time axis can be predicted. In order to determine the mean concentration of dye by the standard logarithmic (Stewart-Hamilton replot) method, the descending limb of the curve must be redrawn and extrapolated to zero. This is done by plotting the time-concentration curve on semi-log paper with indicator concentration on the logarithmic axis and the descending limb thus becoming a straight line (Fig. 1, Right). The point at which indicator concentration is 1% of the peak concentration is taken as the disappearance time, and the indicator dilution curve is extrapolated to this point. Determining mean concentration of dye from the redrawn curve is done by measuring the area under the curve by planimetry and di-

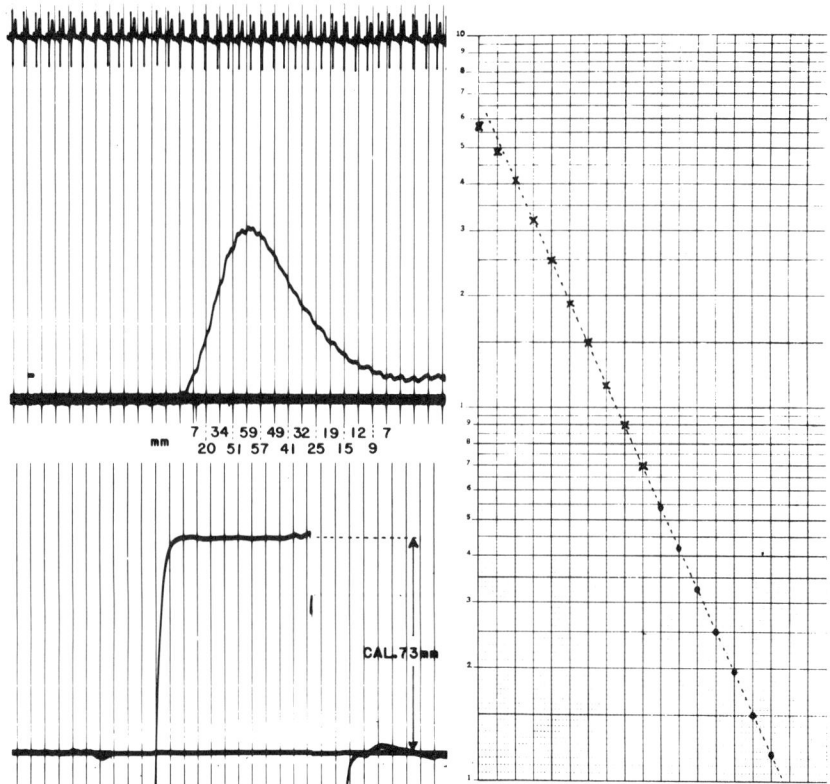

Figure 1. Dye dilution curve #1. Cardiac output calculated by the Stewart-Hamilton method. Left (top): Actual curve. Numbers represent the height of the curve at 1-sec intervals. Left (bottom): Calibration (see text). Right: Logarithmic replot. x = actual points obtained from the curve before recirculation; dots = points determined by extrapolation of the slope of the actual data points (x).

viding the value obtained by the length of the duration of the curve.

Mean concentration of dye also can be estimated by an integration method. The height of the curve (in mm) is measured from the corrected curve at 1-sec intervals. The sum of these values is then an estimate of the area of the curve (mm.sec) (Fig. 1):

$$7 + 20 + 34 + 51 + 59 + 57 + 49$$

$$+ 41 + 32 + 25 + 19 + 15 + 12 + 7$$

$$+ 5.4 + 4.2 + 2.5 + 1.9 + 1.5 + 0.4$$

$$= 441 \text{ (mm.sec)}.$$

A calibration factor is then necessary to convert the calculated curve area (mm.sec) into mean concentration in mg dye/L of blood. The calibration curve is obtained by adding 20 lambda (0.020 mL) of dye to 10 mL of blood. This is equivalent to a concentration of 2 mL of dye/L of blood (5 or 10 mg of dye/L depending upon the concentration of Cardiogreen that is used.) The calibration blood is then withdrawn through the densitometer and a calibration curve is obtained (Fig. 1, Left bottom). Thus, if 5 mg/mL of dye was used for the injection, the 2 mL of dye/L of blood calibration would be 10 mg dye/L of blood. Thus

Calibration Factor (K) mg/L

$$= \frac{\text{Indicator Concentration (mg/L)}}{\text{mm deflection}}.$$

Therefore

Calibration Factor (K) mg/L

$$= \frac{5 \times 2}{73} = \frac{10}{73} = 0.137.$$

Then

C.O. (L/min)

$$= \frac{I \text{ (mg)} \times 60 \text{ (sec/min)}}{Area \text{ (mm.sec)} \times K \text{ (mg/L/mm)}}$$

C.O. (L/min)

$$= \frac{5 \text{ (mg)} \times 60 \text{ (sec/min)}}{441 \text{ mm.sec} \times 0.137} = 4.97.$$

The Fore 'n Aft Triangle method has greatly simplified this calculation by eliminating replotting and planimetry or integration. This method, described by Bradley and Barr, shows excellent correlation with the logarithmic extrapolation method (Fig. 2). It estimates the area under the curve by measuring the height of the peak of the curve (PC) and the width of the curve at half its peak height (T_{50}). Using an empirical constant (0.856) derived from a regression analysis correlating areas calculated by logarithmic extrapolation and the Fore 'n Aft Triangle method, the equation for determining cardiac output becomes

$$\text{Cardiac Output (L/min)} = \frac{I \text{ (mg)} \times 60 \text{ sec/min} \times 0.856}{Area \times K}$$

$$= \frac{I \text{ (mg)} \times 51.4 \text{ (sec/min)}}{PC \text{ (mm)} \times T_{50} \text{ (sec)} \times K}$$

$$\text{Calibration Factor (K) mg/L} = \frac{5 \times 2}{50} = \frac{10}{50} = 0.2$$

then

$$\text{Cardiac Output (L/mm)} = \frac{5 \text{ mg} \times 51.4 \text{ sec/min}}{144 \text{ mm} \times 2.8 \text{ sec} \times 0.20} = 3.19.$$

The reliability of the indicator dilution method has been demonstrated in a number of studies comparing indicator dilution and Fick (oxygen consumption) cardiac outputs (Hamilton et al. 1948; Miller et al. 1962; Grenvik 1966). The indicator dilution method has some advantages over the Fick method in that it determines cardiac output over a shorter interval and is therefore not as dependent upon maintaining a steady state for an extended period. Also, it is independent of the composition of respiratory gases, and an immediate readout can be obtained by computerized methods.

It has been claimed that there is considerable variability of duplicate determinations, but this has not been our experience. Theoretically, one might expect the indicator dilution method to be relatively inaccurate with the low and prolonged curves of low cardiac output or valvar insufficiency. A number of investigators have suggested that in the presence of valvar regurgitation, cardiac output by indicator dilution will be underestimated if the injection was made proximal to the regurgitation (Rahimtoola and Swan 1965). This has subsequently been refuted by Samet (1966) and by Reddy (1976). Lastly, error can be introduced if injection and sampling sites are too close for complete mixing of the injected dye to take place before it is sampled (Shepherd et al. 1972). The limitation on the number of determinations that can be performed has been overcome with the introduction of Cardiogreen.

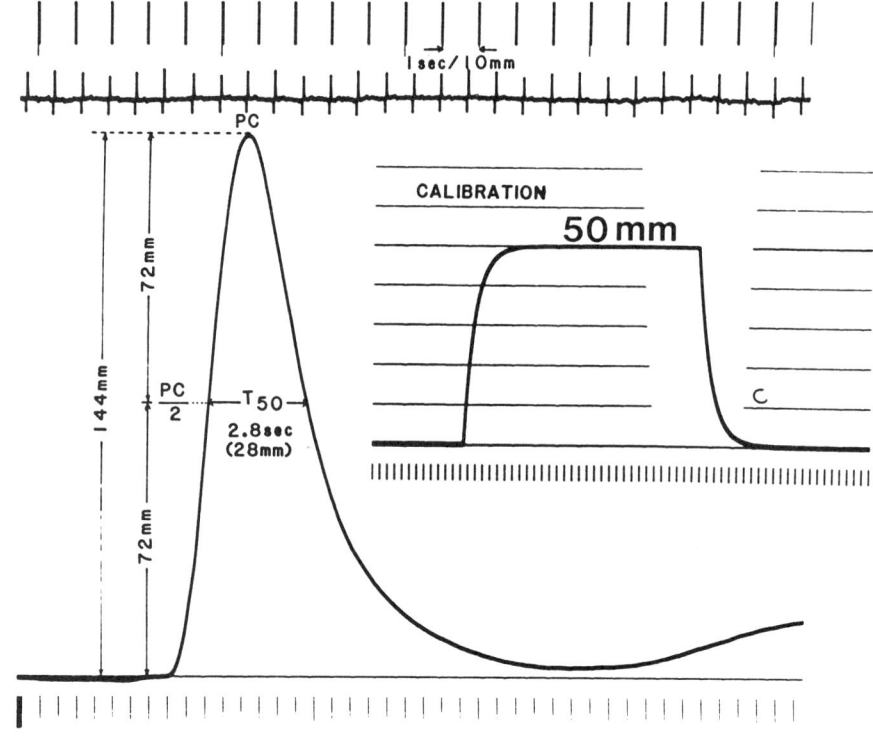

Figure 2. Dye dilution curve #2. Cardiac output calculated by the fore 'n aft triangle method (see text).

Thermodilution

Determination of cardiac output by thermodilution is useful in the catheterization laboratory and in the setting of the intensive care unit. The indicator dilution principle is the same. An indicator, cold saline, is injected into the right atrium and the resultant temperature change is recorded by a thermistor on the tip of a catheter in the pulmonary artery. Double-lumen thermodilution catheters are available in sizes ranging from #5 French upward. These catheters are flexible and are flow-directed with the distal lumen connected to a balloon and there is a proximal lumen for injection of the cold saline.

Thermal dilution cardiac output is measured by the following equation:

$$C.O. = \frac{(T_b - T_i) \times (V) \times (60) \times (1.08) \times (0.825)}{D_6 (t) dt}$$

where $D_6 (t) dt$ = area under curve registered; T_b = body temperature; T_i = injectate temperature; V = volume of injectate; 1.08 = ratio of products of specific heat of 0.9% saline and blood; 60 = 60 sec/min; 0.825 = factor to correct for loss of heat during injection.

In most instances, cardiac output is determined by a computer coupled to the thermistor that records the temperature changes following injection of the cold saline. Other variables such as height and weight are entered manually using dials or a keypad on the front of the computer.

There are several advantages of this method. The injected fluid equilibrates with body temperature during passage through the peripheral capillaries so there is no recirculation curve. Also, mixing of the cold fluid with blood is rapid, and multiple determinations can be performed within a short period. Lastly, determination of cardiac output can be accomplished without violating a peripheral artery.

A number of studies have been published indicating that thermodilution outputs are as reliable as indicator dilution and Fick-determined cardiac outputs (Weisel et al. 1975; Enghoff et al. 1970). In our experience, indocyanine green dye and thermodilution cardiac outputs have correlated well in the older child. Several centers have reported good correlation between thermodilution and dye dilution cardiac outputs even in small subjects (Callaghan et al. 1976; Moodie et al. 1978). However, we have found a considerable difference between indocyanine green dye and thermodilution methods in infants and small children. Sequential determinations of thermodilution cardiac output in these small patients have a 10%–25% variability from one determination to the next (Freed and Keane 1978). We have not found this inconsistency with the green dye method. This variability of thermodilution might be explained by fluctuation in pulmonary arterial temperature with the respiratory cycle which may approach the 1–2° C temperature change seen following injection of the cold saline, or by heat loss of the injectate between the injection port and the right atrium (Maruschak et al. 1982).

References and Suggested Reading

Bradley EC, Barr JW. Fore 'n aft triangle formula for rapid estimation of area. Am Heart J 1969; 78:643–648.

Callaghan ML, Weintraub WH, Coran AG. Assessment of thermodilution cardiac output in small subjects. J Pediatr Surg 1976; 11:629–634.

Cournand AJ, Riley FL, Breed ES, Bladwin EF, et al. Measurement of cardiac output in man using the technique of catheterization of the right auricle or ventricle. J Clin Invest 1945; 24:106–116.

Enghoff E, Michaelsson M, Pavek K, Sjogren S. A comparison between the thermal dilution method and the direct Fick and the dye dilution methods for cardiac output measurements in man. ACTA Soc Med 1970; 73(3):157–170.

Freed MD, Keane JK. Cardiac output measured by thermodilution in infants and children. J Pediatr 1978; 92:39–42.

Grenvik A. Errors of the dye dilution method compared to the direct Fick method in determination of cardiac output. Scand J Clin Lab Invest 1966; 18:492–496.

Hamilton WF, Moore JW, Kinsman JM, et al. Studies on the circulation IV. Further analysis of the injection method and of changes in hemodynamics under physiological and pathological conditions. Am J Physiol 1932; 99:534–551.

Hamilton WF, Riley RL, Attyah AM, Cournand AJ, et al. Comparison of the Fick and Dye injection methods of measuring the cardiac output in man. Am J Physiol 1948; 153:309–321.

La Farge CG, Mienttinen OS. The estimation of oxygen consumption. Cardiovasc Res 1970; 4:23–30.

Maruschak GF, Potter AM, Schauble JF, et al. Overestimation of pediatric cardiac output by thermal indicator loss. Circulation 1982; 65:380–383

Miller DE, Gleason WL, McIntosh. A comparison of the cardiac output by the direct Fick method and the dye-dilution method using indocyanine green dye and a cuvette densitometer. J Lab Clin Med 1962; 59:345–350.

Moodie DS, Feldt RH, Kaye MP et al. Measurement of cardiac output by thermodilution. Development of accurate measurements at flows applicable to the pediatric patient. J Surg Res 1978; 25:305–311.

Rahimtoola SH, Swan HJC. Calculation of cardiac output from indicator-dilution curves in the presence of mitral regurgitation. Circulation 1965; 31:711–718.

Reddy PS, Curtiss EI, Bell B, O'Toole, JD, et al. Determinants of variation between Fick and indicator dilution estimates of cardiac output during diagnostic catheterization. Fick vs dye cardiac outputs. J Lab Clin Med 1976; 87:565–576.

Samet P, Bernstein WH, Castillo C. Validity of indicator-dilution determinations of cardiac output in patients with mitral regurgitation. Circulation 1966; 33:410–416.

Samet P, Castillo C, Bernstein WH. Validity of indicator-dilution determinations of cardiac output in patients with mitral regurgitation. Circulation 1966; 33:609–619.

Shepherd RL, Higgs LM, Glancy DL. Comparison of left ventricular and pulmonary arterial injection sites in determination of cardiac output by indicator dilution technique. Chest 1972; 62:175–178.

Stewart GN. Researches on the circulation time and on the influences which affect it. IV. The output of the heart. J Physiol 1897; 22:159–183.

Visscher MB, Johnson JA. The Fick Principle. Analysis of potential errors in its conventional application. J Appl Physiol 1953; 5:635–638.

Weisel RD, Berger FL, Hechtman HB. Current Concepts: Measurements of cardiac output by thermodilution. N Engl J Med 1975; 292:682–684.

Wood EH, Bowers D, Shepherd, Fox EJ. Oxygen content of 'mixed' venous blood in man during various phases of the respiratory and cardiac cycles in relation to possible errors in measurement of cardiac output by conventional application of the Fick method. J Appl Physiol 1955; 7:621–628.

Yang SS, et al. (eds). From Cardiac Catheterization Data to Hemodynamic Parameters. 3rd ed. Philadelphia, PA, FA Davis Co. 1988.

9

Angiocardiography

Sang C. Park, M.D.

Angiocardiography is an essential part of the diagnostic cardiac catheterization and plays a major role in defining precise anatomy, particularly in complex cardiac anomalies. Proper angiocardiographic technique is important in obtaining diagnostic information and is also essential for patient safety, since some serious complications of cardiac catheterization are related to angiocardiography. Good equipment is obviously required as is skill in its operation.

Radiographic Equipment

In recent years, there have been substantial improvements in radiographic equipment. The "C arm" (used generically for multiangle radiographic equipment) removes some of the limitations of fixed vertical and lateral units. The desired standard projection or compound angled view can then be obtained without moving the patient and thus often without awakening a sleeping child.

Two types of apparatus are available: cut or roll film changers and image intensifiers with cinecamera attachments. In the cut film changer, a cassette is transported into position for the x-ray exposure and then rapidly conveyed out of the way as the next cassette is moved into position. Sanchez-Perez and Picker-Amplatz are examples of changers of this type. In a Schoenader roll film changer, film is transported from a feeding magazine into the exposure field and after exposure the film is ejected into a receiving magazine. Roll film changers are made by Elema-Franklin and Picker-Amplatz. Changers of this type can expose up to 12 frames/sec in two planes.

The major advantage of the large film technique is that a larger field is visualized. There are, however, several major drawbacks to large film changers. Patients must be positioned over the film changer without the fluoroscopic monitoring that is often needed for centering the patient or repositioning the catheter. The films are recorded without continuous fluoroscopic visualization or simultaneous videotape recording, and the results of angiocardiography are not known until the film is developed. In addition, some information is lost due to the slow speed of filming (12 frames/sec vs 60 frames/sec in cineangiography). For these reasons, cineangiography is the preferred approach for the evaluation of most patients with congenital heart disease.

Cineangiograms are usually recorded at 60 frames/sec, although speeds exceeding this are available. Currently available image intensifiers are capable of producing high-quality cinefilms that are almost equivalent to large film in resolution. Cineangiographic units are generally equipped with a 35-mm camera and some units are also capable of recording 70-mm spot films. The image intensifier is connected both to a video screen for viewing and to a video recording device. This enables cineangiograms to be reviewed before the film has been developed and is an essential requirement for any cardiac catheterization laboratory. Over the last few years, digital subtraction cineangiographic units have become available in some laboratories. These use high-speed minicomputers to digitize video information at rates as high as 30 frames/sec and to store the acquired images for subsequent evaluation. Prior to angiography, the plain film or "background" video image is digitized and similarly stored. Once the study has been completed, the background image is subtracted from the images acquired during angiography, thus resulting in a much clearer picture of the angiographic information. This technique provides a satisfactory image with the use of much less contrast material, even with a peripheral venous injection.

Contrast Media and Catheters

Contrast Material

Most contrast media used in angiography are either sodium or methylglucamine salts of the organic iodine compounds diatrizoate or iothalamate. In some cases, a combination salt is used. The viscosity of the various contrast media is variable and is dependent upon the type of salt used (Table 1). The viscosity of contrast material is also significantly influenced by temperature, with viscosity at 37° C about two-thirds of that at 25° C. Some power injectors are equipped with a sleeve heater around the injector syringe so that contrast is heated to body temperature and can be delivered at lower pressure for any given flow rate. One drawback, however, is that a high concentration of sodium may be detrimental in patients with congestive heart failure. In our laboratory, a combination salt is used (Renografin-76). Although the viscosity is high, there is a low sodium content, a low incidence of side effects, and excellent contrast quality. Recently, low ionic and nonionic contrast media have become available that avoid problems of high sodium and osmolality. Since these contrast media are more expensive, we usually reserve their use for specific indications such as in neonates and in patients with severe congestive heart failure or renal disease.

Table 1
Physical Properties of Selected Contrast Media

Commercial brand	Iodine content mg/mL	Sodium meq/mL	Sodium mg/mL	Viscosity (CPS) 37°C	Osmolality (mOsm/kg H₂O)
Mallinckrodt					
Conray 60%	282	0.0014	0.04	4.0	1,400
Conray 400	400	1.05	24.2	4.5	2,300
Hexabrix*	320	0.15	3.48	7.5	600
Squibb					
Renografin-60	293	0.16	3.76	3.9	1,420
Renografin-76	370	0.19	4.48	8.4	1,940
Isovue 370**	370	0.0002	0.040	9.4	796
Winthrop					
Hypaque sodium 50%	300	0.8	18.1	2.3	1,515
Hypaque Meglumin 60%	282	0.001	0.02	4.1	1,415
Hypaque Meglumin 75%	385	0.39	9.0	8.35	2,105
Omnipaque 350**	350	0	0	14.4	844

* low Ionic contrast media.
** nonionic contrast media.

Power Injectors

A power injector is essential for the rapid delivery of contrast media into the cardiovascular system. Early models of pressure injectors were designed so that volume of contrast and delivery pressure could be controlled, but not the rate of delivery. Both total volume and rate of injection can be controlled on currently available injectors, which generate the pressure necessary to deliver a selected amount of contrast at a selected rate (mL/sec). There is also an automatic cutoff when the pressure in the injector reaches a preselected level. Injectors such as these made by Cordis, Viamonte-Hobbs, Medrad, and others can be synchronized with the patient's electrocardiogram and can be programmed to inject a preset amount of contrast material during selected portions of the cardiac cycle. Theoretically, a synchronized injection during diastole should improve visualization of coronary artery anatomy with an aortic root injection and avoid dysrhythmia during ventriculography. However, we have not found synchronized injections to be particularly useful.

Catheters

A variety of catheters are available for angiocardiography and are made from woven Dacron, Teflon, polyethylene, or polyurethane. The choice of catheter size for angiocardiography is influenced by a number of factors. The pressure drop during laminar flow of a homogenous fluid through a rigid tube of constant caliber is directly proportional to the length of the tube, the volume of delivery fluid (actually the flow rate), and the viscosity of the fluid, and is inversely proportional to the fourth power of the radius (Poiseuille's law). Therefore, a catheter with the largest internal diameter and shortest length possible should be used, particularly when delivery of a large volume of contrast is necessary. Obviously, a thin-walled catheter provides a relatively large internal diameter. Double-lumen catheters,

such as balloon-tipped catheters, always have a smaller internal diameter for a given external diameter, and for fluid delivery these catheters are satisfactory only when smaller amounts of contrast are needed.

Ideally, an angiographic catheter should deliver 1 mL/kg/sec of contrast medium without exceeding a pressure of 800 lbs/square inch (PSI). In patients with large left-to-right shunts, a delivery rate of 1.5 mL/kg/sec may be required. In the venous system, catheter size is usually not limiting, even in the newborn period. In retrograde arterial catheterization, however, the use of a large catheter may result in vascular compromise and thus there may need to be compromise between the quality of angiograms and patient safety. Recommendations for the choice of catheter based upon size of the patient are discussed in Chapter 3.

General Considerations

A good angiocardiographic study requires careful planning with appropriate modifications of that plan during the procedure as new information becomes available. The most important diagnostic angiocardiograms should usually be obtained first. Should there be some unexpected complication, such as a severe allergic reaction to the contrast material, the major diagnostic information will already have been obtained. Ideally, angiography should be performed after completion of the hemodynamic evaluation since it may alter resting hemodynamics. During pediatric cardiac catheterization, however, a catheter may enter an unusual site or one that may be difficult to reenter prior to completion of the hemodynamic evaluation. When this occurs, the necessary angiogram should be performed before removing the catheter from that site. For example, if the catheter is passed out into the ascending aorta from the right ventricle in an infant with a ventricular septal defect, an aortogram should be performed to rule out a patent ductus arteriosus or a coarctation of the aorta before the catheter is withdrawn to the ventricle. Whenever possible, angiocardiographic views that cause the least maneuvering of the patient should be done first, especially in smaller children. Anteroposterior and lateral views require no movement of the patient but a four-chamber or sitting up view may awaken a sedated child. This is not a problem if a C-arm radiographic unit is available.

A sufficient volume of contrast material and an adequate rate of contrast delivery should be used. Unnecessarily large doses of contrast should be avoided, however, since there is a relationship between the volume of contrast used and the incidence of complications. In general, the total volume of contrast should not exceed 5 mL/kg. It is thus imperative to set the priority of each angiographic view and then proceed until adequate information is obtained or until the maximum volume of contrast medium is reached. It should be reemphasized that a few well-planned angiocardiograms are more informative than multiple poorly selected ones.

Selection of Projection

The precise visualization of the anatomy of complex cardiac malformations is an essential part of the evaluation of patients with congenital heart disease. With single or double C-arm equipment, most projections can be obtained without moving the patient. However, some laboratories are equipped only with fixed anteroposterior and lateral radiographic units. The necessary positions for the various views or projections will be discussed for both the fixed biplane and C-arm arrangements.

The primary objectives in selecting a projection are to delineate the area of interest as clearly as possible and to avoid overlapping of other opacified structures. The introduction of axial angiography by Bargeron, et al. (1977, 1981) has greatly improved pediatric angiocardiography. Axial views are designed to visualize the heart in its long axis rather than using the long axis of the body or thorax as the reference point. The axial views minimize the superimposition of adjacent structures that is often such a problem in conventional views. Although axial views require more radiation because of the inclusion in the field of abdominal organs such as the liver, the increase in diagnostic information justified their use.

The standard biplane radiographic unit has a fixed angle between the vertical and horizontal (lateral) tubes. However, movable radiographic arms are capable of rotation as well as cranio-caudal angulation of the beam. Also, movable biplane units are not necessarily at right angles to one another, as they are with fixed units. To facilitate description of the tube positions for various projections, two imaginary planes are established through the crux of the heart (the posterior junction of the atrial and ventricular septa). One is at right angles to the long axis of the table (Fig. 1) and identifies the degree of "rotation." The other plane is parallel to the long axis of the table and identifies cranial "angulation" of the x-ray beam. To simplify the orientation of the radiographic unit, only the location of the image intensifier, and not the x-ray tube, will be identified. Two numbers (e.g., 30/15) will be used to describe rotation and angulation of the image intensifier within these planes. The first number indicates the degrees of *rotation* (side to side) within the vertical plane, with 0° being perpendicular to the horizontal plane (standard anteroposterior image intensifier position) and 90° being parallel to it (standard lateral tube image intensifier position). These numbers will be preceded by an *R* or *L* to indicate rotation of the image intensifier to the patient's right or left (Fig. 1). The second number indicates the *angulation* in the cranial direction of the image intensifier. The notation "0°" indicates no cranial angulation with the long axis of the table and the number increases as the image intensifier is angled more cranially.

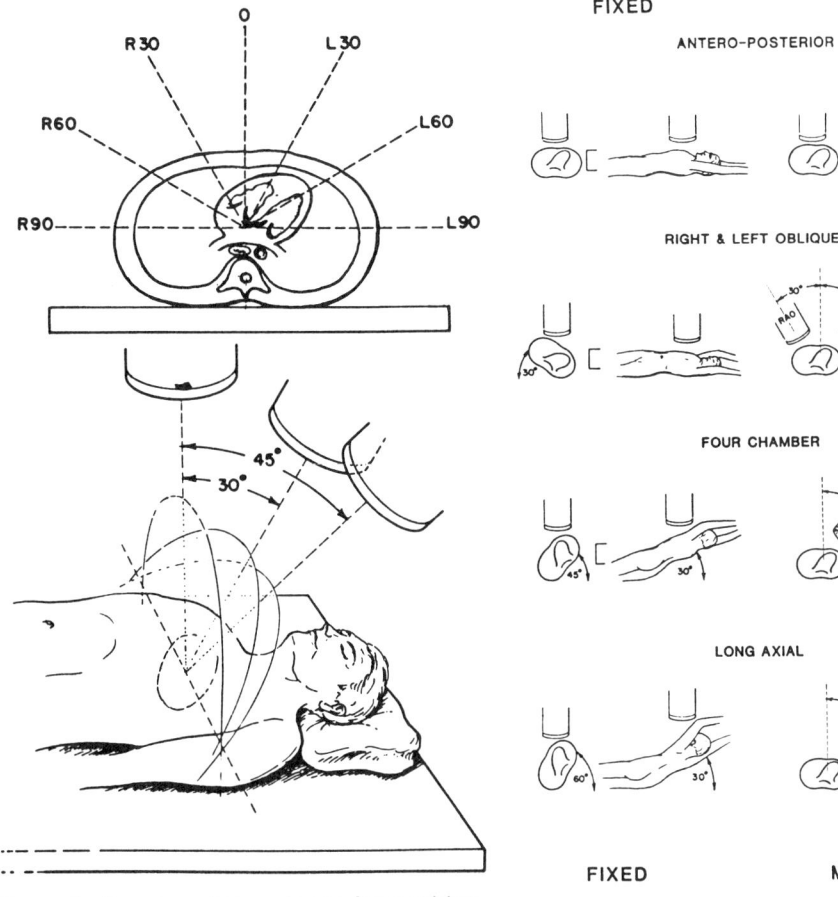

Figure 1. Two imaginary planes for positioning of C-arm image intensifier for angiography. Top: Transverse plane rotation. Bottom: Cranial angulation.

The following descriptions of projections and recommendations for positioning are based on normal cardiac location. However, variables such as the level of the diaphragm, presence of a rotational anomaly, or an unusual body habitus may significantly alter the "optimal" projections. The various views using fixed or movable radiographic units are summarized in Figure 2. A summary of the different projections and their advantages is found in Table 2, while the suggested views for various cardiac lesions are found in Table 3.

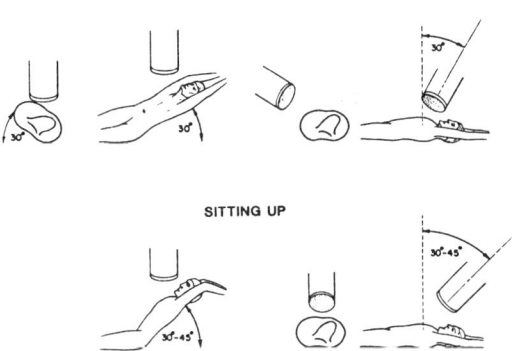

Figure 2. Summary of various views using fixed or movable radiographic units.

Table 2

A Summary of Various Projections

Projection	Radiographic unit	
	Fixed (patient's position)	Movable (II position)
Anterior-posterior	V: Supine	0/0
Lateral	L: Supine	L90/0
Right anterior oblique	V: 30°–45° RAO	R30–45/0
Left anterior oblique	Only V: 60° LAO	L60/0
	Only L: 30° RAO	
4-chamber	V: 45° LAO	L45/30
	+30° elevation	
Long axial	Only V: 60° LAO	L60/30
	+30° elevation	
	Only L: 30° RAO	
	30° slant to left	
Elongated right anterior oblique	V: 30° RAO	R30/30
	+30° elevation	
Sitting up	V: 30°–45° elevation	0/30°–45°

II, image intensifier; L, lateral radiographic unit; LAO, left anterior oblique view; RAO, right anterior oblique view; V, vertical radiographic unit.

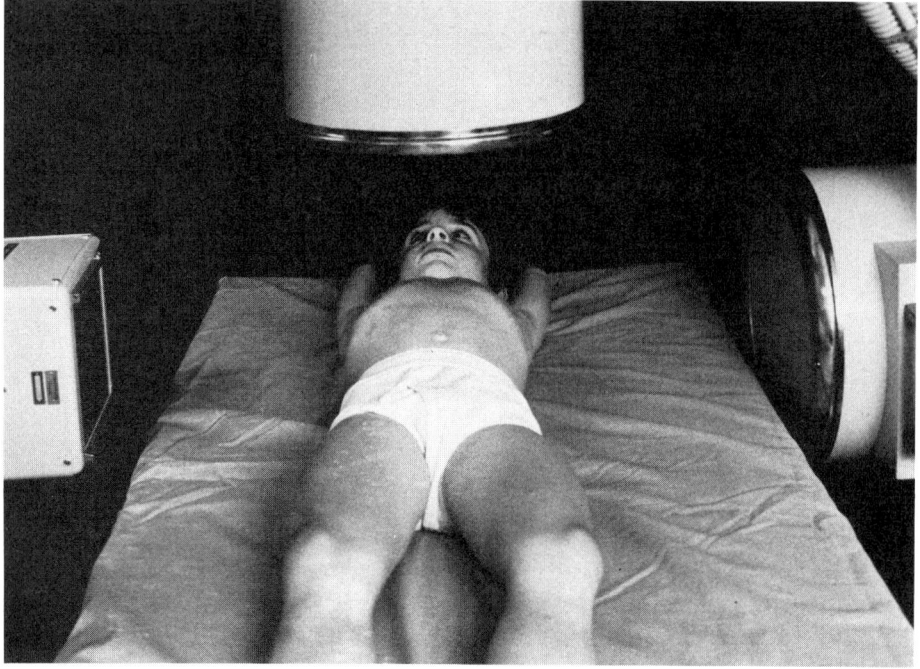

Figure 3. Patient positioned for AP and lateral views using fixed cameras.

Table 3
Essential Angiographic Sites and Views for Various Cardiac Lesions

Type of cardiac abnormality	Site	View Selection
A. *Septal defect*		
Ventricular septal defect	LV	4-C or LA
Atrial septal defect	RUPV	4-C
Atrioventricular septal defect	LV	4-C
B. *Valvar disease*		
Mitral	LV	RAO
Tricuspid	RV	RAO or AP
Aortic		
valvar stenosis	LV & Ao	4-C or LA
subvalvar stenosis	LV & Ao	AP & LA
regurgitation	Ao	4-C or LA
Pulmonic		
stenosis	RV	ERAO & LT
regurgitation	PA	LT
C. *Conotruncal abnormality*		
Tetralogy of Fallot	RV	ERAO & LA or LT
Double outlet RV	RV	AP & LT or ERAO & LT
	LV	4-C or AP & LT
Transposition (TGA)	LV	LA
	RV	AP & LT
Corrected TGA	LV (R. sided)	AP & LT or SU & LT
	RV (L. sided)	AP & LT
Truncus arteriosus	Truncus	AP & LT or RAO & LAO
	LV	4-C
D. *Miscellaneous*		
TAPVR	PA	AP
Coarctation of aorta	Ao	AP & LAO or LT
Patent ductus arteriosus	Ao	AP & LT or RAO & LT

Ao, aorta; AP, anteroposterior; ERAO, elongated right anterior oblique; LA, long axial; LAO, left anterior oblique; LT, lateral; LV, left ventricle; PA, pulmonary artery; RAO, right anterior oblique; RV, right ventricle; SU, siting up; TAPVR, total anomalous pulmonary venous return; TGA, transposition of the great arteries; 4-C, four-chamber view.

Standard Anteroposterior and Lateral Views

In the above notational system, these views are 0/0 and 90/0, respectively (Figs. 2, 3, 4, and 5). They are excellent for determining side-to-side and anteroposterior relationships of cardiac structures and great arteries. The anteroposterior pulmonary angiogram is useful in determining pulmonary artery size and distribution of peripheral pulmonary arteries. Pulmonary venous return usually can be defined on the levo-

phase. In the patient with a complex cardiac malformation and/or a rotational anomaly, anteroposterior and lateral views provide useful information and help in the selection of subsequent injection sites and views. Anterorposterior and lateral views are reproducible and are usually adequate for volumetric studies and functional evaluation of the ventricles. Although these views are not usually ideal for visualization of the ventricular and atrial septa, the anteroposterior view can be ideal for delineating the interventricular septum in patients with

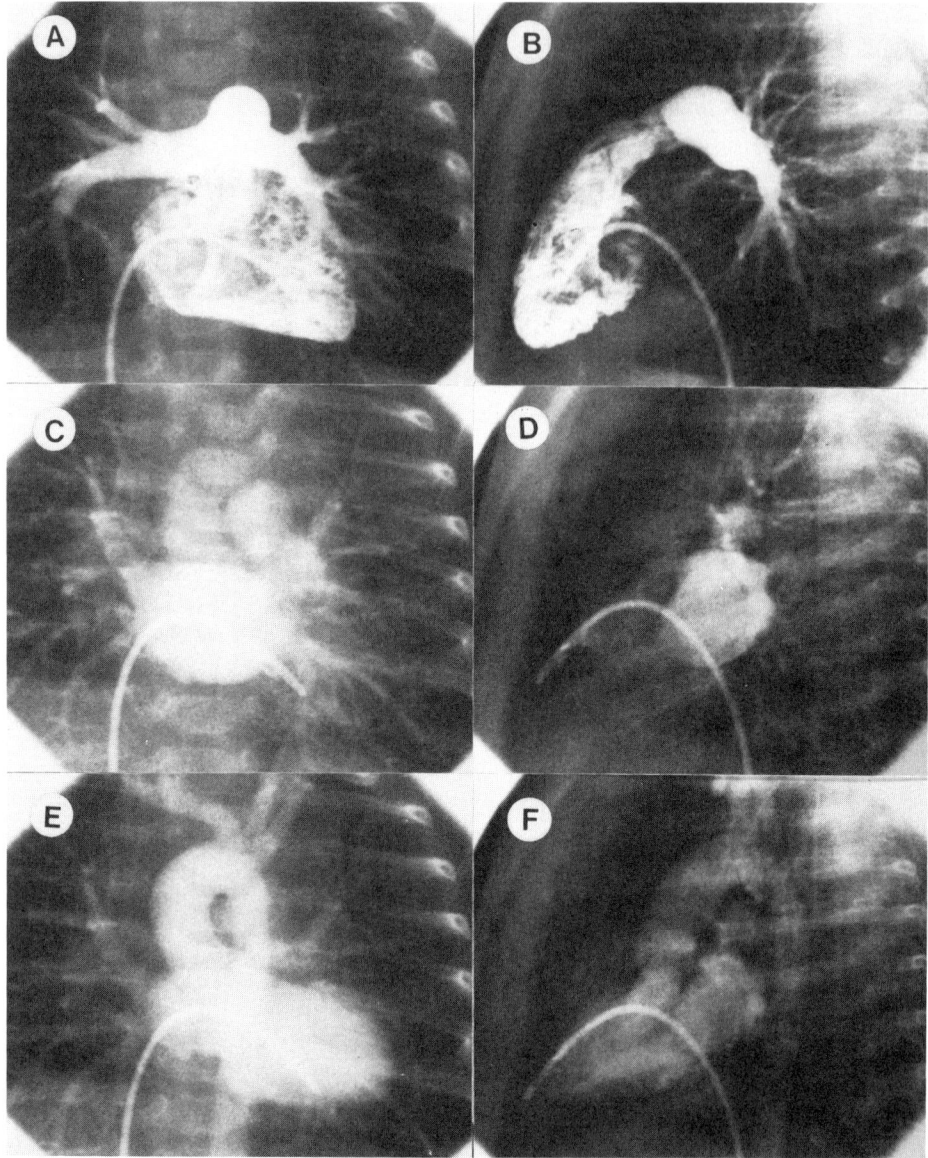

Figure 4. Selective right ventriculogram. A: AP view. B: Lateral view. C: Early levophase (AP). D: Early levophase (lateral). E: Late levophase (AP). F: Late levophase (lateral).

corrected transposition of the great arteries.

Oblique Views (Right and Left Anterior Oblique Views)

When a fixed, right-angle, biplane radiographic unit is employed, the patient is rotated by raising the right shoulder and back 30° to 45° above the horizontal using a radiolucent sponge wedge (Figs. 2, 6, and 7). In this position, the anteroposterior camera records the right anterior oblique view and the lateral camera records the left anterior oblique view. When two movable C-arms are used, the anteroposterior image in-

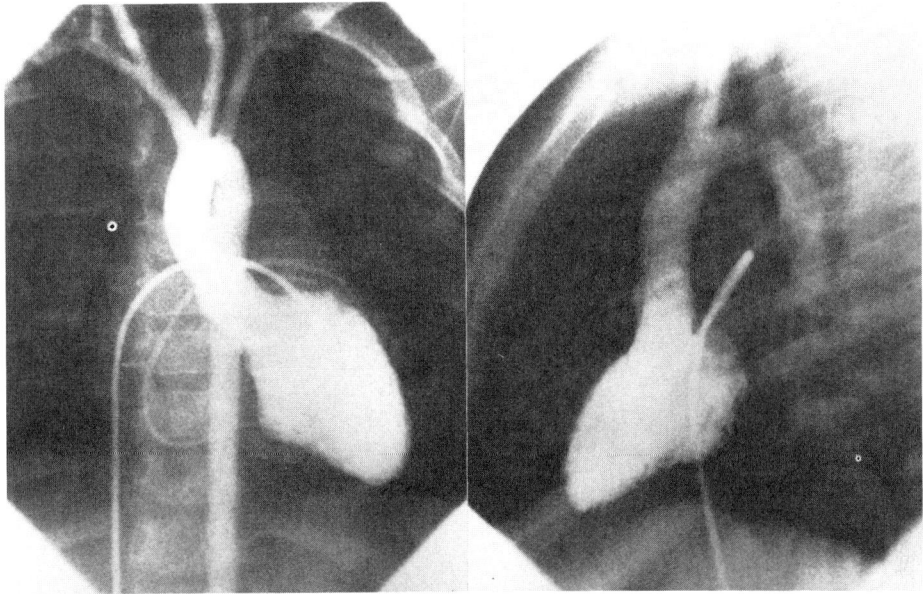

Figure 5. Selective left ventricular angiogram. Left: AP view. Right: Lateral view.

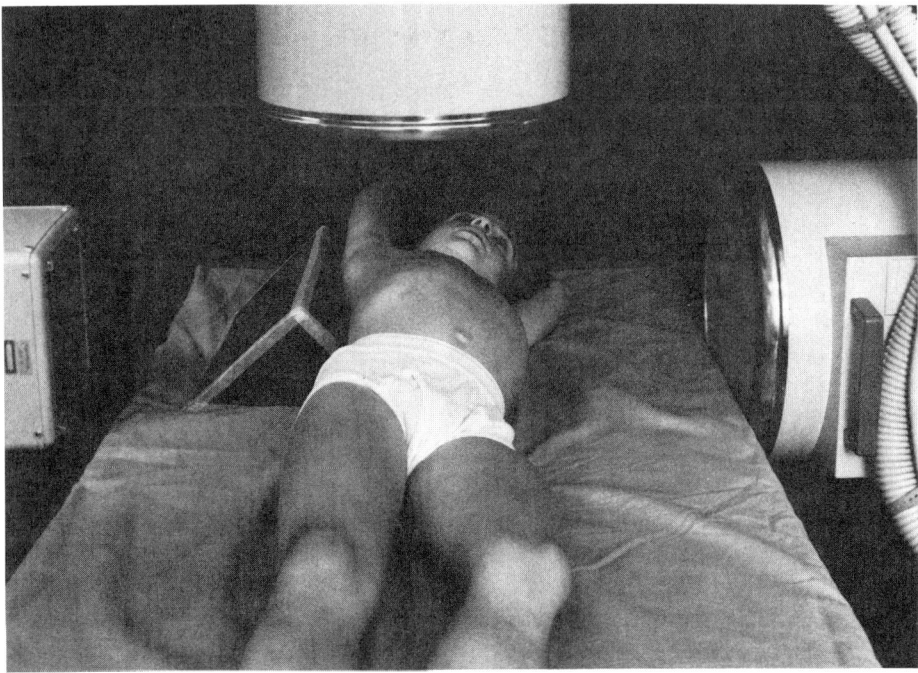

Figure 6. Patient positioned for simultaneous right and left anterior oblique views using fixed radiographic units.

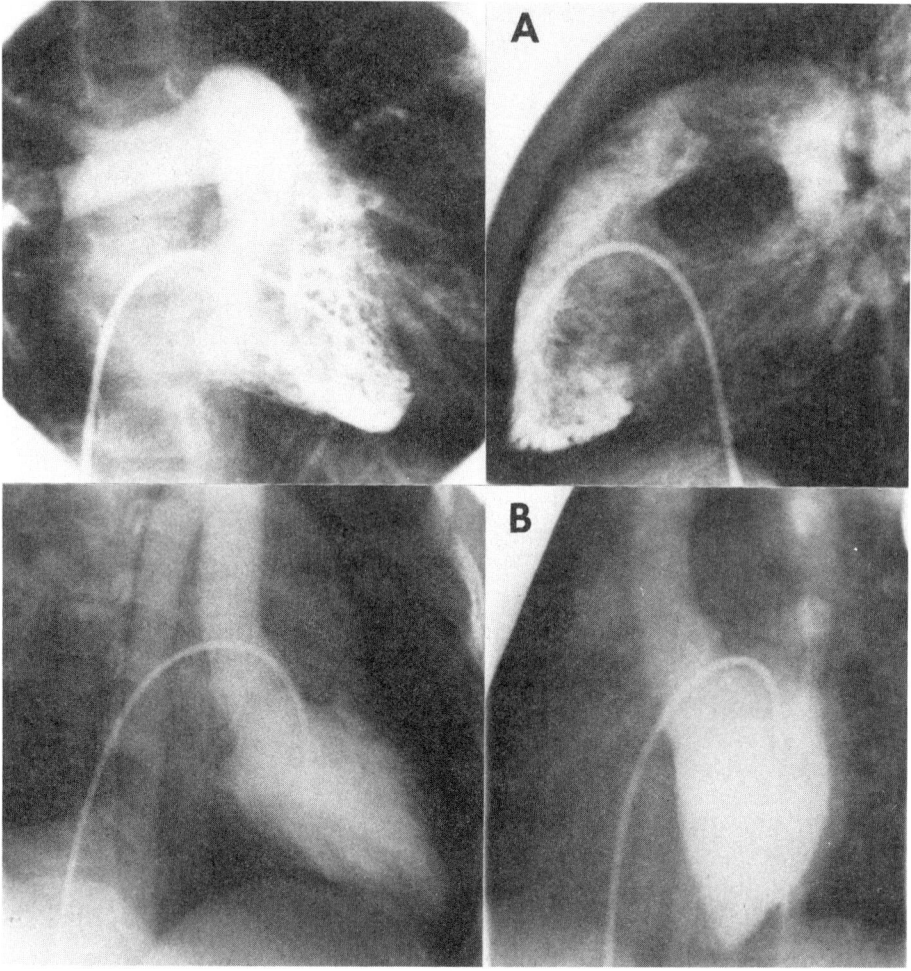

Figure 7. Right and left anterior oblique projections. A: Right ventricle. B: Left ventricle.

tensifier is positioned R30–45/0 and the lateral at L60/0. The right anterior oblique view is usually perpendicular to the plane of the atrioventricular orifices and is therefore valuable in defining abnormalities of the atrioventricular valves. The left anterior oblique view traditionally has been used to visualize the interventricular septum, but this structure is more adequately seen by the axial views described below. In patients with a left aortic arch, the left oblique view is perpendicular to the plane of the arch and coarctation of the aorta, and other arch anomalies are well visualized. The anatomy of the aor-

tic valve and of the coronary arterial system is usually well defined in the oblique views.

Axial Four-Chamber, or Hepatoclavicular, View

To obtain this projection with a fixed vertical image intensifier, the patient's upper trunk is elevated 30° from the table and the patient is rotated approximately 45° by elevating the left shoulder (Figs. 2, 8A, 8B, and 9). When a movable vertical image intensifier is used, the tube is rotated 45° to

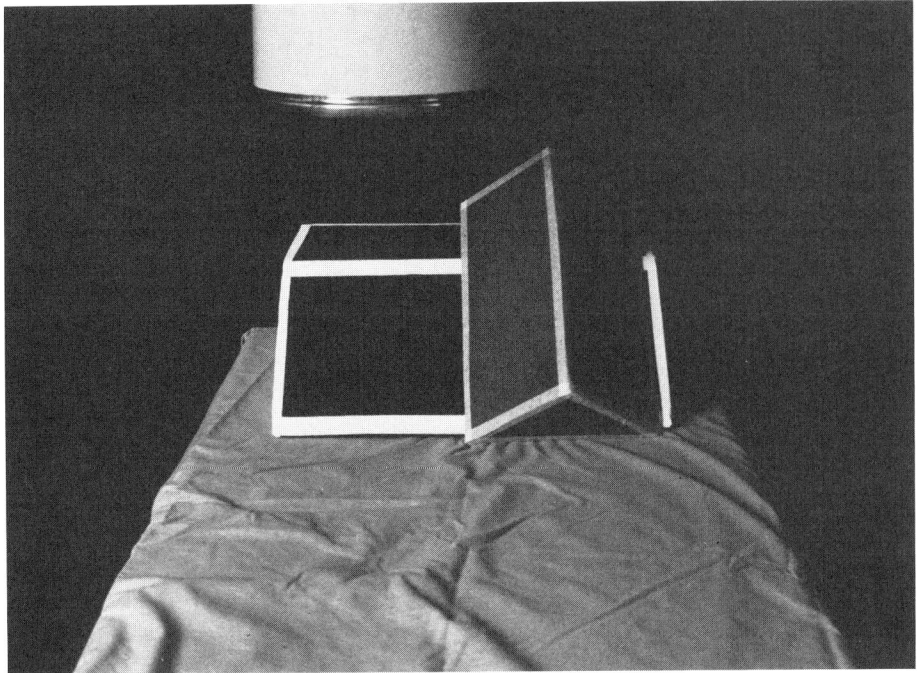

Figure 8A. Four-chamber view. Sponge layout.

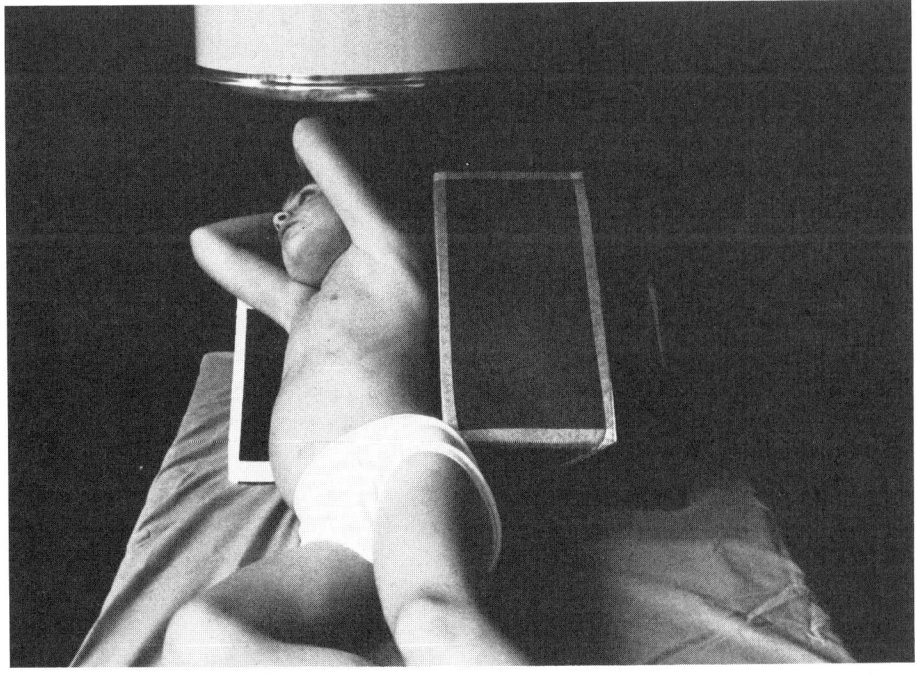

Figure 8B. Four-chamber view. Patient in position using an AP fixed unit.

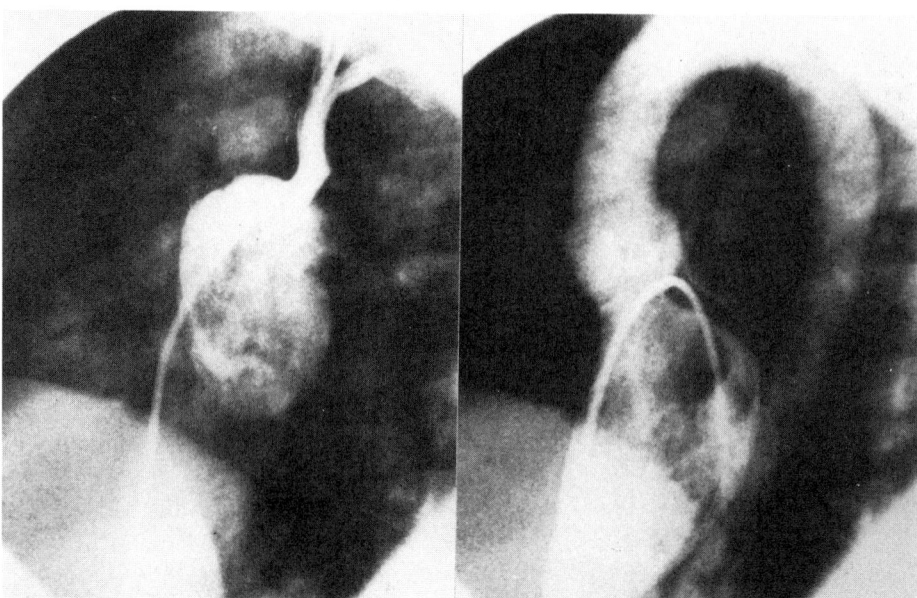

Figure 9. Four-chamber view. Left: Pulmonary vein, left atrial injection. Right: Left ventricle selective injection.

the patient's left (L45) and then cranially angulated 30° (L45/30). If a complimentary view (elongated right anterior oblique) is to be obtained along with the four-chamber view, using two movable arms, the lateral unit should be used for the four-chamber view, positioned at L45/30. The vertical unit is positioned at R45/30 (or R45/0 if a standard, rather than elongated, right anterior oblique view is desired). In any technique, both of the patient's arms are raised above the head to remove them from the radiographic field.

The four-chamber view enables visualization of all four cardiac chambers, the interatrial septum, the posterior interventricular septum, and both atrioventricular valves. This view is useful for defining atrial and ventricular septal defects and other abnormalities of the septa, and is particularly useful for visualizing the morphology of atrioventricular septal defects (endocardial cushion defects). It also provides an excellent view of the left ventricular outflow area in patients with transposition of the great arteries. It is valuable in demonstrating aortico-mitral valve continuity or its lack in patients with cono-truncal abnormalities such as double-outlet right ventricle or the Taussig Bing anomaly.

Long Axial Oblique View

To obtain the long axial projection with a fixed lateral image intensifier, the patient's upper trunk is rotated by elevating the right shoulder 30° and the upper body is positioned obliquely across the table at 30° (head toward the image intensifier tube) (Figs. 2, 10, and 11). For a single C-arm, the projection should be L60/30. The long axial view is rotated about 15° greater (closer to the standard lateral) than the four-chamber view and demonstrates the anterior portion of the interventricular septum, the left ven-

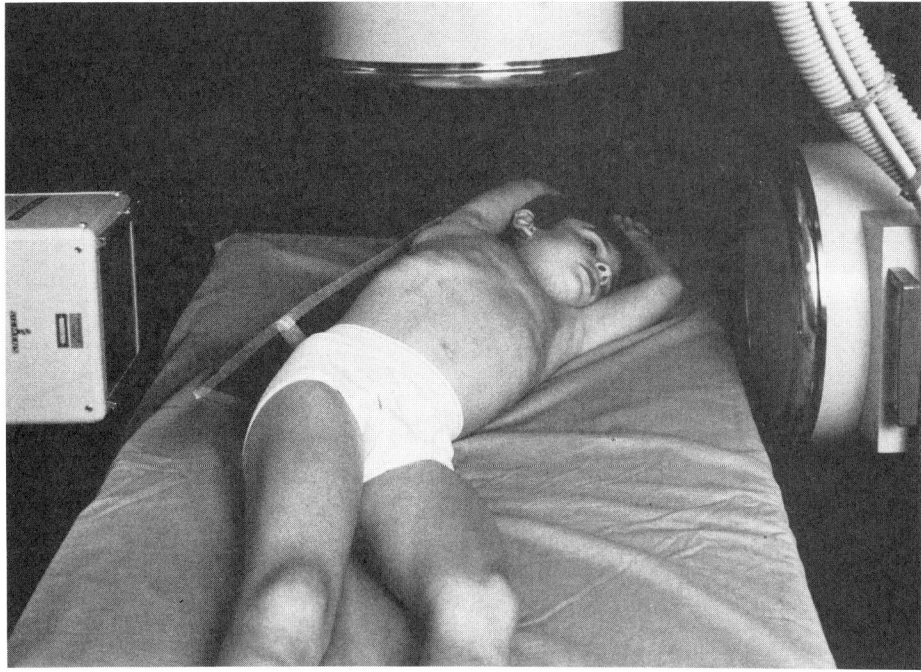

Figure 10. Long axial view. Patient in position using both AP and lateral fixed units.

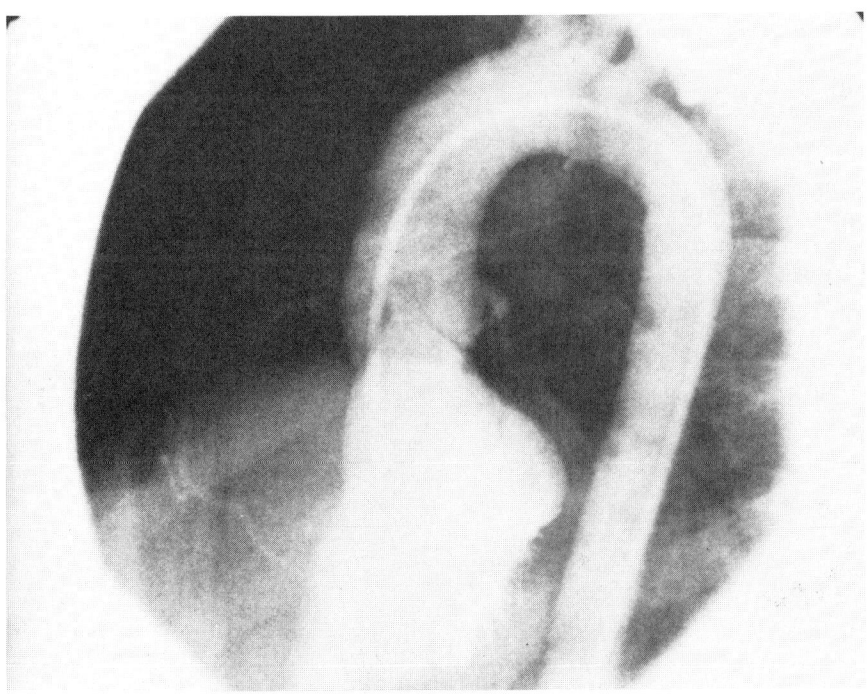

Figure 11. Long axial oblique-left ventricular injection.

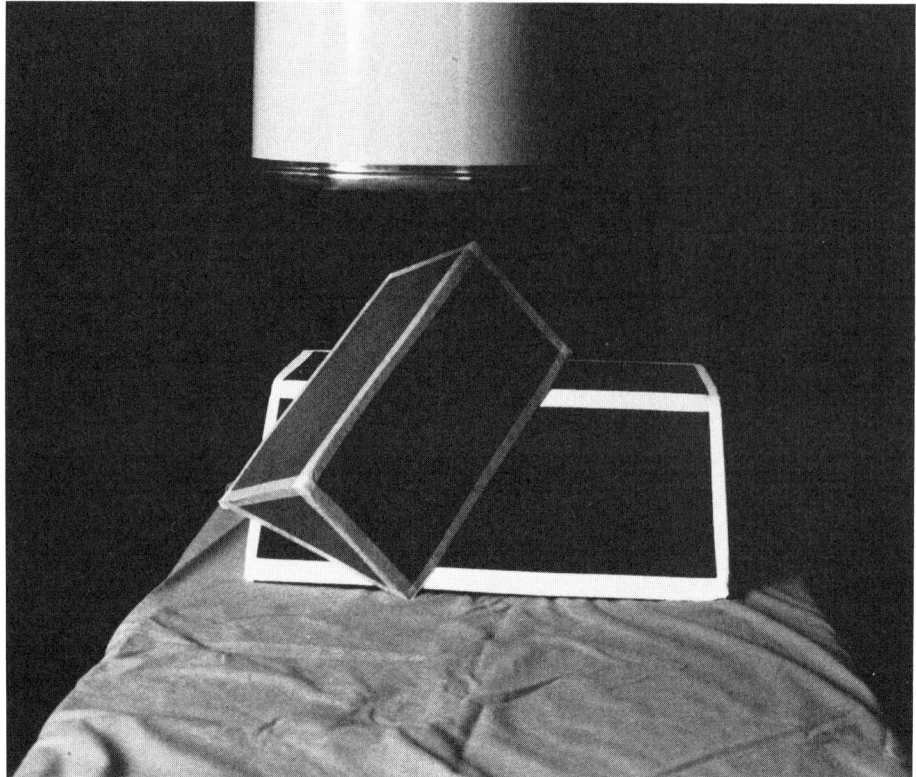

Figure 12A. Elongated right anterior oblique view. Sponge layout.

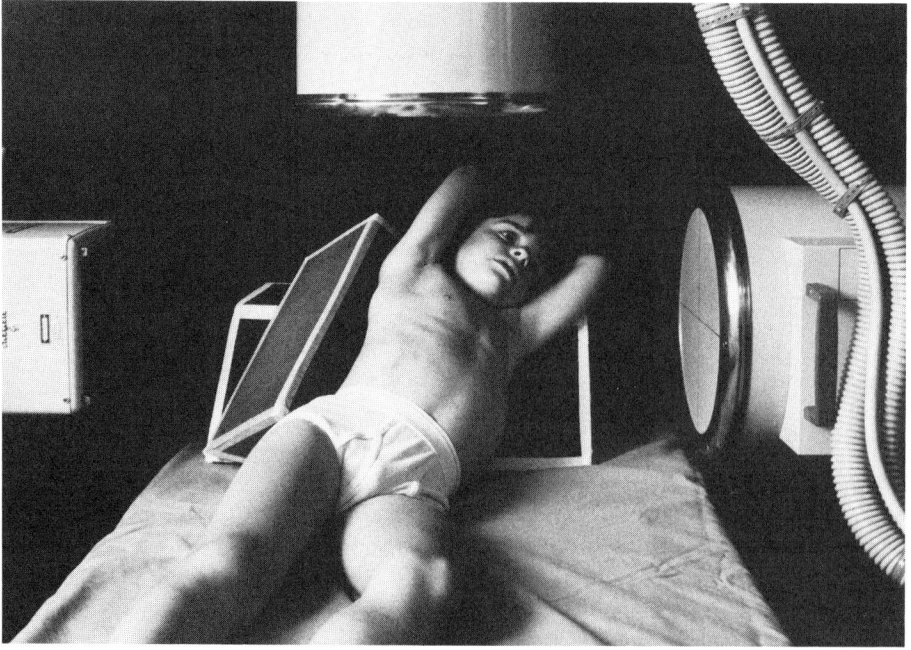

Figure 12B. Elongated right anterior oblique view. Patient in position using fixed units.

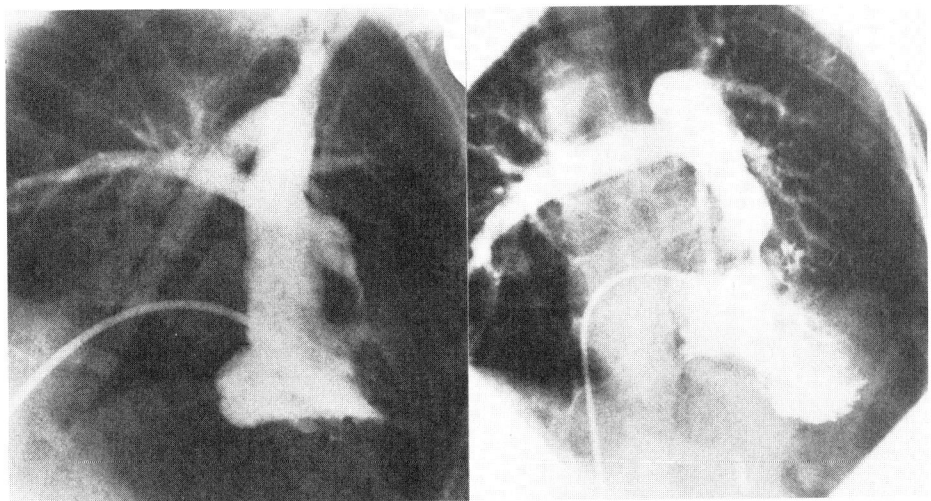

Figure 13. Elongated right anterior oblique view-right ventricular injection. Left: Tetralogy of Fallot. Right: Abnormal muscle bundle.

tricular outflow tract, and the muscular interventricular septum. It is quite helpful for the estimation of interventricular septal thickness.

Elongated Right Anterior Oblique View

To obtain this view using a fixed vertical image intensifier, the patient's upper trunk is elevated 30° from the table and rotated in the right anterior oblique position (Figs. 2, 12A, 12B, and 13). When a movable unit is used, the vertical tube is positioned to R30/30. This additional cranial tilt provides an excellent visualization of the right ventricular outflow tract and the pulmonary arterial tree. This view is useful for tetralogy of Fallot, double-chambered right ventricle in association with an abnormal muscle bundle, and Ebstein's malformation of the tricuspid valve.

Simultaneous use of the lateral unit perpendicular to the vertical unit provides a long axial view (L60/30).

Sitting Up (Cranio-Caudal) View

For the position known as the sitting up view, the patient's upper body is elevated 30° to 45° (0/30 to 0/45 with a movable C-arm) (Figs. 2, 14A, 14B, 14C, and 15). This view is primarily used to demonstrate the main pulmonary artery and its branches and in particular the area of the pulmonary artery bifurcation. A slight left anterior oblique view (L10°–15°) may be useful to visualize the proximal left pulmonary artery, since this area is often obscured by the overlap of the main pulmonary artery. This especially occurs when the main pulmonary artery is dilated.

Some movable C-arm radiographic units have limited cranial angulation. When more angulation is required, this can be achieved by elevating the patient's shoulders using a rolled towel or wedge-shaped radiolucent sponge. This can provide as much as 25° initial angulation and further angulation can then be obtained by moving the image intensifier.

Complications of Angiocardiography

Complications of angiocardiography are of two major types. The first type is me-

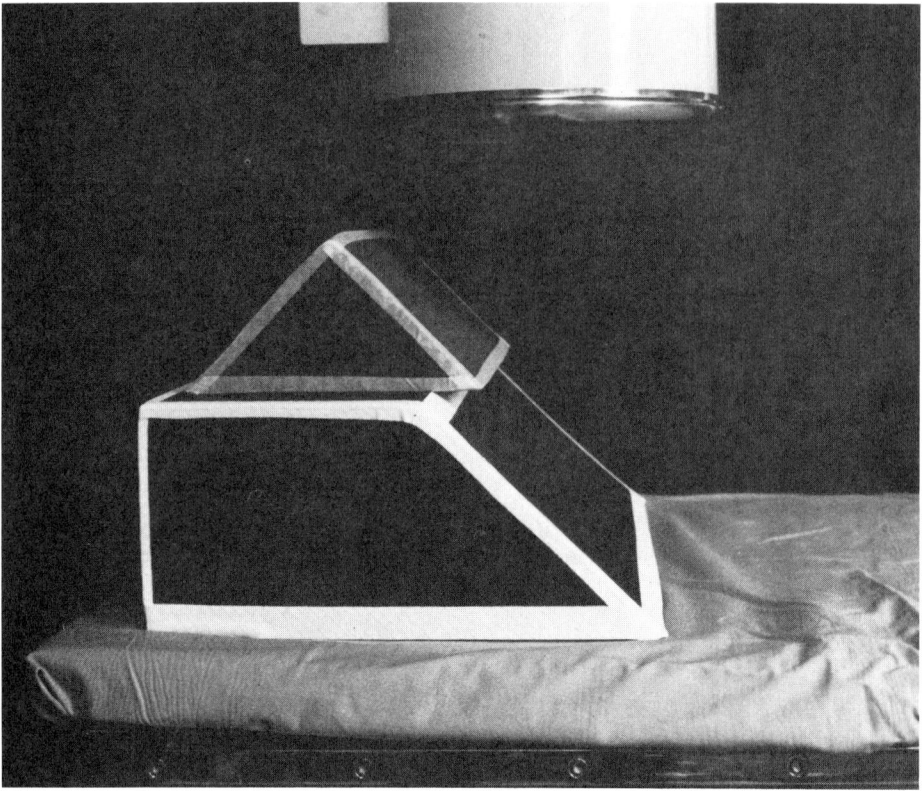

Figure 14A. Sitting-up view. Sponge layout.

chanical trauma due to catheter manipulation, which may result in damage to cardiovascular structures. The second is related to injection of contrast media. When the tip of the catheter is inappropriately positioned prior to angiography, infiltration of contrast material into the myocardium or even perforation by the catheter may occur. This complication is more likely when an endhole or a combined end- and side-hole catheter is used, or when a relatively large quantity of contrast material is delivered at a rapid flow rate. It is less likely if a side-hole catheter is used. After the catheter has been positioned for the angiocardiogram, a small amount of contrast material (0.5 to 2 mL) should be injected manually using fluoroscopic monitoring to evaluate the appropriate position of the catheter.

Complications may result from the con-

trast media itself. Contrast material is not a physiologic solution and can alter physiology, especially when infused into the cardiovascular system rapidly and in a large amount. All patients experience a "hot flush" sensation immediately after injection of contrast material. This reaction is due to the vasodilator effect of the contrast and subsides within a few seconds. There may be a transient elevation of the systemic arterial pressure followed by a drop in systolic and diastolic pressures. Transient tachycardia is common but the heart rate usually returns to baseline within minutes. Some patients experience nausea, vomiting, salivation, or lacrimation. Contrast material is a hyperosmolar solution and may cause an increase in the central blood volume that may be deleterious to patients with congestive heart failure. Coronary angiography often results

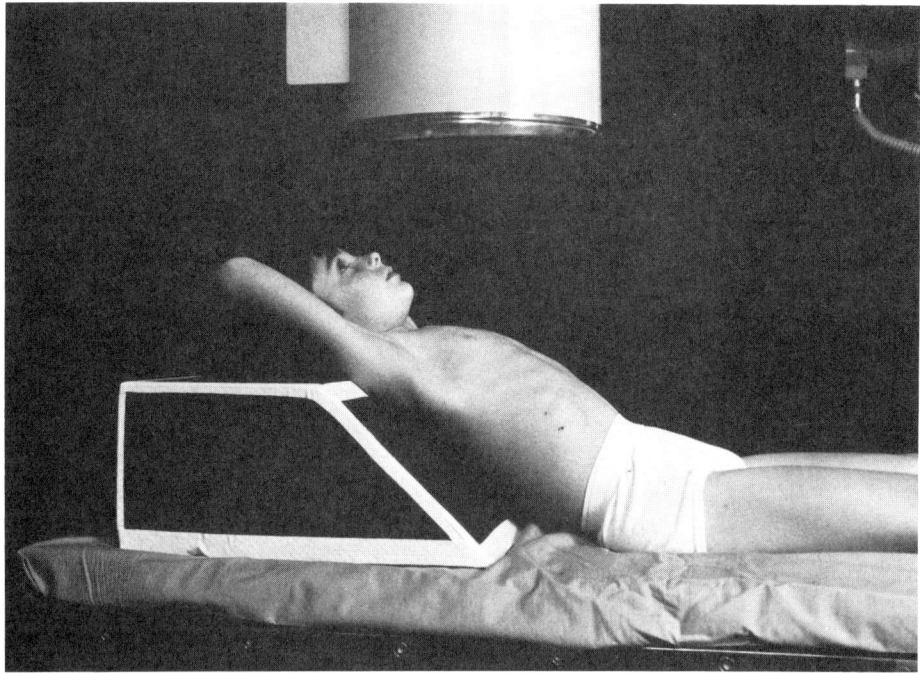

Figure 14B. Sitting-up view. Patient in place using an anteroposterior fixed unit.

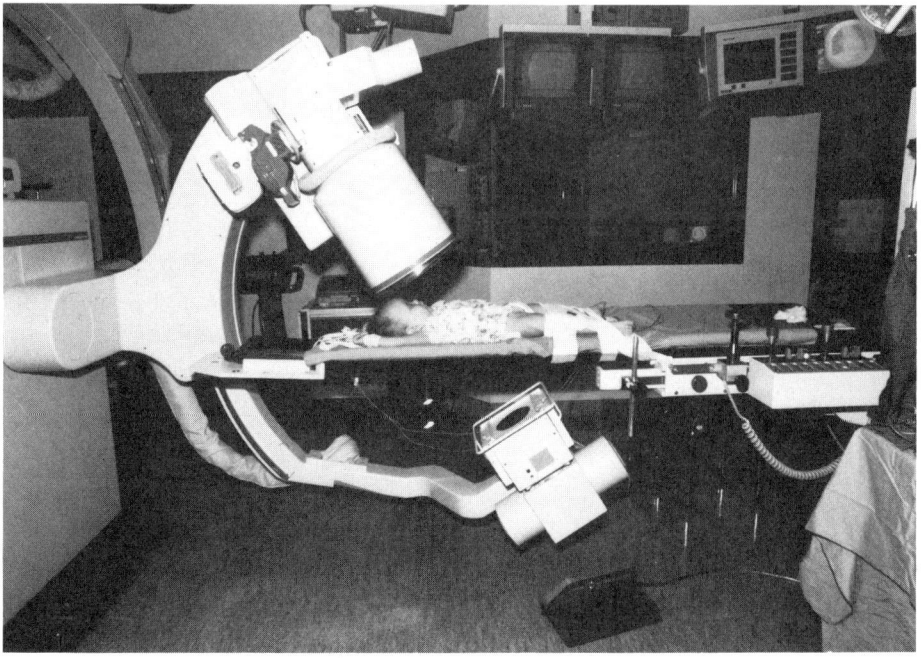

Figure 14C. Patient using a movable C-arm unit.

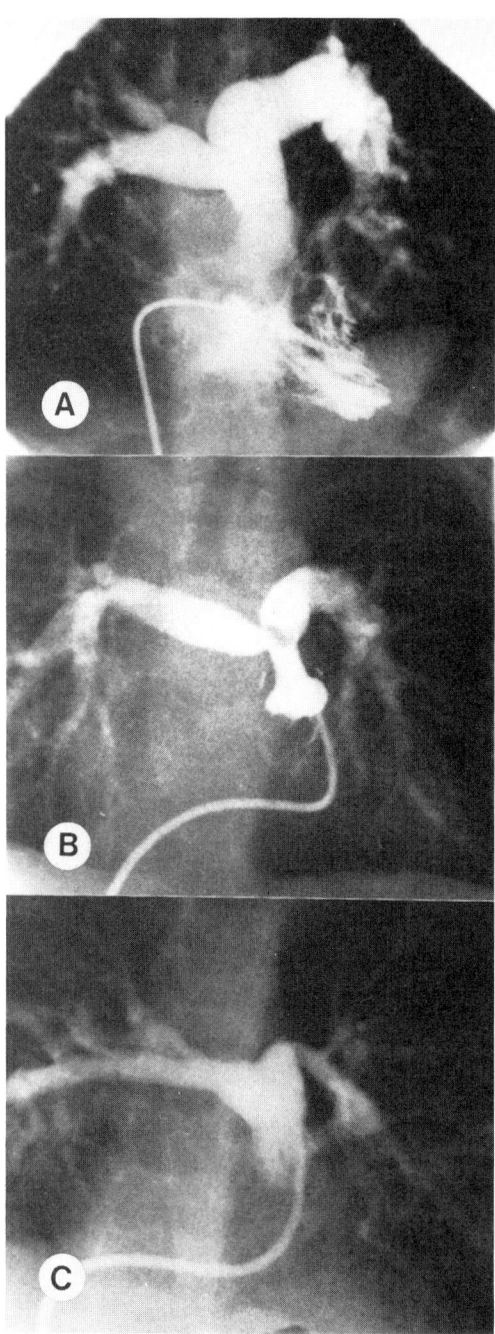

Figure 15. Sitting up view. A: Normal. B: Pulmonary artery banding. C: Pulmonary artery stenosis.

in bradycardia and may cause transient prolongation of PR, QRS, and QT electrocardiographic intervals. There is also a high incidence of ventricular arrhythmias. Popio et al. (1978) have studied the mechanism of cardiac toxicity of contrast material in animals and have suggested that the arterial hypotension, increased left ventricular end diastolic pressure, and decreased left ventricular contractility are due to calcium chelating properties of the contrast material.

There may be a transient pause in respiration after administration of contrast, followed by an increased depth of respiration for a short period. Pulmonary artery wedge or pulmonary venous wedge angiograms almost always induce coughing and a pulmonary arteriogram may do so as well. In patients with pulmonary hypertension, particularly of the "essential" variety, pulmonary angiography is extremely hazardous and may lead to profound vascular collapse and even sudden death.

When a large amount of contrast material is injected into the cerebral vascular system, it may cause headache, a convulsion, hemiplegia, or syncope. These neurologic problems are probably related to direct irritation or to the hyperosmolarity of the media and are usually transient, although occasionally permanent damage may result.

Contrast material is excreted through the kidneys and should be used with caution and in low doses in patients with renal failure.

Contrast media occasionally causes minor allergic reactions. The most common is urticaria, which can appear on any part of the body but generally is found on the trunk and face. The rash is usually pruritic and can persist from a few minutes to several hours. Fortunately, serious reactions are extremely rare. The Hospital for Sick Children in Toronto reported two serious reactions in over 4,000 pediatric cardiac catheterizations. Treatment with diphenhydramine (Benadryl) 2 mg/kg (maximum 50 mg) intravenously usually suffices. Rarely, the

Occasionally, a patient known to be allergic to iodine and/or contrast material requires angiographic study. Sensitivity testing is of little use. Deaths have been reported following administration of even small amounts of contrast media and, in addition, a negative reaction to a sensitivity test does not assure that a severe reaction will not occur. Steroids have been used to prepare such patients for angiography. Zweiman et al. (1975) reported the successful use of oral corticosteroids as a prophylactic measure in adult patients with a previous history of allergic reaction to contrast material. These were continued for 24 hours after angiographic study. In the reported study, even patients who had previously experienced a severe reaction to contrast media underwent angiographic study without serious reaction.

References and Suggested Reading

Bargeron LM, Elliott LP, Soto B, Bream PR, Curry GC. Axial cineangiography in congenital heart disease: Section I. Concept, technical and anatomic considerations. Circulation 1977; 56:1075–1083.

Bargeron LM. Axial cineangiography in congenital heart disease. In: Engle M (ed), Pediatric Cardiovascular Disease. Philadelphia, PA, FA Davis Co. 1981, pp 275–291.

Ceballos R, Soto B, Bargeron LM. Angiographic anatomy of the normal heart through axial angiography. Circulation 1981; 64:351–359.

Eliott LP, Bargeron LM, Bream PR, Soto B, Curry GC. Axial cineangiography in congenital heart disease. II. Specific lesions. Circulation 1977; 56:1084–1093.

Moes CAF. Angiocardiography. In: Keith JD, Rowe RD, Vlad P (eds), Heart Disease in Infancy and Childhood. 3rd ed. New York, NY, MacMillan Publishing Co. 1978. pp 116–128.

Popio KA, Ross AM, Oravec JM, Ingram JT. Indentification and description of separate mechanics for two components of renografin cardiotoxicity. Circulation 1978; 58:520–528.

Swartz RD et al. Renal failure following major angiography. Am J Med 1978; 65:31–37.

Zweiman B, Mishkin MM, Hildret EA. An approach to the performance of contrast studies in contrast material—reactive persons. Ann Intern Med 1975; 83:159–162.

10

Intracardiac Electrophysiology

Lee B. Beerman

Most arrhythmias occurring in the pediatric population can be diagnosed accurately by evaluation of the standard surface electrocardiogram. There are circumstances, however, when this evaluation proves inadequate. For example, to make a rational therapeutic decision, the pediatric cardiologist should be able to differentiate between supraventricular and ventricular origin of a wide QRS tachycardia, or to determine the site of block in disturbances of atrioventricular conduction. In addition, the remarkable strides that have been made in the surgical treatment of congenital heart disease have led to a need for accurate postoperative evaluation of conduction disturbances, bradyarrhythmias, and tachyarrhythmias. Invasive electrophysiology, along with exercise electrocardiography and ambulatory cardiac monitoring, have become valuable tools in the evaluation and management of these problems. Techniques for recording intracardiac electrograms and programmed electrical stimulation of the heart have greatly enhanced the understanding of rhythm disturbances and the ability to deal with them effectively. In recent years, certain intractable arrhythmias, such as atrial ectopic or atrioventricular reciprocating tachycardias, have proven amenable to operative intervention and cure. To define the mechanism and to localize abnormal sites or pathways involved in these and other arrhythmias, multiple catheter intracardiac electrophysiologic studies are essential. This chapter will provide an overview of the approach to this subject. For more detail, there are excellent reference sources available to the reader with specific interests (Gillette and Garson 1981; Josephson and Seides 1979; and Roberts and Gelband 1983).

Indications

The indications for intracardiac electrophysiologic studies vary somewhat among institutions, depending upon their experience and familiarity with the techniques. Some of the major situations in which intracardiac recordings and pacing can prove to be of great value are shown in Table 1 and are discussed below.

Advanced Atrioventricular Block

It is usually unnecessary to resort to electrophysiologic studies in patients with first degree or Mobitz type I second degree atrioventricular block. However, Mobitz type II block, 2:1 atrioventricular block, and third degree atrioventricular block may be caused by abnormalities of the intra- or infra-Hisian conduction system and therefore have a more serious prognosis. The management of a postoperative patient with complete heart block that has persisted more than 2 weeks is greatly aided by knowing if the block is above, within, or below the bundle of His. The site of block can be confirmed by His bundle studies (Fig. 1). These investigations also provide valuable information in asymptomatic patients with third degree atrioventricular block (either congenital or acquired) in whom there is a

Table 1

Indications for Electrophysiologic Studies in Children

1. Advanced atrioventricular block
2. Wide QRS tachycardia of uncertain etiology
3. Recurrent supraventricular tachycardia
4. Preexcitation syndrome associated with serious or refractory arrhythmia
5. Recurrent ventricular tachycardia
6. Sycope of uncertain etiology
7. Assessment of conduction disturbances related to cardiac surgery
8. Therapeutic pacing

decrease in ventricular rate or change in the QRS morphology on the surface electrocardiogram.

Wide QRS Tachycardia of Uncertain Etiology

Tachycardias with abnormal or prolonged QRS morphology may be due to a ventricular focus, a supraventricular site with aberrant conduction, or anterograde conduction of a supraventricular impulse through an atrioventricular bypass tract. The origin of such wide QRS tachycardias may be obscure and can be elucidated by determining the relationship of atrial and His bundle depolarizations to the ventricular complexes.

Recurrent Supraventricular Tachycardia

The mechanism of the tachycardia (automatic vs reentry) as well as the response to drug therapy can be assessed with programmed pacing techniques. Accurate localization of a reentrant or ectopic site may allow an operative approach to an intractable arrhythmia.

Preexcitation Phenomenon Associated with Serious or Refractory Arrhythmias

The location and electrophysiologic properties of an atrioventricular bypass pathway can be determined and the efficacy of drug therapy evaluated. This is particularly important in patients who have pharmacologically intractable supraventricular tachycardia or a rapid wide QRS tachycardia due to atrial fibrillation associated with the preexcitation phenomenon. These patients may be at risk for sudden death because of a short refractory period of the bypass tract. Thorough intracardiac studies are an essential first step when surgical intervention is considered for division or ablation of the accessory pathway.

Recurrent Ventricular Tachycardia

Although this is a much less common problem in the pediatric population than in adults, recurrent sustained ventricular tachycardia does occur and is a clear indication for intracardiac electrophysiologic studies. An intracardiac tumor or hamartoma must be considered in an infant with this abnormality, while a small subset of older children or adolescents who have had operative repair for tetralogy of Fallot or other lesions are prone to develop complex ventricular arrhythmias. If the clinical tachycardia can be reproduced reliably by ventricular extrastimulus studies, a reentrant mechanism can be inferred and the site of origin determined by endocardial mapping. Serial drug studies allow more directed antiarrhythmic therapy and surgical intervention can be considered in selected cases.

Syncope of Uncertain Etiology

When sinus node dysfunction, occult atrioventricular conduction disease, or paroxysmal tachyarrhythmias are suspected, electrophysiologic studies can help to determine if there is an electrical cause for the syncope. The index of suspicion would be

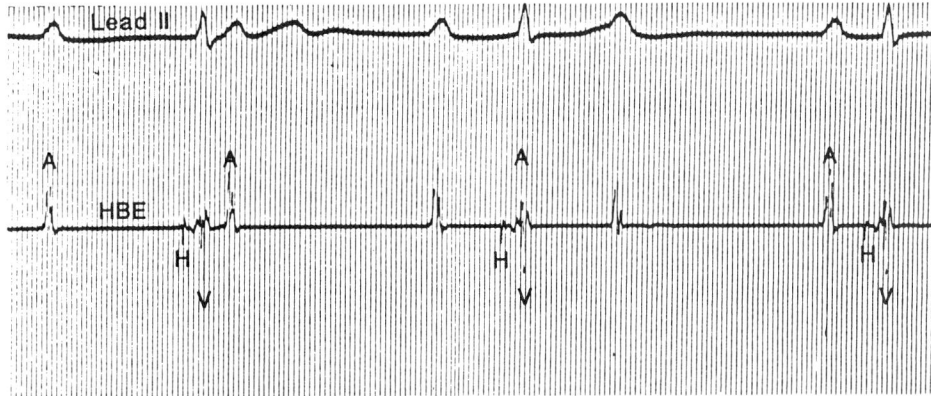

Figure 1A. Intracardiac His bundle recording (HBE) allowing determination that the site of complete atrioventricular block is above the bundle of His. Note that each ventricular electrogram (V) is preceded by a His deflection (H) while atrial activity (A) is not associated with either the His or ventricular electrograms.

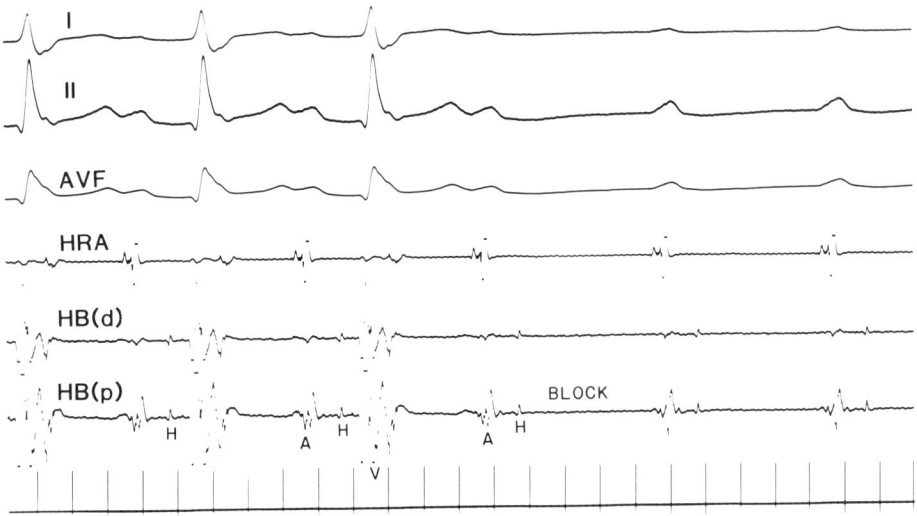

Figure 1B. Spontaneous onset of block below the His bundle shows His deflection is associated with each atrial electrogram.

increased by the presence of any baseline electrocardiographic abnormality such as atrioventricular block, bifascicular or trifascicular block, or marked sinus bradycardia with or without junctional escape rhythms. Attempts to induce ventricular tachyarrhythmias by ventricular stimulation may be indicated in some patients even in the absence of any documented spontaneous ventricular ectopy. The presence of the Wolff-Parkinson-White syndrome on the electro-

cardiogram in an individual with otherwise unexplained syncope is a strong indication for an electrophysiologic study.

Assessment of Conduction Disturbances Related to Cardiac Surgery

Pre- and postoperative studies in patients with defects that have a high risk of postoperative arrhythmias and/or conduction abnormalities can give valuable prognostic information as well as help in evaluating surgical techniques. Some of these high-risk defects include tetralogy of Fallot, transposition of the great arteries, and congenitally corrected transposition of the great arteries.

Therapeutic Pacing

Severe symptomatic bradycardia requires emergent placement of a temporary transvenous pacemaker. In the infant or small child, this can be done most safely and expeditiously in a setting where fluoroscopy is available. At the other end of the spectrum of rhythm disorders, persistent supraventricular or ventricular tachycardia may be amenable to overdrive atrial or ventricular pacing, respectively.

Equipment

A variety of types and sizes of electrode catheters are available for bipolar stimulation and recording at intracardiac sites. The most commonly used are bipolar, tripolar, and quadripolar electrode catheters in French sizes 5, 6, or 7. Interelectrode distance varies from 1 to 10 mm, but 2- to 5-mm spacing for use in infants and smaller children and 5- to 10-mm spacing for adolescents and adults are most acceptable. The quadripolar catheter is used most frequently at our institution. Other catheters that are available include those with three or more electrode pairs for more detailed endocardial mapping studies (particularly useful when positioned in the coronary sinus), specialized mapping catheters with internal tip-deflecting stylets, and electrode catheters with an end-hole lumen or an inflatable balloon.

A junction box (switch box) should be available to permit easy selection of any pair of leads for stimulating or recording. Recording apparatus consisting of signal processors (filters and amplifiers), an oscilloscope, and a recorder are needed, and these are usually combined into a single unit. Ideally, at least seven or eight amplifiers should be available so that three or four surface electrocardiographic leads and four or more intracardiac leads can be recorded. The surface leads should be standardized to include leads I, aV_F, and V_1. In many cases, it is helpful to include V_6 as well.

Each amplifier should be equipped with a low-band and high-band pass filter. Special additional filters for multiples of 60 Hz are available for ECG amplifiers and are quite helpful in eliminating 60-cycle interference. His bundle and other intracardiac electrograms are most clearly defined in the range from 40–500 Hz. For safety reasons, the amplifiers and cables must be completely patient-isolated to minimize the chance of current leakage while using multiple catheters. The recorder must have a high-frequency response and provide hard copy, which can be either photographic or direct writing. Paper speeds of up to 250 mm/sec should be available, although speeds of 50–100 mm/sec are acceptable for most studies. Ongoing analysis of the data while the study is in progress is facilitated by a freeze-screen oscilloscope. If desired, paper usage can be conserved by using a magnetic tape recorder and limiting paper printouts to pertinent sequences.

An electrical stimulator must be available. Although a simple temporary pacing unit is all that is required for rapid atrial pacing and sinus node recovery times, a programmable stimulator is necessary for determination of refractory periods and for the performance of more sophisticated procedures utilizing atrial or ventricular extrastimulus studies. The stimulator should be capable of pacing at cycle lengths from <50 to >2,000 msec. It should also be able to provide up to at least three extrastimuli synchronized with either intrinsic or paced rhythms and provide output of variable milliamperage and pulse duration. Generally, rectangular pulses of 1- to 2-msec duration with an output of 1–4 mA (twice the diastolic threshold) are used for atrial or ventricular pacing.

General Techniques

Since electrophysiologic studies in pediatric patients are often part of a complete hemodynamic and angiographic evaluation, routine premedications are required. Chlorpromazine (Thorazine) should be omitted because of the vagolytic affects of the phenothiazines. However, the other standard medications used in the pediatric laboratory such as meperidine (Demerol), promethazine (Phenergan), and ketamine are acceptable. Ketamine transiently enhances sympathetic tone, but this effect is brief, which allows this drug to be useful in providing supplemental sedation for long or difficult studies. Electrophysiologic studies should be performed prior to angiography since the stress of contrast media injection may alter autonomic tone. However, they may be done either before or after hemodynamic studies, depending on the relative importance of the data to be obtained.

In most laboratories, the percutaneous femoral technique is used for routine electrophysiologic studies. When more than one catheter is required, a second sheath can be inserted into the same femoral vein (approximately 1 cm proximal or distal to the original site) if the patient is at least 7–10 kg. In a smaller child, it is preferable to utilize the contralateral femoral vein. In adolescents or adults, up to three sheaths may be inserted into the same femoral vein. An upper extremity approach from an antecubital vein (either percutaneous or cutdown) may be desirable or necessary in certain situations, such as iliofemoral vein thrombosis, studies requiring four or more catheters, or to facilitate catheterization of the coronary sinus, which is most easily approached from the left arm. In institutions familiar with percutaneous internal jugular or subclavian venous techniques, these approaches are very useful. In older children, either #5 or #6 French electrode catheters can be used, but for children less than 6 months of age or if a second catheter is used in the same vein, the #5 French size is preferred.

Recording Sites

Depending on the goals of the study, obtaining various recording sites in the heart may be essential or desirable. The most important site required for almost all studies is that of the His bundle. Other sites that are often recorded include the high right atrium, right ventricular apex, right ventricular outflow tract, and coronary sinus or left atrium. The His bundle potential can be most easily recorded from the femoral venous approach, using an electrode catheter with two or more poles. A tripolar or quadripolar catheter allows recordings from multiple paired electrode combinations in the vicinity of the His bundle and facilitates having a stable His electrogram throughout the study. A gently curved catheter is advanced to the right atrium and then passed across the tricuspid valve under fluoroscopic guidance. Once oscilloscopic monitoring of the intracardiac electrograms indicates that the recording electrodes are within the ventricle, reflected by a large ventricular deflection (V) with a small or absent atrial deflection (A), the catheter is pulled back slowly with clockwise rotation until the typical His bundle electrogram (H) is obtained (Fig. 2). In general, this occurs when relatively equal-sized atrial and ventricular electrograms are present. A relatively small atrial deflection may indicate that the presumed His spike is actually an electrogram from the proximal right bundle. An unusually short HV interval also suggests the deflection is not a valid His electrogram (Fig. 3). When the upper extremity approach is used, it is often difficult to record the His bundle electrogram, as the catheter must be looped and rotated in the right atrium to gain proximity to the posterior superior aspect of the tricuspid valve

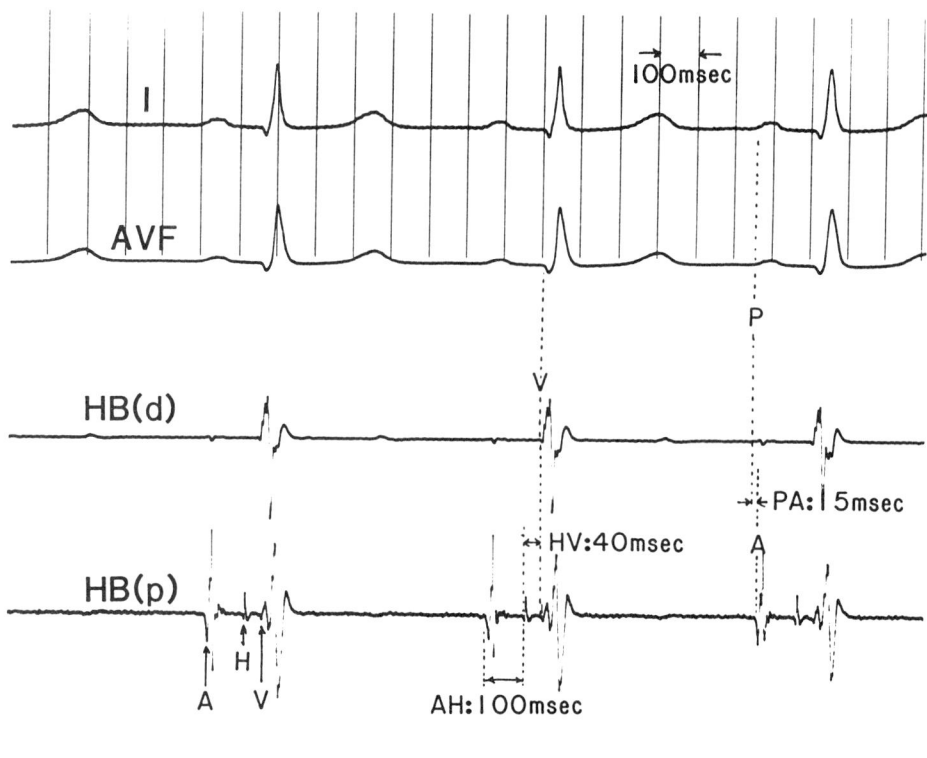

Figure 2. His bundle recording using a single quadripolar catheter. The AH interval is measured from the onset of low septal right atrial electrogram (A) to the onset of the His deflection (H). The HV interval is measured from the His spike to the earliest onset of ventricular activity (V) recorded either from intracardiac leads or from the Q wave of a surface lead. Note the nearly identical amplitude of the atrial and ventricular electrograms confirming validity of the His deflection. The PA interval is measured from the onset of the surface P wave (P) to the onset of the low septal right atrial electrogram. The following abbreviations are used in this and other figures: AH = AH interval; HB (d) = His bundle recording (distal); HB (p) = His bundle recording (proximal); HV = HV interval; PA = PA interval.

ring. In certain situations when the His bundle recording is not obtained by either of these routes, it may be obtained via the arterial side of the circulation. In patients with normally connected great arteries, this is accomplished by positioning the catheter in either the posterior aortic sinus or just below the aortic valve and angling it toward the interventricular septum. For patients with transposition of the great arteries who have had a Mustard or Senning operation, the His bundle may be recorded by a retrograde arterial catheter passed across the aortic valve into the right ventricle and then rotated anteriorly and rightward so as to point toward the tricuspid annulus.

An electrogram from the high right atrium is frequently useful, as it provides a point of reference near the sinus node. This is recorded from the high posterior lateral right atrium near the superior vena caval junction. Recordings from the right ventricular apex and outflow tract can be obtained by passing the catheter across the tricuspid valve and positioning the tip in the apex of the right ventricle or in the outflow tract just proximal to the pulmonic annulus, respectively. Recordings from these sites allow the

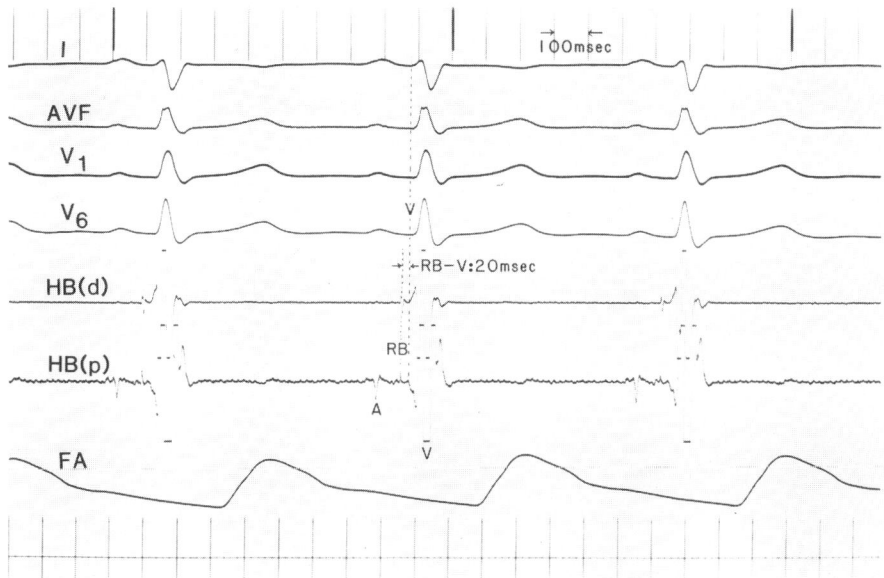

Figure 3. Recording of a right bundle electrogram (RB). Note small amplitude atrial deflection (A) compared to ventricular activity (V) and short RB-V interval. FA = femoral artery pressure tracing. See legend for Figure 2 for additional abbreviations.

mapping of ventricular activation sequences and determining whether a right bundle-branch block is central or peripheral. A left atrial electrogram is a necessary component of any study of supraventricular tachycardia or Wolff-Parkinson-White syndrome and can be obtained directly from the left atrium or from the coronary sinus. The former may be entered via a patent foramen ovale or by the transseptal approach. The latter site can be obtained most easily by an approach from the left antecubital fossa, left subclavian vein, or left internal jugular vein. If one of these sites is used, the catheter is curved against the low lateral right atrial wall so as to direct the tip posteriorly and leftward toward the mouth of the coronary sinus, which lies in the medial inferior wall of the right atrium. It is also possible to enter the coronary sinus from the femoral venous approach by creating a large loop within the right atrium and directing the tip as just described.

The fluoroscopic appearance of cathe-

ters at various recording sites is shown in Figure 4.

Baseline Conduction Intervals

In general, measurements for timing intracardiac events are made from the onset of the first rapid deflection from the baseline obtained at the site of interest. To be certain that the His bundle and not the proximal right bundle-branch activity is being recorded, the A and V spikes should be of approximately equal amplitude and the longest HV interval that can be obtained is used. The atrial activity on this recording represents a low septal right atrial electrogram. The intervals measured generally include PA, AH, HV, and QRS duration. The PA interval gives a crude and clinically not very useful approximation of intra-atrial conduction and is measured from the earliest deflection of the surface P wave to the earliest rapid atrial deflection on the His bundle

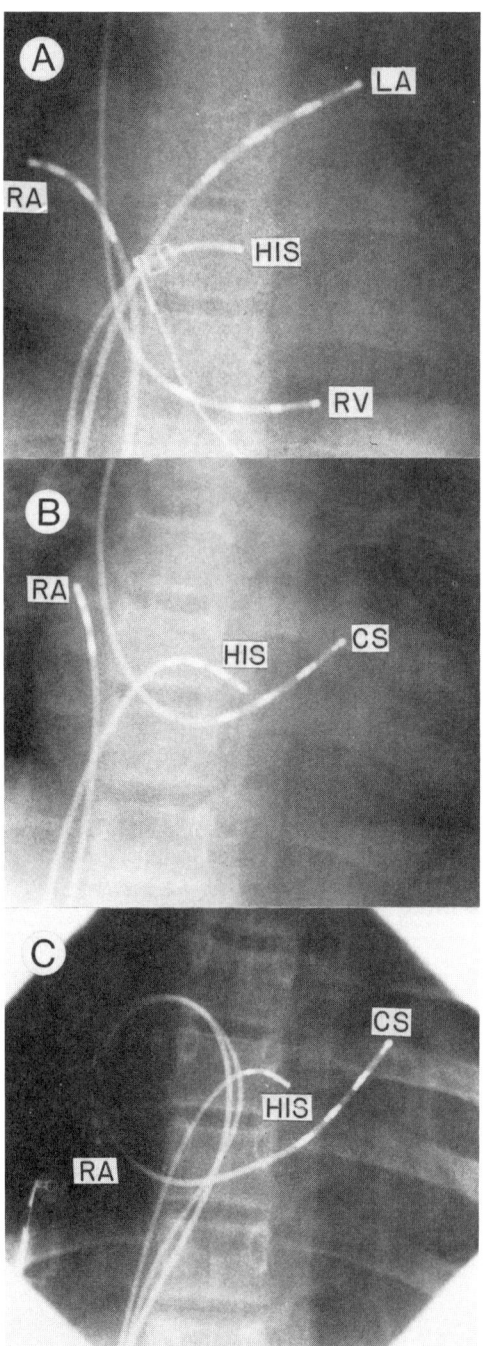

tracing. Intra-atrial conduction is better estimated by recording a high right atrial electrogram and measuring the interval between it and the low septal right atrial activity. The AH interval, measured from the earliest rapid atrial deflection on the His recording to the onset of the His spike, represents primarily AV nodal conduction time. The HV interval, from the His spike to the earliest evidence of ventricular activation from either the surface or intracardiac recordings, measures conduction in the His-Purkinje system from the proximal His bundle to the ventricular myocardium. The QRS duration indicates the time required for ventricular depolarization. Measuring the interval from the onset of the QRS deflection to activation of the right ventricular apex presumably reflects the conduction time of the proximal right bundle. Although its validity has recently been questioned, this measurement may allow a central right bundle-branch block to be differentiated from a peripheral one, since the Q to RV apex time is prolonged in a central block. The atrial and ventricular activation sequences can be determined by simultaneously recording from multiple sites within the atria and ventricles. This technique is called endocardial mapping. Examples of intracardiac recordings and measurements are shown in Figure 5. Normal values for these intervals in children and adults are given in Table 2.

Atrial Pacing

Programmed stimulation of the atrium allows assessment of sinus node, atrial muscle, and AV nodal function. These pacing studies are generally performed from the high lateral right atrium near the superior vena caval junction, which is a site contig-

Figure 4. A: Multiple intracardiac catheters positioned to record from the high right atrium (HRA), left atrium (LA), His bundle (HB), and right ventricle (RV). B: A catheter from a left antecubital vein maneuvered into the coronary sinus (CS). C: The coronary sinus can also be entered from the femoral

vein approach by looping the catheter in the right atrium. See legend for Figure 2 for additional abbreviations.

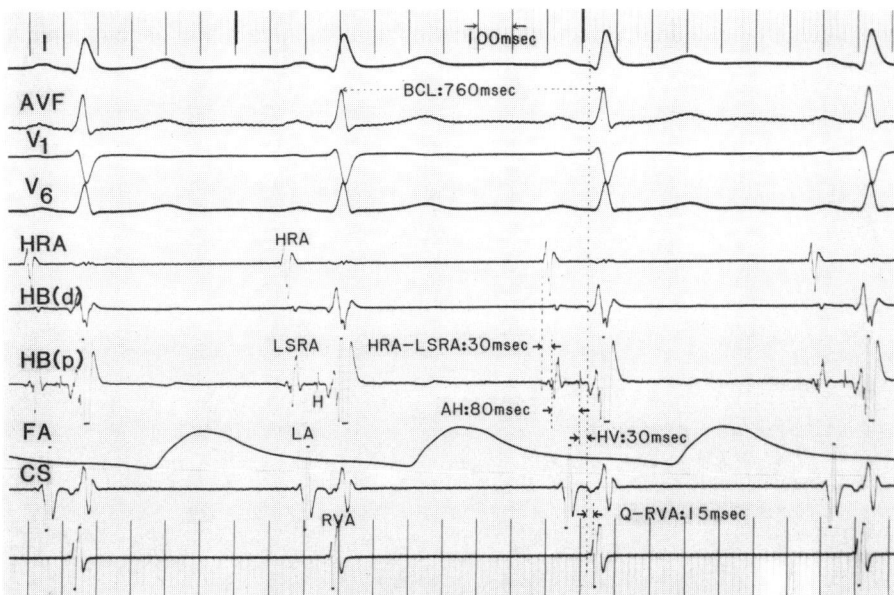

Figure 5. A multiple catheter recording allows measurement of conduction intervals. Note the normal atrial activation sequence with onset at the high right atrium (HRA), followed by low septal right atrium (LSRA), and lastly the left atrium (LA) as recorded from a coronary sinus (CS) catheter. The activation time of the right ventricular apex (RVA) is the interval from the onset of the surface Q wave to the RVA electrogram. FA = femoral artery pressure tracing; BCL = basic cycle length. See legend for Figure 2 for additional abbreviations.

uous to the normal sinus node. The format of atrial pacing may include one or all of the following: burst rapid pacing for up to 30 seconds at progressively faster rates, introduction of premature atrial stimuli into sinus rhythm, or introduction of progressively premature atrial beats into a paced atrial rhythm faster than the sinus rate (usually a train of 8 stimuli at cycle lengths ranging from 600–400 msec).

Assessment of Sinus Node Function

The electrophysiologic function of the sinus node and perinodal tissue can be assessed by rapid atrial pacing or by the introduction of premature atrial beats into either sinus or paced atrial rhythms. The most widely used approach is to measure sinus node recovery time after overdrive atrial pacing. The high right atrium is paced for at least 30 seconds at progressively faster

pacing rates, starting just above the sinus rate. After abrupt termination of pacing, the time for recovery of the sinus node is measured from the last paced atrial beat to the first sinus beat (Fig. 6). This measurement is repeated at each paced rate, allowing at least a 30-sec interval between pacing sequences to allow the sinus rate to return to its baseline level. The longest sinus node recovery time, which generally occurs at rates of 120–140 beats/min, is used for analysis. Since this interval normally varies with the resting sinus rate, a corrected sinus node recovery time (CSNRT) should be calculated. This CSNRT is the difference between the measured sinus node recovery time and the resting sinus cycle length. For example, if the resting cycle length is 500 msec and the SNRT is 700 msec, the CSNRT is 200 msec. Normal values for CSNRT in children are ≤275 msec. Corrected sinus node recovery times can also be expressed as a percentage of the resting sinus cycle length

Table 2
Normal Electrophysiologic Values

	Children (<15 yrs)	Adults
Conduction intervals (msec)		
PA	10–50	10–60
HRA-LSRA	10–40	10–50
AH	50–120	60–150
HV	22–55	35–55
Q-RVA	15–35	—
Sinus node function		
CSNRT	≤275 msec or <166% BC	≤550 msec or <150% BC
Total SACT (msec)	≤200	≤250
Atrioventricular conduction		
Onset of Wenckeback AV block with rapid arial pacing (dependent upon vagal tone)	≥170 BPM or Pacing CL ≤350 msec	≥120 to 170 BPM or Pacing CL ≤500 to 350 msec

		Mean ± 1 SD	
	Pacing CL	FRP	ERP
Refractory periods (msec)			
Atrium			
(Children)	280–459	200 ± 35	165 ± 37
	460–599	234 ± 43	199 ± 43
	600–850	247 ± 53	206 ± 80
(Adults)	—	—	330
AV Node			
(Children)	280–459	299 ± 46	219 ± 45
	460–599	354 ± 66	260 ± 55
	600–850	427 ± 74	303 ± 81
(Adults)	—	525	425

AV, atrioventricular; BCL, basic cycle length; BPM, beats per minute; CL, cycle length; CSNRT, corrected sinus node recovery time; ERP, effective refractory period; FRP, functional refractory period; HRA, high right atrium; LSRA, low septal right atrium; RVA, right ventricle apex; SACT, sinoatrial conduction time; SD, standard deviation.

(sinus node recovery time ÷ resting cycle length × 100), with a normal range in children of 100%–166%. On occasion, there may be an abnormal recovery focus rather than the sinus node following cessation of atrial pacing. This can be considered an abnormal response only if the recovery time is prolonged (e.g., >275 msec).

Sinus node function may also be assessed by the determination of sinoatrial conduction time (SACT) utilizing the introduction of progressively premature atrial beats into either sinus rhythm or a paced atrial rhythm of 8 beats. The Strauss technique uses the former approach of coupling premature atrial beats to sinus beats. A "reset" zone is determined where the paced atrial beat is premature enough to depolarize the sinus node. A total (SACT) conduction time into and out of the sinus node is determined by subtracting the sinus cycle length from the interval between the paced atrial beat and the first sinus recovery beat. The upper limit of normal in the pediatric population is 200 msec. For a more detailed explanation of the performance of this study,

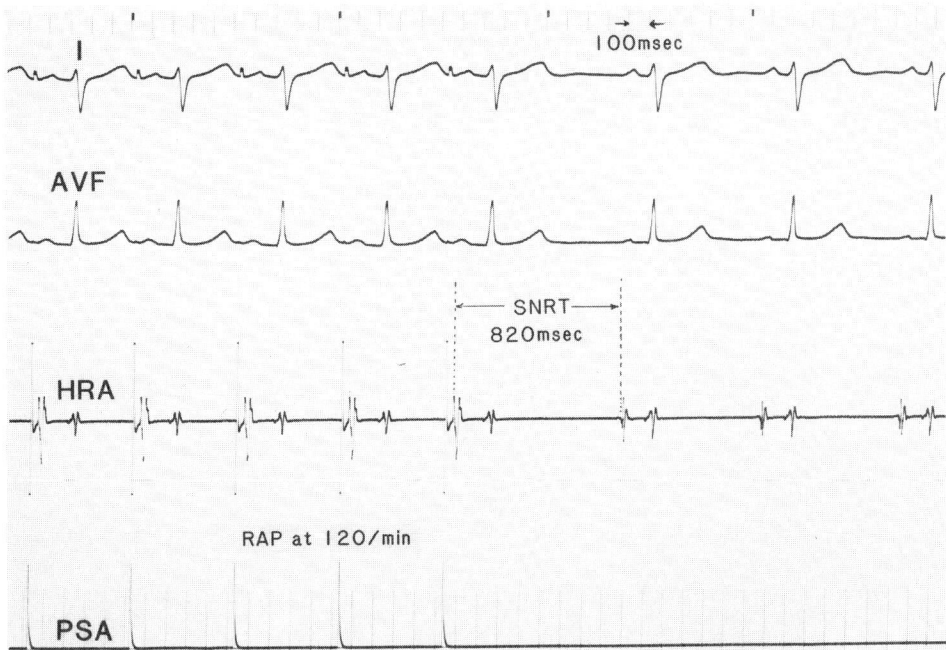

Figure 6. Sinus node recovery time (SNRT) is determined by measuring the interval from the onset of the last paced atrial activity to the onset of the first spontaneous sinus beat following a period of rapid atrial pacing (RAP). HRA = high right atrium; PSA = pacing stimulus artifact. See legend for Figure 2 for additional abbreviations.

the reader is referred to other reference sources (Strauss et al. 1973; Kugler et al. 1974). The Narula method uses a simplified approach of inserting progressively premature atrial beats into a paced atrial rhythm at a pacing rate just greater than the sinus rate. Normal values in children are not well standardized with this technique. It also has the additional problem of possibly causing overdrive suppression of the sinus node, which would introduce considerable error into the SACT calculation (Narula et al. 1978).

Assessment of Atrial Muscle Function

In addition to the measurements of intra-atrial conduction times that were discussed previously, the electrophysiologic function of the atrial muscle itself may be assessed by determining atrial refractory periods, using the introduction of premature atrial beats into a paced atrial rhythm. This will be discussed further in the following section.

Assessment of AV Node Function

The assessment of AV nodal response to rapid atrial pacing is very useful in testing the integrity of atrioventricular conduction. This can be combined with the determination of sinus node recovery times as previously discussed. The high right atrium is paced for 30 seconds at progressively increasing atrial rates, starting at a rate 10–20 beats/min greater than the resting sinus rate. The pacing rate is incrementally increased by 10–20 beats/min until AV block develops or until a rate of 220–240 beats/min is reached. Normally, the AH interval gradually increases with increasing pacing rates until Wenckebach second degree AV block (Mobitz type I) develops within the AV node. In a normal child, this usually occurs at rates of 180 beats/min or above and rarely is seen at pacing rates less than 170 beats/min. Therefore, Wenckebach block is considered abnormal at pacing rates less than 170 beats/min. On the other hand, in the normal adult, the rate at which Wenckebach block develops has a range between 120 and 170 beats/min, depending on vagal tone.

Further electrophysiologic data about the AV node and other intracardiac sites can be obtained by determining refractory periods of the various components of the conduction system. At least two catheters must be used, one positioned to record the low septal right atrium, His bundle, and right ventricle and another to pace and record from the high right atrium in the proximity of the sinus node. The atrium is paced for 8 beats at one or more constant cycle lengths, generally 600, 500, or 400 msec. The pacing stimulus artifacts of these 8 beats are designated as S1 with the cycle length being the S1-S1 interval. Progressively premature atrial beats are then introduced at 10–20 msec shorter cycle lengths until the atrium can no longer be captured (that is, atrial refractoriness occurs). The premature pacing stimulus is designated as S2. The effective refractory period of the AV node is reached when the atrial impulses are no longer conducted to the His-Purkinje system. The AV node effective refractory period is defined as the longest A1–A2 interval (where A1 and A2 represent atrial depolarizations following S1 and S2 respectively) which fails to result in a His bundle depolarization. The functional AV node refractory period is defined as the shortest H1-H2 interval (H1 and H2 refer to His bundle depolarizations following A1 and A2, respectively) that can be obtained during the extrastimulus study. In children, most commonly the AV node is the earliest site in the conduction system to develop block. Therefore, once the AV nodal refractory periods have been determined, atrial refractoriness can be assessed by introducing even more premature stimuli. The atrial effective refractory period is the longest S1-S2 interval that fails to result in atrial capture, while the functional refractory period of the atrium is the shortest A1-A2 interval that can be obtained. Occasionally, in the pediatric population, atrial refractoriness will be encountered before it occurs in the AV node, precluding determination of refractory periods for the latter site. Rarely, block may occur first below the His bundle in children allowing the measurement of the refractory periods of the His-Purkinje system. The effective refractory period of this tissue would be defined as the longest H1-H2 interval that fails to depolarize the ventricles. Examples of the use of atrial extrastimulus studies to measure refractory periods are shown in Figure 7. Normal values for refractory periods in children were established in a study by Dubrow et al. and are shown in Table 2.

Ventricular Pacing

The major role of ventricular pacing is in the study of tachyarrhythmias, whether supraventricular or ventricular in origin. However, valuable basic information about the electrophysiologic function of the ventricle and AV node can be obtained safely by a simple pacing protocol consisting of single premature ventricular beats introduced into either sinus rhythm or a paced ventricular rhythm (8 beats at a constant cycle length of 600, 500, or 400 msec). Ventricular refractory periods can be determined by this approach with the effective refractory period being the longest S1-S2 not capturing the ventricle, and the functional refractory period defined as the shortest V1-V2 obtainable. The presence or absence of retrograde conduction through the AV node can also be established. More sophisticated and potentially risky programmed stimulation of the ventricle is necessary for evaluation of ventricular arrhythmias and will be discussed later.

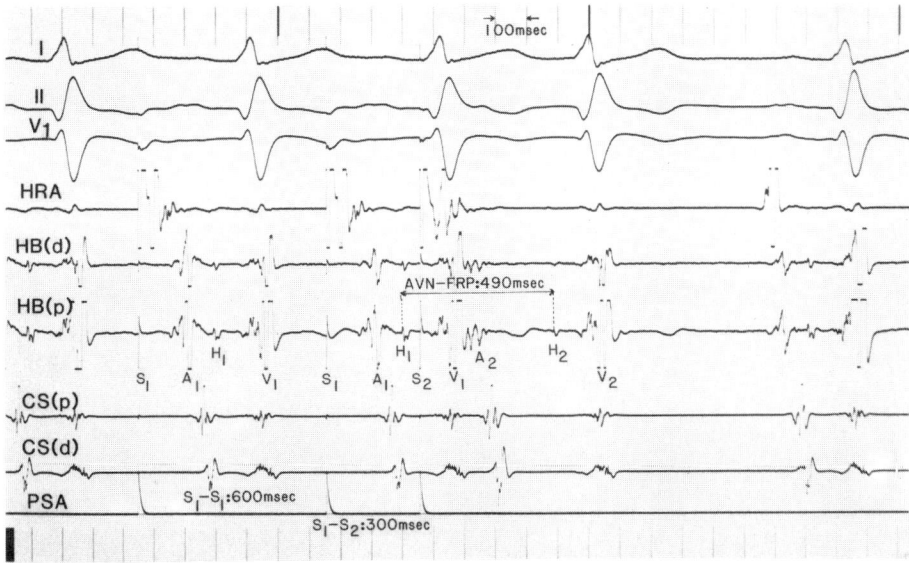

Figure 7A. Determination of atrial and AV nodal refractory periods by atrial extrastimulus technique. The AV node functional refractory period (AVN-FRP) is the shortest H1-H2 produced by progressively premature atrial beats (S2) introduced into a paced atrial rhythm at a fixed cycle length (S1-S1). CS (d) = coronary sinus recording (distal); CS (p) = coronary sinus recording (proximal). See legend for Figure 2 for additional abbreviations.

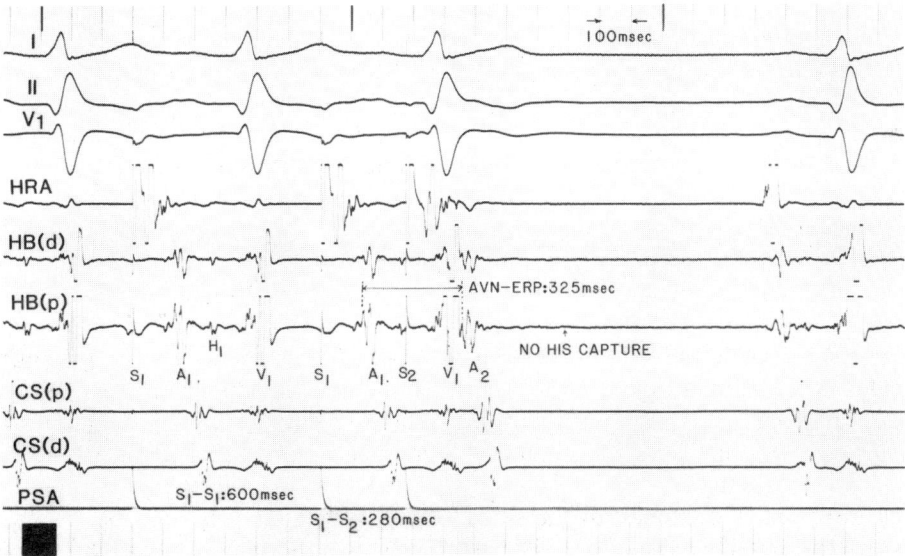

Figure 7B. Determination of atrial and AV nodal refractory periods by atrial extrastimulus technique. The AV node effective refractory period (AVN-ERP) is the longest A_1-A_2 that blocks in the AV node. Note the absence of a His deflection following A_2. CS (d) = coronary sinus recording (distal); CS (p) = coronary sinus recording (proximal). See legend for Figure 2 for additional abbreviations.

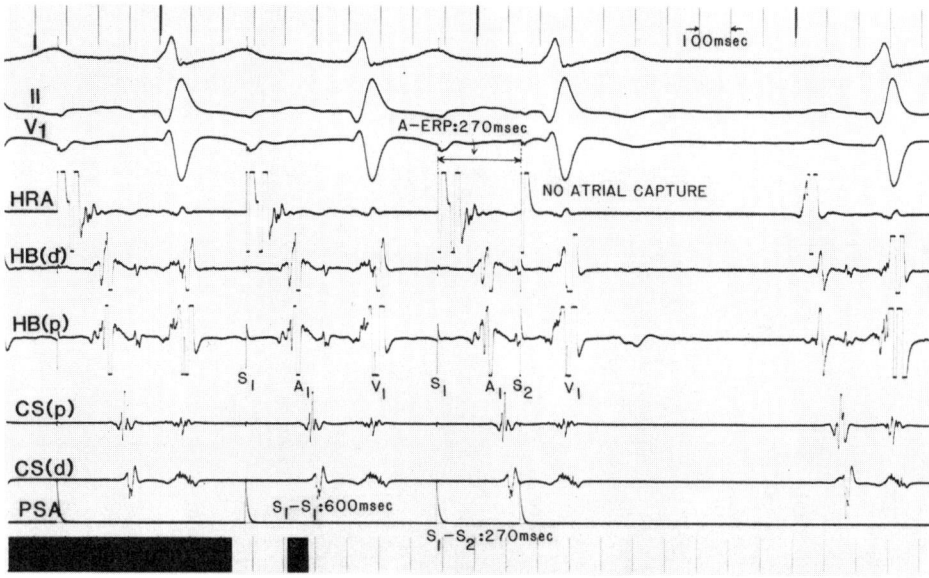

Figure 7C. Determination of atrial and AV nodal refractory periods by atrial extrastimulus technique. The atrial effective refractory period (A-ERP) is the longest S1-S2 interval that fails to capture the atrium. The atrial functional refractory period (not shown) is the shortest A_1-A_2 interval that can be elicited. CS (d) = coronary sinus recording (distal); CS (p) = coronary sinus recording (proximal). See legend for Figure 2 for additional abbreviations.

Investigation of Supraventricular Arrhythmias

The essential requirements for an effective evaluation of supraventricular tachyarrhythmias include reproducibly initiating the clinically relevant arrhythmia by programmed stimulation (if it does not occur spontaneously), while recording stable simultaneous intracardiac recordings from the His bundle, right and left atria, and right ventricle. Ideally, four catheters should be inserted and positioned to record the (1) high right atrium in proximity to the sinus node, (2) His bundle along with electrograms from the low septal right atrium and right ventricle, (3) left atrium obtained via an atrial communication or preferably the coronary sinus, and (4) right ventricular apex. It may be necessary during the course of the study to move the right and left atrial catheters to record various sites within

these chambers. However, the His bundle catheter should remain in place to provide a reliable reference point throughout the study. Recording of four surface leads (I, aV_F, V_1 and V_6) is extremely useful in defining the morphology of the arrhythmia and relating it to clinically documented rhythm disturbances.

The mechanism of rhythm disturbances can be defined as being in one of the two broad categories of reentry or automatic. The former has the characteristics of being readily inducible and terminated by programmed stimulation, with a tendency to start and stop suddenly. Furthermore, reentrant arrhythmias have a nearly constant cycle length other than slight oscillation from beat to beat. On the other hand, automatic (or ectopic) rhythms tend to occur spontaneously, are not influenced by pacing, and have a "warm-up" phenomenon characterized by gradual acceleration of the rate at the onset of the tachycardia. A third mechanism known as triggered automaticity has been postulated to exist, but its relevance to clinical arrhythmias is uncertain. Reentrant tachyarrhythmias can be further defined as those arising from totally within the AV node (AV node reentry), those that utilize an accessory atrioventricular connection (preexcitation phenomena including Wolff-Parkinson-White syndrome), or those that occur due to reentry within a localized area of atrial muscle or the sinus node. Automatic rhythms may arise from anywhere in either atria or from the AV junction itself.

The following steps are taken during the investigation. Baseline intervals are obtained and basic atrial pacing studies including rapid atrial pacing and the introduction of single premature atrial beats into sinus and paced atrial rhythms are performed. This allows evaluation of sinus node function, as well as the determination of the refractory periods of the various intracardiac sites. In addition, supraventricular tachycardia may be initiated during this phase of the stimulation protocol. If there is no induction of arrhythmia, further stimulation should be performed. Double, or even triple, progressively premature atrial beats are introduced into sinus rhythm or paced atrial rhythms at various cycle lengths. In some instances, ventricular pacing, either burst ventricular pacing at cycle lengths from 600–200 msec for 8–10 beats or the introduction of single premature ventricular beats into sinus or paced rhythms, may result in initiation of a supraventricular arrhythmia. Another maneuver that may be helpful is to repeat the atrial pacing at a second site, preferably in the left atrium. If the above extensive protocol still does not succeed in initiating an appropriate arrhythmia, pacing should be repeated after the administration of intravenous atropine (0.02 mg/kg) or isoproterenol (intravenous drip beginning at 0.05 μg/kg/min with upward titration based on heart rate), if necessary. Even if an arrhythmia cannot be induced with these maneuvers, evidence of the presence of an accessory atrioventricular connection

may be obtained by eliciting a delta wave with rapid atrial pacing or when pacing an atrial site remote from the sinus node. Other evidence for such a connection would include documenting an anomalous retrograde atrial activation sequence during ventricular pacing (i.e., an atrial site other than the low septal right atrium being the earliest atrial electrogram obtained following ventricular stimulation).

Once the tachycardia is present, there are several important observations that should be made. The relationship of atrial and ventricular depolarizations is of utmost importance. Atrioventricular dissociation most often indicates the rhythm is ventricular in origin. However, if the ventricular rate exceeds the atrial rate and a His bundle electrogram precedes the ventricular depolarization, or if the QRS morphology is narrow or identical to that present in sinus rhythm, then the etiology is probably a junctional ectopic tachycardia. When the atrial rate is greater than the ventricular rate and AV block is present, it is evident that the AV junction is not necessary for maintenance of the tachycardia. This indicates the etiology is an atrial ectopic tachycardia, atrial flutter, atrial muscle reentry, or sinoatrial node reentry. If there is a 1:1 relationship between atrial and ventricular activity during the tachycardia, then the atrial activation sequence and proximity of the atrial and ventricular depolarizations must be determined. An atrial deflection following that of the ventricle with a short ventriculoatrial interval and with the earliest atrial activation site being the low septal right atrium, followed by the high right atrial depolarization, suggests the presence of AV nodal reentry. A longer ventriculoatrial interval with an anomalous atrial activation sequence (i.e., some left or right atrial site preceding the low septal right atrium with late activation of the high right atrium) is virtually pathognomonic for the Wolff-Parkinson-White syndrome, with an accessory atrioventricular connection. A high to low atrial depolarization pattern with the atrium preceding the ventricle indicates the presence of an atrial tachycardia with 1:1 AV conduction.

The mode of initiation and termination of the tachycardia are important to document. As already stated, a reentry mechanism is suggested when burst pacing or single premature beats can reliably initiate or terminate the tachycardia.

If Wolff-Parkinson-White syndrome is present, further studies should be done to localize the accessory connection, as well as to determine its refractory period. The former is done by mapping the right and left atria around the atrioventricular ring as much as possible to determine the earliest site of atrial activation during orthodromic supraventricular tachycardia (anterograde conduction through the AV node with retrograde conduction through the bypass tract)

or ventricular pacing (Fig. 8). Since pacing in proximity to the atrial insertion of the accessory connection enhances ventricular preexcitation, the atrial pacing site that results in the largest delta wave at any given rate also helps to localize the bypass pathway. The refractory period of the bypass tract is determined by introducing single premature atrial beats into paced rhythm and by the induction of atrial fibrillation. The latter rhythm usually can be initiated by pacing the atrium briefly at very rapid rates with cycle lengths of 50–150 msec. The longest A1-A2 interval that results in loss of the delta wave is the refractory period of the bypass tract as determined by programmed atrial premature beats, while the shortest RR interval between consecutive preexcited beats during atrial fibrillation provides another

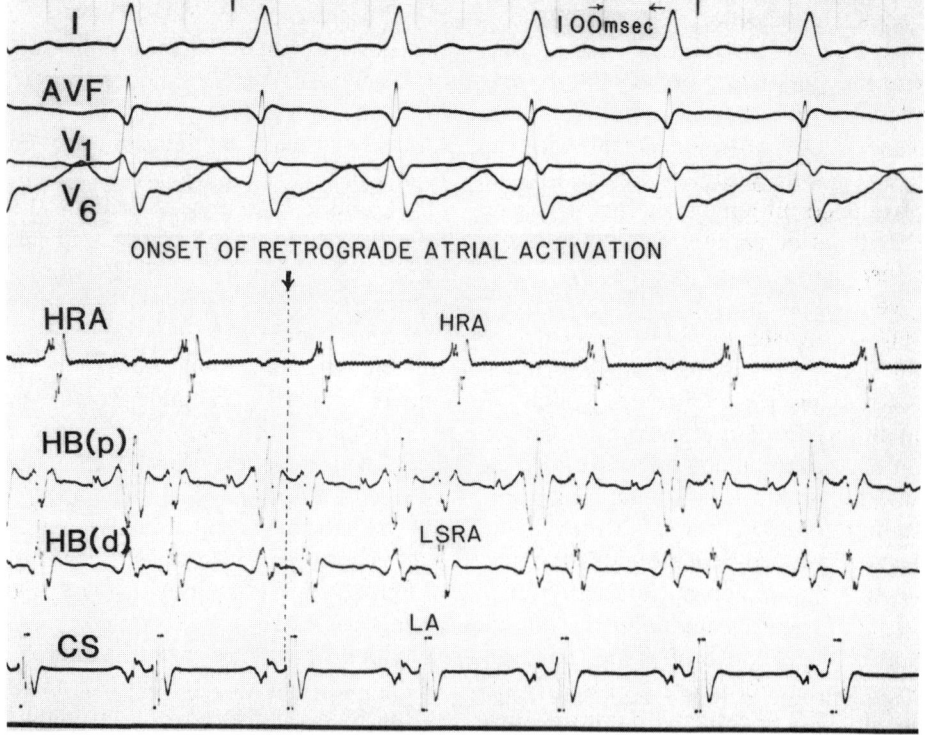

Figure 8. Tracing from a patient with Wolff-Parkinson-White syndrome and a left-sided bypass tract during orthodromic supraventricular tachycardia. Note the earliest site of retrograde atrial activation occurs in the left atrium (LA) as recorded by a catheter in the coronary sinus (CS). See legend for Figure 2 for additional abbreviations.

measure of the refractory period. Serial drug studies to assess potential efficacy can be performed if the supraventricular tachycardia is reproducibly started and stopped by pacing. Furthermore, the effect of drugs on the refractory period of the accessory connection also can be determined. For further information concerning the electrophysiologic evaluation of supraventricular arrhythmia, numerous excellent references are available.

Investigation of Ventricular Arrhythmia

A protocol of ventricular programmed stimulation can be carried out safely, but the possibility of inducing ventricular fibrillation or a hemodynamically unstable ventricular tachycardia is always present and appropriate precautions must be taken. These include monitoring of arterial pressure, facilities for immediate cardioversion or defibrillation, and the ready availability of resuscitation and intubation equipment should they be needed. Furthermore, careful attention to an accepted pacing protocol is essential, including the use of stimuli of appropriate strength (i.e., 1- to 2-msec pulse width and an amplitude of twice the diastolic threshold). The stimulation protocol used in our laboratory consists of burst ventricular pacing of 8–10 beats at cycle lengths ranging from 600–200 msec or until ventricular refractoriness occurs. Single, double, and triple, progressively premature ventricular beats are then introduced into a paced ventricular rhythm of 8 beats. Ventricular pacing is done at the right ventricular apex and the extrastimuli are introduced into a paced ventricular rhythm of at least two different cycle lengths (usually 500 and 400 msec) (Fig. 9A). Some protocols also include introducing the premature beats into sinus rhythm. If these maneuvers fail to induce significant ventricular ectopy, the pacing should be performed at a second site, usu-

ally the right ventricular outflow tract. In cases where the clinical suspicion for the presence of ventricular arrhythmia is high and the above maneuvers have not initiated abnormal ventricular rhythms, repeating the pacing study after isoproterenol infusion or pacing of the left ventricle should be considered. A stable ventricular tachycardia can most often be terminated by overdrive pacing (Fig. 9B). However, some ventricular arrhythmias may be electrically or hemodynamically unstable and require immediate defibrillation.

The site of origin of a stable ventricular tachycardia can be localized by recording ventricular electrograms from multiple sites within the ventricles at paper speeds of at least 100 mm/sec. The major benefits of ventricular pacing studies are (1) confirmation of the presence of a substrate for significant ventricular arrhythmias and (2) allowing serial drug studies to assess efficacy if the ventricular arrhythmia can be reproducibly initiated by pacing. In cases of ventricular tachycardia resistant to medical therapy, accurate endocardial localization of the site of origin allows consideration of surgical ablation. For more details regarding these studies, the reader is again referred to other sources.

Therapeutic Pacing

Placement of a temporary ventricular pacemaker for life-threatening bradycardia can best be performed in the electrophysiologic laboratory, using fluoroscopy. The temporary pacing catheter may be introduced via a sheath using an approach from the femoral vein, antecubital fossa, subclavian or internal jugular vein. The catheter tip should be positioned at the right ventricular apex, if possible, for greatest stability.

Sustained supraventricular tachycardia, unresponsive to noninvasive maneuvers, can be treated effectively in many cases by overdrive pacing. The atrium is

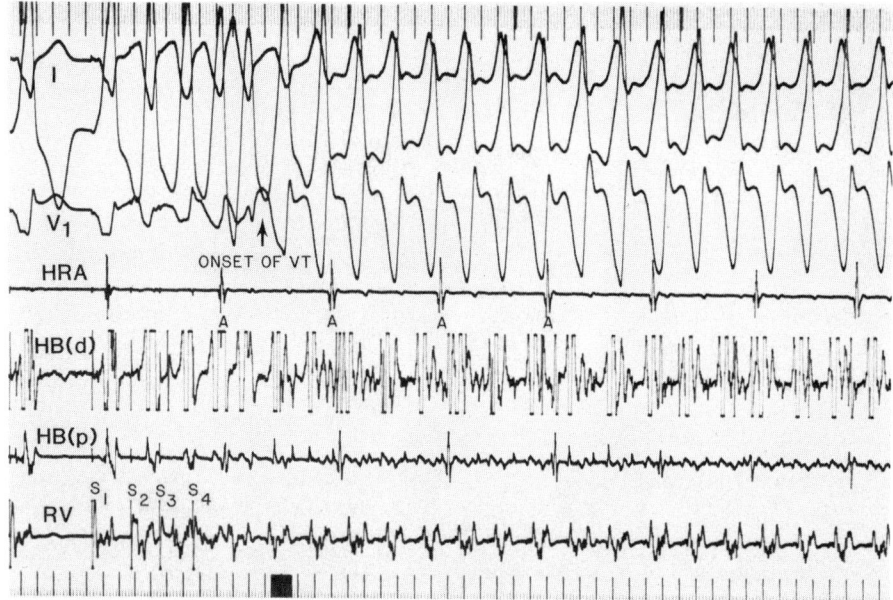

Figure 9A. Induction of sustained ventricular tachycardia (VT) by the introduction of triple premature ventricular beats (S2, S3, S4) into a paced ventricular rhythm (S1-S1). Note atrioventricular dissociation during VT with atrial activity (A) recorded from a catheter at the high right atrium (HRA). CL = cycle length. See legend for Figure 2 for additional abbreviations.

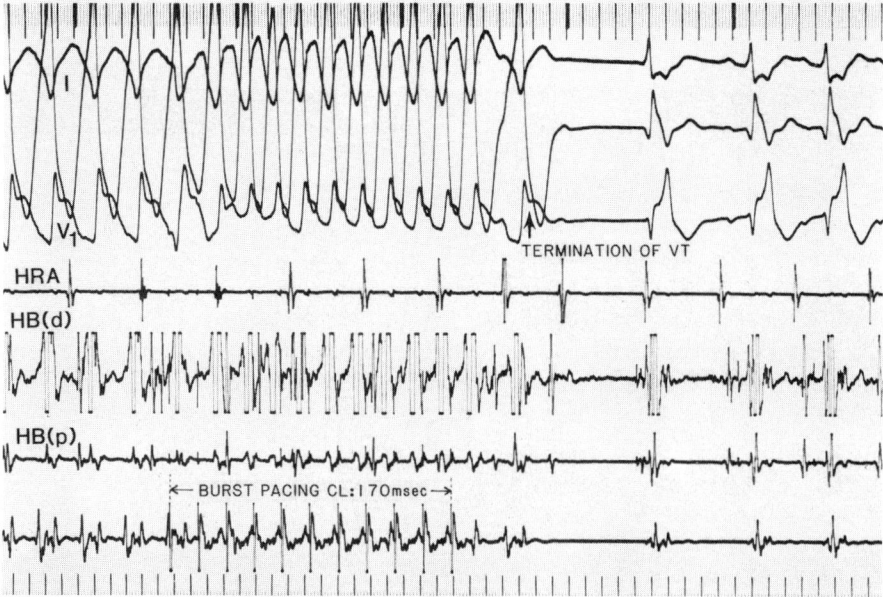

Figure 9B. Tachycardia successfully overdriven by burst ventricular pacing. CL = cycle length. See legend for Figure 2 for additional abbreviations.

paced at a rate greater than the tachycardia (rates of 110%–130% of the tachycardia rate are most likely to be effective) for 30 seconds or more. Once the tachycardia is entrained, the sudden termination of pacing often results in conversion to sinus rhythm. This is not always successful and synchronized cardioversion may be necessary. For intractable, rapid supraventricular tachycardias persisting after the termination of overdrive pacing, improved hemodynamic stability may be obtained by continued atrial pacing. Pacing the atrium at a high enough rate to produce a 2:1 or greater AV block will effectively decrease the ventricular rate.

Complications

The risks and complications of an electrophysiologic study are generally the same as for a routine cardiac catheterization as long as care is taken to insure that the equipment is properly maintained and the patient is isolated from electrical current leaks. Sustained, hemodynamically compromising arrhythmias may be induced in this setting, either by design or as an unsuspected consequence of intracardiac stimulation. These should be controllable by overdrive pacing, synchronized DC cardioversion, or defibrillation. The electrode catheters used are stiffer than standard cardiac catheters and therefore require cautious manipulation, particularly in smaller children. There is also some increased risk of thromboembolism if a prolonged study is required and the use of anticoagulation is therefore recommended.

References and Suggested Reading

Dubrow IW, Fisher EA, Amat-y-Leon F, et al. Comparison of cardiac refractory periods in children and adults. Circulation 1975; 51:485–491.

Garson A, Gillette PC. Electrophysiologic studies of supraventricular tachycardia in children. I. Clinical-electrophysiologic Correlations. Am Heart J 1981; 102:233–250.

Garson A, Porter CJ, Gillette PC, et al. Induction of ventricular tachycardia after repair of tetralogy of Fallot. J Am Coll Cardiol 1983; 16:1493–1502.

Gillette PC. The mechanism of supraventricular tachycardia in children. Circulation 1976; 54:133–139.

Gillette PC, Garson A. Pediatric cardiac dysrhythmias. New York, NY, Grune & Stratton. 1981.

Josephson ME, Seides SF. Clinical cardiac electrophysiology. Philadelphia, PA, Lea & Febiger. 1979.

Klein GJ, Guiravdon GM, Sharma AD, et al. Surgical treatment of tachycardia: Indications and electrophysiologic assessment. Prog Cardiol 1987; 15:139–153.

Kugler VD, Gillette PC, Mullins CE, et al. Sinoatrial conduction in children: An index of sinoatrial node function. Circulation 1974; 59:1266–1276.

Narula OS, Shanth N, Vasques M, et al. A new method for measurement of sinoatrial conduction time. Circulation 1978; 58:706–714.

Roberts NK, Gelband H. Cardiac arrhythmias in the neonate, infant and child. Norwalk, CT, Appleton-Century-Crofts. 1983.

Strauss HC, Saroff AL, Bigger JT, et al. Premature atrial stimulation as a key to understanding of sinoatrial conduction in man. Circulation 1973; 47:86–93.

Yabek SM, Jarmakani JM. Sinus node function in children. Circulation 1976; 53:485–491.

11

Intracardiac Phonocardiography

J. R. Zuberbuhler, M.D.

Intracardiac phonocardiography, the recording of cardiac sounds and murmurs within the heart and vascular system, came into use in the mid 1950s. In 1954, Yamakawa et al. published tracings obtained from dogs and Lewis (1956), 2 years later, recorded sounds and murmurs from the right heart of humans using a barium titanate transducer. Since the frequency response of this system was poor, below 10 Hz, simultaneous intracardiac pressures could not be obtained. Luisada et al. (1965), utilizing standard fluid-filled catheters, were able to obtain pressure frequencies in the same range as sound and thus recorded simultaneous intracardiac sound and pressure. A high-fidelity micromanometer developed by Allard and Laurens (1962) eliminated the transmission delay inherent in fluid-filled systems, and because of its broader range of frequency response, the precise correlation of pressure and sound became possible. The micromanometer, subsequently developed by Millar and now in wide use, is a sensitive and relatively durable transducer that is capable of recording high-fidelity pressure and sound.

Heart Sounds

The most important application of intracardiac sound recording has been in the investigation of the genesis of heart sounds and in the alteration of their intensity and timing in different hemodynamic states; in the process, making auscultation of the heart a more rational exercise. Only a few examples of this application will be cited. The genesis of the first heart sound has been extensively investigated using intracardiac phonocardiography and high-fidelity pressure tracings, sometimes combined with echocardiography or flow velocity recordings. Piemme (1966) showed that the first major component of the first heart sound coincided with the left atrial C wave and with the onset of isometric left ventricular contraction. This component occurred after crossover of the atrial and ventricular pressure tracings. It also occurred simultaneously with mitral valve closure on echocardiogram and with the cessation of mitral flow by flow velocity recording. Similar recordings in the right heart have demonstrated a tricuspid component to the first heart sound, sometimes occurring with or close to the mitral component and sometimes following it at a considerable interval. The loud early systolic sound so commonly heard in patients with Ebstein's anomaly was shown by Fontana and Wooley (1972) to be a loud and delayed tricuspid closure sound, which they dubbed the "sail sound."

The second heart sound has also been extensively studied by intracardiac phonocardiogram techniques. One of the most important recent investigations elegantly demonstrated that the widely split second heart sound associated with an interatrial septal defect, with mild pulmonic stenosis, and with idiopathic dilatation of the pulmonary artery is caused, not by prolonged right ventricular mechanical systole, but by a separation of the descending pulmonary artery pressure curve from the right ventricular curve. The pulmonary artery incisura thus "hangs out" from the descending limb of the ventricular tracing (Fig. 1) (Shaver et al. 1974). The pulmonary artery closure sound, the high-frequency counterpart of the incisura, is delayed because the inertia of the right ventricular ejectate prolongs the ejection phase beyond right ventricular mechanical systole. As a last example, the early systolic ejection sounds of valvar aortic and pulmonic stenosis have been shown to be related to maximal opening, and therefore sudden tensing, of the doming aortic and pulmonic valves (Shaver et al. 1975; Martino

et al. 1975). The simultaneity of the acoustical and mechanical events can be shown by combined intracardiac phonocardiography and echocardiography.

Evaluation of Murmurs

In the early years of intracardiac phonocardiography, there was a tendency to overestimate its value as a diagnostic tool. In fact, it has less value in diagnosis than in investigation, but there are certain instances where it has considerable diagnostic value. These include the confirmation of tricuspid

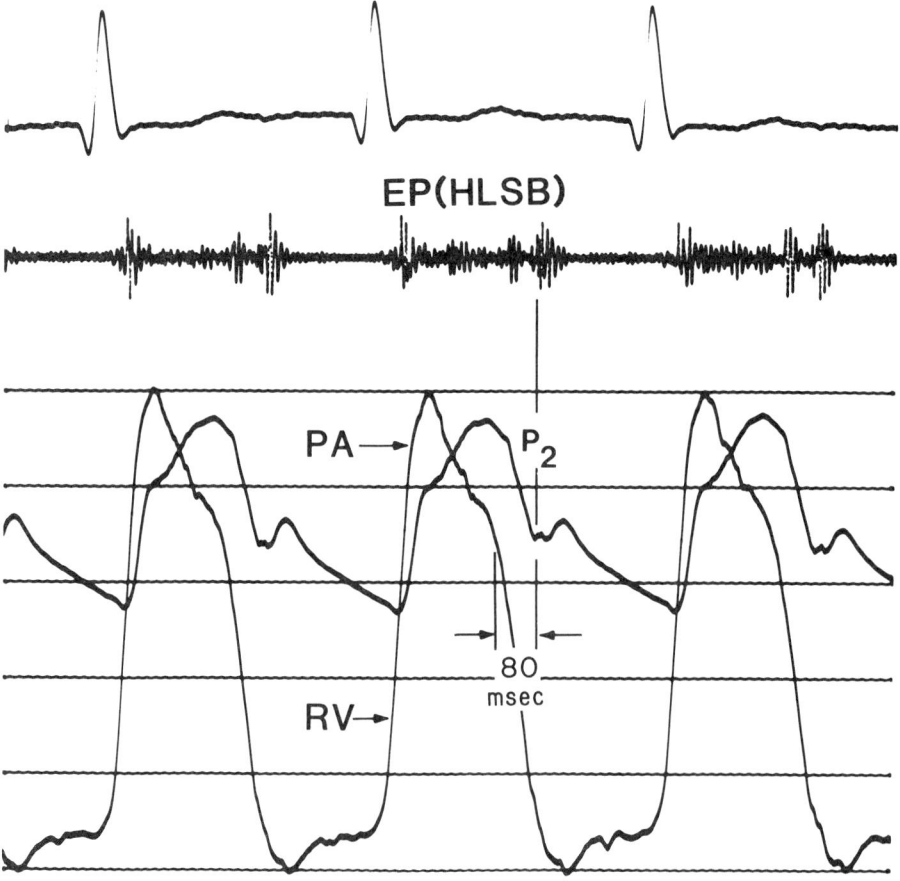

Figure 1. Simultaneous recording of an external phonocardiogram (EP) and a high-fidelity intracardiac pressure recording, showing "hangout" of the pulmonary artery incisura. HSLB = high left sternal border; PA = pulmonary artery; P_2 = pulmonary closure sound; RV = right ventricle.

regurgitation, pulmonic regurgitation, and a left ventricular–right atrial shunt. Tricuspid regurgitation is uncommon in the pediatric age group. When it occurs with high right ventricular pressure, the resulting low left sternal border murmur is usually high pitched and pansystolic and may simulate a small interventricular septal defect. When tricuspid regurgitation occurs with low right ventricular pressure, the murmur tends to be shorter and less high pitched and may seem quite unimpressive. The confirmation of tricuspid regurgitation may be difficult, even at cardiac catheterization, since regurgitation of contrast media to the right atrium during right ventriculography may be catheter- or arrhythmia-induced. Trivial, physiologic tricuspid regurgitation is usually seen with color Doppler echocardiography in most patients. The demonstration of a systolic murmur in the right atrium near the tricuspid valve is strong evidence of tricuspid regurgitation, providing the murmur is absent or at least much attenuated in the right ventricular inflow tract (Fig. 2). It must

be noted that the murmur of tricuspid regurgitation is usually rather localized within the right atrium. It is recordable near the tricuspid valve or along the path of the jet of regurgitation if one is present, but may be very faint or unrecordable at other right atrial sites.

Intracardiac phonocardiography is a very sensitive method of detecting pulmonic regurgitation. Normotensive regurgitation is relatively easily recognized clinically; the murmur is maximal at the high left sternal border, is crescendo-decrescendo, and is of medium pitch. The murmur is characteristically louder in the recumbent than in the upright position. The diastolic murmur of hypertensive pulmonic regurgitation, on the other hand, may be more difficult to diagnose confidently "at the bedside." It is also a left sternal border murmur, but may closely resemble the murmur of aortic regurgitation. Indeed, it has been stated that the classical Graham-Steele murmur, presumably representing hypertensive pulmonic regurgitation, is usually really aortic

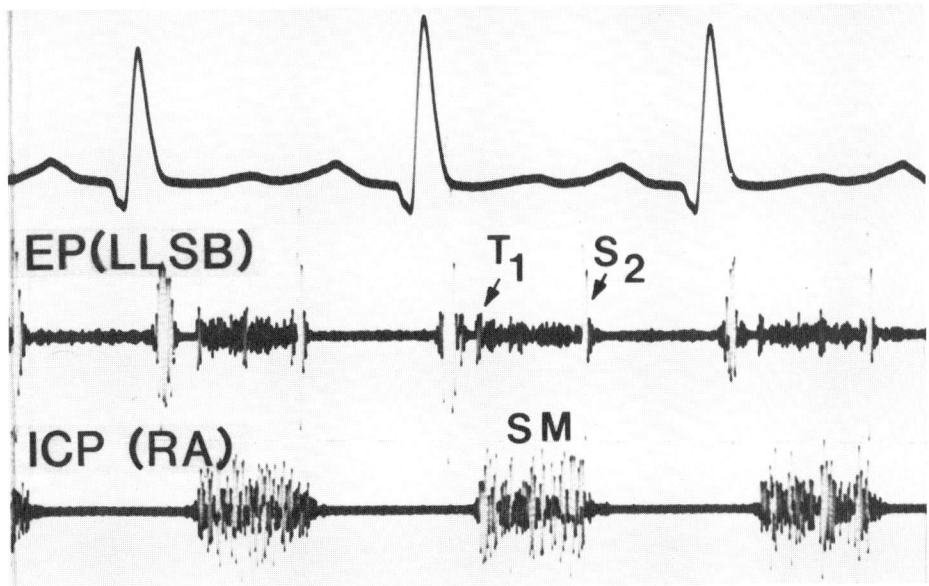

Figure 2. Simultaneous external phonocardiogram (EP) at the lower left sternal border (LLSB) and intracardiac phonocardiogram (ICP) in the right atrium (RA), showing the systolic murmur (SM) of tricuspid regurgitation. S_2 = second heart sound; T_1 = tricuspid valve closure component of the first heart sound.

regurgitation. Again, mild physiologic pulmonary regurgitation is often seen by color Doppler echocardiography. The cineangiographic demonstration of pulmonic regurgitation suffers from the same limitations as that of tricuspid regurgitation; if no regurgitation is seen cineangiographically, there is certainly no regurgitation. However, if regurgitation is present with injection of contrast into the pulmonary artery, it may be catheter-induced. In addition, pulmonary artery injection may be quite hazardous in the presence of advanced pulmonary vascular disease. When pulmonic regurgitation is suspected, intracardiac phonocardiography is a very useful diagnostic tool, since the

murmur of pulmonic regurgitation, whether normotensive or hypertensive, is readily recorded in the right ventricular outflow tract (Fig. 3). Lack of a diastolic murmur at this site makes pulmonic regurgitation extremely unlikely and another source for the diastolic murmur must be sought.

Lastly, intracardiac phonocardiography is useful in documenting the presence of a left ventricular–right atrial communication. This is a very rare congenital cardiac anomaly and consists of a defect in the atrioventricular portion of the membranous septum. During systole, blood flows from the high-pressure left ventricle to the low-pressure right atrium, and the resultant systolic mur-

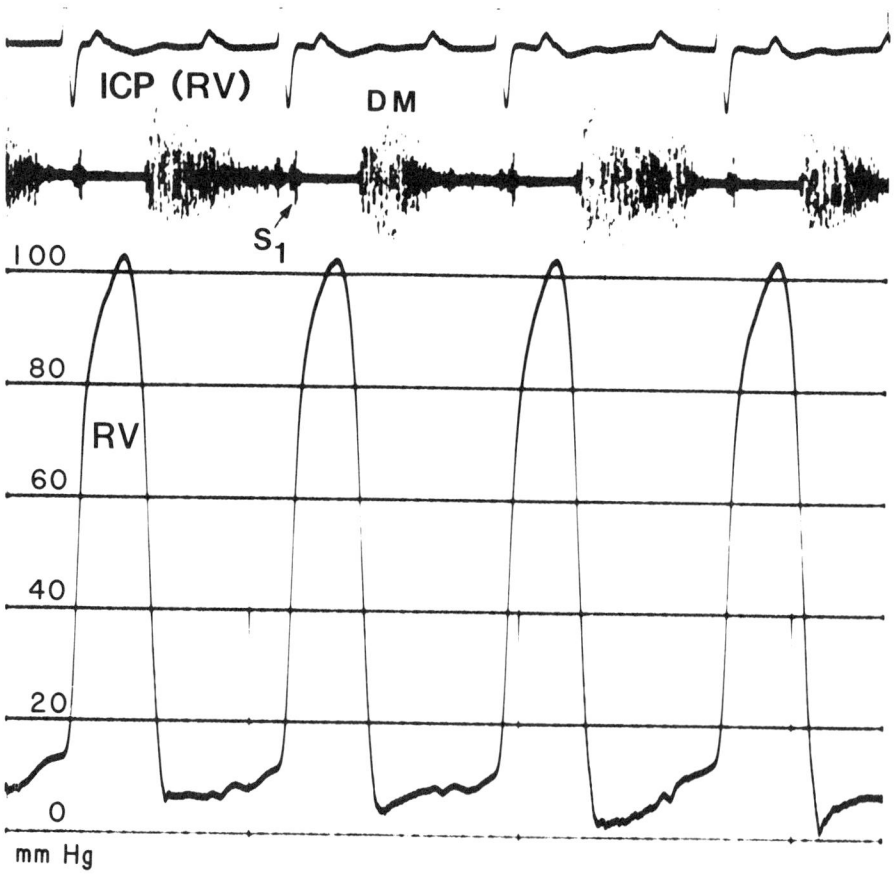

Figure 3. Simultaneous recording of pressure and intracardiac phonocardiogram (ICP) in the right ventricle (RV) using a high-fidelity, micromanometer-tipped catheter in a patient with hypertensive pulmonary regurgitation. DM = diastolic murmur; S_1 = first heart sound.

mur is indistinguishable from the murmur of an interventricular septal defect. A true left ventricular–right atrial communication must be distinguished from the more common combination of an interventricular septal defect and tricuspid regurgitation. It may be difficult to do this echocardiographically, and thus the diagnosis may be only established at cardiac catheterization. In both entities, there is an oxygen step-up at right atrial level and, in each, the right atrium fills promptly after injection of contrast into the left ventricle. However, in the patient with a true left ventricular–right atrial communication, the murmur is absent or at least much less loud in the right ventricular inflow tract, while there is a prominent right ventricular inflow tract systolic murmur in the patient with a ventricular septal defect and tricuspid regurgitation.

Intracardiac phonocardiography is not a difficult technique, but unfortunately the Millar catheters are stiffer and more difficult to maneuver than standard fluid-filled catheters. Catheter positioning is less difficult if a variety of catheter tip curves are available. Although relatively durable, the Millar catheters must be treated with care. The tip must be protected and gas sterilization is required. We routinely soak the catheters overnight in a detergent solution following use. The connection between the catheter and the connecting wire should be kept dry during the catheterization procedure, and this can be accomplished by wrapping the connection with a 4 x 4 gauze strip. The transducer is balanced prior to introduction with the tip immersed in fluid. (Whatever catheterization flush solution is used is acceptable.)

References and Suggested Reading

Allard EM. Sound and pressure signals obtained from a single intracardiac transducer. IRE Trans Bio-Med Elec BME-9, Number 1, 1962.

Fontana ME, Wooley CF. Sail sound in Ebstein's anomaly of the tricuspid valve. Circulation 1972; 46:155–164.

Franke ED. Physiologic pressure transducers. Meth Med Res 1966; 11:132.

Lewis DH, Deitz GW, Wallace JD, Brown JR. Intracardiac phonocardiography in man. Circulation 1957; 16:764–775.

Luisada AA, MacCannon DM, Slodki JD. Intracardiac phonocardiography: Description of a new simplified system. Circulation 1965; 32:563–569.

Martin CE, Shaver JA, O'Toole JD, Leon DF, Reddy PS. Ejection sounds of right-sided origin. Am Heart Assoc Monograph, no. 46, 1975; 35–44.

Piemme TE, Barnett GO, Dexter L. Relationship of heart sounds to acceleration of blood flow. Circ Res 1966; 18:303–315.

Shaver JA, Griff FW, Leonard JJ. Ejection sounds of left-sided origin. Am Heart Assoc Monograph, no. 46, 1975; 27–34.

Shaver JA, Nadolny RA, O'Toole JD, Thompson ME, Reddy PS, Leon DF, Curtiss EI. Sound pressure correlates of the second heart sound: An intracardiac sound study. Circulation 1974; 49:316–325.

Yamakawa K, Shionoya Y, Kitamura K, Nagai T, Yamamoto T, Satoshi O. Intracardiac phonocardiography. Am Heart J 1954; 47:424–431.

12

Atrial Septostomy

Sang C. Park, M.D.

Balloon Atrial Septostomy

Balloon atrial septostomy was the first major therapeutic technique utilized during pediatric cardiac catheterization. Since Rashkind and Miller introduced the technique in 1966, it has been widely used with great success. The technique is designed to enlarge an already existing interatrial opening without thoracotomy, utilizing a catheter with an inflatable balloon tip. It is used in anomalies in which a large interatrial communication is hemodynamically advantageous. Transposition of the great arteries is the most common indication, but the technique also may be useful in patients with tricuspid atresia, mitral atresia, total anomalous pulmonary venous return, or pulmonary atresia with intact interventricular septum. The technique is most effective in the newborn period and is rarely successful beyond the first month of life.

Preparation

The usual premedication for cardiac catheterization is sufficient. In our laboratory, no sedation is used in newborn infants. The procedure can be done either by saphenous or femoral vein cutdown or percutaneously via the femoral vein. In a newborn, the umbilical vein also can be used successfully. Despite the difficulty of maneuvering the balloon catheter via the umbilical vein (the Fogarty catheter is better for this approach), balloon septostomy can be performed as effectively and safely as from the femoral route (Newfeld et al. 1974; Rosuin et al. 1984). There are several types of balloon atrial septostomy catheters available (Fig. 1). The Rashkind catheter (USCI) is available as a #6 French catheter with a recessed balloon. The #5 French Fogarty septostomy catheter (American Edwards Laboratory) has a single lumen for balloon inflation. The capacity of the balloon in most of the septostomy catheters is approximately 2 mL, but a larger Fogarty septostomy catheter with a capacity of 4 mL and diameter of 16 mm is available (Miller septostomy catheter, American Edwards Laboratory). When the procedure is to be performed by the percutaneous technique, a #6 French sheath is used for the Rashkind catheter, while the introducer or the sheath must be #7 French size for the Fogarty catheter in order to accommodate the balloon tip. A side-port sheath with a back bleed prevention gasket is therefore necessary to prevent blood loss around the catheter.

Procedure

Prior to balloon atrial septostomy, both left and right atrial pressure should be recorded and systemic saturation determined. The balloon catheter is introduced into the left atrium with the location of the catheter tip confirmed by lateral fluoroscopic examination. Ideally, the atrial defect should be sized before the therapeutic septostomy is performed. To do this, the balloon is inflated gradually with diluted con-

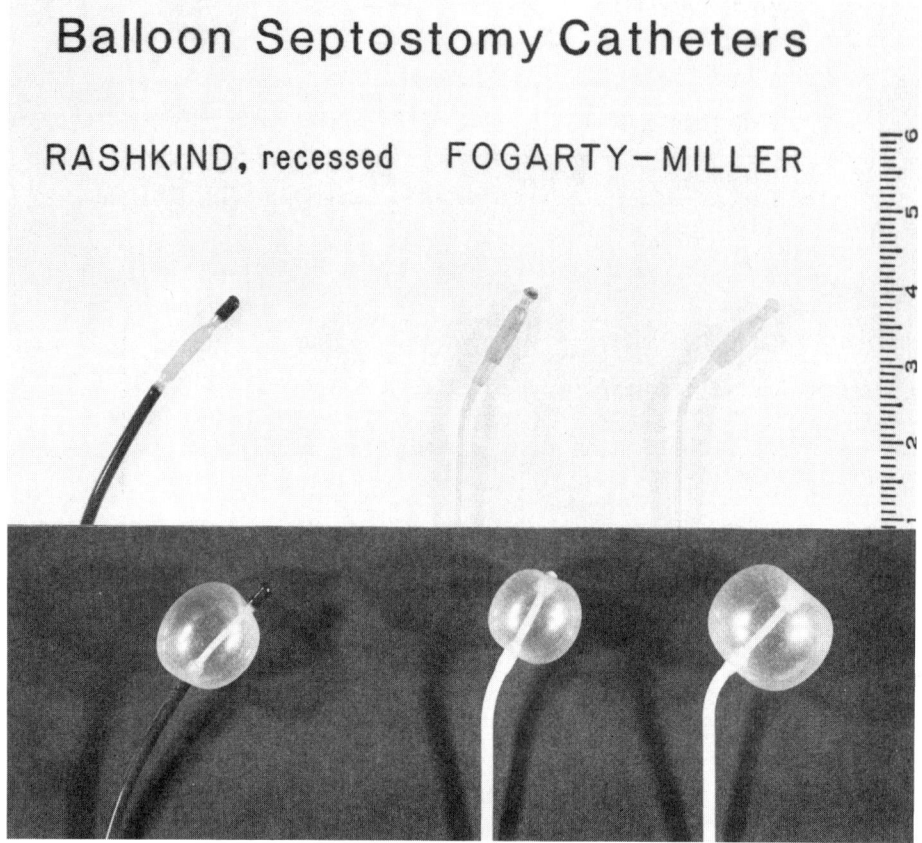

Figure 1. Balloon septostomy catheters.

trast material, making sure that it is not in a pulmonary vein or in the left atrial appendage. The balloon size should be about the width of one vertebra. The balloon is then gently withdrawn until it engages the septum. The balloon is deflated, maintaining gentle traction on the catheter, until the balloon "pops" into the right atrium. The procedure is recorded on videotape and/or cinefilm. A calibration grid should be in the field or recorded subsequently for calculating the size of the defect. The defect size is estimated by the diameter of the balloon at the time it pops across the septum.

To now perform the actual balloon septostomy, the catheter is again placed in the left atrium and inflated as before, and drawn back against the septum. The catheter is then pulled back into the right atrium with a quick, short jerk (Fig. 2). The excursion should be less than 5 cm. At the end of the jerk, the hand should be returned to the original site to return the balloon to the mid portion of the right atrium. The balloon is then deflated. The balloon septostomy should be repeated two or three times, although the first withdrawal of the balloon is the most important and crucial part of the procedure. The defect can then be sized again as described above. A measured defect > 12 mm is considered an excellent result, while a defect < 8 mm is considered inadequate. In the last few years, balloon septostomy also has been performed by means of echocardiographic guidance (Allan et al. 1982; Baker et al. 1984; Steeg et al. 1985; Lin et al. 1986).

It should be mentioned that lack of a substantial interatrial gradient does not

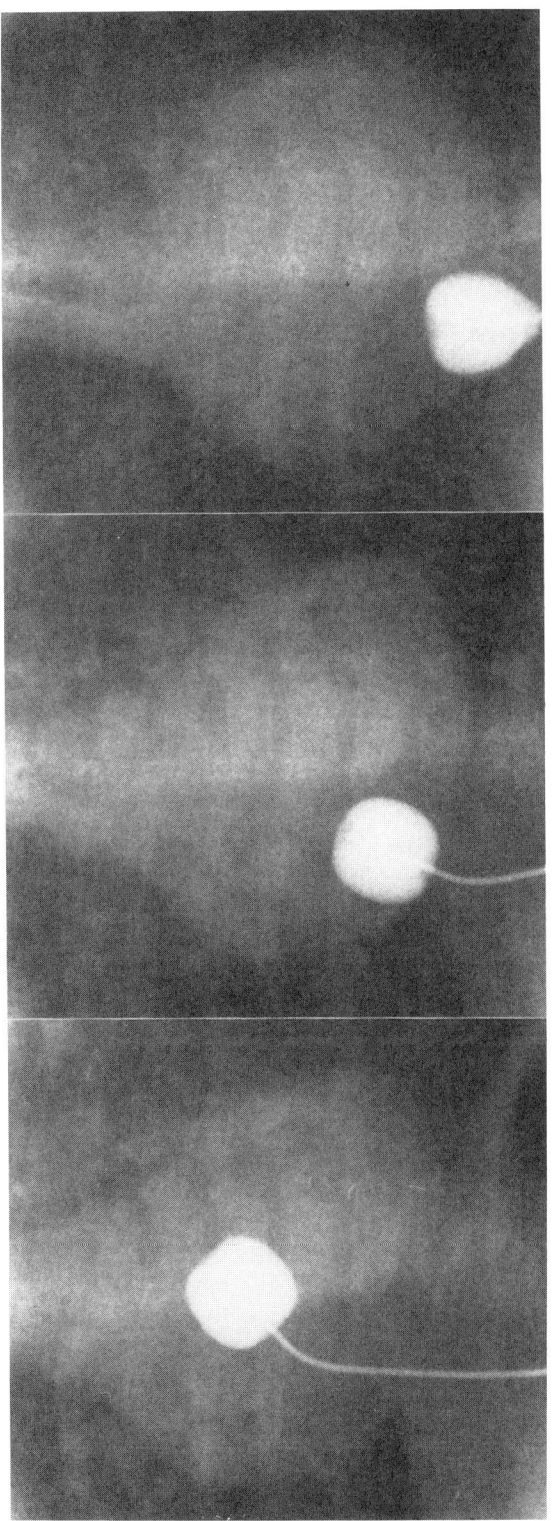

Figure 2. Sequence of balloon atrial septostomy. Three consecutive cineframes recorded at 60 frames/sec.

guarantee a large interatrial defect. Measurement of the defect with the balloon, before and after balloon septostomy, both radiographically and echocardiographically, is very useful in the assessment of the success of the procedure. In some patients, interatrial mixing is not satisfactory for a day or so even after substantial enlargement of the interatrial opening by balloon septostomy. Infusion of prostaglandin E_1, or volume expansion, may be helpful to promote increased atrial mixing (Beitzke and Suppan 1983; Weldon et al. 1983). In others, interatrial mixing may not improve at all and, in such patients, surgical septectomy may be equally ineffective. Knowing that the interatrial defect is large (> 12 mm) should lessen enthusiasm for surgical septectomy.

Complications

In the early days of balloon septostomy, complications were usually related to rupture and fragmentation of the balloon. The fragmented latex caused systemic embolization, usually to the central nervous system or kidneys. Recently, improved materials and construction have minimized this problem. Another early complication was inability to deflate the balloon after the procedure. This was due to slippage of the balloon back over the opening between the catheter lumen and the balloon itself. Probably the most devastating complication of balloon septostomy is accidental rupture of the tricuspid valve, occurring when the pullback is inadvertently begun in the right ventricle rather than in the left atrium. This is unlikely to occur if a lateral fluoroscopic unit is used to confirm a proper posterior location of the balloon catheter. If only anteroposterior fluoroscopy is available, it is helpful to advance the catheter tip gently into a left pulmonary vein to confirm proper positioning. Even in the unusual case where a pulmonary vein is not easily entered, the lack of PVCs when the catheter contacts the lateral wall of the heart is reassuring. Echocardiography is also quite valuable for localizing the position of the balloon catheter in the left atrium.

Rapid inflation of the balloon in a pulmonary vein instead of in the left atrium may cause damage. Therefore, balloon inflation should always be done slowly and with fluoroscopic monitoring. Arrhythmias may occur immediately following balloon atrial septostomy, but are usually transient. Advanced atrioventricular block is rare and is usually associated with damage to the tricuspid valve. Bradycardia may also be seen when the balloon is pulled against the interatrial septum for an extended period of time. Bradycardia is also noted when the balloon almost completely fills a small left atrium and interferes with pulmonary venous return.

Since the balloon is larger than the shaft of the catheter, blood loss occurs at the venotomy site or through the sheath unless proper precautions are taken. With the cutdown technique, a double loop of thread placed proximal the venotomy and secured with a hemostat is helpful. A gasket seal type introducer is available with the percutaneous technique. Appropriate replacement of blood loss with packed cells or whole blood is, of course, recommended.

Blade Atrial Septostomy

Balloon atrial septostomy is usually not successful in older infants and in children with a thickened interatrial septum. Repeat balloon atrial septostomy in an infant, after an initially apparently successful procedure, is usually ineffective (Baker et al. 1971; Neches et al. 1973). In 1973, a catheter with a built-in surgical blade was developed to enlarge the interatrial opening in such patients, and experiments in animals demonstrated its efficacy and safety (Park et al. 1975, 1978). Subsequently, this technique has been successful in patients with various congenital heart defects in whom a large interatrial opening is beneficial (Park et al. 1982).

Components and Construction of Blade Catheter

The catheter is made of #6 French radiopaque polyethylene tubing (Cook Incorporated) (Fig. 3). The standard size blade catheter tip consists of a 3.5-cm section of stainless steel tubing with a 2.5-cm slit in its long axis. The metal tubing contains a small blade that is linked to a lever whose distal end pivots at the catheter tip. The proximal portion of the blade is linked to a solid guidewire that passes through the entire catheter and exists at the hub. Advancing the wire extends the blade and the lever through the slit to form a triangle. There is a Y connector at the proximal portion of the catheter; one side branch is for fluid infusion and pressure measurement and the other is for the wire that controls the blade. Currently, in addition to the standard size 12-mm blade component, 16-mm (#6 French) and 21-mm (#8 French) blade catheters are available for use in older children or adults.

Preparation

The procedure can be performed by cutdown or percutaneous technique through either the saphenous or femoral vein. A biplane image intensifier for rapid access to lateral fluoroscopy without moving the patient is essential. Patients receive standard premedication for cardiac catheterization, and general anesthesia is not re-

quired. When the procedure is done percutaneously, it is necessary to use a sheath that is large enough to accommodate both the blade septostomy and the balloon septostomy catheters. Although the blade septostomy catheter shaft is #6 French, a #7 French introducer should be used to accommodate the slightly larger catheter tip. A special sheath with a device to control back bleeding, such as Hemaquet (USCI), is recommended to prevent blood loss due to mismatch between the size of the sheath and the smaller size catheter. Selective left atrial angiocardiography is done before blade septostomy, to evaluate the size of the left atrium and the interatrial opening. In infants with mitral atresia, angiocardiographic evaluation of left atrial size is particularly important, since the left atrium is often small.

Procedure

The catheter system (Fig. 3) is checked before introduction. The locking device (D) is loosened from the wire holder (E), and the locking device and wire holder are moved toward the gasket (B) so that no gap is present between the locking device (D) and the gasket (B). The locking device is then tightened to prevent inadvertent protrusion of the blade during the manipulation of the catheter. The flexible plastic tubing is connected between the port (C) and a pressure transducer or an infusion line. The catheter system is flushed with heparinized solution.

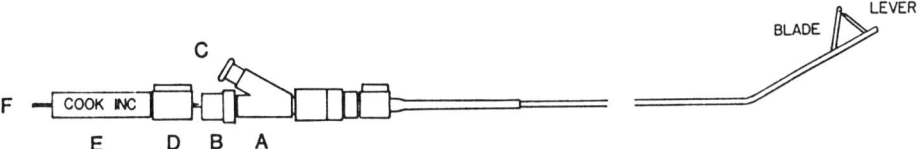

Figure 3. Blade septostomy catheter and assembly components. A = Y connector; B = gasket to prevent leakage; C = side arm for fluid infusion and pressure measurement; D = locking device for wire holder; E = blade control wire holder; F = blade control wire.

The catheter is introduced into the left atrium (Fig. 4A). Because the side arm is in the same plane as the curve of the catheter tip, passage of the catheter into the left atrium can be facilitated by maintaining the side arm in a posterior and leftward orientation. The location of the catheter in the left atrium is confirmed by lateral fluoroscopy and pressure measurement.

After the position of the catheter tip in the left atrium is confirmed, the locking device is loosened from the control wire and pulled backward until the gap between the gasket and the locking device is 12 mm; the holder is then tightened. Next, the blade is extended by advancing the blade control wire holder gently toward the catheter tip under fluoroscopic control (Fig. 4B). If resistance is met or if the blade cannot be fully extended, the catheter tip may be positioned in the left atrial appendage or in a pulmonary vein. In this situation, the control wire holder is withdrawn to fold the blade back into the catheter. Then, the entire catheter system is slightly withdrawn and the same maneuver repeated. Once the blade has been extended, the gasket and the locking device are held together with the thumb and index finger. The catheter is then slightly rotated counterclockwise until the blade is facing somewhat anteriorly as seen by lateral fluoroscopy (Fig. 4C).

The entire catheter system is slowly withdrawn to the right atrium using both hands to maintain the same catheter orientation (Fig. 4D). Resistance of the interatrial septum is usually encountered in the middle or lower portion of the cardiac silhouette. Gentle, but firm, force is maintained to withdraw the catheter from the left atrium to the right atrium until a sudden decrease in resistance is felt. Continued resistance may be felt despite withdrawal of the catheter to the level of the diaphragm or even lower, especially if the left atrium is large or if the interatrial septum is quite thick. *Under*

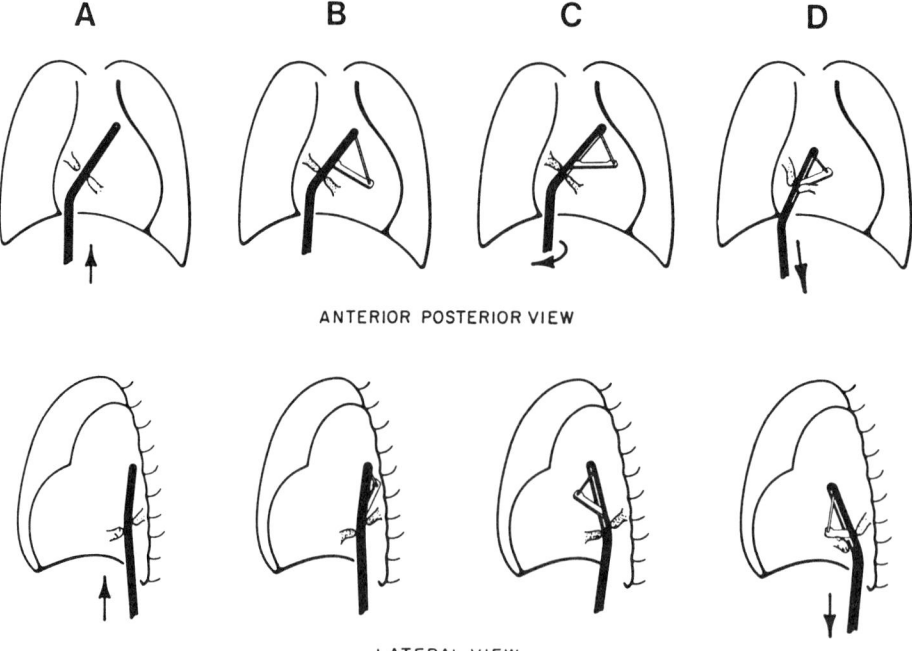

ANTERIOR POSTERIOR VIEW

LATERAL VIEW

Figure 4. Sequence of the blade atrial septostomy procedure. A: Catheter tip positioned in the left atrium. B: Blade extended. C: Blade is facing anteriorly, inferiorly, and to the left. D: Pullback to the right atrium.

no circumstances should rapid withdrawal be attempted.

Once the blade septostomy catheter has been withdrawn across the interatrial septum, the catheter is advanced to the mid right atrial position and the blade is folded back into the catheter lumen by withdrawing the locking device and blade control wire holder. Although one passage of the blade across the interatrial septum usually suffices, the procedure should be repeated if moderate resistance was encountered during the initial withdrawal. The angulation of the blade should be changed slightly on subsequent withdrawals to ensure adequate incision of the atrial septum. When the interatrial septum is unusually thick and the interatrial opening is very small (< 4 mm in diameter or with a transseptal approach), the first withdrawal of the catheter is done with only a partially extended blade. This is followed by withdrawal with a fully extended blade. This facilitates initial withdrawal of the blade across a thickened interatrial septum and causes less stress on the delicate blade assembly. Using a Rashkind septostomy catheter or a Fogarty septostomy catheter, balloon atrial septostomy is performed to further enlarge the interatrial opening.

Blade atrial septostomy can be performed with a transseptal technique in patients with an intact interatrial septum. The introduction of the long percutaneous sheath has made transseptal blade atrial septostomy possible. (The transseptal technique is described in more detail in Chapter 14.) A long percutaneous transseptal sheath (Mullins transseptal catheter introducer, USCI) is used to introduce the blade catheter into the left atrium. Initially, the long sheath is passed into the left atrium with a Brockenbrough needle and the Mullins introducer set. The introducer sheath can also be used in patients with a restrictive interatrial communication in whom it is difficult to maneuver the stiff blade septostomy catheter into the left atrium (Fig. 5). The long sheath is initially introduced into the left atrium over a regular catheter, which can be more easily

maneuvered (Fig. 5B and 5C). Once the sheath is properly positioned in the left atrium, the catheter is replaced with the blade catheter (Fig. 5D). Before the blade septostomy procedure, the tip of the sheath is withdrawn to the inferior vena cava (Fig. 5E). As the septostomy is performed, the sheath must be withdrawn simultaneously with the blade catheter to prevent possible cutting of the sheath. In a similar manner, balloon atrial septostomy is subsequently performed after repositioning the long sheath in the left atrium (Figs. 5F, 5G, and 5H).

Complications

Major complications have included laceration of the left atrial posterior wall by the blade and a perforation of the right ventricular outflow tract by the catheter tip. Fortunately, these complications have been rare (Park et al. 1982). Seizures have rarely occurred following this procedure, possibly related to blood loss and/or air embolism. Blood loss is no longer a problem since the introduction of sheaths with a bleeding control device. These devices also minimize the risk of air embolism, a potential hazard during cardiac catheterization of patients with cyanotic cardiac malformations.

Prerequisites and Cautions

Because blade atrial septostomy is performed from the femoral approach, bilaterally thrombosed femoral or iliac veins or an absent intrahepatic segment of the inferior vena cava preclude using this technique. A superior vena cava approach has not been attempted. If the left atrium is exceedingly small (< 2 cm in diameter) extension of the blade component may not be feasible since the metal component is 2.5 cm in length. The maximal height of the extended blade of the standard blade septostomy catheter is 12–13 mm. Thus, when the diameter of the interatrial opening is > 10 mm, it is unlikely

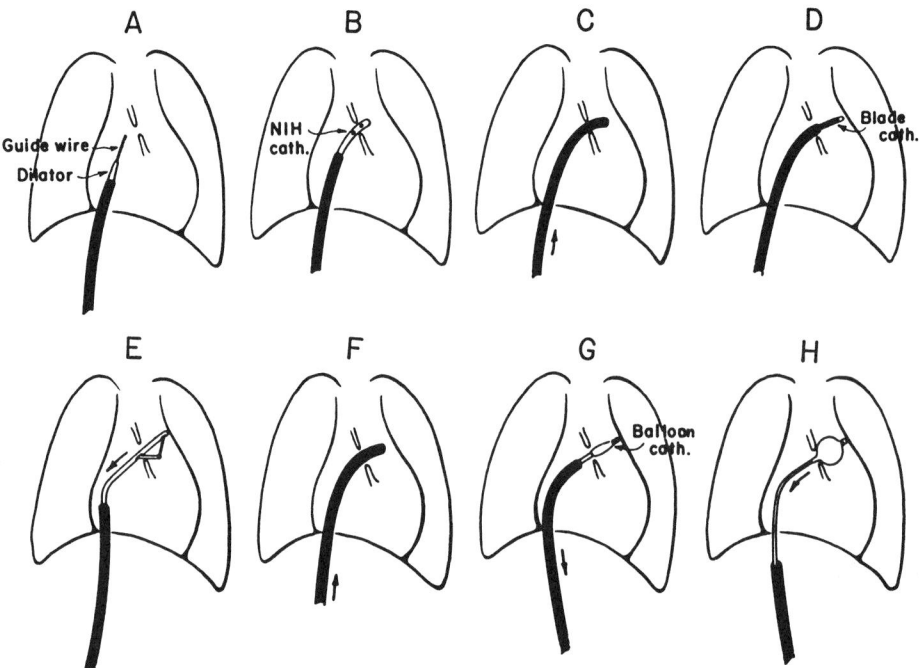

Figure 5. Use of the Mullins transseptal long sheath for blade and balloon atrial septostomy. A: The long sheath is advanced into the right atrium using a guidewire and dilator. B: The preformed NIH catheter is passed into the left atrium. C: The sheath is advanced over the catheter into the left atrium. D: The blade catheter is passed into the left atrium after withdrawal of the NIH catheter. E: Blade atrial septostomy is performed after the sheath has been withdrawn into the inferior vena cava. F: The long sheath is repositioned into the left atrium as in B and C. G: The balloon catheter is positioned in the left atrium. H: Balloon atrial septostomy is performed.

that the blade will effectively engage the interatrial septum. Larger blade catheters have become available and should be used in those patients with a borderline interatrial opening. Generally, several withdrawals of the blade across the interatrial septum with variable angulation of the blade are recommended.

References and Suggested Reading

Allan LD, Leanage R, Wainwright T, et al. Balloon atrial septostomy under two dimensional echocardiographic control. Br Heart J 1982; 4:41–43.

Baker F, Baker L, Zoltun R, Zuberbuhler JR. Ef-fectiveness of the Rashkind procedure in transposition of the great arteries in infants. Circulation 1971; 43 & 44(Suppl I):1–6.

Baker EJ, Allan LD, Tynan MJ, et al. Balloon atrial septostomy in the neonatal intensive care unit. Br Heart J 1984; 51:337–338.

Beitzke A, Suppan CH. Use of prostaglandin E_2 in management of transposition of the great arteries before balloon atrial septostomy. Br Heart J 1983; 49:341–344.

Lin AE, Di Sessa TG, Williams RG. Balloon and blade atrial septostomy facilitated by two-dimensional echocardiography. Am J Cardiol 1986; 57:273–277.

Neches WH, Mullins CE, McNamara DG. Balloon atrial septostomy in congenital heart disease in infancy. Am J Dis Child 1973; 125:371–375.

Newfeld EA, Purcell C, Paul MH, et al. Transumbilical balloon atrial septostomy in 16 infants with transposition of the great arteries. Pediatrics 1974; 54:495–497.

Park SC, Zuberbuhler JR, Neches WH, et al. A new

atrial septostomy technique. Cathet Cardiovasc Diagn 1975; 1:195–201.

Park SC, Neches WH, Zuberbuhler JR, et al. Clinical use of blade atrial septostomy. Circulation 1978; 58:600–606.

Park SC, Neches WH, Mullins CE, et al. Blade atrial septostomy: Collaborative study. Circulation 1982; 66:258–266.

Rashkind WJ, Miller WW. Creation of an atrial septal defect without thoracotomy: Palliative approach to complete transposition of the great arteries. JAMA 1966; 196:991–992.

Rosuin N, Sujov P, Montag J. Transumbilical balloon atrial septostomy for transposition of the great arteries in infants under the age of 60 hours. Am Heart J 1984; 107:174–176.

Steeg CN, Bierman FZ, Hordof AJ, et al. Bedside balloon septostomy in infants with transposition of the great arteries: New concepts using two-dimensional echocardiographic techniques. J Pediatr 1985; 107:944–946.

Weldon CS, Hartmann AF, Jr., Kelly JP. Current management of transposition of the great arteries: Immediate septostomy, occasional prostaglandin infusion, and early Senning operations. Ann Thorac Surg 1983; 36:10–18.

13

Balloon Angioplasty and Valvotomy

José A. Ettedgui, M.D.

Historical Developments

The development and application of balloon angioplasty was pioneered by Gruentzig in the 1970s. Initially, the application of this technique was confined to the treatment of coronary artery disease, but after extensive animal experimentation, it was utilized in the treatment of congenital heart disease. In 1982, Kan and coworkers (Kan et al. 1982) reported the first successful application of percutaneous balloon valvotomy in the treatment of pulmonary valve stenosis. Since then, balloon angioplasty and valvotomy have been used successfully in the treatment of a wide variety of congenital anomalies. These modalities have become the initial treatment of choice in pulmonary valve stenosis and recoarctation of the aorta. The use in lesions such as native coarctation of the aorta, aortic valve stenosis, pulmonary artery stenosis, and other various malformations is still under investigation and in some cases remains controversial. In this chapter, balloon dilation will be used to refer to balloon angioplasty and/or valvotomy.

General Principles

Balloon dilation can be performed by an experienced physician in any well-equipped cardiac catheterization laboratory. Biplane fluoroscopy is desirable, but not essential. At least two experienced operators are required for the dilation procedure. It can be performed safely in the vast majority of patients if the basic principles regarding patient selection, indications, and careful catheterization technique are followed. Although there is always an inherent risk with any invasive therapeutic procedure, meticulous attention to detail will minimize this risk. Complications related to balloon dilation range from transient bradycardia at the time of balloon inflation to patient death. The risks vary with the underlying lesion and will be considered separately.

The basic mechanism of balloon dilation is to produce damage to the abnormal cardiovascular structures, while avoiding damage to normal tissue. This is achieved by the exertion of circumferential and linear wall stress at the site of inflation. When applied to stenotic valves, the predominant effect is splitting of fused commissures (Ettedgui et al. 1987), although on some occasions, the valve leaflets may be torn and/or the valve insertion partially avulsed. When applied to stenotic vessels, balloon dilation produces intimal and medial tears that will then heal in the open position. Even though these techniques have not been employed long enough to compare the long-term results adequately against those of surgical treatment, the intermediate term beneficial effects are comparable.

Procedures

Prior to any balloon dilation procedure, a diagnostic catheterization is required, with accurate hemodynamic and angiographic assessment of the lesion to be dilated. Percutaneous femoral vessel access is preferred since it is much easier to introduce the dilation balloon through this approach than through a cutdown. Angiographic measurements are used for selection of an appropriate size balloon even though accurate echocardiographic measurements can be obtained in patients with aortic and pulmonary valve stenosis. It is important to measure cardiac output before and after balloon dilation to allow proper evaluation of the effectiveness of the procedure. A drop in cardiac output can account for a reduction in the gradient across a dilated lesion and lead to a false interpretation of success. The hemodynamic and angiographic evaluation should also be repeated after dilation. Since the cardiovascular structures at the site of balloon inflation have been weakened by this procedure, this dilated area should never be crossed by an unguided catheter. Failure to observe this principle can lead to cardiac or vascular perforation.

Once the decision to proceed with balloon dilation has been made, there are a series of technical considerations regarding the equipment to be used (Lock 1987; Keane and Lock 1987; Tynan 1988). A wide variety of angioplasty balloons are commercially available and the appropriate device needs to be carefully selected. We have mostly used single-balloon catheters in the treatment of various lesions. However, the large-diameter, single-balloon catheters tend to have a very slow inflation-deflation time. In some lesions, two balloons positioned side by side and inflated simultaneously have been used when a larger dilating area was required. Catheters with two and even three balloons mounted on the same shaft have been designed for this purpose and are mainly used in adults for dilating mitral valve and aortic valve stenosis, respectively. The main concern about the use of multiple balloons is the uneven distribution of wall stress upon inflation. Technological advances in catheter design have led to the

development of larger diameter balloons mounted on smaller shafts. This has particular advantage in the application of dilation techniques to small infants, in addition to reducing the incidence and extent of injury to the vessel through which the balloon catheter has been introduced. The recommended balloon diameter varies according to the lesion that is being dilated and will be addressed separately. It ranges from a diameter smaller than that of the valve ring in aortic stenosis to three to four times the diameter of the narrowed segment in pulmonary artery stenosis. In general, the use of a balloon that is too small will not produce the desired effect, whereas balloons that are too large are more likely to injure normal neighboring structures. The length of the balloon is another important factor. In the majority of lesions, short balloons are preferred. This minimizes the risk of damaging adjacent structures as the inflated balloon straightens. In long, straight vessels and in older children with aortic valve stenosis, longer balloons may be preferred.

Balloon-dilation catheters are delivered to the desired area over a guidewire. Teflon-coated wires with a J tip have a low incidence of vascular injury. Prior to balloon insertion, the wire is anchored in an appropriate position (left pulmonary artery in pulmonary valve stenosis, left ventricular apex in aortic valve stenosis, etc.). The wire is introduced through an end-hole catheter and this catheter is then removed carefully while leaving the guidewire in place. The size of the guidewire will depend on the lumen of the angioplasty catheter that has been selected. In general, the largest diameter wire that will fit should be used. This facilitates manipulation and delivery of the catheter at the desired site together with reducing the risk of causing damage with the catheter tip.

Prior to inserting the balloon catheter, it is advisable to reinfiltrate the groin with 1% lidocaine in order to reduce discomfort. If the arterial approach is being used, we administer 100 units/kg of heparin. Additional sedation may also be required at this point. Our preference is intravenous ketamine (Ketalar) in 1 mg/kg aliquots. Prior to the first bolus of ketamine, a single dose of atropine (10–20 μg/kg) is given to minimize the risk of laryngospasm.

Once the catheter used to position the guidewire and the introducing sheath have been withdrawn, continuous pressure is applied to the puncture site to avoid the development of a large hematoma. Some of the newer angioplasty catheters are mounted on a shaft small enough to allow their introduction and removal through a sheath, thus simplifying this step. The selected balloon catheter is wiped and flushed with a heparinized solution prior to introduction. The balloon may be primed with fluid to minimize the presence of air bubbles before insertion; however, this may increase the difficulty of passage through the skin. Most balloon catheters have a tapered tip, which facilitates introduction. We generally perform a small skin incision of approximately 2–3 mm and dissect the subcutaneous tissue with a hemostat to further aid this process. Occasionally, it is necessary to stretch the femoral vessels with progressively larger dilators before the balloon catheter can be introduced. Continuous rotation of the catheter also eases its passage through the skin and subcutaneous tissue.

The balloon can be flushed free of air after insertion into the femoral vessels, using carbon dioxide initially, followed by a heparinized solution. The catheter is then advanced gently over the guidewire until the radiopaque markers at both ends of the balloon are straddling the narrowed segments. An initial inflation with diluted contrast is performed to assess the appearance of a "waist" (hourglass-like narrowing) on the balloon produced by the stenotic segment. Ideally, the catheter should be positioned so that the waist is located over the central portion of the balloon, the area in which the maximum inflation diameter is achieved. The highest recommended inflation pressures vary with the type of balloon that is used. A special pressure gauge should be used to monitor these pressures and this gauge is interposed between a syringe filled with diluted contrast and the port connecting to the balloon. In general, the balloon is inflated until the maximal pressure is achieved or until the waist is obliterated. Even though current angioplasty catheters are designed so that the balloons tear longitudinally rather than circumferentially, care should be taken to avoid overinflation and bursting. Inflation/deflation cycles of 10–20 sec are safe and effective in most lesions. Usually, it is the first inflation that produces the greatest therapeutic effect; however two to three inflations are generally performed.

Following balloon dilation, the angioplasty catheter is removed, taking care not to dislodge the guidewire. The balloon needs to be fully deflated in order to withdraw it through the skin. Continuous catheter rotation in the same direction used for introduction, together with sustained negative pressure on the balloon, may facilitate this process. Firm pressure on the puncture site in the groin is required to avoid hematoma formation. A valved sheath of the same diameter as the shaft of the angioplasty catheter (to avoid excessive bleeding from the puncture site) is then advanced over the guidewire along with an end-hole catheter. The catheter is then advanced to the angioplasty site and a repeat hemodynamic and angiographic evaluation are performed. As mentioned earlier, the site of balloon inflation should never be crossed with an unguided catheter (except during withdrawal) to avoid perforation of the weakened area. At the end of the procedure, the catheter and sheath are removed and hemostasis is achieved by firm pressure on the puncture site in the groin. Afterwards, we routinely apply a pressure dressing over this area. The majority of patients return directly to their room and are discharged the following day. Intensive care monitoring is not usually necessary.

Pulmonary Valve Stenosis

Balloon valvotomy has become the initial treatment of choice for "typical" pulmonary valve stenosis. It produces effective relief of the stenosis in the majority of patients with this lesion and has been used in all age groups, from newborns to adults. The "ideal" valve for balloon valvotomy has relatively thin, mobile leaflets that dome during systole. On auscultation, these patients usually have an ejection click. In these patients, stenosis is mainly due to fused commissures, that are split by balloon dilation. In pulmonary valve dysplasia, stenosis is due to thick, immobile pulmonary valve leaflets rather than to commissural fusion. In these patients, balloon valvotomy usually is not effective.

Procedure

A diagnostic catheterization is performed for hemodynamic evaluation of the severity of the pulmonary stenosis. We favor introducing a cannula in the femoral artery for comparison of right ventricular pressure to systemic pressure as well as for monitoring the systemic pressure throughout the inflation/deflation cycle. There are no established guidelines as to when pulmonary valvotomy should be performed. We proceed with balloon dilation if the right ventricular pressure is more than two-thirds of the systemic pressure or if the gradient across the pulmonary valve is greater than 40 mm Hg. Right ventricular cineangiography is performed to evaluate the anatomy of the pulmonary valve as well as to establish the presence of other potential areas of obstruction. The pulmonary valve "ring" is measured from the lateral projection of the right ventricular angiogram at the level of insertion of the valve leaflets (Fig. 1). This measurement can also be obtained echocardiographically.

Once the decision for balloon dilation is made, an appropriate size angioplasty catheter is selected. In the early days, an angioplasty catheter with a balloon diameter 1–2 mm smaller than the pulmonary valve ring was used. The general experience has been that larger diameter balloons produce more effective dilation and can be employed

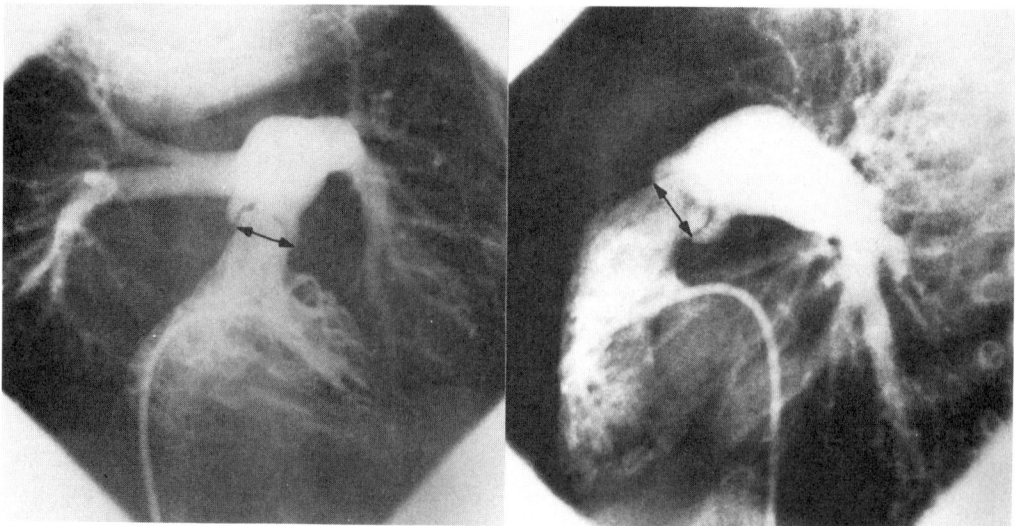

Figure 1. Measurement of the pulmonary valve annulus from a right ventricular angiogram. Left: Anteroposterior view. Right: Lateral view.

safely. Therefore, a catheter (or combination of two catheters) with a balloon diameter between 20% and 40% larger than the pulmonary valve ring is currently recommended (Radtke et al. 1988). When a second balloon catheter is used, it is introduced through the contralateral femoral vein. The use of two catheters in tandem tends to be very awkward. However, two balloons can be inflated and deflated more rapidly than a single balloon of equivalent effective diameter. Also, the smaller diameter balloon catheters have smaller shafts, thus minimizing vascular trauma. Catheters with short balloon lengths are preferred in order to reduce the potential damage to the pulmonary artery bifurcation distally or to the tricuspid valve proximally by the ends of the balloon as it straightens with inflation.

The groin is reinfiltrated with 1% lidocaine and additional intravenous sedation is given if necessary. We also administer 100% oxygen through a face mask. An end-hole catheter is positioned in a branch pulmonary artery and a heavy gauge (0.035- to 0.038-inch diameter) exchange guidewire is anchored in a stable position. The right and left lower lobe arteries provide the most stable wire placement. In the newborn, it may be difficult to enter the branch pulmonary arteries and the wire may have to be passed through the ductus arteriosus into the descending aorta. In these infants, with critical pulmonary stenosis, patency of the ductus arteriosus is usually being maintained with intravenous prostaglandin E_1. The catheter and sheath are carefully removed, while ensuring that the guidewire remains in the desired position. The selected angioplasty catheter is flushed, wiped, and introduced in the femoral vein. The balloon is freed of air bubbles. The catheter is then advanced gently over the guidewire until the radiopaque markers on either side of the balloon are straddling the position of the pulmonary valve (Fig. 2). In some patients, it is difficult to manipulate the stiff balloon catheter from the right atrium to the desired position in the right ventricular outflow tract. A combination of clockwise rotation, while advancing the catheter along with gentle withdrawal of the guidewire, may allow adequate positioning. On occasion, the catheter is too large to pass through the stenotic pulmonary valve orifice. In these cases, initial dilation with a smaller diameter balloon may be necessary before the desired diameter balloon catheter can be used. Upon obtaining a satisfactory position, the balloon is inflated until the waist produced by the stenotic valve is obliterated (Fig. 2). Several inflation/deflation cycles of 10- to 20-sec duration are usually performed. The balloon needs to be fully deflated and withdrawn slightly into the right ventricle between inflations in order to avoid prolonged occlusion of pulmonary blood flow. With an adequate inflation, there is a transient reflex bradycardia with reduction in systemic blood pressure that resolves with balloon deflation. Interestingly, the degree of bradycardia is much less in patients with a foramen ovale, presumably as a result of decompression of the right atrium.

Following balloon valvotomy, the catheter is withdrawn, while leaving the guidewire in position. An end-hole catheter is advanced over the guidewire to the distal pulmonary artery, and a withdrawal pressure recording across the pulmonary valve is performed to assess the residual gradient. An angiographic catheter is then used for a repeat right ventricular angiogram to exclude extravasation of contrast material as well as to determine any angiographic changes of the pulmonary valve.

The care post-balloon pulmonary valvotomy does not differ from that of other cardiac catheterizations and most patients are discharged the following day.

Complications

Complications related to balloon pulmonary valvotomy are isolated and are rarely serious. Deaths related to this procedure have not been reported. Inflation of

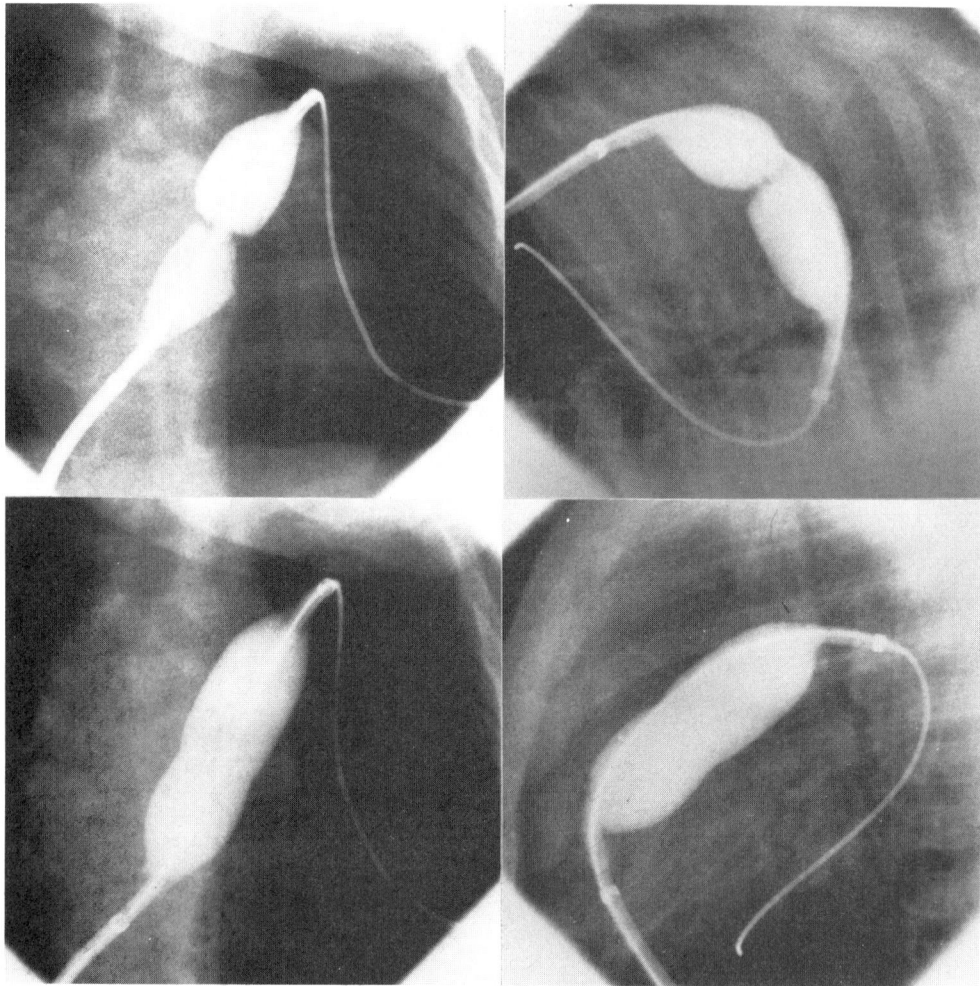

Figure 2. Dilation of valvar pulmonary stenosis. Left: Anteroposterior view. Right: Lateral view. Top: Balloon catheter inflated, showing the "waist" indentation at the level of the pulmonary valve. Bottom: Balloon catheter maximally inflated with disappearance of the waist.

the balloon usually produces a transient hypotensive and bradycardic response that disappears with balloon deflation. This is due to the transient interruption of pulmonary blood flow and is presumably accompanied by a vagal reflex. Transient loss of consciousness and convulsions have also been reported. Other complications such as reactive infundibular outflow tract obstruction and supravalvar stenosis secondary to hematoma formation in the pulmonary artery have been described. Pulmonary insufficiency is a common finding following valvotomy but is rarely of any clinical significance.

Critical Pulmonary Stenosis in the Newborn

Balloon valvotomy has been used effectively in the treatment of severe pulmonary stenosis in newborns. In some of these infants, right ventricular pressure may be at suprasystemic level. Patency of the ductus arteriosus usually is maintained by intravenous administration of prostaglandin E_1. Occasionally, the ductus arteriosus is widely patent and the pulmonary artery pressure is equal to the aortic pressure. As a result, in these latter patients, there may be no gradient across the pulmonary valves, and the decision to proceed with valvotomy may depend on the angiographic appearance of the valve.

There are several variations to the valvotomy technique that can be applied in this subgroup of patients (Tynan 1988). In some patients, it may prove very difficult to cross the stenotic pulmonary valve. Steerable guidewires may be particularly useful for this purpose. The presence of a widely patent ductus arteriosus often makes it difficult to manipulate an end-hole catheter into a branch pulmonary artery. We have performed pulmonary valvotomy effectively and safely with the guidewire positioned in the descending aorta through the ductus arteriosus. In this situation, care must be taken to avoid inflating the balloon within the duct itself. An angioplasty catheter with as short a balloon as possible should be employed. Assessment of initial success may be difficult since there may be little change in the pressures. However, antegrade flow across the right ventricular outflow tract improves leading to an increase in systemic oxygenation. Occasionally, patients have subsequently required ductal ligation because of heart failure secondary to excessive pulmonary blood flow. In some patients, the appropriate size dilation balloon may be too large to fit across the stenotic valve. Therefore, initial dilation with a small-diameter balloon will allow introduction of the desired diameter balloon catheter.

Although the results of balloon valvotomy are not as good in neonates with critical pulmonary stenosis compared to the results obtained in older children, it is certainly a therapeutic option in these seriously ill, cyanotic newborns.

Aortic Valve Stenosis

Balloon dilation has been used in the treatment of aortic valve stenosis. The results are less satisfactory than in children with pulmonary valve stenosis and the procedure is, at best, palliative. It carries a higher morbidity and mortality and is technically more demanding. Some patients have developed significant aortic regurgitation that has led to urgent valve replacement, and several deaths have been reported (Keane and Lock 1987; Sholler et al. 1988).

Procedure

A left-heart catheterization is performed for hemodynamic and angiographic assessment of the severity of the aortic stenosis. The left ventricle can be entered antegradely across the atrial septum and through the mitral valve or retrogradely across the stenotic aortic valve. The antegrade approach requires the presence of a patent foramen ovale or a transseptal puncture. We only recommend balloon valvotomy if the severity of the obstruction would otherwise require surgical treatment. The operating room is on standby throughout the procedure, and at least two units of blood are available for transfusion. The patient must have secure venous access as well as a separate monitoring line in the femoral artery. All patients are given 100 units/ kg of heparin.

Once the decision is made to proceed with balloon valvotomy, an appropriate size catheter is selected. The diameter of the dilation balloon should not exceed that of the aortic valve ring. We prefer a balloon with a diameter 1 mm smaller than the aortic annulus. The annulus can be measured from the left ventricular angiogram or from an echocardiogram. Balloons with a diameter larger than the annulus can severely disrupt the aortic valve or tear a leaflet, leading to severe aortic regurgitation.

Most of the experience with balloon aortic valvotomy is with the retrograde approach. An end-hole catheter is advanced into the left ventricle across the aortic valve, and a heavy-gauge (0.035–inch), J-tipped, Teflon-coated, exchange-length guidewire is introduced. The guidewire can be curled in the apex of the left ventricle and serves to provide a stiffer support for the balloon catheter. The end-hole catheter and the introducing sheath are removed while maintaining the guidewire in a stable position in the left ventricular apex. Firm pressure on the puncture site in the groin is required to avoid hematoma formation while the catheters are being exchanged. The balloon catheter is flushed and wiped prior to introduction. The balloon is then flushed free of air using carbon dioxide or dilute contrast. The catheter is advanced over the guidewire and positioned with the balloon straddling the aortic valve. In smaller children, adequate positioning can be difficult due to the tight curve around the aortic arch. Gentle, slight withdrawal of the guidewire while rotating and advancing the catheter is often useful. Adequate positioning of the balloon is ascertained by the presence of a balloon waist upon gentle inflation with dilute contrast. A rapid inflation/deflation cycle of 10–15 sec is performed with obliteration of the waist being the desired effect (Fig. 3). Left ventricular contractions tend to eject the inflated balloon, and therefore, firm forward pressure of the catheter is required to counteract this and to keep the balloon in the proper position across the valve. In this particular situation, the use of longer balloons can be advantageous. On the other hand, the longer balloons tend to have a slower inflation/deflation time. As in pulmonary valvotomy, the actual number of inflations required to adequately relieve the obstruction is not known, but we usually perform two to three inflations.

After completion of a series of inflation/deflations, if the waist lesion is obliterated using an appropriate size balloon, then an effective result can be anticipated. The angioplasty catheter is exchanged for an end-hole catheter through a valved sheath, taking care not to dislodge the guidewire. The

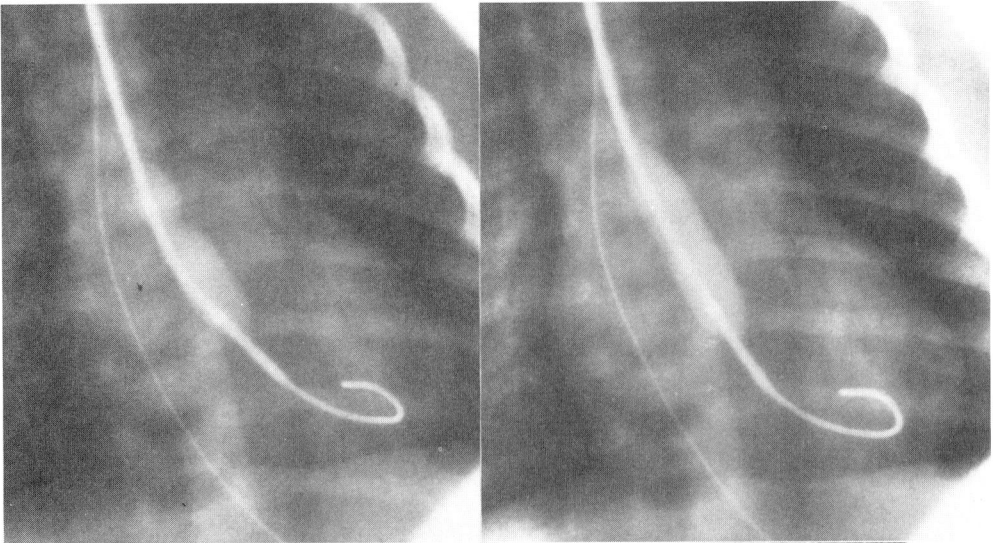

Figure 3. Balloon dilation of valvar aortic stenosis in the newborn (carotid approach). Left: Balloon catheter inflated, showing the "waist" indentation at the level of the aortic valve. Right: Balloon catheter inflated with disappearance of the waist.

left ventricular pressure following valvotomy can be compared to the femoral artery pressure, and if the gradient has not been effectively reduced, a repeat series of dilations with a larger diameter balloon can be considered. We emphasize avoiding the use of balloons with a diameter larger than the aortic annulus. A left ventriculogram may be repeated, but is not essential. Withdrawal pressures are obtained from the left ventricle to the ascending aorta, and an aortogram is performed to assess the presence and severity of aortic insufficiency. We prefer to use an NIH angiographic catheter to avoid the possibility that the sharp tip of the pigtail might damage the dilated area. It is useful to measure cardiac output before and after valvotomy to determine the effect of changes in output on the residual gradient. All catheters and sheaths are removed upon completion of the procedure, and patients do not leave the catheterization laboratory until hemostasis has been achieved. A pressure dressing is applied to the groin, and the patients return to their room. Intensive care monitoring is usually not required. Apart from those with loss of femoral pulses, the majority of patents are discharged the following day.

Complications

As mentioned earlier, morbidity and mortality related to balloon aortic valvotomy are much higher than for pulmonary valvotomy. Deaths related to severe disruption of the valvar apparatus with acute aortic insufficiency and aortic wall tears have been reported. Some patients develop significant aortic insufficiency and require valve replacement. Ventricular arrhythmias requiring cardioversion and varying degrees of atrioventricular block can also occur. Damage to the femoral artery leading to transient, or occasionally permanent, loss of femoral pulses is a well-recognized complication and is initially treated with intravenous heparin. The availability of lower pro-

file catheters with larger diameter dilating balloons, mounted on smaller shafts, should reduce the incidence of many of these complications.

Critical Aortic Stenosis in the Newborn

Newborns with critical aortic stenosis have a very high surgical mortality. Balloon valvotomy in this group has had varying degrees of success when the conventional femoral artery approach has been used. The major difficulty is related to manipulation of the angioplasty catheter around the aortic arch and into the left ventricle. Intraoperative balloon valvotomy through an apical left ventriculotomy has also been attempted. In a small series of these patients, we have overcome the problems of catheter manipulation around the arch and through the aortic valve by performing balloon dilation through a right carotid artery cutdown (Fischer et al. 1989). The babies are intubated and ventilated throughout the catheterization procedure. A #6 French valved sheath is introduced into the right carotid artery by surgical cutdown and advanced to the aortic arch. Through this sheath, an end-hole catheter can be easily advanced across the aortic valve into the left ventricle. A long, heavy-gauge, J-tipped guidewire is curled in the apex of the left ventricle, and the catheter is removed and replaced with a balloon catheter. Catheters with up to an 8-mm diameter balloon mounted on a #5 French shaft (Meditech) are currently available. These catheters have the advantage that they can be introduced and withdrawn through a #6 French sheath. Balloon dilation is performed as described for the femoral approach (Fig. 3).

Following valvotomy, the sheath in the carotid artery is removed and the arteriotomy repaired. In the five patients in whom this approach has been used, effective relief of the gradient was obtained in four. There have not been any neurologic complications and the only perioperative death occurred in an infant with very poor left ventricular systolic function.

Coarctation of the Aorta

Balloon angioplasty for the treatment of native coarctation of the aorta remains a highly controversial topic. In neonates and infants in whom isthmal hypoplasia is a common component of the coarctation syndrome, the likelihood of balloon angioplasty being successful is very low. The development of aortic aneurysms at the site of balloon angioplasty is a recognized complication. In general, we do not recommend this technique for the treatment of native coarctation of the aorta, since surgical results are better in the vast majority of patients. However, there may be a place for balloon angioplasty as a subset of this group. On the other hand, some centers advocate the use of balloon dilation as the initial treatment of native coarctation and have reported good results.

The technique for balloon angioplasty in unoperated coarctation of the aorta is very similar to that in other vessels (Lock, 1987). A diagnostic left heart catheterization is performed for hemodynamic and angiographic assessment. All patients receive 100 units/kg of heparin. A monitoring line is placed in the contralateral femoral artery and secure venous access is obtained. The narrowest portion of the coarctation is measured from the aortogram and a catheter with a balloon 2.5 to 3 times the diameter of the narrowest portion is selected. An exchange guidewire is positioned in the ascending aorta, and the end-hole catheter and sheath are exchanged for the angioplasty catheter. The balloon is flushed free of air after introduction into the femoral artery in order to minimize the possibility of air embolization. The balloon is positioned so that it is straddling the narrowest segment guided by the presence of a waist upon gentle inflations of the balloon with dilute contrast. Upon obtaining a satisfactory position, a full inflation to the maximum recommended pressure is performed with a 10- to 20-sec inflation/deflation cycle. It is advisable to withdraw the catheter into the descending aorta to avoid occlusion of systemic blood flow between inflations. The number of inflations is variable and the end point is complete obliteration of the waist (Fig. 4). A non-pigtail angiographic catheter, along with a valved sheath, is then exchanged for the angioplasty catheter. Pressures proximal to the coarctation can be compared to those recorded through the distal monitoring line. A postdilation aortogram is obtained, and pullback pressures across the dilated segment are recorded. At the end of the procedure, firm pressure on the groin is required to prevent development of a hematoma. Damage to the femoral artery with transient or permanent loss of the pulses are recognized complications.

The use of balloon angioplasty for the treatment of recoarctation of the aorta following previous surgical coarctectomy is less controversial. It is the preferred treatment modality when restenosis occurs. It appears to be more successful when the initial operation has been a primary resection with end-to-end anastomosis rather than a subclavian flap repair. The technique is identical to that described above except that the recommended balloon diameter is up to twice that of aorta proximal to the obstruction.

Pulmonary Artery Stenosis

Balloon dilation has been used for the treatment of congenital as well as acquired branch pulmonary artery stenosis (Ring et al. 1985). The underlying anatomy is usually a combination of pulmonary artery hypoplasia with multiple stenotic segments. This treatment modality has a low success rate (50%–60%) and a mortality of approximately 2%. This combination is conducive

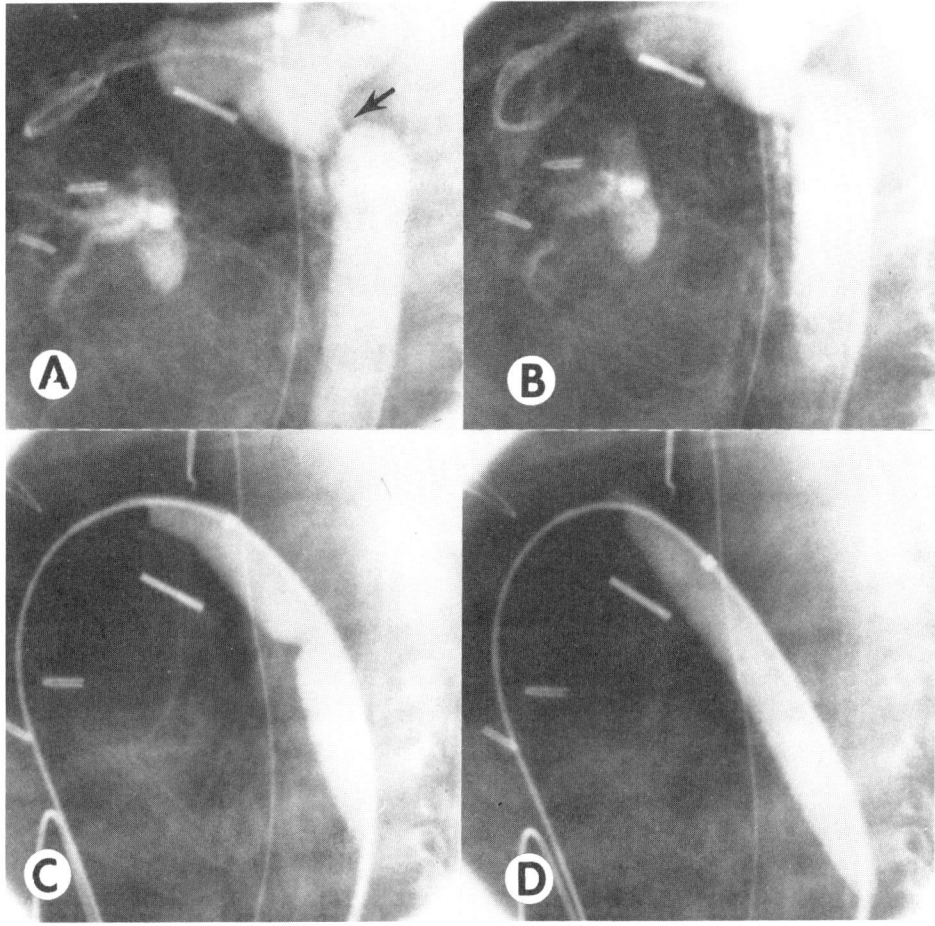

Figure 4. Balloon dilation of coarctation of the aorta. A: Angiogram in the lateral view demonstrating a recurrent coarctation (arrow). B: Angiogram following balloon dilation demonstrating increased diameter of the aortic segment. C: Balloon catheter inflated, showing "waist" indentation at the site of the coarcted segment. D: Balloon catheter inflated with disappearance of the waist.

towards careful patient selection. It has the advantage over surgery in that distal lesions as well as multiple stenoses are amenable to treatment. In many patients, it is the only available therapeutic modality.

A diagnostic right heart catheterization is performed. The pressure in the pulmonary artery proximal to the obstruction should be significantly elevated and close to, or above, systemic levels before balloon dilation is considered. Since pulmonary artery stenoses tend to be multiple, selective injections in the vessels that are going to be dilated

are necessary. For this same reason, reduction in proximal pulmonary artery and right ventricular pressures are not suitable indicators for success. The main criteria for success is an increase in the diameter of the stenotic vessel by at least 50%. The most severe and distal lesions should be attempted first. Extreme care should be taken not to recross a balloon-dilated area with an unguided catheter if more than one lesion is to be dilated in the same session. The diameter of the angioplasty balloon should be three to four times that of the stenotic seg-

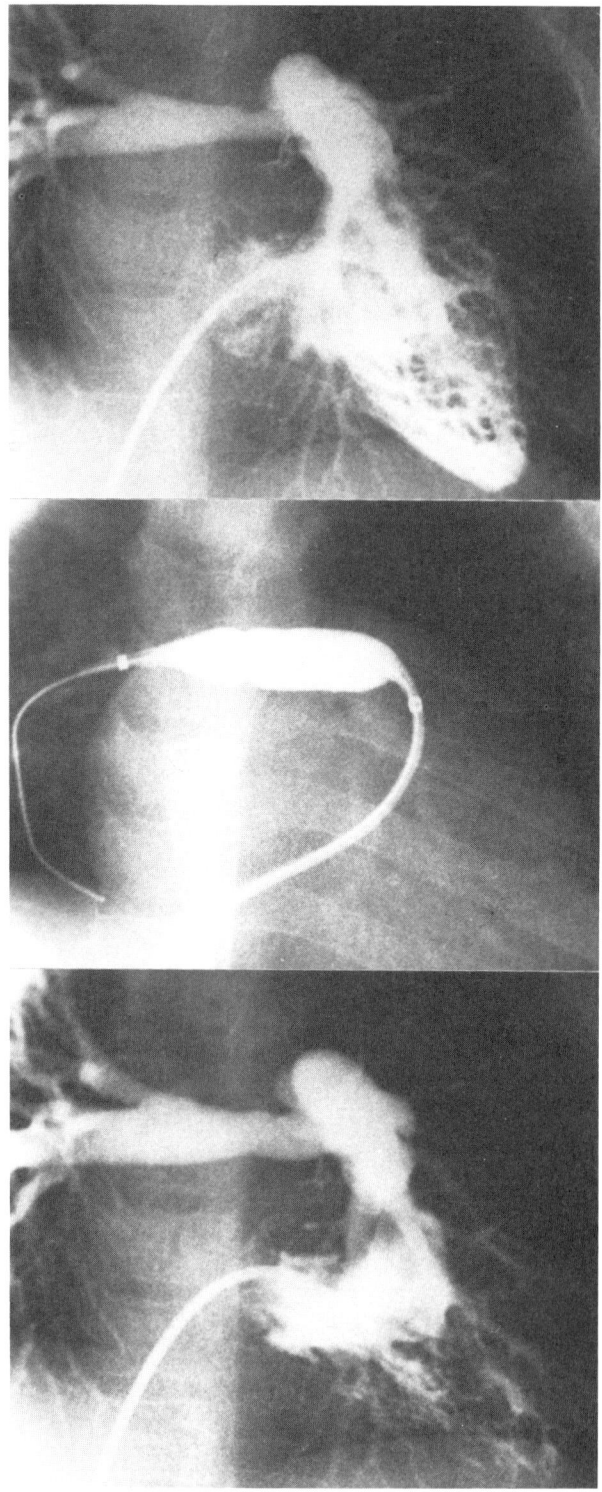

Figure 5. Balloon dilation of pulmonary artery stenosis. (Top): Right ventricular angiogram demonstrating right pulmonary artery stenosis (arrows). (Middle): Balloon catheter inflated, showing the "waist" indentation at the site of pulmonary artery stenosis. (Bottom): Angiogram following balloon dilation, demonstrating increased diameter of the stenotic segment.

ment, but not to exceed twice the diameter of the normal pulmonary artery on each end of the obstruction (Fig. 5). Since these lesions are more rigid, higher inflation pressures are required. Only a small portion of the pulmonary vasculature is occluded during each inflation and therefore these are well tolerated.

The main complications related to balloon pulmonary arterioplasty are pulmonary artery thrombosis, rupture, or aneurysm formation at the site of angioplasty.

Mitral Valve Stenosis

Percutaneous balloon mitral valvotomy is an experimental procedure. It has been used for the treatment of rheumatic mitral stenosis and in isolated cases of congenital mitral stenosis (Kveselis et al. 1986). This procedure requires large-diameter dilation balloons. This can be achieved with single-balloon catheters, catheters with two balloons mounted on the same shaft, or with two separate single-balloon catheters. The most common approach is antegrade from the femoral vein through a transseptal atrial puncture. An end-hole catheter is introduced in the long transseptal sheath and advanced across the mitral valve. A heavy-gauge exchange guidewire is then positioned in the apex of the left ventricle, but some investigators advance it across the aortic valve into the ascending aorta. Dilation of the atrial septum with a smaller angioplasty catheter may be required to allow passage of the desired diameter balloon catheter. There are no clear indications as to when balloon mitral valvoplasty should be performed or what diameter balloon should be used. This procedure should be limited to patients with severe stenosis and only minimal, if any, regurgitation. Most investigators recommend that the balloon diameter not exceed that of the mitral valve ring. Although uncommon, significant mitral regurgitation can occur. An atrial septal de-

fect as a result of dilation of the atrial septum is a recognized complication.

Miscellaneous Lesions

A wide variety of congenital and acquired obstructed lesions have been treated with balloon dilation. These include systemic venous obstructions following atrial redirection operations for transposition of the great arteries, stenotic Blalock-Taussig shunts (Fischer et al. 1985), bioprosthetic valves, etc. Angioplasty of stenotic pulmonary veins has been attempted unsuccessfully, and in many centers, this lesion is not considered suitable for balloon dilation.

References and Suggested Reading

Ettedgui JA, Ho SY, Tynan MJ, Jones ODH, Martin RP, Baker EJ, Reidy Jr. The pathology of balloon pulmonary valvoplasty. Int J Cardiol 1987; 16:285–294.

Fischer DR, Park SC, Neches WH, Beerman LB, Fricker FJ, Mathews RA, Zuberbuhler JR, Wedemeyer AL. Successful dilation of a stenotic Blalock-Taussig anastomosis by percutaneous transluminal balloon angioplasty. Am J Cardiol 1985; 55:861–862.

Fischer DR, Ettedgui JA, Siewers RD, Park SC. Carotid arterial approach for balloon valvotomy of aortic stenosis in neonates (Abstr). Am J Cardiol 1989; 64:421.

Kan SS, White RI, Mitchell SE, Gardner TJ. Percutaneous balloon valvuloplasty: A new method for treating congenital pulmonary valve stenosis. New Engl J Med 1982; 307:540–542.

Keane JF, Lock JE. Catheter intervention: Balloon valvotomy. In: Lock JE, Keane JF, Fellows KE (eds), Diagnostic and Interventional Catheterization in Congenital Heart Disease. Boston, MA, Nijhoff. 1987, pp 111–122.

Kveselis DA, Rocchini AP, Beekman R, Snider AR, Crowley D, Dick M, Rosenthal A. Balloon angioplasty for congenital and rheumatic mitral stenosis. Am J Cardiol 1986; 57:348–350.

Lock JE. Catheter intervention: Balloon angioplasty. In: Lock JE, Keane JF, Fellows KE (eds), Diagnostic and Interventional Catheterization in Congenital Heart Disease. Boston, MA, Nijhoff. 1987, pp 91–110.

Lock JE, Bass JL, Amplantz K, Castaneda Zuniga WR. Balloon dilation angioplasty of coarctations in infants and children. Circulation 1983; 68:109–116.

Radtke W, Keane JF, Fellows KE, Lang P, Lock JE. Percutaneous balloon valvotomy of congenital pulmonary stenosis using oversized balloons. J Am Coll Cardiol 1986; 8:909–915.

Ring JC, Bass JL, Marvin W, Fuhrman BP, Kulik TJ, Foker JE, Lock JE. Management of congenital branch pulmonary artery stenosis with balloon dilation angioplasty. Report of 52 procedures. J Thorac Cardiovasc Surg 1985; 90:35–45.

Sholler GF, Keane JF, Perry SB, Sanders SP, Lock JE. Balloon dilation of congenital aortic valve stenosis. Results and influence of technical and morphological features on outcome. Circulation 1988; 78:351–360.

Tynan M. Balloon angioplasty in congenital heart disease. Herz 1988; 13:59–70.

14

Special Procedures

Sang C. Park, M.D.

Transseptal Catheterization

Since the initial introduction of transseptal left heart catheterization technique by Cope and Ross et al.—independently—in 1959, the procedure has been used primarily in adult cardiac catheterization. In recent years, however, the technique has begun to be used more frequently in the pediatric patient as well (Duff and Mullins 1978). This technique provides access to the left atrium and from the left atrium to the left ventricle in the presence of an intact interatrial septum. Transthoracic needle puncture of the left ventricle or transbronchial puncture of a left atrium via the bronchoscope are historically interesting techniques that are no longer in use.

Indications

The most common indication for transseptal cardiac catheterization is lack of another, easier access to the left ventricle, as in patients with severe aortic stenosis or prosthetic aortic valve, or in patients with severe coarctation of the aorta who have no suitable artery in the right arm. It is useful in the rare pediatric patient with mitral stenosis or with pulmonary vein stenosis.

As a result of the orientation of the atrial septum, transseptal catheterization is done from an inferior approach. Therefore, certain venous anomalies, such as absent inferior vena cava with azygos continuation to the superior vena cava or bilateral ileofe-moral or inferior vena caval thrombosis, make such an approach impossible. Other relative contraindications that make transseptal catheterization more difficult or dangerous include severe scoliosis, rotational anomalies of the heart, a very small left atrium, or suspected left atrial thrombosis or tumor. A large left aortic root or a large atrium also increases the risk of transseptal catheterization. Anticoagulation is another relative contraindication.

Equipment

Both Ross and Brockenbrough transseptal needles are used for transseptal catheterization, but the former is very stiff and is difficult to use in the pediatric age group. Brockenbrough needles are more suitable in pediatric practice and are available in two different sizes. The adult Brockenbrough transseptal needle is 71 cm long and has an 18-gauge shaft tipped with a 15-mm long, 21-gauge needle. The proximal portion of the needle is attached by an arrow-shaped metal flange that points in the same direction as the needle curve (Fig. 1). The children's size is 56 cm long and has a 19-gauge shaft with a 22-gauge needle. Two different types of transseptal catheters are available for use with the transseptal needles. A #8.5 French, 69-cm long, Teflon catheter is used in conjunction with the adult type of needle and a #7 French, 55-cm long catheter with the pediatric needle. These transseptal catheters have an end hole and multiple side holes. There is a simple flange without the usual

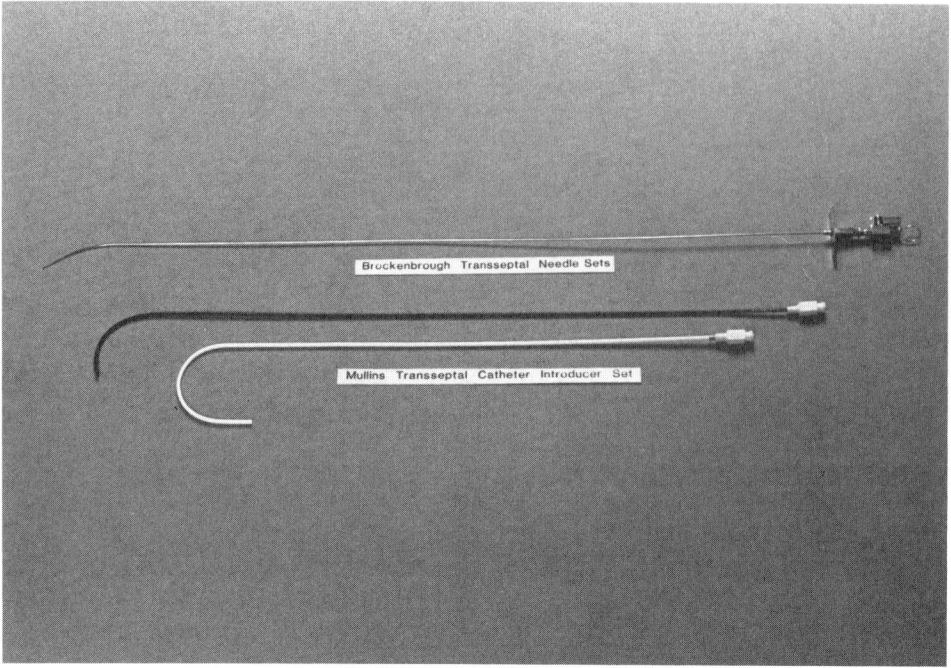

Figure 1. Transseptal catheterization set.

metal hub on the proximal end of the catheter and a special adaptor (male and female metal portions) is necessary to form a hub. The distal portion of the catheter is shortened to facilitate passage into the left ventricle and is available with a number of different radii. The distal curve ranges from 2–3.5 cm in adult catheters and from 1.5–2 cm in the pediatric catheters. A curved #3 French Brockenbrough tip occluder is available for occluding the catheter tip hole during angiographic studies and is also useful in positioning the catheter in the left atrium. In our laboratory, we use the Mullins transseptal catheter introducer set (USCI) exclusively. This provides a long sheath to enable introduction of a variety of catheters and devices transseptally (Fig. 2). These are available in 44- and 59-cm lengths and in sizes #6 to #8 French.

Preparation

Patients must be adequately sedated for transseptal catheterization. Routine pre-medication (meperidine hydrochloride 2 mg/kg, promethazine 0.5 mg/kg, and chlorpromazine 0.5 mg/kg) is used, and in addition, the patient often receives ketamine hydrochloride 1 mg/kg intravenously just prior to the procedure. If ketamine is used, atropine or scopolamine are given prior to its administration to prevent laryngeal spasm.

Selective biplane right ventriculography or a pulmonary arteriogram is routinely performed prior to transseptal catheterization to evaluate the left atrium, left ventricle, and aorta. The size and location of the left atrium is of particular importance. A small amount of contrast should also be injected in the left innominate vein to rule out a persistent left superior vena cava draining to the coronary sinus.

If the patient's weight is more than 20–25 kg (usually over 7 years of age), an adult needle and catheter are used. In smaller children, pediatric sets are employed. After the appropriate catheter and needle are selected, they are assembled to be sure the catheter is the appropriate length for the

the direction of the metal arrow. The catheter tip is threaded through the female adapter.

Introduction of the Catheter

The sequence of transseptal puncture technique is demonstrated in Figure 3. (The numbers in parenthesis in the following paragraphs refer to the numbered sequences in the figure.) The catheter used for the right heart catheterization is withdrawn and the dilator is replaced in the sheath. A 125-cm long, 0.035-inch, coil-spring guidewire with a flexible tip is advanced into the high superior vena cava (1), and then the sheath and dilator are withdrawn. The transseptal catheter is passed over the guidewire to the high superior vena cava (2), and the guidewire is removed. After placing the male adapter over the female adapter, the catheter is aspirated to eliminate bubbles and clots within the catheter. The transseptal needle is filled with heparinized solution, and the stylet is inserted. The needle with the stylet is advanced into the catheter until it is positioned about 1 cm before the catheter tip (3). The needle is allowed to rotate spontaneously as it advances to avoid perforation of the catheter wall or damage to the needle tip. The stylet is removed and the needle is then attached to the pressure transducer using flexible connecting tubing. The stopcock is opened and the pressure tracing is observed.

Puncture of the Interatrial Septum

The needle and catheter together are gradually withdrawn inferiorly (4) while the needle tip is directed posteromedially, 45° to 65° from the horizontal plane (Fig. 4). Upon entering the right atrium, some atrial arrhythmia is usually seen. The operator will often notice a sensation of the catheter slipping medially as the catheter tip engages the fossa ovalis. If no such sensation is felt, other landmarks should be used. The ideal puncture site in the interatrial septum corre-

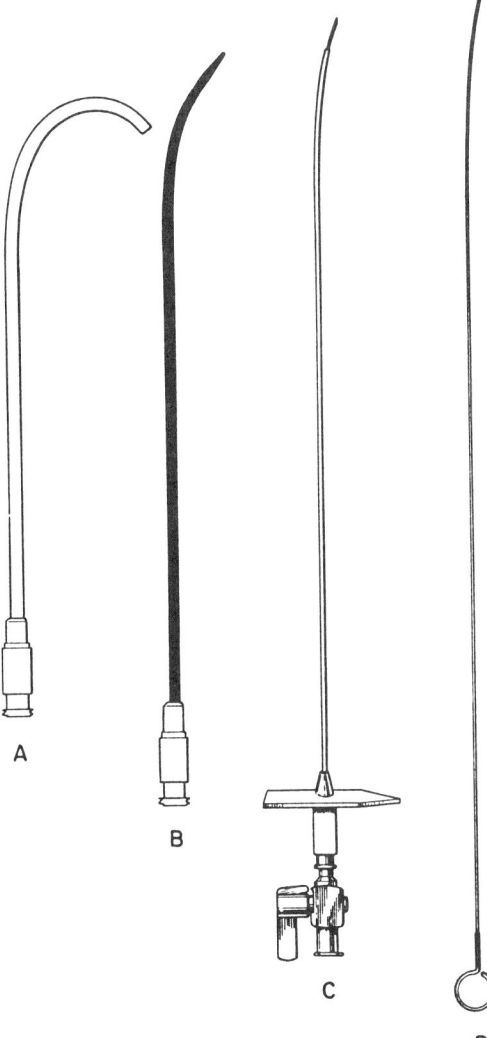

Figure 2. Transseptal catheterization set diagram. A: Mullins long sheath. B: Mullins sheath introducer/dilator. C: Brockenbrough needle. D: Stylet for Brockenbrough needle.

needle. The distance between the proximal end of the catheter and the metallic arrow is noted, first with the needle tip just inside the catheter tip and then with the needle fully exposed outside of the catheter tip. The distance should be gauged by finger width of the operator so that this distance can be maintained during the procedure without the need to watch the proximal end of the catheter. The needle curve is matched with

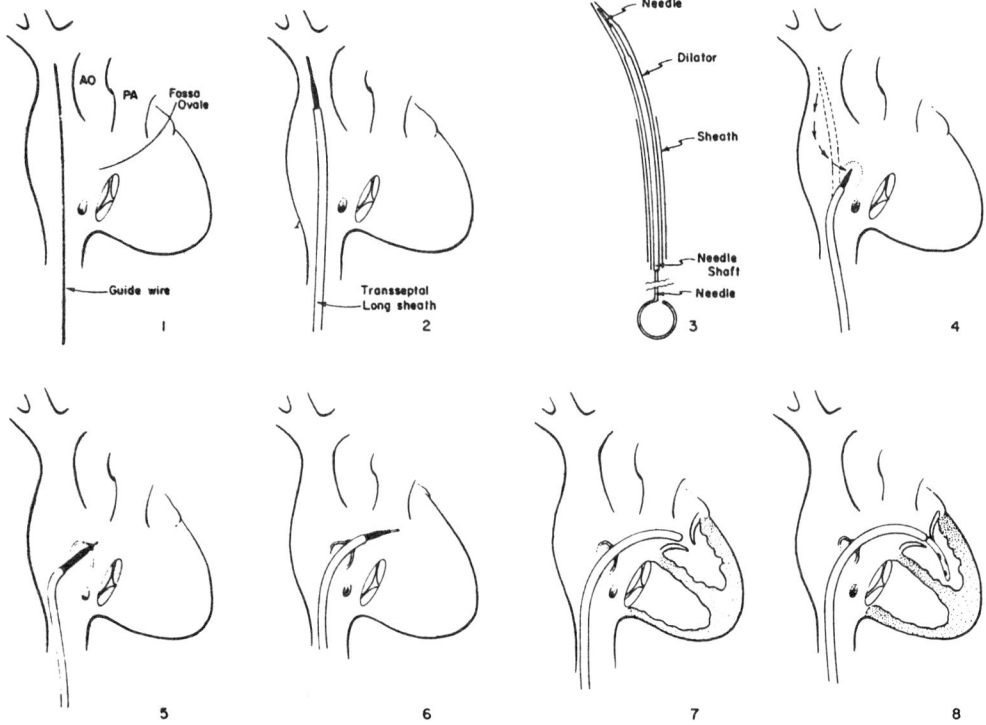

Figure 3. Transseptal puncture technique (see text).

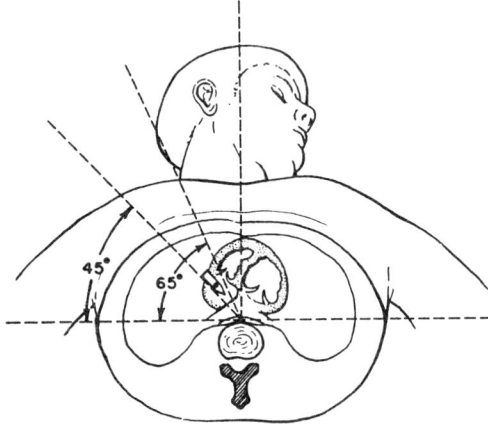

Figure 4. Cross-section diagram of thorax at the level of the atria. The arrow-shaped metal flange of the transseptal needle (superimposed on the diagram) is directed posteriorly and toward the left.

sponds to the lower margin of the left atrium as seen in the posteroanterior angiogram. Therefore, the needle entry point in the patient with a large left atrium should be lower than in a patient with a normal-sized left atrium. Both anteroposterior and lateral fluoroscopy should be used to direct the needle posteriorly and leftward. Once the catheter is appropriately positioned, the needle is advanced against the interatrial septum (5). Atrial pressure becomes damped as the needle tip touches the septum. When the needle is advanced through the septum, a "popping" sensation is noted and a left atrial pressure contour appears. If an adequate pressure contour is not seen, the needle is held in the same position and a small amount of contrast medium (0.5–1 cc) is slowly injected into the needle. If the contrast freely flows into the left atrium, one can be assured of its proper position. If the contrast forms a myocardial plaque, however, the puncture should be repeated. When one is sure the needle is in the left atrium, gentle but steady pressure is applied to both needle and catheter under fluoroscopic and pressure monitoring. Good phasic left atrial pressure should be observed throughout this maneuver. When the catheter crosses the interatrial septum (6), another "popping" sensation will be appreciated by the operator. The needle is now slightly withdrawn and the catheter is advanced further into the left atrium (7). The needle is then removed. The curved tip of the catheter facilitates passage into the left ventricle (8), but if the pass is difficult, a J-tipped flexible guidewire or a curved occluder wire can be used. Care must be taken when advancing the stiff curved-tip wire through the catheter, since accidental withdrawal of the catheter from the left atrium may occur. Now pressure and oxygen saturation data can be obtained through the catheter.

Since the catheter has a large lumen, is short, and has multiple side holes it is usually not necessary to use the end-hole occluder for angiography. If end-hole occlusion is desired, a wire adapter (Touhy) is required: one branch for the wire and the other for the injection of contrast medium.

The Long-Sheath Technique

The above described transseptal technique does not permit catheter change during the procedure or the use of other than end-hole catheters. However, a technique has been developed to allow use of more than one type of catheter. The Mullins transseptal catheter introducer set (USCI) consists of a long percutaneous sheath and dilator that are used in conjunction with a conventional transseptal needle. After puncture of the septum by the needle, both dilator and sheath are advanced across the septum. The dilator is withdrawn and a succession of catheters can be advanced through the sheath into the left atrium. There are two different lengths of sheaths

depending upon the type of needle to be used. For the adult transseptal needle the dilator is 63 cm long and the sheath, 59 cm. For the pediatric patient, a 49-cm dilator and 43-cm sheath are used. Sizes range from #6 to #8 French for both adult and pediatric sets.

The Transseptal Technique via the Superior Vena Cava

In 1960, Bevegarg et al. described a method of transseptal technique via the right jugular vein. Subsequently, Loskot et al. (1965) introduced a method using direct puncture of the right subclavian vein. Transseptal catheterization by the superior vena cava has thus far been used only in adults but the approach should be feasible in the pediatric age group.

Complications of Transseptal Cardiac Catheterization

There are only a few reports of transseptal cardiac catheterization experience in the pediatric age group. However, the complications in children seem to be similar to those reported in adults. The most serious complication is perforation of the right atrium, left atrium, or aortic root. Duff and Mullins (1978) reported 80 cases of pediatric transseptal catheterization, with 40% of patients being under 5 years old or weighing less than 20 kg. There were no fatalities but two patients (2.5%) had cardiac perforation. Fortunately, there were no serious consequences. Two other patients had intramyocardial infiltration during injection of contrast medium in the left ventricle. Other complications include thrombus formation at the site of the transseptal puncture noted on post mortem examination following a transseptal procedure (Pinkerson et al. 1963). Another rare complication is persistence of a defect in the atrial septum at the site of the puncture (Ross et al. 1964; Libanoff 1965). Systemic embolization has also been seen following the transseptal procedure in adults (Libanoff 1965).

Although complications are relatively uncommon, careful selection of patients, meticulous preparation of instruments, and observance of proper procedure should improve the safety of the procedure.

Endomyocardial Biopsy

Major indications for endomyocardial biopsy include monitoring of immunosuppressive therapy in the cardiac transplant patient, differentiating acute inflammatory myocarditis from congestive cardiomyopathy, and monitoring Adriamycin toxicity. In the patient with a transplanted heart, the intensity of immunosuppressive therapy is altered when there is evidence of rejection. At this writing, histologic abnormalities on the endomyocardial biopsy are the most reliable indicators of rejection, and in our institution, endomyocardial biopsy is done routinely and repeatedly in the cardiac transplant patient.

Equipment

A Cordis disposable bioptome with a long introducer sheath is most frequently used in our institution (Fig. 5). The Cordis instrument is #5 French in diameter and comes in 50-cm and 110-cm lengths. Alternatively, the Cava-Shultz bioptome can be used. The standard bioptomes of this type are #6.5 and #9 French and are available in a variety of lengths. The introducer sheath has a bleeding control gasket and a side arm for flushing. This type of sheath must be used to prevent inadvertent aspiration of air and/or excessive blood loss.

Procedure

Endomyocardial biopsy can be performed at the conclusion of a standard diagnostic catheterization or as an independent procedure, usually with measurement of right heart pressures. The biopsy can be performed from the femoral vein approach using a long sheath or from the percutaneous internal jugular approach. This latter technique is described in detail in Chapter 4. If the femoral or internal jugular approach is used, the distal end of the bioptome is curved by slowly withdrawing the distal shaft over a round syringe barrel. This distal end must be curved to facilitate passage of the bioptome across the tricuspid valve and toward the apex of the right ventricle. If the bioptome is being passed from the internal jugular vein, it is important to be sure that the catheter is in the right ventricle and not in the coronary sinus. When the long sheath is used from the femoral vein approach, the tip of the sheath is positioned near the apex of the right ventricle. The bioptome is advanced through the sheath and the sheath is then withdrawn about 3 cm to expose the bioptome tip. Once positioned in the right ventricle, the bioptome is rotated so that the tip is against the right ventricular septal surface (Fig. 6). The jaws are opened and the catheter is advanced to engage the myocardium. The jaws are closed and the catheter is withdrawn. A sudden release of tension indicates that the biopsy has been obtained. The sheath is then advanced back over the bioptome into the original position to facilitate the subsequent biopsy. The bioptome is removed and the specimen secured. A total of three to five specimens are obtained, each usually measuring 1–2 mm in diameter.

The femoral artery also can be utilized for percutaneous introduction of the instrument to biopsy the left ventricle if a long sheath and disposable Cordis bioptome are used. For a left ventricular biopsy, we prefer to use the venous approach via an existing interatrial communication or by transseptal technique. In the small infant with an interatrial communication, it may be safer to biopsy the left, rather than the right, ventricle. Perforation of the thin-walled right ventricle is a greater risk in a small infant compared to an older child or adult.

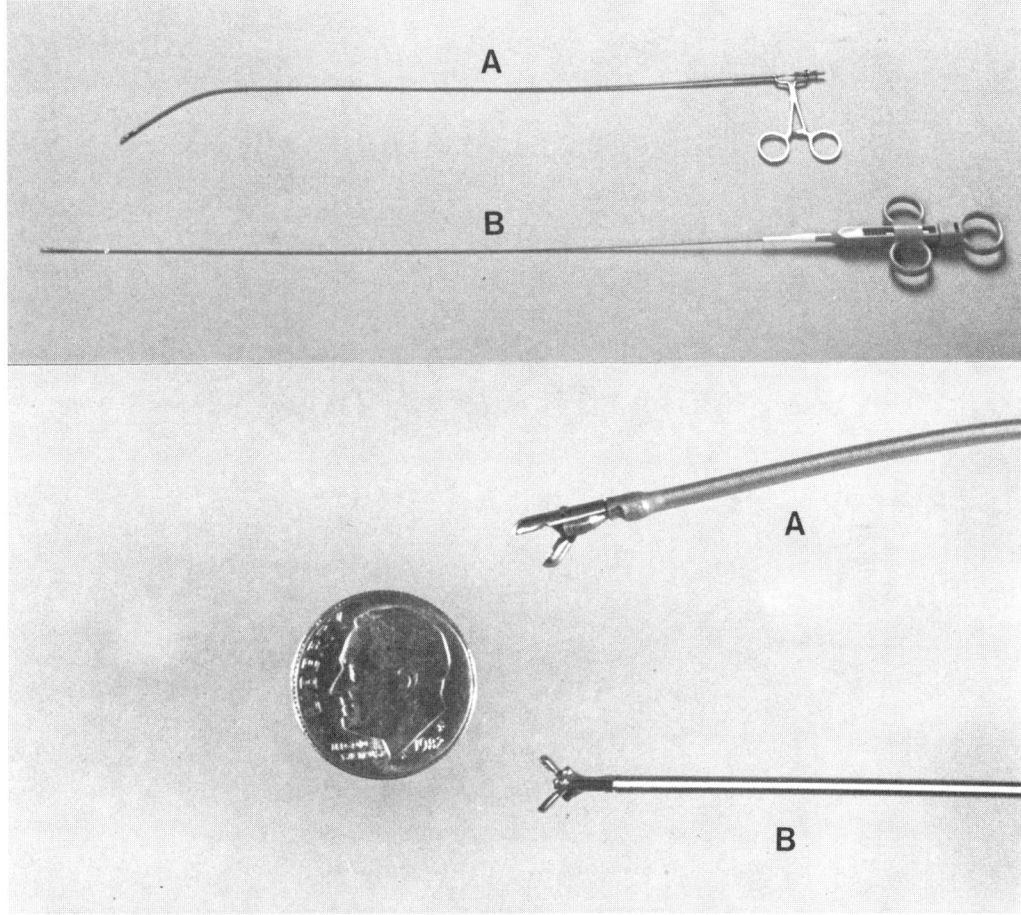

Figure 5. Bioptomes for endomyocardial biopsy. Top: View of entire catheter. Bottom: Magnified view of the catheter tip. (A) Cava-Shultz bioptome. (B) Cordis disposable bioptome.

Complications

There have been no serious complications in our series of over 200 endomyocardial biopsies. In a much larger series of adult posttransplant patients, no mortality was reported. Possible complications include cardiac perforation, pneumo- or hemothorax, and air embolism.

Pericardiocentesis

Pericardiocentesis can be a diagnostic or therapeutic procedure, or both. Excessive pericardial fluid may be produced by either infectious or noninfectious processes and their differentiation is sometimes possible only after examination of the pericardial fluid. Most commonly, pericardiocentesis is done to relieve cardiac tamponade.

Confirmation or Suspicion of Pericardial Effusion

The presence of pericardial effusion is usually evident either by clinical examination (e.g., pulsus paradoxus) or by echocardiography. The cross-sectional echocardiogram is especially useful and provides information as to the amount and location of the pericardial effusion. If echocardio-

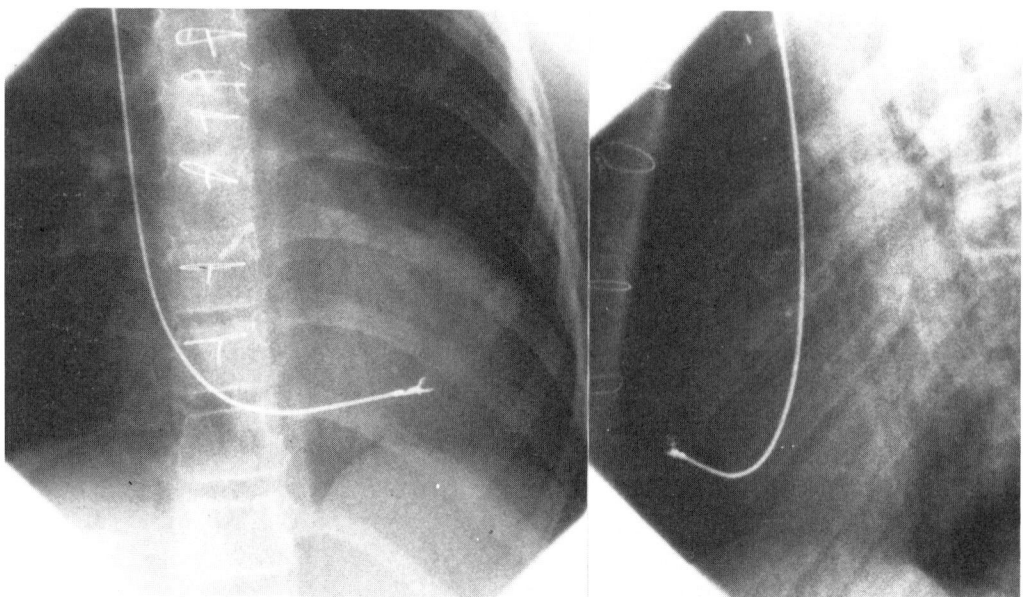

Figure 6. Bioptome positioned in the right ventricle with jaws opened. Left: Anteroposterior view. Right: Lateral view.

graphy is not possible or is technically poor, it is usually wise to do a central venous or right atrial angiogram prior to pericardiocentesis. Blind pericardiocentesis without angiographic or echocardiographic study is not justified unless the patient is critically ill.

Preparation

Ideally, pericardiocentesis should be performed in the cardiac catheterization laboratory where fluoroscopy and resuscitation equipment are available. Occasionally, the procedure is performed on the ward on an emergency basis without the aid of fluoroscopy. Critically ill patients may not require premedication, but in most patients, a short-acting sedative such as parenteral Valium or ketamine is advisable shortly before the procedure.

Procedure

The patient is placed in the supine position or in a partially sitting position (re-

verse Trendelenburg) if orthopneic. The ECG is monitored and all four extremities are restrained. The subxiphoid area and the adjacent left anterior chest are prepped using an iodine containing antiseptic (Betadine) and 70% alcohol. Lidocaine (1%) is infiltrated 0.5 cm below the left costoxiphoid angle using a 25-gauge, 1.5-inch long needle. The infiltration is extended posteriorly and slightly superiorly.

Since the nature of the pericardial fluid is usually not known and since a thick, viscous fluid may be encountered, a large needle is preferred for pericardiocentesis. A 16-gauge Intracath (Deseret Pharmaceutical Company) is adequate. It has three components: the needle, a 20-cm long radiopaque Teflon catheter, and a plastic needle clamp. Unfortunately, the Teflon catheter has only an end hole, which is easily occluded when advanced against the pericardial or epicardial surface. Two or more additional side holes facilitate the withdrawal of pericardial fluid. A scalpel can be used to make these holes 1–2 cm from the tip. Care must be taken to avoid weakening the tubing by making the holes too large. Alternatively, a new device has been developed specifically for pericardiocentesis (Pericardiocentesis Set; Cook, Inc.) (Fig. 7). This is available in an #8.3 French size. The set consists of a short bevel needle, J-tipped guidewire, dilator, and a soft, flexible pigtail catheter with an end hole and multiple side holes. Since this catheter is too large and stiff for use in a small infant, a #5 French catheter has been designed and is being tested in our laboratory.

Insertion of the Catheter

The needle is attached to a small syringe containing a small amount of flushing solution. The needle is introduced into the previously anesthetized area in the left costoxiphoid space, aiming toward the left ax-

illa with the needle angled 30° from the horizontal plane. If the needle is inserted at a lower angulation (more parallel to the chest wall), it may fail to enter the pericardial space. The operator can usually feel the needle entering the pericardial space. Also, if gentle suction is applied with the syringe as the needle is advanced, the fluid will be aspirated readily into the syringe as soon as the pericardial space is entered. Once pericardial fluid has been obtained, the syringe is then removed, being careful to keep the needle tip in the pericardial space. If an Intracath is used, the catheter is inserted through the needle under fluoroscopic guidance until it is well within the pericardial space (Fig. 8). The needle is then withdrawn over the catheter until the needle tip is outside of the skin. The plastic clamp is now applied to both the catheter and needle to prevent damage to the catheter by the needle tip.

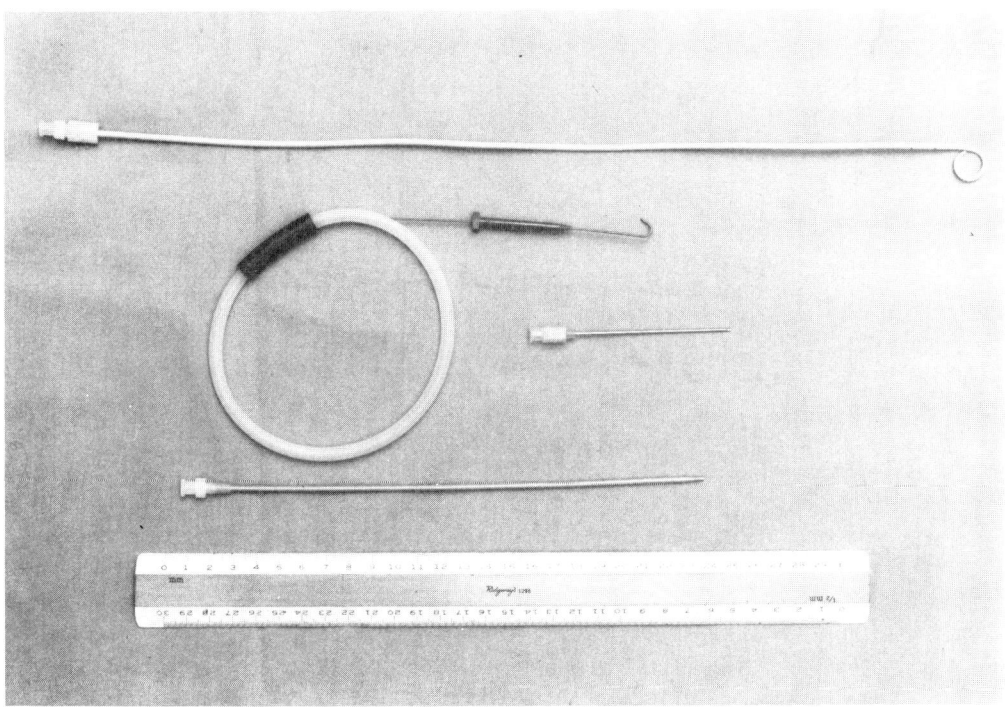

Figure 7. Pericardiocentesis Set (Cook Inc., Bloomington, IN).

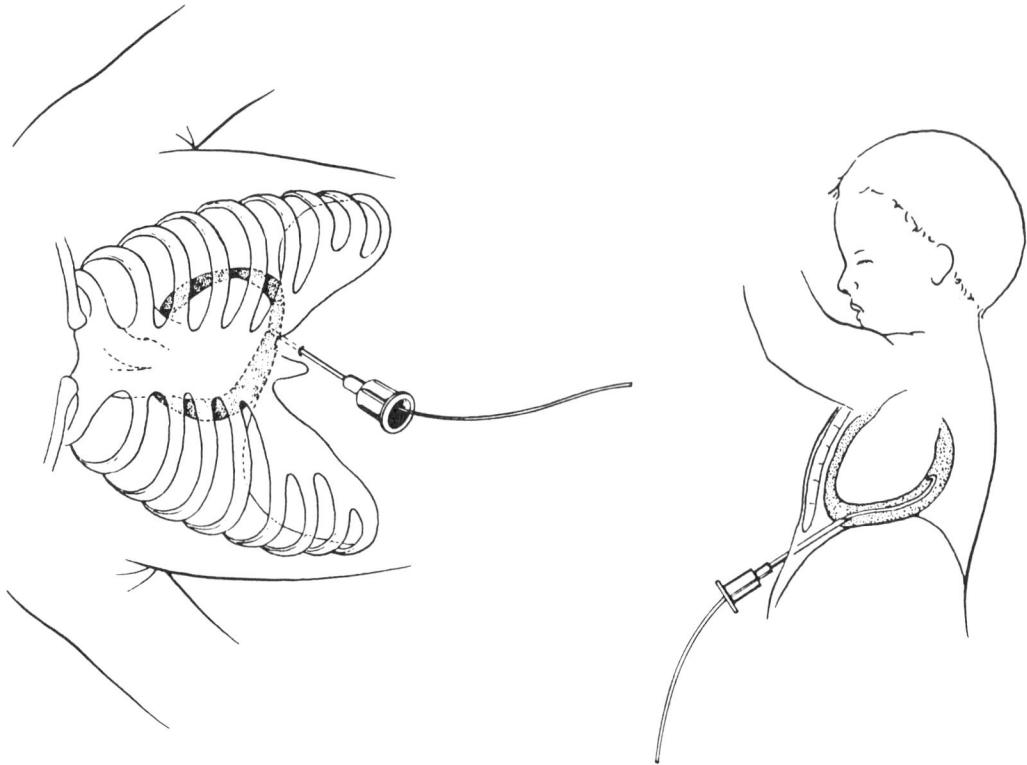

Figure 8. Pericardiocentesis technique (see text).

If the Pericardiocentesis Set is used, the guidewire is advanced through the needle into the pericardial space. The needle is withdrawn with the wire remaining in place. The dilator is then used to enlarge the opening in the subcutaneous tissue. After this has been accomplished, the dilator is then withdrawn, the special catheter is inserted over the wire, and the wire is then removed.

The proximal portion of the catheter is now linked to a three-way stopcock and a 30-ml or 50-ml syringe is attached and pericardial fluid aspirated. Pericardial fluid is promptly sent to the laboratory for cell count, protein, and culture. Prior to removal of the catheter, 2 or 3 ml of contrast media can be injected into the pericardial space to evaluate the amount of residual fluid. Echocardiographic evaluation should be also performed.

Indwelling Pericardial Drainage

The pericardial catheter is usually removed at the termination of the pericardiocentesis. Sometimes, patients with recurrent, rapidly accumulating, noninfectious pericardial effusion may require temporary continuous drainage. There are no specific guidelines as to how long the catheter can safely be left in place for continuous drainage, but Wei et al. (1978) and Lock et al. (1984) have reported successful chronic drainage via an indwelling pericardial catheter.

Alternative Method

The subxiphoid approach is the standard method for pericardiocentesis. Occasionally, this approach is not successful because of an unusually high diaphragm, a rotational anomaly of the heart, or a thoracic deformity. In such situations, venous angiography is essential. If the cardiac silhouette is simply unusually high, pericardiocentesis can be performed through the 4th or 5th intercostal space along the left sternal border by pointing the needle directly posteriorly and slightly leftward. This approach can be used in patients with an unusually large liver or spleen.

Emergency Pericardiocentesis

Rarely, pericardiocentesis must be performed outside the cardiac catheterization laboratory and without fluoroscopy. Usually, such patients require no premedication, but proper restraints should be applied. Skin preparation and local anesthesia are the same as outlined above. In general, the procedure can readily be performed in this setting with echocardiographic assistance. If echo also is not available, an ECG lead may be helpful. To use this technique, a sterile wire with an alligator clip at each end is attached to the hub of the needle and to an ECG precordial lead. As the needle is inserted, the ECG is continuously monitored for an epicardial injury current pattern, (ST segment shift), which can appear if the needle enters the myocardium. Such ECG monitoring is helpful in preventing inadvertent myocardial damage (Sobol et al. 1975).

Complications

Complications of pericardiocentesis are unusual, but include cardiac perforation or laceration of a coronary artery. Improper insertion of the needle may damage adjacent abdominal organs such as the liver or spleen, and puncture of a lung may cause pneumothorax. Pneumoperitoneum also has been reported as a complication. Improper

antiseptic technique during the procedure may lead to infection. Costochondritis has also been reported (Kwasnik et al. 1978).

Foreign Body Retrieval

Embolization of a catheter fragment is a rare complication of a number of diagnostic and therapeutic procedures, including cardiac catheterization, placement of a central venous line, or a neurosurgical ventriculoatrial shunt. Loss of a catheter fragment into the cardiovascular system may result from poor technique or from material failure.

Probably the most common clinical setting for embolization is the use of a central venous line for monitoring or for infusion of fluid. Lines that have been in place for long periods of time may become brittle and fracture spontaneously. Commonly, the lines are sheared accidentally by the needle used for insertion or become detached from a poorly secured needle inserted into the proximal lumen. When embolization complicates diagnostic cardiac catheterization, it most often results from fracture of a catheter, usually at the site of a side hole. A guidewire can be sheared while being withdrawn through a percutaneous needle, and an introducer sheath may become dislodged from the hub. At one time, the inner portion (dilator) of some introducer sets could inadvertently be inserted completely through the outer sheath and into the vein. This is no longer a problem since the distal end is flared or has a fitting attached and thus cannot traverse the sheath. Arterial embolization occurs less frequently, but has been reported from left atrial monitoring lines and during diagnostic cardiac catheterization.

After embolization from a systemic vein, the catheter fragment may lodge in a peripheral vein, the superior or inferior vena cava, the right atrium, right ventricle, or pulmonary artery. A long fragment may extend through several of the above sites.

Although embolic fragments may remain in a vein, a cardiac chamber, or a pulmonary artery for several years without difficulty, the danger of infection, perforation, or thrombosis usually make retrieval of the fragment mandatory (Aldridge and Lee 1977). This can be accomplished surgically, but cardiopulmonary bypass is required if the fragment lies beyond the venae cavae. Nonoperative removal can be attempted by several techniques, including the use of forceps, snares or hooks, and wire baskets.

Technique

Forceps are quite stiff and practical only if the fragment is in a vena cava or the right atrium (King et al. 1976). The most commonly used technique is a simple loop snare, constructed from an end-hole catheter and a loop of guidewire extending from the end hole (Massumi and Ross 1967). The major

advantage of the loop snare is its simplicity. It can be constructed "on the spot," permitting an early attempt at removal if no other device is available (Fig. 9). A #7 or #8 French catheter and a 0.021- or 0.025-inch guidewire more than two times the length of the catheter are usually used (King et al. 1974). (It is very difficult to move the wire in and out to enlarge or tighten the loop if a catheter with a smaller bore is used.) The catheter is advanced to a position just proximal or distal to a free end of the fragment, the loop is enlarged by advancing the wire, and an attempt is made to maneuver the loop around the fragment. If the fragment can be engaged, the loop is tightened and the catheter is withdrawn, pulling the fragment with it (Fig. 10). It is sometimes impossible to completely withdraw the assembly and in this circumstance, a cutdown must be done proximal to the catheterization site and the fragment removed through a venotomy. It should be noted that the tech-

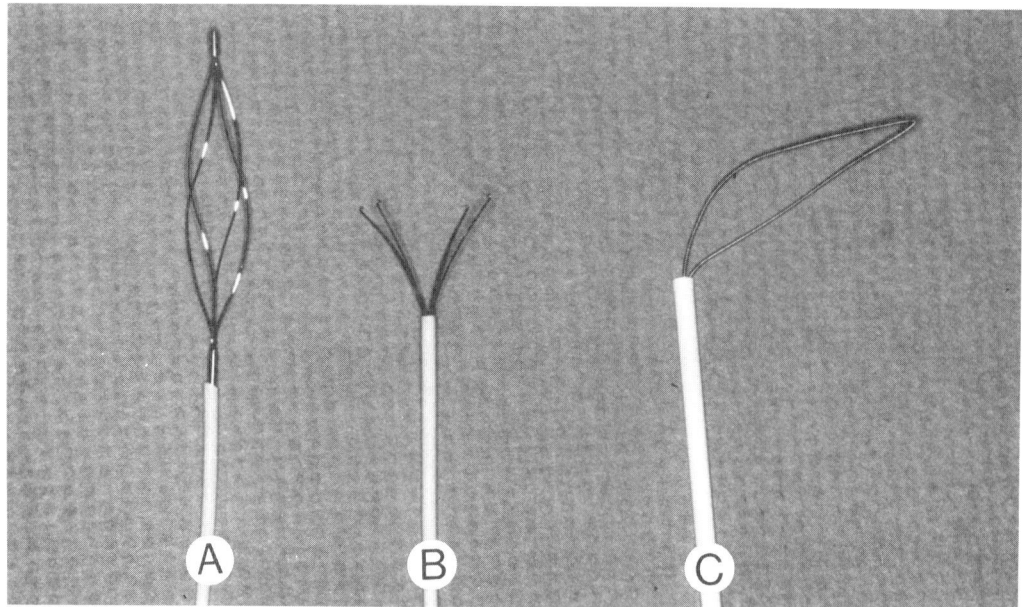

Figure 9. Various retrieval devices. A: Basket snare (#6 French, 5.5-cm) (Meditech, Watertown, MA). B: Grasping forceps (#6 French, 120-cm) (Meditech). C: Snare loop using a 0.018-inch guidewire in a #7 French catheter.

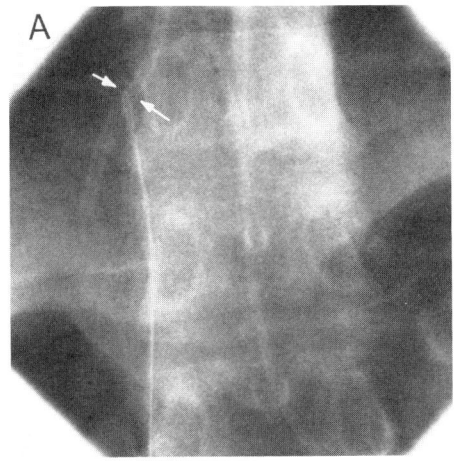

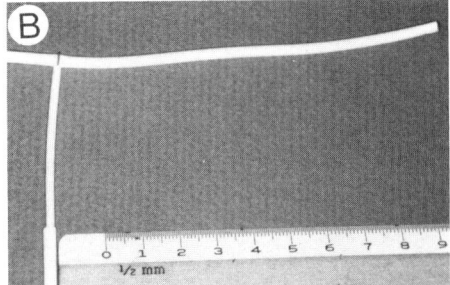

Figure 10. (A) Fractured Hickman subcutaneous port line lodged in the right atrium is snared by a loop of guidewire that has been passed through a catheter. (B) The retrieved line was secured by the guidewire loop that had been withdrawn tightly against the catheter tip.

nique requires that at least one end of the fragment be free-floating; if both ends are impacted in the wall of a vessel or chamber, the loop cannot engage the fragment of catheter.

One variation of the snare technique involves prebending each end of the wire into a Z shape before insertion, supposedly creating a more effective loop (Leth et al. 1973). In another variation (Hyman 1972), the soft end of a guidewire is attached to the exterior of the tip of the catheter with fine wire and epoxy glue. The other end of the wire is threaded through the catheter, creating the loop.

Catheter deflector systems have been used to "hook" catheter fragments (McSweeney and Schwartz 1971). The deflector wire may be inserted through an end-hole catheter positioned near the fragment, or the wire may be encased in a polyethylene tube. In either case, the technique is useful only if the fragment is relatively long. It is probably the method of choice if neither end of the fragment is free-floating. If the deflector system is not available, a sharp hook can be "cooked" into the tip of a standard catheter using a hot sterile water bath or steam. The sharp curve is lost as the catheter is withdrawn into a peripheral vein, but the fragment may then be secured by a loop or basket snare. A grasping forceps (Fig. 9) also can be used for this purpose.

The basket snare (Lassers and Pickering 1967; Dotter et al. 1971) consists of a helical array of wires that form a "basket" as the wires are advanced beyond the catheter tip (Fig. 9). The #8 French Dotter system is quite stiff and is usually not suitable for children. The Bean-Smith-Mahorney biliary stone removal set may be useful (Alridge and Lee 1977), but is only 50 cm long. A special 100-cm set can be ordered, or the wire from a second basket can be soldered to the first to obtain a wire 100 cm long. In the basket technique, the delivery catheter is placed just proximal or distal to the fragment and the basket is protruded. By repeatedly advancing and withdrawing the catheter and by rotating it in the process, the fragment may be encompassed by the basket, which is then tightened around the fragment by withdrawing the wire. Removal of fragments in the right or left pulmonary artery may be attempted by the snare technique. If this is not possible, a basket method may be tried, preferably the smaller, more flexible Bean-Smith-Mahorney device. If the fragment is not radiopaque, retrieval is much more difficult. Cineangiography or echocardiography may be useful in locating the fragment, but engaging it in a snare or basket is by trial and error.

References and Suggested Reading

Aldridge HE, Lee J. Transvascular removal of catheter fragments from the great vessels and heart. Can Med J 1977; 1117:1300–1304.

Bevegard S, Carlens E, Jonsson B, Karlof I. A technique for transseptal left heart catheterization via the right external jugular vein. Thorax 1960; 15:299.

Brockenbrough EC, Braunwald E. A new technique for left ventricular angiocardiography and transseptal left heart catheterization. Am J Cardiol 1960; 6:1062–1064.

Cope C. Technique for transseptal catheterization of the left atrium. Preliminary report. J Thorac Surg 1959; 37:482.

Dotter CT, Rosch J, Bilbao MK. Transluminal extraction of catheter and guide fragments from the heart and great vessels: 29 collected cases. Am J Roentgenol Radium Ther Nucl Med 1971; 1111:467–472.

Duff DF, Mullins CE. Transseptal left heart catheterization in infants and children. Cathet Cardiovasc Diagn 1978; 4:213–223.

Enghoff E, Cullhed I. Experiences with transseptal left heart catheterization. A review of 454 studies. Am Heart J 1971; 81:398–407.

Epstein EJ, Couloshed N. Transseptal catheterization via the right subclavian vein. Br Heart J 1971; 33:658–663.

Hyman AL. An improved snare catheter for retrieving embolized fragments of polyethylene tubing. Chest 1972; 62:98–99.

Kossowsky WA, Bleifer SB. Fatal cerebral embolism complicating transseptal left heart catheterization. Circulation 1965; 65:811–813.

Krikorian JG, Hancock EW. Pericardiocentesis. Am J Med 1978; 65:808–814.

Kwasnik EM, Koster K, Lazarus JM, et al. Conservative management of uremic pericardial effusions. J Thorac Cardiovasc Surg 1978; 76:629–632.

Lassers BW, Pickering D. Removal of an iatrogenic foreign body from the aorta by means of a ureteric stone catheter. Am Heart J 1967; 73:375–378.

Leth A, Ehlers D, Jensen G, Lauridsen P. Removal of a catheter fragment from the right atrium by a new catheterization technique. Scand. J Thorac Cardiovasc Surg 1973; 7:171–174.

Limbanoff AJ, Silver AW. Complications of transseptal left heart catheterization. Am J Cardiol 1965; 16:390–393.

Lock JE, Bass JL, Kulik TJ, Fuhrman BP. Chronic percutaneous pericardial drainage with modified pigtail catheters in children. Am J Cardiol 1984; 53:1179–1182.

Loskot F, Michaljanic A, Musil J. Right and left heart catheterization via the subclavian veins. Cardiologia 1965; 46:114–128.

Massumi RA, Ross AM. Atraumatic non-surgical technic for removal of broken catheters from cardiac cavities. N Engl J Med 1967; 277:195–196.

McSweeney WJ, Schwartz DC. Retrieval of a catheter foreign body from the right heart using a guide wire deflector system. Radiology 1971; 100:61–62.

Owens WC, Schaefer RA, Rahimtoola SH. Pericardiocentesis: Insertion of pericardial catheter. Cathet Cardiovasc Diagn 1975; 1:317–321.

Pinkerson AL, Kelser GA, Jr, Adkins PC. Mural thrombus in the left atrium secondary to transseptal catheterization of the left side of the heart. N Engl J Med 1963; 268:367–368.

Ross J, Jr, Braunwald E, Morrow AG. Transseptal left atrial puncture: New technique for the measurement of left atrial pressure in man. Am J Cardiol 1959; 3:653–655.

Sobol SM, Thomas HM, Jr, Evans RW. Myocardial laceration not demonstrated by continuous electrocardiographic monitoring occurring during pericardiocentesis. N Engl J Med 1975; 292:1222–1223.

Wei JY, Taylor GJ, Achuff SC. Recurrent cardiac tamponade and large pericardial effusions: Management with an indwelling pericardial catheter. Am J Cardiol 1978; 42:281–282.

Wong B, Murphy J, Chang CJ, et al. The risk of pericardiocentesis. Am J Cardiol 1979; 44:1110–1114.

Transcatheter Vascular Occlusion

William H. Neches, M.D.

It has now become possible to occlude undesirable or unwanted vascular structures in the cardiac catheterization laboratory. Occlusion can be accomplished with a number of different devices and techniques, which include polyurethane foam plugs, coils, balloons, glue materials, and umbrella-like devices. The types of vascular structures that can be occluded include a patent ductus arteriosus, systemic-to-pulmonary artery collaterals, systemic-to-pulmonary artery shunts, various anomalous arterial or venous connections, or even the vascular supply to an entire organ. Regardless of the technique employed or the vessel involved, the goal is to provide a safe, easy to use and effective method that avoids the necessity and risk of general anesthesia, a surgical procedure, and also shortens the patient's hospitalization. This chapter is divided into two categories: techniques used for closure of a patent ductus arteriosus and techniques used for occlusion of other vascular structures.

Catheter Occlusion of the Ductus Arteriosus

Polyurethane Foam Plug

The first device used for catheter occlusion of the ductus arteriosus was a polyurethane foam plug described by Porstmann (1971) and also used by others in Japan (Sato 1975). We have no experience with the use of this device but will briefly describe the technique as reported by Porstmann and Sato. A variety of different sized foam plugs are available with the selection of the appropriate plug based upon the size of the ductus arteriosus determined from angiography. This techniques requires both arterial and venous access. On the arterial side, a long catheter is introduced either percutaneously or under direct vision by means of a cutdown on the left femoral artery. The catheter is then advanced from the aorta into the ductus arteriosus. With one technique (Porstmann 1974), this catheter is manipulated from the ductus arteriosus, through the right heart, down the inferior vena cava, and out through the corresponding femoral vein. With another method (Sato 1975), a "catching" venous catheter is introduced either by cutdown or percutaneously into a femoral vein and advanced in prograde fashion into the main pulmonary artery. The arterial catheter is then snared in the right heart by the catching wire and catheter and is withdrawn through the right heart, down the inferior vena cava, and out the femoral vein.

Once the catheter has passed from the femoral artery, through the heart, and out the femoral vein, a long, 400-cm guidewire is passed into the retrograde arterial catheter and advanced through the catheter until it exits the body through the right femoral vein. The catheter is then removed, and the guidewire now remains in a continuous pass from the femoral artery to the thoracic aorta, through the ductus arteriosus, the main pulmonary artery, the right side of the heart, the inferior vena cava, and exiting through the femoral vein. A catheter is inserted over the wire on the venous side and advanced to the pulmonary artery to serve as a stop point for the pulmonary artery side of the plug. At this point, the cone-shaped foam plug is introduced, tapered end first, over the guidewire and into the femoral artery. An end-hole "pushing" catheter is also introduced over the wire behind the plug. The wire is then held at a fixed point on the table and the catheter is used to advance the plug over the wire and into the ductus arteriosus. The plug should become seated in the ductus arteriosus with its larger end wedged in the mouth of the duct on the aortic side. The plug is held in place by the higher aortic pressure and thrombus formation that occurs quite rapidly. The guidewire is then removed from the venous side, and closure of the ductus arteriosus is confirmed by angiography and/or echocardiography. Although this technique has been used successfully in over 200 cases by Porstmann, Sato, and others, it may require direct exposure of the femoral artery and/or vein and requires a vessel large enough to accept the foam plug (> 3 mm). It thus cannot be used in infants and small children and has been used only in older children or adults.

Rashkind PDA Occluder

The first clinical use of the Rashkind PDA occluder was performed in 1977 in a 3.5-kg infant (Rashkind 1979). The initial occluder consisted of a single circular piece of flat foam mesh that was sutured to a three-pronged, umbrella-like wire device, with fish hook-like prongs on the ends of each of the ribs of the device. This occluder could be collapsed into a small enough size to fit within a #5 or #6 French sheath. The small collapsed size of the device enabled its use even in infants. Although it was used successfully in a number of patients, the rate of successful closure was low, and the hooked end of the device prevented further manipulation once it had been extruded from the

catheter. Subsequent modifications and redesign of the catheter and delivery system over the next decade resulted in the double-disc Rashkind PDA occluder system that is now commercially available (USCI, Angiographic Systems Div., Tewksbury, MA).

Catheter System Design

The Rashkind PDA occluder system consists of two components, an implantable prosthesis and a catheter delivery system. The prosthesis consists of two small discs of polyurethane foam that are sutured to two opposing spring-arm assemblies (Fig. 1). The two opposing sets of arms are attached to a central spring mechanism and resemble two small umbrellas. The arms are arranged perpendicular to the long axis of the prosthesis. The implantable prosthesis comes in two sizes: the 12-mm prosthesis, which collapses into an #8 French loading catheter, has three arms arranged 120° apart; and the large, 17-mm prosthesis, which has four arms 90° apart and is used with an #11 French loading catheter. The ends of each spring arm are fashioned into a small coil or eyelet that serves as a point to which the foam mesh is sutured. This eyelet also serves as a rounded contact point against the wall of the vessel at the time of implantation thus minimizing the possibility that the spring arm will pierce the vessel wall. On the long axis of the prosthesis, the proximal end is fashioned into a small loop or eye and serves as a point of attachment to the catheter delivery system. A black suture is passed through the eyelet loops on the distal side of the prosthesis (Fig. 1B), and the ends of that suture are passed through a clear plastic loading device.

The catheter delivery system consists of an 85-cm, #8 French delivery catheter with a thin-walled, stainless steel, 1.7-cm long tubular pod. This metal tip area will contain the prosthesis that is to be deposited into the vascular system. The 12-mm prosthesis can be collapsed and inserted into a

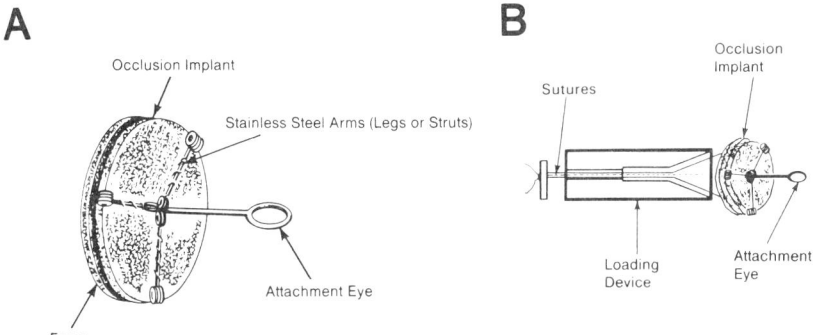

Figure 1. Close-up of view of the Rashkind PDA occluder. A: Occluder prosthesis. B: Prosthesis with loading device.

pod that is #8 French in diameter, while the 17-mm prosthesis requires an #11 French delivery pod that is also attached to an #8 French catheter. A back bleed prevention assembly with a side port for infusion of flushing solution is attached to the opposite or back end of the catheter shaft (Fig. 2). The inner mechanism of the delivery system is a double guidewire that consists of an inner stainless steel guidewire surrounded by an outer coil-spring wire. The inner wire can slide back and forth within the outer core.

Both wires pass through a locking collar and are threaded through the catheter shaft with the tip emerging through the steel pod at the distal end. A stainless steel control clamp is attached to the back end of the wire. This clamp has a knuckle-control locking spring that will prevent movement of the central core wire once it has been attached to the prosthesis. The distal end of the core wire is fashioned in the shape of a knuckle-like protrusion. The distal end of the coil spring outer wire ends in a small tubular metal

The USCI˙ Rashkind˙ PDA Occlusion System

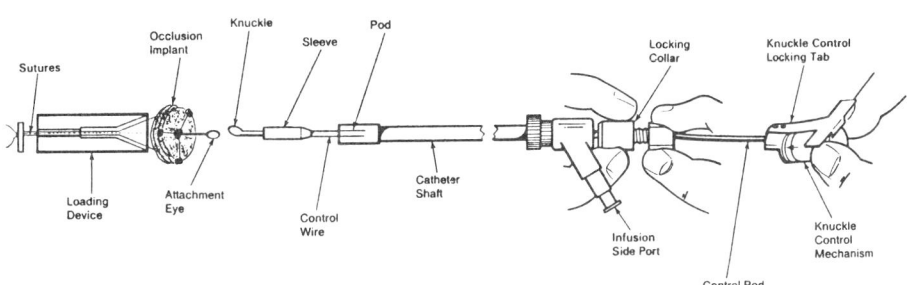

Figure 2. The Rashkind PDA occlusion system.

sleeve into which the knuckle of the central core wire can be withdrawn. The function of this knuckle and sleeve arrangement will be described in the paragraphs below.

Loading the Catheter

The size of the vessel to be occluded is estimated from angiography. The smaller, 12-mm prosthesis can be used for vessels up to 4 mm in diameter, whereas the larger, 17-mm prosthesis is used for vessels 4 mm in diameter or larger. Vessels that have a diameter greater than 10 mm probably cannot be closed with a Rashkind PDA occluder unless they are long and tortuous with a smaller distal segment. Once the appropriate size occluder and catheter have been selected, the prosthesis is soaked in normal saline solution for a period of about 30 minutes. It is recommended that the loading of the prosthesis into the pod of the catheter delivery system should take place as close as possible to the time of insertion into the patient. This will minimize the time that the prosthesis is collapsed and compressed within the catheter delivery system.

The inner core guidewire is first advanced until the knuckle at the tip is protruding from the sleeve at the end of the outer wire (Fig. 2). This is accomplished by moving the knuckle-control locking spring upward so that the metal tab is released from the round portion of the knuckle-control clamp. The rear round portion of the knuckle-control clamp can then slide forward, thus advancing the tip of the central core wire. Using a hemostat or syringe, a gentle curve is formed at the distal few centimeters of the coil guidewire. The knuckle of the inner core wire should point toward the concavity of the curve. This curve will allow the system to follow the natural position through the pulmonary artery and into the ductus, thereby producing less tension on the prosthesis while it is being positioned. The remainder of the steps for loading catheter require two people, one to work

the knuckle-control locking mechanism and the other to perform the loading at the tip of the catheter. The small loop, or attachment eye, on the shaft of the prosthesis is placed over the knuckle at the tip of the central core wire. It is held in this position the person working the knuckle-control locking mechanism slowly withdraws the rear portion of the knuckle-control clamp. As this maneuver is performed, the central core guidewire is withdrawn into the outer wire and the knuckle protrusion with the attachment eye of the prosthesis resting on the knuckle is withdrawn into the sleeve at the tip of the outer wire. If the knuckle and loop are positioned properly, they should slide easily together into the sleeve. If this does not occur easily, *DO NOT* try to force the loop into the sleeve, since this will likely result in damage to this mechanism. Instead, check to be sure that the loop is placed over the protruding end of the knuckle and again try to withdraw this coupling together into the sleeve. Once this has been accomplished, the tab of the knuckle-control locking spring will slip into the groove on the control locking clamp from which it was removed earlier. Once this tab has locked in place, the prosthesis will be securely fastened to the central core wire and cannot be accidentally released. The knuckle-eye locking mechanism that is contained within the sleeve at the tip of the outer wire is carefully machined to very narrow tolerances. As a result, the eye of the prosthesis cannot slide over the knuckle while it remains locked within the sleeve at the tip.

Once the prosthesis has been successfully attached to the core wire, the entire loader assembly and prosthesis should be immersed in sterile saline solution and wet thoroughly again prior to loading the prosthesis into the catheter. This maneuver will serve to minimize the friction of the device during loading. The prosthesis is now withdrawn into the loader device (Fig. 3). To accomplish this, the delivery sleeve is held in one hand while the loader and loader handle are held in the other. Gentle traction on the

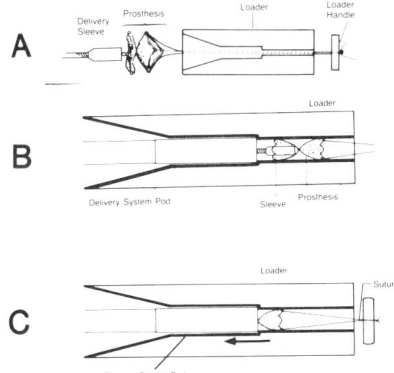

Figure 3. Sequence (A-C) of loading the Rashkind PDA occluder prosthesis into the delivery catheter (see text).

loader handle will bend the distal ribs of the prosthesis toward the loader (Fig. 3A). The distal end of the prosthesis is then withdrawn into the funnel of the loader, making certain that the distal ribs are pointing toward the loader while the proximal ribs are folded backward toward the back end of the catheter (Fig. 3B). Once the prosthesis has been collapsed and advanced into the front portion of the loader, the catheter delivery pod is advanced into the loader and held tightly in position. The person who is assisting the loading of the catheter then slowly withdraws the prosthesis from the distal end of the loader into the pod at the tip of the catheter (Fig. 3C). Once the prosthesis is fully retracted into the catheter, the suture attaching it to the loader handle is cut and withdrawn. The locking collar nut is now advanced on the shaft of the catheter until it abuts against the side-port collar. This is then locked in place and will prevent the prosthesis from being accidentally advanced during catheter manipulation. The catheter delivery system is then flushed carefully with saline solution, being certain to remove all air bubbles prior to insertion of the catheter into the patient.

Occlusion Technique

The following steps of catheterization and placement of the long sheath should all be performed prior to the loading of the prosthesis into the catheter that has just been described. In this way, the loaded delivery system can be inserted immediately into the sheath and advanced to the region of the ductus arteriosus in a minimum amount of time. As was stated earlier, the size, configuration, and location of the ductus arteriosus are determined angiographically and will govern the size of the prosthesis selected and whether the vessel is suitable for catheter occlusion. Once this has been performed and the appropriate prosthesis selected, an appropriate size, long sheath (either #8 or #11 French) is selected and inserted into the venous system. A long catheter is manipulated into the pulmonary artery and through the ductus arteriosus into the descending aorta. The long sheath is then advanced over the catheter and positioned with its tip in the descending aorta just beyond the ductus arteriosus, and the catheter is removed. Alternatively, an end-hole catheter can be positioned in the descending aorta via the ductus arteriosus. An exchange guidewire is passed through the catheter and the catheter is then removed. The long sheath is then passed over the guide wire, through the heart, and into the descending aorta.

Once the sheath has been properly positioned in the descending aorta, the occluder delivery system is inserted into the sheath and advanced to just beyond the level of the tricuspid valve. The delivery system catheter is extremely stiff and, as a result, it will be impossible in most cases to manipulate this catheter into the region of the ductus arteriosus. This problem is eliminated by using a technique described by Bash and Mullins (1984) that uses the sheath as an extension of the delivery system pod (Fig. 4). With the catheter positioned just beyond the tricuspid valve, the locking collar at the back of the catheter is loosened and the guidewire assembly slowly advanced, while fluoroscopically monitoring the position of the prosthesis in the long sheath. The prosthesis is gradually advanced into the long

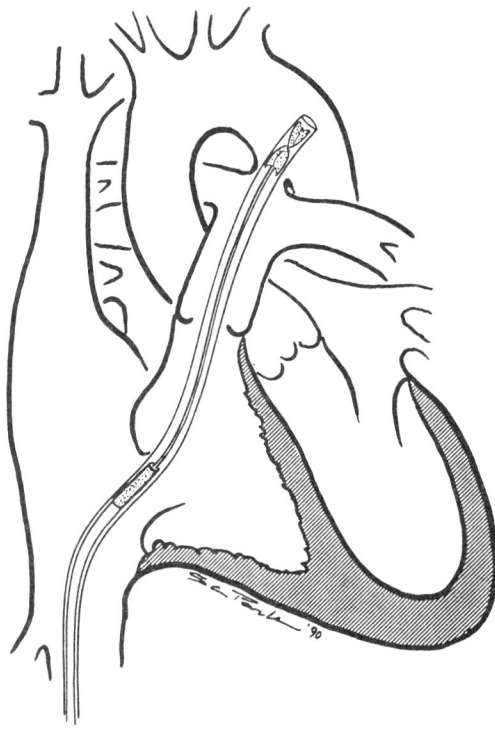

Figure 4. Diagram showing the Rashkind PDA occluder within the long sheath just prior to delivery.

sheath until the prosthesis is positioned in the proximal pulmonary artery. Occasionally, it may be difficult to advance the prosthesis past the bend in the right ventricle where the sheath turns cephalad toward the pulmonary artery. If this occurs, the entire system, including the sheath, is slowly advanced forward simultaneously. This will usually advance the prosthesis past the kink in the sheath. The delivery system then can be advanced forward slightly followed by slight withdrawal of the sheath. This series of steps is repeated until the tip of the sheath is again positioned in the aorta just past the ductus arteriosus and the prosthesis is positioned in the pulmonary artery but still within the sheath.

It is suggested that the patient be sedated with ketamine just prior to insertion of the catheter delivery system into the sheath. Although general anesthesia is not

required, a brief period of heavy sedation with ketamine will prevent patient movement during placement of the prosthesis. At the time of angiography, it is helpful to define a landmark that identifies the aortic end of the ductus arteriosus and this will be used as a guide during placement of the prosthesis. This landmark is often the posterior wall of the trachea as visualized in the straight lateral projection. The site of constriction at the pulmonary artery end of a conical ductus will be at the anterior wall of the trachea. The position of the tip of the sheath in relationship to these landmarks is now carefully noted prior to advancing the prosthesis. The tip of the sheath should be localized in the aorta near the mouth of the ductus arteriosus. The prosthesis is then slowly advanced a millimeter at a time using careful fluoroscopic guidance. As soon as the distal arms of the prosthesis are delivered from the sheath, they will spring outward while the proximal arms still remain collapsed within the sheath (Fig. 5A). The operator tightly grasps the sheath and catheter assembly, which are withdrawn together slowly as a single unit. As soon as the operator visualizes the ribs of the prosthesis begin to move toward each other in the funnel of the aortic end of the ductus arteriosus, withdrawal is stopped (Fig. 5B). Although this is not a crucial maneuver in the case of a long tortuous vessel, in the case of a vessel that is quite short, it is essential that the prosthesis not be withdrawn any further, since this might result in the distal arms of the prosthesis being pulled back into the pulmonary artery. Once the distal arms of the prosthesis have been properly positioned in the aortic end of the ductus arteriosus, the guidewire portion of the delivery catheter assembly is fixed at a point on the table a few centimeters from the end of the sheath. It is now important not to move the wire that, in turn, might move the prosthesis and result in its dislodgement. The sheath is now slowly withdrawn while maintaining the wire in the fixed position. The proximal arms of the prosthesis will now pop free and

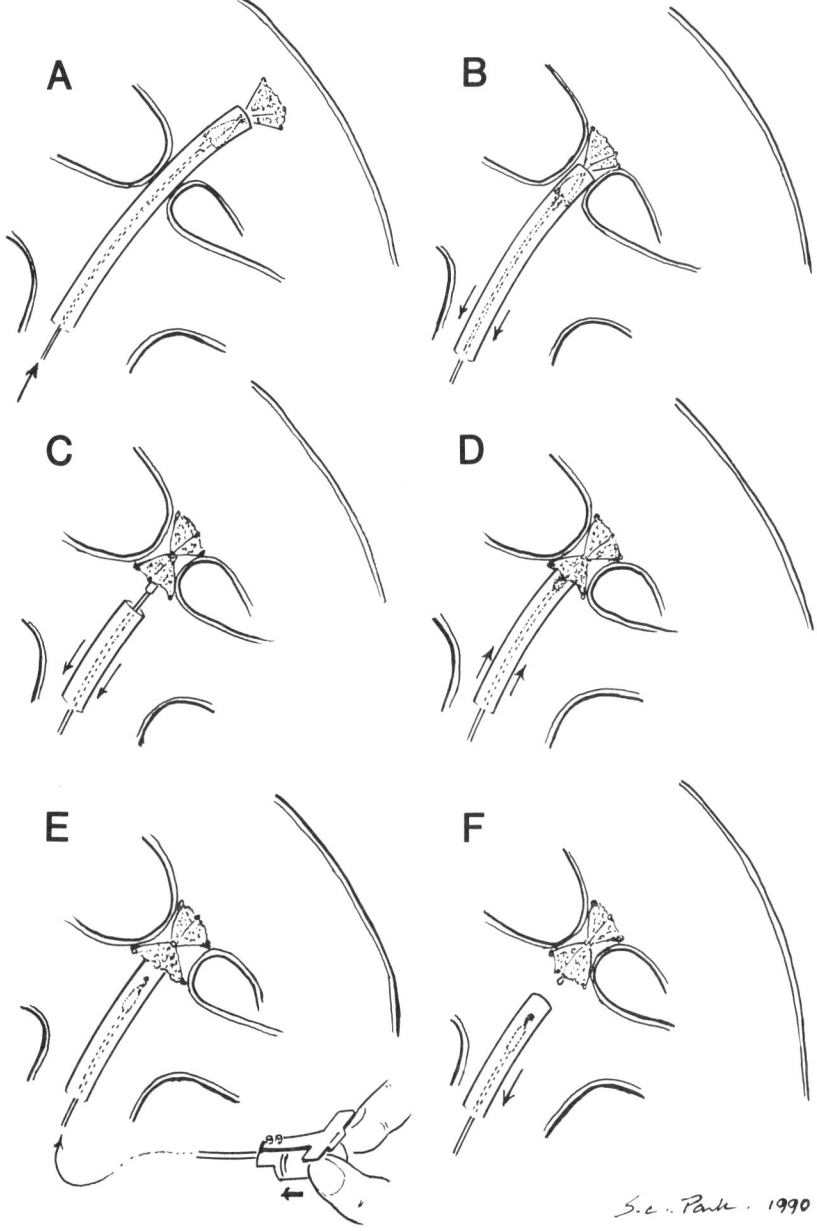

Figure 5. Diagram illustrating the sequence (A-F) of maneuvers for inserting the occluder prosthesis into the ductus arteriosus.

the prosthesis will be visualized to be properly positioned in the region of the ductus arteriosus (Fig. 6A and 6B).

Once the operator is certain that the prosthesis has been properly positioned in the ductus arteriosus, the occluder is then released from the delivery system. This maneuver is accomplished very slowly and very carefully. If you think back to the loading of the delivery catheter, you will remember that the release of the knuckle-control locking mechanism advances the knuckle at the

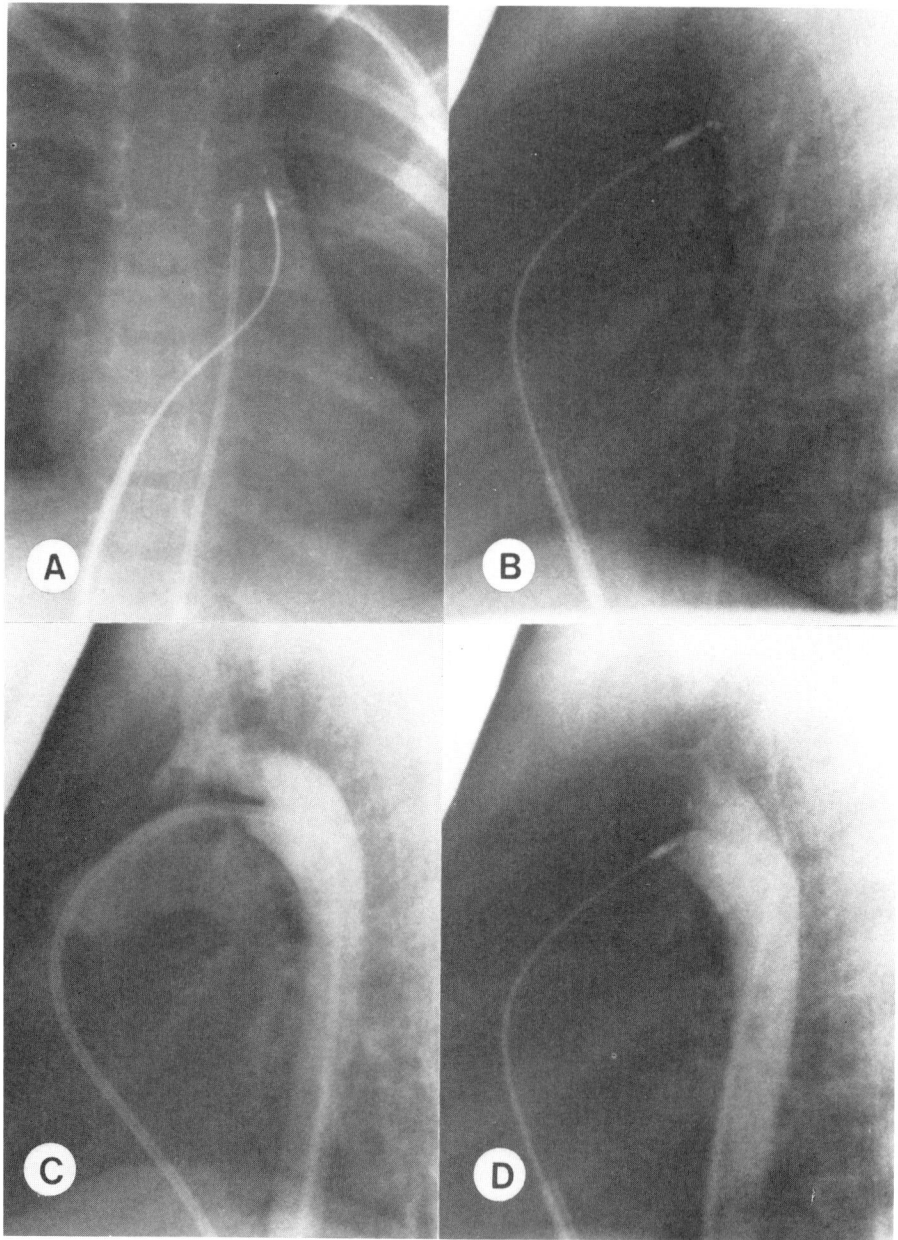

Figure 6. Cineangiogram demonstrating PDA occlusion. A: Occluder positioned in the ductus arteriosus (anteroposterior view). B: Occluder positioned in the ductus arteriosus (lateral view). C: Angiogram before occlusion demonstrating a patent ductus arteriosus (lateral view). D: Angiogram after occlusion (lateral view).

tip of the core wire out of its containing sleeve. If this is done with the entire assembly in the position shown in Figure 5C, then the knuckle may catch in the mesh of the prosthesis and accidentally pull the prosthesis out of the ductus during attempted withdrawal. To avoid this potential problem, the catheter assembly is held at a fixed point on the table while the long sheath is advanced slowly until it abuts against the prosthesis (Fig. 5D). Once this is accomplished, the knuckle-control locking tab is elevated to release the round portion of the knuckle-control mechanism. The rear portion of the pin-locking mechanism is held in the right hand and fixed to a point in the table. The front portion of the locking mechanism, which is held in the left hand, is now moved slowly toward the rear portion held in the right hand (Fig. 5E). As soon as the knuckle has advanced past the end of the sleeve, the catheter will release the prosthesis. The catheter and sheath, together as a single unit, should be immediately withdrawn a few centimeters to avoid hitting the prosthesis and accidentally dislodging it from the position in the ductus. If the prosthesis appears to be appropriately positioned, the delivery system is then withdrawn and the long sheath aspirated to remove any clots or air that may have been introduced into the system. Again, care must be taken to be certain that the tip of the long sheath has been withdrawn to at least the proximal pulmonary artery and is not near the region of the prosthesis. We generally prefer, at this point, to withdraw the long sheath back to the region of the right atrium. After a period of approximately 15 minutes, the position of the prosthesis is again verified fluoroscopically and the extent of occlusion of the ductus arteriosus verified with an injection of contrast in the thoracic aorta (Fig. 6C). When angiography is performed with a retrograde catheter, it must again be remembered to keep the catheter tip far enough away from the prosthesis to prevent the catheter from accidentally hitting the prosthesis and possibly dislodging it.

Following the procedure, after adequate hemostasis is obtained, the patient is returned to his room for routine postcatheterization care. Doppler echocardiographic evaluation should be performed after the procedure and again the following day to confirm occlusion of the ductus arteriosus.

Complications

Embolization of the prosthesis is the major risk or disadvantage to catheter occlusion of the ductus arteriosus. This risk occurs only at the time of implantation and not at some future time. Once the prosthesis has been seated properly in the ductus arteriosus, thrombus formation and subsequent endothelialization serve to "cement" the occluder prosthesis in its position permanently. On the other hand, at the time of implantation, the occluder device must be seated exactly within the ductus arteriosus. If the device is too far toward the side of the aorta, then the distal arms of the prosthesis will protrude into the aorta and will not catch on the wall of the ductus arteriosus. Similarly, if the device is too far toward the side of the pulmonary artery, the proximal arms of the prosthesis will be within the pulmonary artery and not against the wall of the ductus arteriosus. If either of these two situations are present, then the occluder prosthesis might embolize into the aorta or the pulmonary artery, respectively. If this occurs, it may be possible to remove the occluder with a snare device. If an embolized occluder cannot be removed during the catheterization, it usually is then necessary for the patient to undergo a surgical procedure, at which time the occluder device is removed from the circulation and the ductus arteriosus is surgically ligated. Thus, if embolization occurs, the patient would basically have an operation similar to that which would otherwise be recommended for closure of the ductus arteriosus (except that in some cases a median sternotomy might be required).

Other risks or complications include the general risks of the cardiac catheterization procedure itself. These include vascular and myocardial trauma or perforation, arrhythmias, infection, etc. These problems are discussed in Chapter 16. Since the ductus occluder device is a foreign body that is being implanted in the circulation, there is an enhanced risk of infectious endocarditis similar to that following a cardiac surgical procedure. It is therefore recommended that the patient receive two to four doses of intravenous antibiotic prophylaxis with cephalosporin or a similar antibiotic.

Catheter Occlusion of Other Vascular Structures

A number of different techniques have been reported for the occlusion of vascular structures such as systemic-to-pulmonary artery collaterals, the arterial supply to tumors or segments of organs, surgically created systemic-to-pulmonary artery anastomoses, or arteriovenous fistula. Transcatheter vascular occlusion has also been performed on the venous side. Techniques include the use of Gianturco coils, Gelfoam, detachable balloons, and tissue adhesive "glue" material.

Gianturco Coils

Coil embolization of unwanted vascular structures has generally been used on the arterial side of the circulation and was first described by Gianturco et al. in 1975. These coils are available commercially (Cook, Inc., Bloomington, IN) and come in a variety of lengths and coiled diameters (Table 1). They resemble small segments of coil-spring guidewires in that they have a central steel core and an outer coil spring. However, these occluder coils tend to assume a circular position when extruded from their delivery tube or from the distal end of a catheter. A series of short, Dacron strands are attached

Table 1

Embolization Coils

Wire diameter (inches)	Coil extruded diameter (mm)	Coil length (mm)
0.018	3	10
	5	15
	7	21
	10	30
0.025	2	12
	2	25
	5	30
	3	40
0.038	3	20
	3	40
	5	50
	8	50
0.052	15	100
	15	150
	20	150

Halal micro coils (0.018 inches);* Occluding spring emboli (0.025, 0.038, and 0.052 inches).*

* Cook Incorporated (Bloomington, IN).

to these wires and it is these strands that make these occluder coils thrombogenic. In addition, the coils can be soaked in topical thrombin to further enhance their thrombogenic properties, especially in high-flow situations such as in arteriovenous fistulae.

Method

The anatomy of the vessel to be occluded is evaluated by selective angiography. The length and diameter of the blood vessel are important considerations in the selection of an appropriate sized coil. The ability to enter the vessel with a catheter and to fix the tip of the catheter within the vessel until the coil has been extruded is key to the success of this procedure. The occluding coils are available as 0.018- to 0.052-inch diameter wires. These coils are relatively stiff and attempt to assume a circular configuration when extruded from the loading tube. As a result, they tend to bend the catheter somewhat as they are advanced toward the tip. If the tip of the catheter is positioned just at the orifice or only slightly further into the vessel, then it is likely that the catheter tip will pull back out of the vessel when the attempt is made to extrude the coil from the distal end of the catheter. This is especially true if the catheter has made a fairly sharp angle to enter the blood vessel. If this occurs while the coil is still within the catheter and being advanced toward the tip, it only necessitates removing the catheter from the patient, extruding the coil from the catheter, and starting over again with an attempt at better positioning of the catheter tip. On the other hand, if the catheter pops out of the vessel after more than one-third to one-half of the length of the coil has been extruded, there is considerable likelihood that the remainder of the coil will advance out of the catheter tip that is now positioned in the aorta. If this occurs, the coil will embolize to the distal aorta and could result in intravascular thrombosis of a crucial area. To avoid this potential problem, it is recommended that the catheter tip be advanced as far out into the vessel as possible and, as was mentioned previously, to avoid any sharp ends in the catheter, especially close to the catheter tip. An end-hole, balloon-tipped catheter may also be helpful to avoid this problem. If the balloon-tipped catheter can be advanced far enough into the vessel, the balloon can be inflated and this will serve to fix the catheter in the blood vessel and also to reduce flow downstream from the inflated balloon. The coil can then be extruded through the end hole of the balloon catheter with less concern about the possibility of dislodgement of the catheter tip during this process.

Another important consideration in the selection of an appropriate sized occluder coil is the distensibility of the blood vessel. If the vessel does not have a site of stenosis distal to the area to be occluded, it is possible that the vessel may become distended proximal to the site of occlusion. If this occurs, the coil may then become inadequate for the diameter of the stretched vessel and

assume its circular configuration. This will result in failure of occlusion since when the coil assumes a circular shape, blood flows through the center opening or if the vessel is large enough, the coil will line up parallel to the long axis of the vessel and flow will occur on either side of it. In either case, the flow passes around or through the coil and vessel occlusion usually does not occur. In addition, distal embolization of the occluder coil is also possible. To avoid this problem, Perry et al. (1989) recommended the use of a balloon-tipped angiographic catheter to determine the stretched diameter of the vessel to be occluded. A balloon-tipped angiographic catheter with proximal side holes is advanced into the blood vessel to the site at which it is expected that the occluder coil will be deposited. Selective angiography to determine vessel diameter is performed both before and after occlusion of the vessel by inflation of the balloon. The larger, dilated diameter of the vessel proximal to the occluding balloon is used as a guide to select an appropriate sized occluder coil. As a general rule, the coiled diameter should be approximately 25% larger than the distended diameter of the vessel to be occluded. It must be remembered that arteries will distend some 10%–20%, while venous structures may increase 30%–50% or more when occluded. Since there is considerable variability, it is strongly recommended that angiographic assessment of stretched diameter be performed by this balloon occlusion technique prior to the selection of the occluder coil to be used.

Once the vessel diameter has been determined, a delivery catheter is selected appropriate to the size occluder coil to be used. Microcoils have extruded diameters of 3–10 mm and can be delivered with a catheter as small as #3 French. The smaller diameter, standard Gianturco wires (0.025-inch) are available with an extruded circular diameter of 2–5 mm and can be used with almost any catheter with an external diameter of #4 French or larger. The larger diameter (0.038-inch) occluder coil is available with an extruded circle diameter of 3–8 mm. This wire, of course, requires a delivery catheter with an internal diameter of at least 0.040 inches. The largest diameter coils (0.052-inch) have an extruded diameter of 15 mm or 20 mm and would be used in only very large vessels in bigger patients. It is preferable that the internal diameter of the catheter be only slightly larger than the wire size of the occluder coil to be used. If the internal diameter of the catheter is much larger than the wire size of the coil, then the occluder coil may curl slightly inside the catheter rather than remaining straight. This may result in the coil wire getting caught inside the catheter at any point of irregularity on the internal wall or at the site of any sharp catheter angle. This would make it extremely difficult, if not impossible, to extrude the occluder coil from this catheter. Polyurethane or other soft catheters are not recommended for use with these coils since they may buckle due to the tendency of the coil to try and assume a circular shape. This will result in jamming of the coil within the catheter. Side-hole catheters may also result in problems and these catheters also should not be used as delivery catheters. If a side-hole catheter is used, the coil may catch in the side hole and may either jam in the catheter or be extruded in a location other than was originally intended. Since the soft, floppy end of a coil-spring guidewire is used to advance the occluder coil through the catheter, it is a good idea to check to be certain that the guidewire will pass easily through the distal end of the delivery catheter to be used.

Once the appropriate sized occluder coil has been selected, the delivery catheter is inserted through the sheath and advanced into the vessel to be occluded. As was described above, the catheter is fixed in position well into the blood vessel and with an attempt to minimize any sharp angulations. The delivery tube, or cartridge, is inserted into that catheter and wedged into the catheter fitting. While the tube is held in this position against the hub of the catheter with one hand, the stiff end of the guidewire to be used as an introducer is inserted into the tube to advance the occluder coil at least 20 cm past the hub and into the catheter. The guidewire is then removed and the delivery tube is discarded. The soft, floppy end of the guidewire is now inserted into the catheter and is used to advance the occluder coil toward the catheter tip. It is important to remember to use the soft end of the guidewire to advance the occluder coil rather than the stiff end. The stiff end will invariably straighten the catheter as it advances and either this may result in the catheter being dislodged from the vessel to be occluded or else it may not be possible to advance the stiff guidewire and coil past any angulations in the catheter.

In some situations, when there is considerable angulation in the catheter, it may be possible to pass the occluder wire past this point of angulation, but not the guidewire being used to push the occluder coil forward. If this happens and the coil has not been extruded from the catheter, the catheter is removed. A further attempt can then be made with the same or another type of catheter that has been positioned differently. On the other hand, if the occluder coil has been partially extruded from the catheter and the catheter tip still remains in the vessel that is to be occluded, the coil can be completely extruded by rapidly flushing the catheter with 1 ml of a saline solution using a tuberculin syringe (Perry et al. 1989). The ability to do this is facilitated by having a catheter whose internal diameter is only slightly larger than the occluder coil. If the delivery catheter has too large an internal diameter, the saline solution will pass around the occluder coil wire and it will not be possible to develop sufficient pressure to extrude the remainder of the occluder coil wire into the blood vessel.

After the occluder coil wire has been positioned in the blood vessel at the desired site, a period of 10–15 minutes should elapse before an attempt should be made to determine if thrombosis has occurred. A hand in-

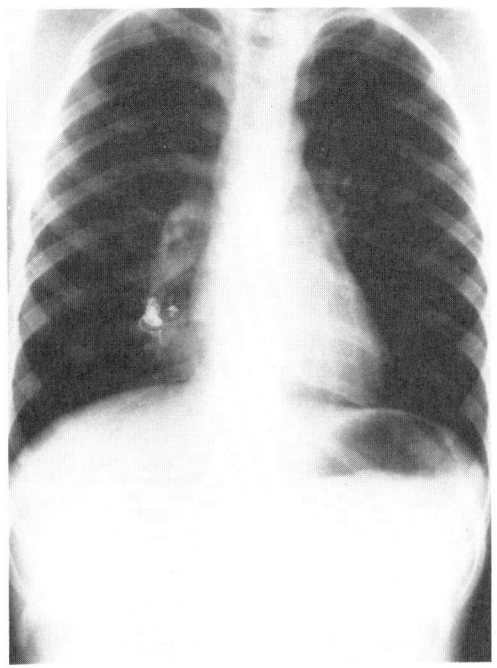

Figure 7. Multiple Gianturco coils embolized in a pulmonary arteriovenous malformation.

jection of a small amount of contrast material will demonstrate the degree of occlusion of the vessel, if any. If the delivery catheter is a balloon catheter and the balloon is still inflated, there may be no forward flow even though the vessel has not been completely occluded. In this case, the balloon should be deflated slowly, and if necessary, the injection of contrast material can then be repeated. If there is incomplete occlusion, the delivery catheter can be left in place to deliver additional occluder coils into the same blood vessel (Fig. 7). Once the vessel has been totally occluded or the physician has decided to discontinue further attempts, the catheters are removed, and adequate hemostasis is achieved. Routine postcatheterization care is provided, and observation in an intensive care setting is unnecessary.

Failure of Occlusion and Complications

It may be necessary to abandon an attempt at vascular occlusion by the coil embolization technique after angiography has demonstrated that a blood vessel is either too small or too large, is a critical source of blood supply to a vital area, or provides a major percentage of pulmonary blood flow in a patient with pulmonary atresia. An attempt at coil embolization may have to be abandoned due to the inability to properly position and fix the delivery catheter far enough into the vessel that is to be occluded or in a situation when it is not possible to deliver the occluder coil through the catheter even though the catheter has been appropriately positioned. In cases where coil embolization had been contemplated prior to cardiac catheterization but where the limit of the amount of contrast material that can be used safely has been reached, it is wise to forego consideration of coil embolization at that catheterization and to defer the vascular occlusion to a separate procedure at a later time.

If incomplete occlusion has occurred, the subsequent management will depend upon the circumstances necessitating the vascular occlusion in the first place. If complete occlusion of the blood vessel was the goal and only partial occlusion has occurred, either a further attempt at transcatheter occlusion by the same or another technique at a subsequent time or a surgical approach for ligation of the blood vessel should be performed. On the other hand, a reduction in the volume of blood flow through an unwanted vessel may be a satisfactory result. For example, a patient with congestive heart failure due to excessive blood flow in large collateral vessels or an arteriovenous malformation may benefit considerably by a reduction of blood flow without complete occlusion. Similarly, in a patient who is to undergo a surgical procedure in a highly vascular area where ligation of feeder blood vessels would normally take place intraoperatively, preoperative reduction of blood flow by even partial occlusion of major arterial feeders may be of great benefit. On the other hand, in patients with arteriovenous malformations or other similar lesions, incomplete occlusion may not provide a satisfactory result and a surgical approach may be necessary.

Complications of transcatheter coil embolization consist mainly of trauma to myocardial or vascular structures as a result of catheter manipulation or inadvertent embolization. This technique usually necessitates lengthy retrograde arterial procedures, sometimes with large catheters. Thus, heparinization with 100 units of heparin/kg at the time of arterial catheter entry may help to lessen the risk of femoral arterial thrombosis. There is also the risk of a vascular tear or perforation as a result of intense catheter manipulation. This is especially true in the case of occlusion of systemic-to-pulmonary arterial collaterals, since these vessels sometimes can be thin and may be easily torn. The other major complication of this procedure is inadvertent distal embolization of the occluder coil. If the vascular occlusion is being attempted in a vessel with a downstream area of dilation just proximal to an area of stenosis, embolization of the loop of coil into that segment will be of little consequence and, in fact, embolization of a few coils may result in the desired occlusion of the vessel. This is also the case in a patient with an arteriovenous malformation. In patients with systemic-to-pulmonary artery collaterals, however, the downstream area is often a segment of true pulmonary artery. Distal embolization of an occluder coil into this area would not be desirable even though, as was mentioned previously, the occluder coil when it forms a loop will often orient itself parallel to the axis of blood flow and thus not result in occlusion.

The aorta would be a site of distal embolization that would be of greater concern because of the risk of thrombosis of an important vascular structure. This usually occurs when the occluder coil is released into an arterial structure too close to its proximal origin from the aorta or if the delivery catheter inadvertently pops back into the aorta at the time that the occluder wire is being delivered into the vessel with resultant release of the occluder coil into the central aorta. Distal embolization into the systemic circulation could also occur during an attempt at occlusion of a persistent left superior vena cava draining to the left atrium. If advertent embolization occurs in the systemic or pulmonary circulation and access to that area is possible with the sheath and/ or catheter, it may be possible to retrieve the occluder coil with a snare device or with the use of a catheter-tip, deflector guidewire advanced through a catheter (Perry et al. 1989). In some circumstances, it may be possible to retrieve the coil through a sheath or to withdraw the coil as close as possible to the point of entry into the circulation where it could be retrieved by means of a cutdown. If these techniques are not successful, it may then be necessary to retrieve the occluder coil with a surgical procedure.

Balloon Embolization

The detachable balloon technique for vascular occlusion (Barth et al. 1982) is useful for the occlusion of a large tortuous vessel with the distal area of stenosis that cannot be occluded by one of the other techniques already described. This might be because the vessel is too large to use one of the other occluder devices and/or because of difficulty in inserting a delivery catheter far enough into the blood vessel. Since these balloons are light and are floated into position, it may be possible to deliver this device into a site that is not accessible by one of the other techniques.

Method

These silicone detachable balloons are commercially available (Becton-Dickinson, Co., Rutherford, NJ) with inflated diameters of 2, 4, or 8 mm. The balloons are attached to small, thin, #2 French polyurethane catheters. As a result of their small size, these inflatable balloons can be inserted through a delivery catheter with an internal diameter of 0.043 inches or larger (#9 French). Once the delivery catheter is positioned as far as possible into the vessel to be occluded, the balloon and its attached #2 French catheter is loaded into a 20–ml syringe or into a delivery device that can contain the coils of the #2 French catheter. This latter device has Luer-Lok fittings on the distal end to attach to the hub of the catheter and on the proximal end, which can be attached to a syringe. In either case, the syringe is filled with normal saline, and the catheter tip with the detachable balloon extends a centimeter or so beyond the end of the syringe. The #2 French catheter is then inserted into hub of the delivery catheter and the syringe or delivery device is slowly advanced until the Luer-Lok end is inserted into the catheter hub. The balloon is then advanced through the delivery catheter and into the blood vessel to be occluded. This is accomplished by slow infusion of saline with an occasional, short-burst infusion, which is necessary to advance the balloon forward if it does not seem to be moving with the slow infusion. A point worth remembering is that the tip of the delivery catheter must be free within the lumen of the blood vessel. If it is positioned against the wall, the saline will infuse without noticeable problem. However, either the balloon catheter will not pass beyond the tip of the delivery catheter, or the tip of the delivery catheter may wedge the #2 French tubing against the wall of the blood vessel and prevent further advancement of the balloon catheter once it has been delivered into the blood vessel.

After the balloon has been positioned appropriately in the vessel to be occluded, the balloon is inflated to its maximal diameter using nonionic contrast material. Hopefully, the balloon will then be wedged in the blood vessel and this will be evident fluoroscopically by the deformation of the side walls of the balloon into a "sausage-like" configuration. Once it is certain that the balloon is wedged in position, the balloon is separated from its attached #2

French catheter by a quick, short, jerking motion. Sometimes, if the #2 French catheter is caught by a sharp angulation in the delivery catheter or is pressed by the catheter tip against the blood vessel, slight withdrawal of the delivery catheter will release the balloon catheter shaft and enable the short, jerking motion to pull it free from the balloon. If this is not successful, further withdrawal of the delivery catheter or possibly a short tug on the delivery catheter while pulling the #2 French catheter simultaneously will facilitate the release. There is a small valve in the detachable balloon that will prevent discharge of contrast material from the balloon after the catheter has been detached.

Thrombosis usually occurs in the blood vessel after it has been occluded with the detachable balloon. It is a good idea to verify complete occlusion with a hand injection of a small amount of contrast material through the delivery catheter approximately 15 minutes after the balloon has been released. If complete occlusion has not occurred, it might be advisable to reduce blood flow in the vessel temporarily by partial or total occlusion with a standard Swan-Ganz, or similar, flow-directed balloon catheter. After an additional period of reduced or occluded proximal flow, if some residual flow is still present around the balloon, it might be worth considering the use of particulate embolization with Gelfoam or the use of a tissue adhesive (see below). If either of these latter techniques is used, the flow in the vessel would again be occluded by means of a proximal balloon catheter, and the additional occluding material would be injected through its lumen. This would allow the injected Gelfoam or tissue adhesive to induce thrombosis in the area of residual flow around the balloon (Fig. 8).

Complications

Distal embolization past the desired site of occlusion is the major complication as-

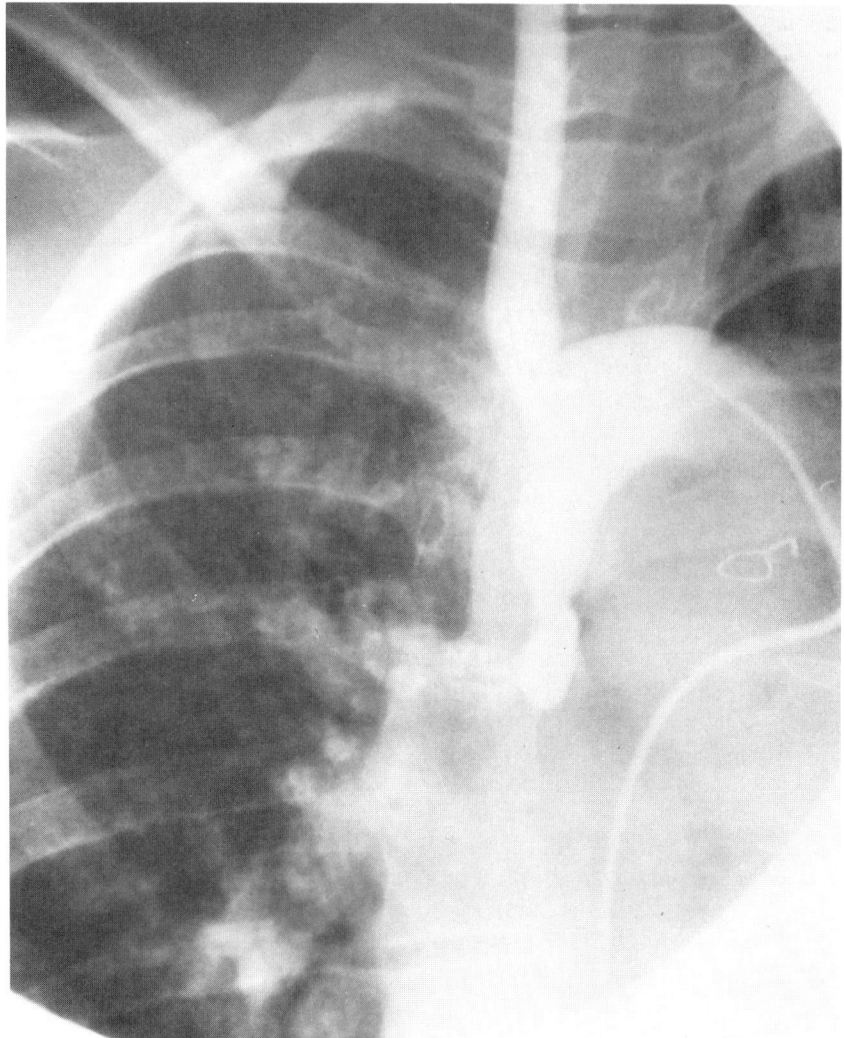

Figure 8. Balloon embolization with additional use of tissue adhesive for occlusion of a residual Blalock-Taussig anastomôsis.

sociated with the use of the detachable balloon technique. The usual site of embolization is into the pulmonary vascular bed where the balloon will lodge into a smaller segmental pulmonary artery. If thrombosis of this vessel occurs and does not extend into a major branch, this will usually not result in any serious complications. If access to that area is possible with a catheter, it may be possible to puncture the thin, silicone balloon using the tip of a guidewire. To do this, the catheter is positioned against the surface of the balloon, and the guidewire advanced to the distal end. If the guidewire is advanced through the tip with a short, jabbing motion, it may be possible to deflate the balloon. Clearly, the balloon would still be present in the circulation but would have a much lower profile, might embolize into a still smaller distal branch, and would be even less of a threat for any major thrombosis.

A problem seen with detachable balloons and not usually with other occluder techniques is a possibility of late embolization. Deflation of the balloon, suddenly or gradually, can occur hours, days, or even weeks following the procedure. In general, if the balloon becomes deflated, proximal thrombosis has already occurred and the vessel remains occluded. If deflation occurs 1 week or later after the procedure, the thrombosis is well organized and the balloon is also fixed in the vessel by fibrous tissue. If deflation occurs within the first few days, however, there would be a greater risk of embolization of the deflated balloon and a partially organized thrombosis.

Particulate Embolization and Tissue Adhesive

Embolization with particles of synthetic material such as Ivalon, Gelfoam, and polyvinyl chloride has been used in a number of circumstances to reduce or occlude blood flow. These include embolization of a pheochromocytoma prior to surgical removal to minimize the outpouring of catecholamine substances that often occurs as a result of manipulation of the tumor (Horton et al. 1983). Preoperative particulate embolization of an extremely vascular tumor would minimize the blood loss that would be expected during resection. This would also be helpful in the management of arteriovenous malformations if at least some reduction of flow could be accomplished by temporary occlusion of the arterial feeders and infusion of particulate emboli prior to operation. Similarly, the tissue adhesive Bucrylate was used in our institution (Zuberbuhler et al. 1974) to close systemic-to-pulmonary artery collaterals during cardiac catheterization preoperatively, postoperatively, as well as intraoperatively, by means of catheters that were inserted in the cardiac catheterization laboratory prior to operation.

The methodology for these techniques will not be described in detail since we have no experience with the particulate embolization techniques and the tissue adhesive is no longer available, thus precluding the use of that technique.

References and Suggested Reading

Barth KH, White RI, Jr, Kaufman SL, et al. Embolotherapy of pulmonary arteriovenous malformations with detachable balloons. Radiology 1982; 142:559–606.

Bash SE, Mullins CE. Insertion of patent ductus occluder by transvenous approach: A new technique. Circulation 1984; 70(Suppl II):285.

Fellows KE, Lock JE. Catheter intervention: Septostomy occlusion techniques, and pericardial drainage. In: Lock JE, Keane JF, Fellows KE (eds), Diagnostic and Interventional Catheterization in Congenital Heart Disease. Boston, MA, Nijhoff. 1987, pp 123–143.

Fuhrman BP, Bass JL, Castaneda-Zuniga W, et al. Coil embolization of congenital thoracic vascular anomalies in infants and children. Circulation 1984; 70:285–289.

Gianturco C, Anderson JH, Wallace S. Mechanical devices for arterial occlusion. Am J Roentgenol 1975; 124:428–435.

Horton JA, Hrabovsky E, Klingberg WG, et al. Therapeutic embolization of a hyperfunctioning pheochromocytoma. Am J Roentgenol 1983; 140:987–988.

Krichenko A, Benson LN, Burrows P, et al. Angiographic classification of the isolated, persistently patent ductus arteriosus and implications for percutaneous catheter occlusion. Am J Cardiol 1989; 63:877–880.

Lock JE, Cocherham JT, Keane JF, et al. Transcatheter umbrella closure of congenital heart defects. Circulation 1987; 75:593–599.

Perry SB, Radtke W, Fellows KE, et al. Coil embolization to occlude aortopulmonary collateral vessels and shunts in patients with congenital heart disease. J Am Coll Cardiol 1989; 13:100–108.

Portsmann W, Hieronymi K, Wierny L, et al. Nonsurgical closure of oversized patent ductus arteriosus with pulmonary hypertension. Report of a Case. Circulation 1974; 50:376–381.

Portsmann W, Wierny L, Warnke H, et al. Catheter closure of patent ductus arteriosus, 62 cases treated without thoracotomy. Radiol Clin North Am 1971; 9:203–218.

Rashkind WJ, Mullins CE, Hellenbrand WE, et al.

Nonsurgical closure of patent ductus arteriosus: Clinical application of the Rashkind
PDA occluder system. Circulation 1987;
75:583–592.

Rashkind WJ, Cuaso CC. Transcatheter closure of
patent ductus arteriosus. Successful use in
a 3.5 kilogram infant. Pediatr Cardiol 1979;
1:3–7.

Sato K, Fujino M, Kozuka T, et al. Transfemoral
plug closure of patent ductus arteriosus. Experiences in 61 consecutive cases treated
without thoracotomy. Circulation 1975;
51:337–341.

Zuberbuhler JR, Dankner E, Zoltun R, et al. Tissue
adhesive closure of aortic-pulmonary communication. Am Heart J 1974; 88:41–46.

16

Complications Associated with Cardiac Catheterization

Sang C. Park, M.D.

Although the first introduction of a catheter into the human heart was performed by Forsman (1929) through his own arm vein over a half century ago, the clinical use of cardiac catheterization for the diagnosis of congenital heart disease in children did not occur until the early 1950s. Since then, there have been many advances in biomedical and electronic technology and many new and innovative devices have been introduced. Special diagnostic or therapeutic techniques such as electrophysiologic studies, transseptal catheterization, myocardial biopsy, balloon atrial septostomy, blade atrial septostomy, nonsurgical closure of atrial septal defect or patent ductus arteriosus, and balloon dilation have added to the dimension and complexity of the cardiac catheterization procedure. Special training and expertise are required to perform these procedures and a host of additional risk factors are now involved.

Mortality

There is general agreement among pediatric cardiologists that no patient is too sick to undergo cardiac catheterization. This aggressive approach has resulted in increased survival of critically ill newborn infants, but has also increased the morbidity and mortality from cardiac catheterization in this age group. Reports in the early 1950s showed a low mortality (0.1%). In those days, studies were mostly right-sided heart catheterizations only. A subsequent collaborative study on cardiac catheterization (Braunwald and Swan 1968) with inclusion of left heart studies showed a higher mortality of 0.44% among the 12,364 cases studied. The mortality under 2 months of age was strikingly high (6%) as compared to the age group between 2 and 59 years of age (0.14%). Another collaborative study from 66 laboratories was performed by the Society for Cardiac Angiography over a 14-month period in 1979–80 (Kennedy 1982). Of the 53,581 patients in the study, 457 were under 1 year of age. The overall mortality was 0.14%, but mortality rates were significantly higher in patients under 1 year of age (1.75%) and over 60 years (0.25%).

A large series of 12,255 studies at the Toronto Hospital for Sick Children showed an overall mortality of 0.95% (Rowe 1978). However, 84% of the deaths occurred in patients under 1 month of age (mortality of 6.7%), while mortality under 1 week of age was 9.6%. Mortality between the age of 1 month and 1 year was 0.5% and beyond age 1 year the rate was only 0.05%. Thus, it is fair to say that cardiac catheterization of children, if one excludes sick newborn infants, involves minimal risk of death.

The relatively high risk in the newborn period is attributable to the precarious status of many of the patients undergoing study. Some are severely hypoxemic or in congestive heart failure and may be acidotic as well. If one defines catheterization mortality as death occurring within 24 hours of the study, some infants will be included who were very sick before the catheterization, survived the procedure, and then died a few hours later.

The morbidity and mortality of cardiac catheterization in the sick newborn and infant can be reduced by accurate clinical diagnosis before the procedure. Cross-sectional and Doppler echocardiography have proven to be effective tools for anatomic diagnosis, eliminating some catheterizations and making others safer by reducing time spent in the laboratory and the amount of contrast agent needed for diagnosis.

A most striking contribution to increased survival of neonates has been the use of prostaglandin E_1. This agent has proven to be of immense value in the management of critically ill neonates with ductus dependent cardiac lesions such as pulmonary atresia or severe coarctation of the aorta. Thus, the combination of newer pharmacologic agents and noninvasive techniques has significantly reduced the mortality of cardiac catheterization in neonates.

Mortality from cardiac catheterization is rare beyond the neonatal period. Nonfatal complications do occur, however, and may be quite serious. (Table 1). Complications related to special procedures or angiocardiography will be discussed separately.

Vascular Complications

The introduction of a catheter always damages the entered vessel and there is always a chance of a vascular complication.

Arterial Complications

Insertion of a catheter into a peripheral artery may lead to arterial spasm or to intimal damage followed by thrombosis. In particular, small patients with relatively small arteries or patients with low cardiac

Table 1

Complications of Cardiac Catheterization

1. *Vascular complications*
   Arterial - spasm, thrombosis
             - dissection, false aneurysm
   Venous - spasm, thrombosis,
             -arteriovenous fistula
2. *Thromboembolic phenomenon*
   Systemic   - cerebrovascular accident
               - arterial embolization
   Pulmonary   - embolism
   Air embolism
3. *Cardiovascular injury*
   Perforation or tear
   Endomyocardial damage
   Ischemia or infarct
   Rupture of atrioventricular valve
     apparatus
4. *Electrocardiographic changes*
   Tachyarrhythmia
   A-V block
5. *Problems with the catheter*
   Kinking of the catheter
   Breakage of catheter or sheath
   Malfunction or rupture of a balloon
   Knotting
   Immobilization of the catheter
6. *Local complication at the site of
     catheterization*
   Hemorrhage
   Hematoma
   Infection
7. *Systemic complication*
   Pyrogenic reaction
   Sepsis and infective endocarditis
8. *Hemodynamic effects*
9. *Reactions to contrast media*
10. *Reactions to premedication*
11. *Radiation hazard*
12. *Electrical hazard*
13. *Neurologic complications*

output have a higher incidence of arterial complications. If there is actual thrombosis at the site of arterial puncture, the involved extremity is cold and pale or mottled. If it seems clear that there is thrombosis rather than spasm, immediate surgical intervention is indicated to restore blood flow. With arterial spasm, the affected extremity is cool and pale, and distal pulses are reduced or absent. This complication usually resolves within several hours as the spasm subsides. A dry, warm compress (rubber glove filled with warm water) placed over the puncture site may hasten relief of the spasm. If the arterial pulse is absent, a Doppler device is helpful to confirm the presence of pulsatile arterial flow. If the vascular compromise is prolonged beyond several hours after the termination of the cardiac catheterization or if distal flow cannot be detected by Doppler, systemic heparinization may be indicated to prevent thrombus formation or extension in the compromised vessel. Heparinization is usually maintained for 24 to 48 hours after the procedure. There is a considerable controversy as to whether patients should routinely be anticoagulated during cardiac catheterization to prevent arterial thrombosis (Miller et al. 1974; Girod et al. 1975; Luepker et al. 1975; Rich et al. 1975). In our laboratory, systemic heparinization is not used routinely. However, it is our impression that systemic heparinization with 100 units of heparin/kg at the initiation of arterial catheterization may be of value in reducing the incidence of arterial thrombosis in high risk patients, those with low cardiac output or high hematocrit ($>65\%$).

Dissection of the arterial wall is another complication that may occur during introduction of a guidewire through a malaligned needle (Fig. 1). If this occurs, the guidewire and needle should be removed and another artery used if at all possible. Another unusual complication is formation of a false aneurysm at the puncture site. An arteriovenous fistula may also occur, presumably due to simultaneous puncture of the artery and vein at the same level during percutaneous cardiac catheterization. If the fistula is small, a bruit over the area is the only manifestation. If the fistula is large (Fig. 2), there is a significant runoff from the artery to the vein, pulses are bounding, and there may be a visible pulsation over the fistula. Most fistulae require surgical intervention.

In addition to immediate arterial compromise, long-term complications of arterial catheterization may occur. Even if there is no apparent difficulty immediately following cardiac catheterization, chronic impairment

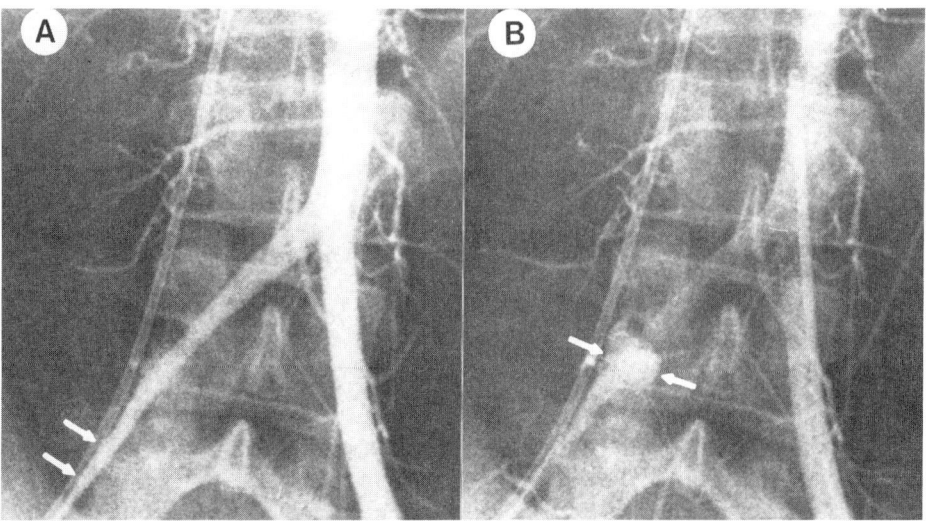

Figure 1. Arterial complications: Dissection and spasm of the right iliac artery following unsuccessful insertion of the percutaneous sheath. A: Angiogram via the left femoral artery demonstrating marked spasm (arrows) of the right iliac and femoral artery. B: Late phase of the angiogram demonstrating a dissecting aneurysm (arrows).

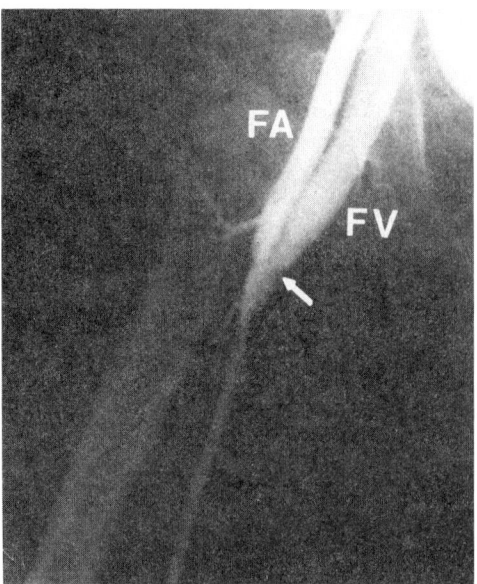

Figure 2. Femoral arteriovenous fistula (arrow) with significant shunt.

of lower extremity blood flow has been noted in children following cardiac catheterization (Skovr Anek and Sam Enek 1979). Hurwitz et al. (1977) angiographically demonstrated arterial occlusion in 3%–8% of patients weighing less than 25 kg at the time of arterial catheterization. Other long-term follow-up studies of patients who underwent femoral artery cardiac catheterization demonstrated that chronic arterial compromise can affect and size and length of a lower extremity (Basset et al. 1972; Rosenthal et al. 1972).

Venous Complications

The problems encountered with venous catheterization differ somewhat from those on the arterial side. Veins are thin and are more fragile structures than arteries and can be damaged easily by insertion and manipulation of the catheter. Tearing of a vein may occur in a newborn infant during a cutdown catheterization, especially during attempts to insert a balloon catheter. During venous cardiac catheterization by the cutdown technique, venous spasm is a rather common occurrence if the vein is small. It results in inability to maneuver the catheter, although the spasm usually disappears within a short time. Use of a smaller catheter may avoid recurrence of spasm, and wiping the catheter with a local anesthetic prior to introduction may also reduce spasm. The percutaneous sheath technique has reduced the incidence of trauma to arteries and veins.

If the venous catheter is inadvertently passed into a small branch of the iliac vein or inferior vena cava, the catheter may be entrapped by severe venous spasm. Forceful withdrawal of the catheter at this point may result in a tear of the vein and retroperitoneal hemorrhage. In this situation, maintenance of continuous gentle traction on the catheter usually is effective in dislodging it.

Ligation of the femoral vein may be necessary at the conclusion of a cardiac catheterization by cutdown technique in a small infant. Edema and cyanosis may be marked, but usually improve within several days, presumably due to establishment of collateral venous drainage.

In recent years, the presence of ileofemoral venous thrombosis after the use of a balloon catheter has been recognized (Mathews et al. 1979). The exact mechanism of this thrombosis is not known, but intimal damage by a large-caliber balloon catheter may initiate the thrombosis. The thrombosis is not limited to the site of puncture, but may extend to the iliac vein and to the inferior vena cava (Fig 3). Unless there is renal vein thrombosis, this complication is generally not recognized until a subsequent cardiac catheterization. In our experience, most patients with this complication have no signs of venous compromise beyond the immediate postcatheterization period. The long-term effect of this venous complication is yet to be determined.

Thromboembolic Phenomena

Thromboembolism is one of the more serious complications of cardiac catheteri-

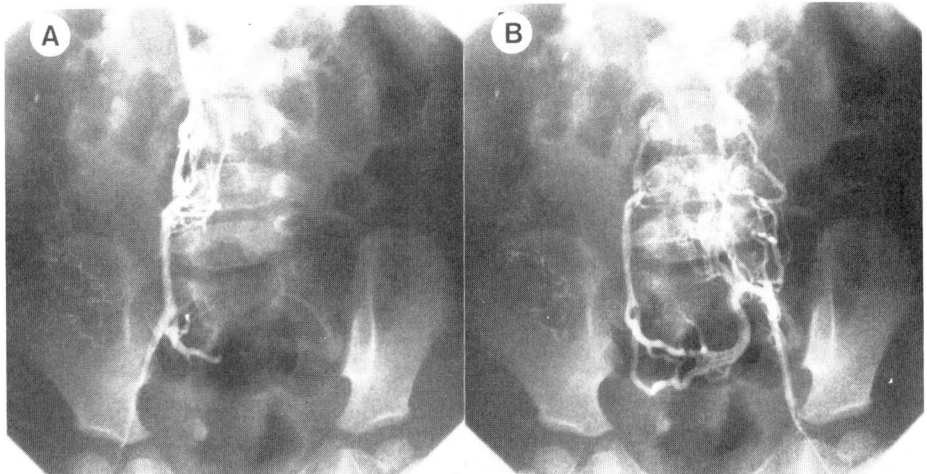

Figure 3. Extensive ileofemoral vein thrombosis. Right (A) and left (B) femoral venous angiogram demonstrating complete obstruction of normal ileofemoral veins and extensive collateral flow via the paravertebral venous plexus and azygos system.

zation. Systemic embolization is most common in patients with a right-to-left shunt such as transposition of the great arteries, tetralogy of Fallot, or tricuspid atresia. Such patients are usually polycythemic and may have an abnormal clotting mechanism. The most common serious complication is a cerebrovascular accident due to cerebral embolism, while embolization to other peripheral arteries may occur. Frequent flushing of the catheter system with heparinized solution minimizes the risk of thrombosis in such patients, but air embolism also must be avoided during flushing. Systemic heparinization of severely cyanotic patients with high hematocrit (>65%) may be helpful in reducing the incidence of such complications.

Pulmonary embolism may also occur during cardiac catheterization, but the incidence is unknown because it is rarely recognized unless it is massive. Tang et al. (1978) reported pulmonary fiber embolism and granuloma in three infants following cardiac catheterization. The emboli originated from the fibrous lining of nondisposable, woven, synthetic-fiber catheters and apparently dislodged during angiography. A significant incidence (12%) of pulmonary perfusion defects has been noted by ventilation—perfusion scans done before and 1 day after cardiac catheterization (Primm et al. 1979). This study suggested that minor pulmonary embolism may be a common complication of routine cardiac catheterization. Fortunately, most are subclinical and appear to cause no sequelae.

Cardiovascular Injury

Perforation of a cardiac free wall or a great artery is rare, but is often fatal, especially if an atrial wall is involved. Such a complication may occur at any cardiovascular site, but the most vulnerable area in the pediatric age group is the right ventricular outflow tract. Prolonged manipulation of the catheter in an attempt to enter the pulmonary artery may result in perforation of this relatively thin area, particularly in patients with right ventricular outflow obstruction. The right and left atrial appendages are also thin and can be easily perforated. Perforation of the left ventricle or a great artery is extremely unusual.

Acute perforation of the myocardium by a catheter during cardiac catheterization can be recognized by the unusual position of the catheter and by the inability to withdraw blood through the catheter. There may also be ST segment and/or T-wave changes on the electrocardiogram. Perforation can be confirmed by injecting a small amount of contrast media through the catheter and into the pericardial space. If the catheter tip is in the pericardial space, the catheter *should not be withdrawn,* because withdrawal may lead to immediate pericardial tamponade. Immediate surgical intervention should be arranged while the catheter remains in situ.

The use of balloon-tipped catheters has resulted in a reduction in the incidence of perforation, particularly with complex defects. Although flow-directed catheters may reduce the incidence of perforation during routine catheterization, they have complications of their own. For example, a Swan-Ganz catheter left in the pulmonary artery for a prolonged period of time for monitoring, at least in adults, may result in pulmonary artery perforation or formation of a pulmonary arteriovenous fistula, hemoptysis (Krantz and Viljoen 1979), and even fatal pulmonary hemorrhage (Pape et al. 1979). Myocardial perforation has also been reported from a pacing catheter in the right ventricle (Hurwitz et al. 1977) and from a central venous line (Dane and King 1975).

Myocardial injury may also be caused by the injection of contrast media into a ventricle, particularly with a power injector (Fig. 4). Improper positioning of the catheter against the chamber wall is usually responsible. Infiltration of contrast media into the myocardium results in transient ST-T changes, which usually resolve spontaneously. The myocardial "staining" may last from a few minutes to hours, depending upon the extent of the infiltration. Rarely, perforation of the myocardial wall occurs during angiocardiography and contrast media is seen in the pericardial space. Such a complication may resolve without development of pericardial tamponade, but may be fatal. An excessive delivery rate of contrast media through a small catheter may cause straightening and whipping of the catheter and may result in myocardial damage.

Dissection of a pulmonary artery or of an aortic aneurysm have been reported in adult cardiac catheterizations.

Electrocardiographic Changes

Arrhythmias are common during cardiac catheterization. The most common are transient premature atrial or ventricular contractions related to catheter manipulation. Occasionally, atrioventricular block or bundle-branch block can be seen, but these usually disappear shortly after cessation of catheter manipulation in the sensitive area. Runs of ventricular tachycardia rarely may lead to ventricular fibrillation. Patients with myocarditis or cardiomyopathy are prone to this arrhythmia during cardiac catheterization. In such patients, the rhythm disorder may be difficult to terminate.

Management depends upon the type and duration of the abnormal rhythm. Premature ventricular contractions (PVCs) and even runs of ventricular tachycardia are usually self-limited and resolve as soon as the catheter is removed from the ventricle. Ventricular fibrillation, of course, requires defibrillation. A bundle-branch block or second or third degree AV block often resolves quickly, but may persist for hours or even days.

Atrial arrhythmias such as paroxysmal atrial tachycardia, atrial fibrillation, or atrial flutter also frequently terminate spontaneously, but can persist. Stimulation of the right atrial wall with the catheter tip may abolish supraventricular tachycardia by inducing a premature beat and interrupting reentry. Occasionally, the introduction of PVCs by stimulating the ventricle may be successful in terminating a supraventricular tachyrhythmia. If none of the above maneu-

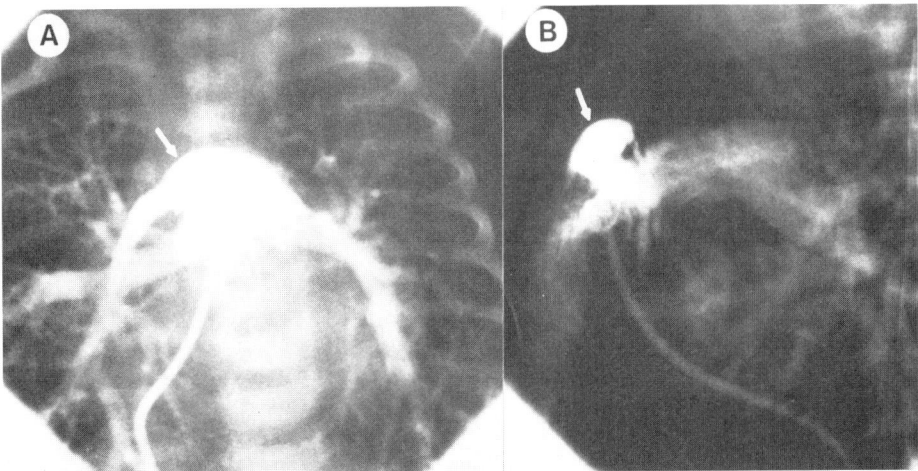

Figure 4. Extensive myocardial infiltration (arrows) of contrast media, which occurred during selective injection in the right ventricular outflow area. A: Anteroposterior view. B: Lateral view.

vers are effective, rapid atrial pacing or electrical cardioversion may be required. Alternatively, the parenteral administration of digoxin or other antiarrhythmic drugs can be used to terminate the arrhythmia.

An electrocardiographic pattern of ischemia or even of infarction may occur during cardiac catheterization. Some instances are related to myocardial injury due to catheter-induced trauma or infiltration of contrast media. At times, there is no apparent reason for such an electrocardiographic change.

Bradycardia without atrioventricular block is an ominous electrocardiographic sign. Its onset can be sudden, but it more frequently appears insidiously. In premature infants or heavily sedated patients, bradycardia may be related to respiratory insufficiency or apnea. Stimulation of such patients often results in resumption of a normal cardiac rate. Occasionally, inhalation of oxygen by face mask is helpful. Other causes of bradycardia are severe myocardial depression or a vagal reflex. Bradycardia may occur spontaneously, may be due to a transient increase of vagal tone, or may be due to a catheter position within the cardiovascular system that causes critical he-

modynamic compromise (such as a catheter pass across a critical semilunar valve stenosis). It should be noted that perforation of the heart with pericardial tamponade also causes bradycardia. Therefore, when bradycardia occurs, prompt assessment and appropriate management are indicated. Once myocardial perforation is ruled out, the catheter should be withdrawn from the heart and corrective measures should be undertaken without delay. It must be emphasized that bradycardia may not be a simple electrical problem, but is often associated with a metabolic derangement or myocardial compromise.

Problems with the Catheter

Kinking of the Catheter

On occasion, a catheter can be sharply bent or looped in the inferior vena cava or in the descending aorta, and it may be quite difficult to straighten it. Usually the loop can be straightened by engaging the catheter tip in a branch vessel (see Chapter 5). Also, the soft end of a guidewire can be introduced to help straighten the catheter. The looped catheter should not be withdrawn into a small peripheral vessel, because this may result in complete fracture of the catheter.

Breakage or Fracture of the Catheter

Rarely, a fractured catheter tip or a piece of a percutaneous sheath can become dislodged and remain in the cardiovascular system. Such fragments have been removed nonsurgically and the technique is discussed in Chapter 14. Open heart surgery may be required to remove a foreign body from the cardiovascular system.

Malfunction or Rupture of a Balloon

Early balloon catheters were sometimes difficult to deflate or ruptured with systemic embolization of rubber fragments. Such problems are rare with current balloon catheters.

Knotting of the Catheter

Flow-directed, flexible, balloon-tipped catheters are now widely used, with or without fluoroscopic guidance. Occasionally, such catheters may knot, prohibiting withdrawal of the catheter from the cardiovascular system. Even woven Dacron catheters may knot during prolonged manipulation. Although it may be possible to loosen the knot by manipulation of the catheter tip after insertion of a guidewire in the proximal portion, in general, it is necessary to withdraw the knotted portion as far as possible and then remove the catheter surgically. Various techniques have been utilized to deal with a knotted catheter (Baldi et al. 1974; Mond et al. 1975; Meister et al. 1977).

Occasionally, the catheter may appear to become knotted during cardiac catheterization. Fortunately, the knot is usually only apparent and is really a superimposition of loops of the catheter. Rarely, when a true knot forms, the knot may be untied by advancing the catheter, the enlarging loop thus freeing the distal end. If this fails, a guidewire can be inserted, *soft end first,* to stiffen the catheter and hopefully free the knot. (However, it must be remembered that the stiff end of a wire may perforate the catheter at one of its sharp curves.) If the knot cannot be undone, it should be withdrawn as far as possible into the extremity and a cutdown and venotomy done. Withdrawal of a loop into a peripheral vein is always painful and may require extra sedation or even general anesthesia.

Immobilization of the Catheter

During manipulation within the cardiovascular system, the catheter may become difficult to move. If a cutdown approach has been used, localized spasm at the entry site may be responsible, or there may be a tight proximal ligature around the vessel. When the percutaneous technique is used, there may be increased friction between the catheter and the sheath due to wrinkling of the sheath or a fibrous deposit within the sheath. True entrapment of catheter within the cardiovascular system usually occurs when the catheter tip is inadvertently lodged in a small branch of a vessel and severe vascular spasm occurs. A common site of entrapment of the catheter is in a small tributary of the inferior vena cava. Forceful withdrawal of the catheter may result in rupture or tear of the vein with retroperitoneal hemorrhage. Gentle and constant traction usually results in release of the catheter. Entrapment of the catheter is the right atrium may be due to a Chiari network (Goldschlager et al. 1972). Also, a balloon catheter may be entrapped within a ventricle, usually due to entanglement in the atrioventricular valve support apparatus. Of course, the balloon should be completely deflated before attempting to withdraw the catheter.

Entrapment of the catheter in the arterial side is not common with the percutaneous technique. If a cutdown is used, however, arterial spasm at the insertion site may be a problem. This may be relieved by local infiltration with a anesthetic and continuous gentle traction on the catheter.

The retrograde approach across a prosthetic valve may result in entrapment of the catheter. Therefore, in this situation, a transseptal approach to the left ventricle is preferred.

Local Complications

A number of local problems can occur at the catheterization site. Inadequate hemostasis or premature release of a pressure dressing after percutaneous catheterization may result in bleeding or formation of a hematoma. Bleeding is more likely to occur and is more prolonged in cyanotic patients with polycythemia and abnormal clotting factors. Infection at the site of a percutaneous catheterization has not been seen in our experience of over 8,000 procedures, but has occurred following cutdown, although rarely. Extensive dissection or an unusually long study predisposes to infection. Proper suture technique and a dry sterile dressing are also important to avoid secondary infection. The groin of an infant is particularly difficult to keep clean and dry and the dressing should therefore be changed frequently until the skin is sealed, usually by 5 days. Routine application of antiseptic ointment over the incision should be avoided, because it may result in delayed granulation. Local treatment of infection usually suffices, but sometimes systemic antibiotic therapy is indicated if the infection is extensive or there are systemic manifestations.

Systemic Complications

Pyrogenic Reaction

Patients occasionally develop a fever to 101° F or 102° F, occasionally to 104° F, a few hours after cardiac catheterization. The fever usually subsides within a few hours without specific treatment. The exact mechanism is unknown, but may be a reaction to foreign protein from the catheters used during the procedure. (Even after meticulous cleansing and sterilization of reusable catheters, a minute amount of foreign protein may remain within the catheter.)

Sepsis and Endocarditis

Sepsis or infectious endocarditis due to cardiac catheterization is extremely rare (Krovetz et al. 1968). Sepsis may be due to direct introduction of bacteria into the cardiovascular system during cardiac catheterization. In addition, trauma to cardiovascular structures during the procedure may predispose those areas to infection should bacteremia occur. A prolonged fever after cardiac catheterization should be considered to be sepsis or endocarditis until proven otherwise and appropriate diagnostic and therapeutic measures should be undertaken.

Hemodynamic Effects

As a general rule, cardiac catheterization does not significantly alter the clinical status of the patient. In some instances, however, volume expansion by flushing solution and/or hypertonic contrast may induce considerable hemodynamic changes. The critically ill infant with congestive heart failure, for example, may be adversely effected by fluid overload. Contrast medium is a potentially cardiotoxic agent and may result in myocardial depression. Excessive blood loss results in hypovolemia and hypotension.

Reactions to Contrast Media

Radiographic contrast media contain organic iodine and hypersensitivity to iodine may result in a allergic reaction. The most common hypersensitivity manifestation is urticaria, appearing within a few minutes after angiography. In most patients there is no great discomfort and no treatment is needed. If the reaction is severe or seems to be progressive, an antihistamine should be given parenterally. Steroids are rarely required. Anaphylactic reactions are extremely rare. Management of hypersensitivity reactions is further discussed in Chapter 9.

Although contrast medium is not usually nephrotoxic, changes in renal function may occur after angiography. Acute renal failure is extremely rare and the mechanism is not known. Myoglobinuria may occur following catheterization and angiocardiography (Donald et al. 1978). Intravascular hemolysis and hemoglobinuria have also been noted following angiocardiography (Cohen et al. 1969). Gastrointestinal complications such as necrotizing enterocolitis (Cooke et al. 1980) and intestinal or hepatic infarcts (Singh et al. 1972) are very rare. Seizures, or even a cerebrovascular accident, may follow injection of a large volume of contrast media, especially directly into the cerebral circulation (Terplan 1973; Dawson and Fischer 1977).

Reaction to Premedication

In our laboratory, premedication for routine cardiac catheterization consists of morphine sulfate in infants between 6 months to 1 year of age and a combination of meperidine, promethazine, and chlorpromazine for patients over 1 year of age (see Chapter 1). There is considerable individual variation in depth of sedation, but no serious adverse reactions have been encountered except for rare instances of respiratory depression. Nalorphrine hydrochloride (Nalline) or naloxone hydrochloride (Narcan) are used if necessary to counteract the respiratory depressant effect of morphine sulfate or meperidine hydrochloride. Ketamine hydrochloride is occasionally used to en-

sure adequate sedation during a transseptal procedure and may induce laryngospasm. A parasympatholytic such as atropine or scopolamine should be given just prior to the ketamine to prevent this adverse reaction.

Radiation Hazard

Cardiac catheterization can not be performed without exposure to radiation. Although there are no immediate manifestations, the long-term effects of this radiation exposure are unknown. A few years ago, a study during cardiac catheterization in pediatric patients indicated radiation exposure to the thorax of about 740 mR (approximately 80% of the radiation was during fluoroscopy). This amount of radiation is equivalent to several hundred chest roentgenographic examinations (Waldman et al. 1981).

It is well known that certain tissues in children are more sensitive to radiation than in adults. The level of radiation exposure to the thyroid gland and gonads during cardiac catheterization has been reported to be low in the pediatric age group (Gustaffsson and Mortensson 1976; Martin et al. 1981; Waldman et al. 1981).

Chromosomal damage has also been reported from cardiac catheterization, due either to radiation or to contrast medium (Adams et al. 1978, Callisen et al. 1979). Patients who require multiple cardiac catheterizations are subject to a cumulative radiation dose, but the long-term effect is unknown.

Radiation exposure during cardiac catheterization can be reduced in two ways. The first is the reduction of exposure time and exposure area. Excessive radiation is usually related to prolonged fluoroscopic examination and exposure time is largely dependent upon the skill of an operator. The inexperienced operator requires more time to maneuver the catheter and may have a "heavy foot." Frequent release of the pedal during fluoroscopic examination substantially reduces the total radiation. Accurate precatheterization clinical evaluation, including two-dimensional echocardiography, minimizes the need for prolonged catheter manipulation in patients with complex cardiac lesions.

It is worthwhile to protect the patient's gonads by using a lead plate under the buttocks and to protect the thyroid by placing a small, malleable lead shield between the primary beam and the neck.

Proper collimation during both fluoroscopy and angiography further reduces the exposure area and the amount of radiation scatter. Pulsed fluoroscopy also promises to reduce radiation (Waldman et al. 1981).

Electrical Hazards

There are a few documented instances of fatal ventricular fibrillation induced by current leaks during cardiac catheterization (Noordijk et al. 1961; Bousvaros et al. 1962). Studies have shown that 60 Hz alternating current as low as 80 μA can produce ventricular fibrillation in humans and this has been observed during cardiac catheterization (Weinberg et al. 1962). However, most instances occurred in the 1960s. Today, electrical monitoring devices currently used in the cardiac catheterization laboratory and in the intensive care unit are quite safe, but must periodically be checked for appropriate grounding and absence of current leaks (Geselowitz et al. 1980).

Neurologic Complications

Central nervous system complications of cardiac catheterization occur in patients with a right-to-left shunt and are related to thromboembolism, either a blood clot, a fragment of the catheter, or fragmented cardiovascular tissue (Phornphutkul 1973; Dawson and Fischer 1977). Occasionally, prolonged hypoxia due to excessive sedation, an anoxic spell, or a prolonged serious ventricular arrhythmia may cause an insult to the central nervous system. An excessive amount of contrast medium may result in a seizure (Terplan 1973).

References and Suggested Reading

Adams FH, Normal A, Bass D, Oku G. Chromosome damage in infants and children after cardiac catheterization and angiocardiography. Pediatrics 1978; 92:312–316.

Baldi J, Fishenfeld MD, Benchimol A. Complete knotting of a catheter and a nonsurgical method of removal. Chest 1974; 62:93–95.

Bousvaros SA, Conway D, Hopps JA. An electrical hazard of selective angiocardiography. Can Med Assoc J 1962; 87:286–288.

Braunwald E, Swan HJC. Cooperative study on cardiac catheterization. Circulation 1968; 37(Suppl III).

Callisen HH, Norman A, Adams FH. Absorbed dose in the presence of contrast agents during pediatric cardiac catheterization. Med Phys 1979; 6:504–509.

Cohen LS, Kokko JP, Williams WH. Hemolysis and hemoglobinuria following angiography. Radiology 1969; 92:329–332.

Cooke RW, Meradji M, de Villeneuve VH. Necrotising entercolitis after cardiac catheterisation in infants. Arch Dis Child 1980; 55:66–68.

Dane TEB, King EG. Fatal cardiac tamponade and other mechanical complications of central venous catheters. Br J Surg 1975; 62:6–10.

Dawson DM, Fischer EG. Neurologic complications of cardiac catheterization. Neurology 1977; 27:496–497.

Donald TG, Cloonan MJ, Wilcken DE. Excretion of myoglobin in urine after cardiac catheterisation. Br Heart J 1978; 40:237–242.

Geselowitz DB, Arzbaecher RC, Barr RC, Briller SA, et al. Electrical safety standards for electrocardiographic apparatus. Circulation 1980; 61:669–670.

Girod DA, Hurwitz RA. Letter: Heparin and arterial thrombosis in children. Circulation 1975; 51:1173–1174.

Goldschlager A, Goldschlager N, Brewster H, Kaplan J. Catheter entrapment in a Chiari network involving an atrial septal defect. Chest 1972; 62:345–346.

Gustaffson M, Mortensson W. Irradiation to the thyroid gland at cardiac catheterization and angiocardiography in children. Br J Radiol 1976; 49:686–689.

Hurwitz RA, Franken EA, Jr, Girod DA, et al. Angiographic determination of arterial patency after percutaneous catheterization in infants and small children. Circulation 1977; 56:102–105.

Kennedy JW. Complications associated with cardiac catheterization and angiography. Cathet Cardiovasc Diagn 1982; 8:5–11.

Krantz EM, Viljoen JF. Haemoptysis following insertion of a Swan-Ganz catheter. Br J Anaesth 1979; 51:457–459.

Krovetz LJ, Shanklin DR, Schiebler GL. Serious and fatal complications of cardiac catheterization and angiography in infants and children. Am Heart J 1968; 76:39–47.

Luepker RV, Bouchard RJ, Burns R, Warbasse JR. Systemic heparinization during percutaneous coronary angiography: Evaluation of effectiveness in decreasing thrombotic and embolic catheter complications. Cathet Cardiovasc Diagn, 1975; 1:35–45.

Martin EC, Olson AP, Steeg CN, Casarella WJ. Radiation exposure to the pediatric patient during cardiac catheterization and angiocardiography. Circulation 1981; 64:153–158.

Mathews RA, Park SC, Neches WH, et al. Iliac venous thrombosis in infants and children after cardiac catheterization. Cathet Cardiovasc Diagn 1979; 5:67–74.

Meister SG, Furr CM, Engel TR, et al. Knotting of a flow-directed catheter about a cardiac structure. Cathet Cardiovasc Diagn 1977; 3:171–175.

Miller HC, Miller GA. Experience with systemic heparinization during cardiac catheterization by brachial arteriotomy. Br Heart 1974; 36:1122–1125.

Mond HG, Clark DW, Nesbitt SJ, Schlant RC. A technique for unknotting an intracardiac flow-directed balloon catheter. Chest 1975; 67:731–733.

Noordijk JA, Oey FTI, Tebra W. Myocardial electrodes and the danger of ventricular fibrillation. Lancet 1961; 1:975–977.

Pape LA, Haffajee CI, Markis JE, et al. Fatal pulmonary hemorrhage after use of the flow-directed balloon-tipped catheter. Ann Intern Med 1979; 90:344–347.

Phornphutkal C, Rosenthal A, Nadas AS, Berenberg W. Cerebrovascular accidents in infants and children with cyanotic congenital heart disease. Am J Cardiol 1973; 32:329–334.

Primm RK, Segall RH, Alison HW, et al. Incidence of new pulmonary perfusion defects after routine cardiac catheterization. Am J Cardiol 1979; 43:529–532.

Rich JM, Cobb TC, Leighton RF. Percutaneous transfemoral coronary arteriography without systemic anticoagulation—A review of 648 consecutive procedures. Cathet Cardiovasc Diagn 1975; 1:275–281.

Rosenthal A, Anderson M, Thompson SJ, et al. Am J Dis Child 1975; 124:240–242.

Rowe R. Cardiac catheterization. In: Keith JD, Rowe RD, Vlad P, eds. Heart Disease in Infancy and Childhood. New York, NY; McMillan Publishing Co., 1978:83.

Rubin SA, Puckett RP. Pulmonary artery-bronchial fisula: A new complication of Swan-Ganz catheterization. Chest 1979; 75:515–516.

Singh HM, Ablett MB. Acute Hemorrhagic intestinal and hepatic infarction and renal insufficiency following cardiac catheterization. J Cardiovasc Surg (Torino) 1972; 13:623–625.

Skovr Anek J, Sam Enek M. Chronic impairment of leg muscle blood flow following cardiac catheterization in children. Am J Roentgenol 1979; 132:71–75.

Tang TT, Chambers CH, Gallen WJ, McCreadie SR. Pulmonary fiber embolism and granuloma. J Am Med Assoc 1978; 239:948–950.

Terplan KL. Patterns of brain damage in infants and children with congenital heart disease. Association with catheterization and surgical procedures. Am J Dis Child 1973; 125:176–185.

Waldman JD, Rummerfield PS, Gilpin EA, Kirkpatrick SE. Radiation exposure to the child during cardiac catheterization. Circulation 1981; 64:158–163.

Part II

Approach to Specific Lesions

17

Atrial Septal Defect

Sang C. Park, M.D.

Anatomy

Atrial septal defects comprise approximately 15% of all congenital heart malformations. There are three relatively common varieties of interatrial communications: ostium secundum, sinus venosus, and ostium primum defects. The most common type is the ostium secundum defect, which involves the region of the fossa ovalis. The sinus venosus defect is located in the upper posterior portion of the atrial septum with the orifice of the superior vena cava immediately above it (Fig. 1). The right upper pulmonary vein often enters the superior vena cava directly. In a rare situation, an inferior sinus venous defect, the communication occurs at the atrial inferior vena caval junction and the right lower pulmonary vein drains directly into the right atrium. The ostium primum defect is a form of atrioventricular septal defect (endocardial cushion defect) and will be discussed in Chapter 19.

In addition to the above, a very rare type of atrial septal defect consists of an interatrial communication in the area usually occupied by the coronary sinus (Fig. 1C). There is no coronary sinus proper and the coronary veins drain into the right atrium. Such defects are commonly associated with a persistent left superior vena cava draining into the left atrium (Raghib et al. 1965). Another form of atrial defect, complete or virtual absence of the atrial septum is known as "common" or "single" atrium. This type of atrial defect is usually associated with an atrioventricular septal defect and will be discussed in Chapter 19.

Hemodynamic Considerations

The major hemodynamic feature of an atrial septal defect is left to right shunting through the defect with resultant increased pulmonary blood flow. The pressure difference between the two atria is usually small and pressures are virtually equal with a large defect. In this latter case, the magnitude and direction of the shunt is dependent upon relative inflow impedance to the right and left ventricles. In the early newborn period, right and left ventricular compliances are nearly equal and atrial shunting is negligible even in the presence of a large defect. Beyond early infancy, right ventricular compliance increases and left ventricular compliance decreases, with a resulting left to right shunt.

Even in early infancy, impedance to left ventricular filling occasioned by high left ventricular end-diastolic pressure from left ventricular volume overload (e.g., ventricular septal defect or patent ductus arteriosus), left ventricular pressure overload (e.g., aortic stenosis or coarctation of the aorta), left ventricular dysfunction (e.g., cardiomyopathy or myocarditis), or by left ventricular inflow obstruction (e.g., mitral valve disease or supravalvular mitral valve ring), will result in interatrial left to right shunting. The shunt can be massive if impedance to left ventricular filling is very high. Under these circumstances the interatrial communication can simply be a stretched foramen ovale. If impedance to right ventricular

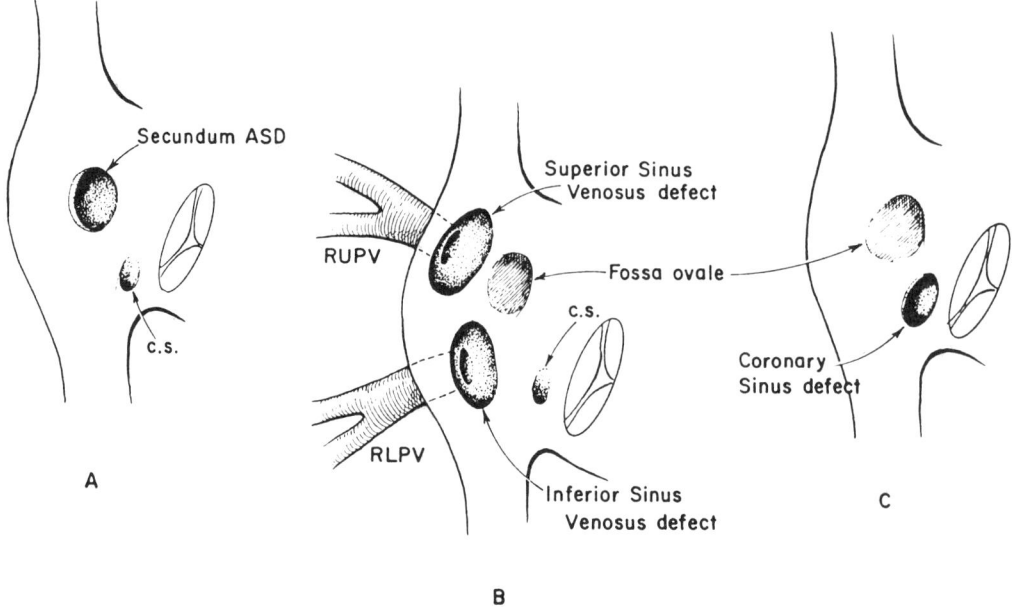

Figure 1. Diagramatic illustration of the types of atrial septal defects. A: Secundum septal defect. B: Sinus venosus defects. C: Coronary sinus defect.

filling is high, usually because of long standing right ventricular hypertrophy, right to left shunting will occur. Right ventricular inflow obstruction or tricuspid regurgitation can also cause right to left shunting across an atrial defect.

Indications for Cardiac Catheterization

Preoperative Indications

Most patients with atrial septal defects are asymptomatic and cardiac catheterization can be deferred until just prior to surgery, usually at 3 to 5 years of age. Because the diagnosis of atrial septal defect can usually be made by noninvasive means and confirmed by echocardiography with color flow mapping, cardiac catheterization today is performed only to evaluate uncommon problems such as pulmonary hypertension or to evaluate associated anomalies such as

anomalous pulmonary venous return, mitral valve abnormalities, etc. In most institutions, including our own, catheterization is not routinely done in patients with typical findings of an atrial septal defect. However, if any unusual finding is present, or if there is a question as to the size of the defect, we still feel more comfortable referring patients for surgery who have had a cardiac catheterization to assess anatomy and hemodynamics, especially because the risk of cardiac catheterization is minimal in this age group. An occasional infant with an isolated atrial septal defect is symptomatic (Dimich et al. 1973) and early catheterization is indicated.

Postoperative Indications

Cardiac catheterization is not usually indicated following surgical repair of an uncomplicated atrial septal defect. Postoperative cardiac catheterization is indicated in the unusual patient with evidence of residual hemodynamic abnormalities. For example,

Neches et al. (1977) reported a patient with an atrial septal defect who developed pulmonary edema following operation. Repeat cardiac catheterization disclosed a previously unsuspected cor triatriatum.

Catheterization Technique

Cardiac catheterization is usually done percutaneously via the femoral approach. Initially, an end-hole catheter is used and oxygen saturations and pressures are recorded in the right heart, including right atrium, right ventricle, pulmonary artery, and pulmonary artery wedge position. Blood samples from the superior vena cava and the left innominate vein are obtained for mixed systemic venous saturation. When the interatrial defect is in the fossa ovale or its environs, the catheter can be passed easily into the left atrium (Fig. 2A) and can then be manipulated into the left ventricle. With a sinus venosus defect passage of the catheter into the left atrium can be much more difficult. However, the catheter tip readily enters the right upper pulmonary vein from the right atrial-superior vena caval junction. A catheter with a sharply curved tip can be helpful in entering the left atrium. Initially, the catheter tip is placed in the superior vena cava and is then rotated counterclockwise as it is withdrawn to the right atrial-superior vena cava junction. As the catheter enters the right atrium it often slips across the defect into the left atrium. Because the passage of the catheter across a sinus venosus defect is high in the atrial septum (Fig. 2B), it is often difficult to advance the catheter into the left ventricle. When an end-hole catheter is used, the flexible tip of a guidewire can be used to guide the catheter into the left ventricle. When a closed end, side-hole (NIH) catheter is used, the sharply curved stiff end of a guidewire can be utilized to direct the catheter tip toward the mitral valve (see Chapter 5).

Whenever possible, pulmonary veins should be probed selectively to rule out abnormal drainage of the pulmonary vein and also to determine pulmonary venous oxygen saturation. The orientation of the catheter tip as it enters the left-sided veins confirms normal drainage to the left atrium. However,

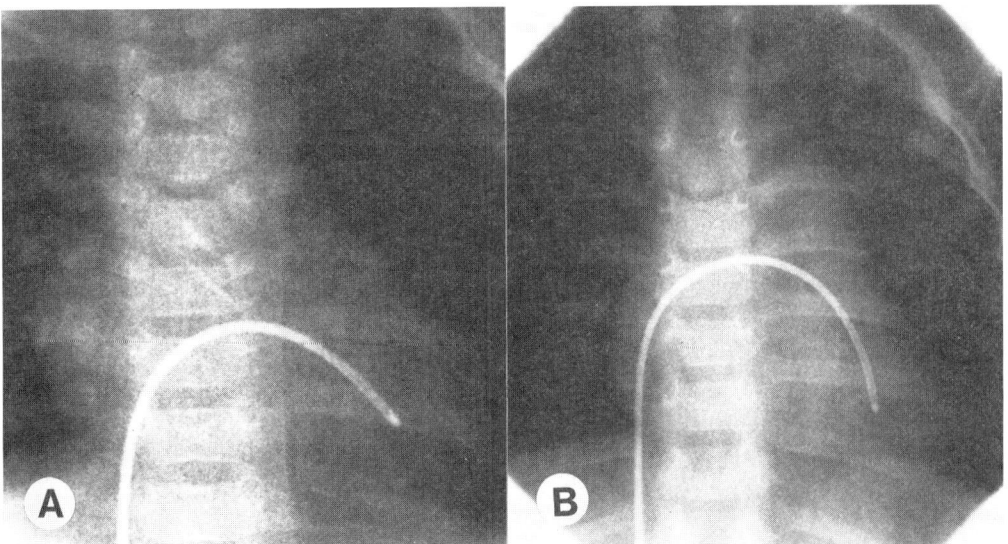

Figure 2. Passage of catheter across various atrial defects. A: Secundum type. B: Sinus venosus type showing high passage of catheter across the defect.

the status of the right-sided pulmonary venous drainage may be more difficult to determine. By catheter passage alone it is usually impossible to determine whether the tip has entered the right upper lobe pulmonary vein directly from the right atrium or has initially traversed the atrial septal defect. Therefore a right upper lobe vein angiogram is helpful in assessing pulmonary venous return. In patients with hypoplasia of the right lung who are suspected of having the scimitar syndrome, an attempt should be made to enter a right lower pulmonary vein at the right atrial-inferior vena cava junction.

If the catheter tip is passed into the coronary sinus during manipulation of the catheter in the right atrium, the catheter tip should be advanced farther to rule out any connection with the left superior vena cava and blood samples should also be obtained to rule out partial anomalous pulmonary venous return to the coronary sinus.

Retrograde arterial catheterization usually is not required in a patient with a typical atrial septal defect unless an associated left sided cardiac anomaly is suspected. Occasionally, an arterial line is placed in the femoral artery for the determination of systemic oxygen saturation, pressure measurement, or indicator dye dilution study.

Hemodynamic Evaluation

Pressure Measurement

In patients with an atrial septal defect pressures are usually normal in the right side of the heart and pulmonary artery, particularly in the pediatric age group. However, a small pressure gradient is common between the right ventricle and pulmonary artery as well as between the main pulmonary artery and the right and left pulmonary arteries. This pressure gradient is related to high flow and not to a demonstrable anatomic obstruction. A pressure difference between the main pulmonary artery and the

right ventricle of 5 to 10 mm Hg is common and occasionally can be as high as 40 mm Hg. Also, a mild pressure gradient is sometimes found between the main pulmonary artery and its branches, more often on the right than the left (Fig. 3).

Right ventricular end-diastolic pressure usually is normal, rarely exceeding 5 mm Hg. Mean pressures in the right and left atrium are often equal when the atrial septal defect is large, but left atrial pressure can exceed the right by 2 or 3 mm Hg. The phasic contour of the pressures are similar and both right atrium and left atrium have prominent "a" and "v" waves. It should be noted that atrial pressures are not always equal in patients with a large left to right shunt, especially if high impedance to left ventricular filling raises left atrial pressures and causes a large flow across a relatively small defect. Systemic arterial and left ventricular systolic and end-diastolic pressures usually are normal.

Children with atrial septal defect almost always have normal or low pulmonary vascular resistance. In adults with chronically increased pulmonary blood flow, pulmonary vascular resistance may be elevated and in this situation, pulmonary arterial pressure increases and may even exceed systemic pressure. In the presence of severe right ventricular hypertrophy or failure, right atrial pressure may exceed left atrial pressure and right to left shunting occurs.

Oxygen Saturation Data

In a typical atrial septal defect an oxygen saturation step-up occurs at right atrial level. If the defect is near the tricuspid valve (ostium primum or coronary sinus variety) there may be considerable streaming and a second oxygen step may be present at right ventricular level, erroneously suggesting an associated ventricular septal defect.

Determination of the oxygen saturation of true mixed venous blood in patients with atrial defects can be difficult because there

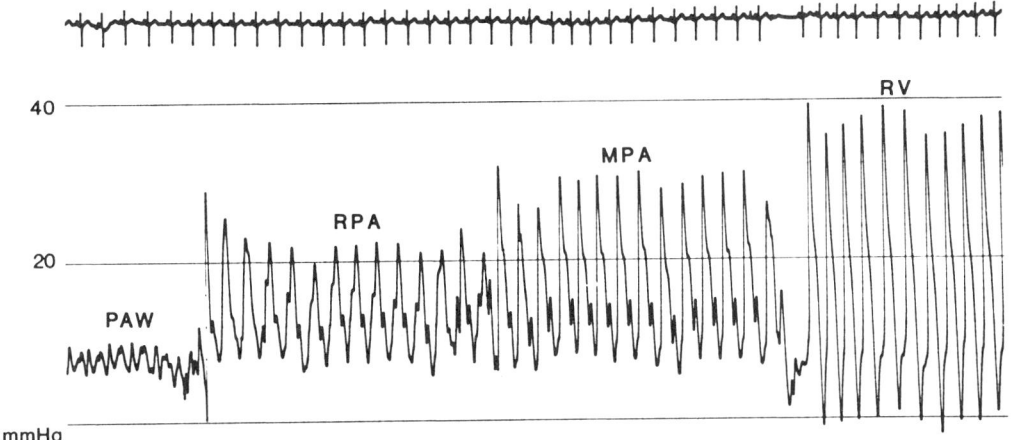

Figure 3. Withdrawal pressure tracing from the right pulmonary artery wedge (PAW) to right pulonary artery (RPA) to main pulmonary artery (MPA) to right ventricle (RV) in a patient with an atrial septal defect. There are mild pressure gradients between right pulmonary artery and main pulmonary artery as well as between main pulmonary artery and right ventricle.

is usually significant reflux of shunted blood into the inferior vena cava and often even into the superior vena cava. This can be demonstrated readily by angiography. In patients with the sinus venosus type of defect the superior vena cava receives highly oxygenated blood from the right upper pulmonary vein directly and in this situation mixed venous saturation should be obtained from the left innominate vein. When the oxygen saturation in the superior vena cava is higher than 80%, the possibility of anomalous pulmonary venous return into the superior vena cava or the innominate vein must be considered. An arteriovenous malformation in the head, neck or upper thorax may also result in similar oxygen saturation findings. Occasionally, oxygen saturations of over 80% can be seen in the superior vena cava without any of the above mentioned anomalies and probably is related to high cardiac output with low arteriovenous difference. For clarification of high oxygen saturation in the superior vena cava, individual blood samples from the jugular and subclavian veins should be obtained. Oxygen saturation of jugular venous blood is considerably lower than subclavian venous blood and a sample taken in the stream of the sub-

clavian vein will be spuriously high. Inferior vena caval blood is not a good measure of mixed venous saturation because of the high oxygen saturation of renal venous blood.

Systemic arterial oxygen saturation in patients with an atrial septal defect is usually normal. When systemic arterial or left ventricular saturation is less than 92%, a few possibilities should be considered. The first is the presence of a pulmonary parenchymal problem with inadequate oxygenation. This can occur unilaterally and thus the blood drawn from pulmonary veins draining the affected lung will be desaturated. Occasionally, pulmonary venous blood can be desaturated simply due to hypoventilation in a heavily sedated patient. Determination of blood gases from different pulmonary veins will be helpful in localizing the site of desaturation. Another cause of systemic arterial desaturation is entry of systemic venous blood into the left side of the heart. It can be either a systemic venous direct anastomosis to the left side of the heart, such as persistent left superior vena cava draining into the left atrium, or a right to left shunt through an atrial defect. The latter condition is usually associated with a tricuspid valve abnormality (such as Ebstein's malformation or tricuspid valve stenosis), right ventricular hypoplasia or severe pulmonary vascular disease.

Other Diagnostic or Therapeutic Procedures

Indicator Dye Dilution Curves

This technique can be used to detect an anomalously draining pulmonary vein. The indicator, usually indocyanine green dye, is injected selectively into right and left pulmonary arteries while systemic arterial blood is sampled. When all veins from one lung drain anomalously, an injection in the ipsilateral pulmonary artery results in a curve with delayed appearance time and low peak (Fig. 4:RPA) similar to a superior vena caval injection (Fig. 4:SVC). However, the curve from the anomalous vein also has a delayed appearance time and a prolonged down slope. In contrast, the curve from the contralateral pulmonary artery is normal (Fig. 4:LPA). However, the diagnosis of anomalies of pulmonary venous return by indicator dilution study alone is not reliable because of preferential left to right shunting from the right pulmonary veins in patients with an isolated atrial septal defect. Furthermore, it is difficult to distinguish whether only one or both pulmonary veins from a given lung are involved unless injections are made far out in the periphery of each of the pulmonary lobes. Thus, the diagnosis of associated partial anomalous pulmonary venous return is best made by selective angiography.

When indicator dye is injected into the right atrium or inferior vena cava, a small early deflection may appear on the curve, indicating minimal right to left shunting (Fig. 5). This usually is present despite the lack of clinical or oximetric evidence of systemic arterial desaturation. Right to left shunting is more common in adults with pulmonary hypertension.

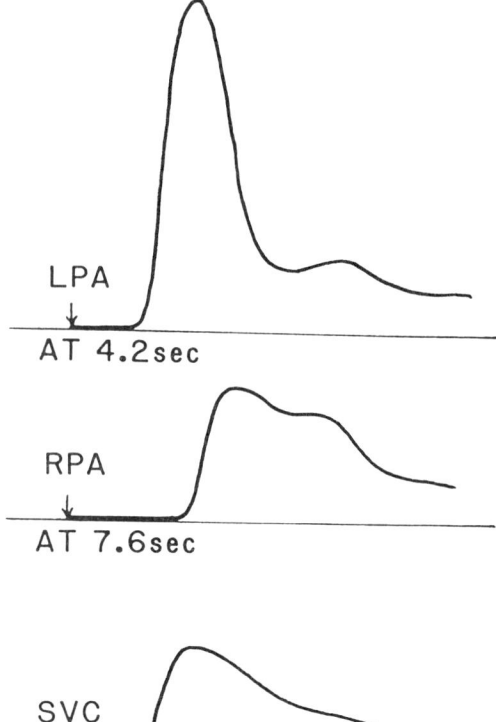

Figure 4. Indicator dilution dye curves in patients with partial anomalous return of the right pulmonary veins (see text). AT = Appearance time; LPA = Left pulmonary artery; RPA = Right pulmonary artery; SVC = Superior vena cava.

Dye dilution study can be helpful in determining the magnitude of the left to right shunt, particularly when a valid mixed venous saturation is difficult to obtain because of associated partial anomalous pulmonary venous return (see Chapter 6).

The Use of a Balloon Catheter

A balloon catheter may be used to measure the size of an interatrial defect and temporarily to occlude it during cardiac catheterization. The balloon-tipped catheter is passed into the left atrium and then the balloon is inflated to larger than the expected

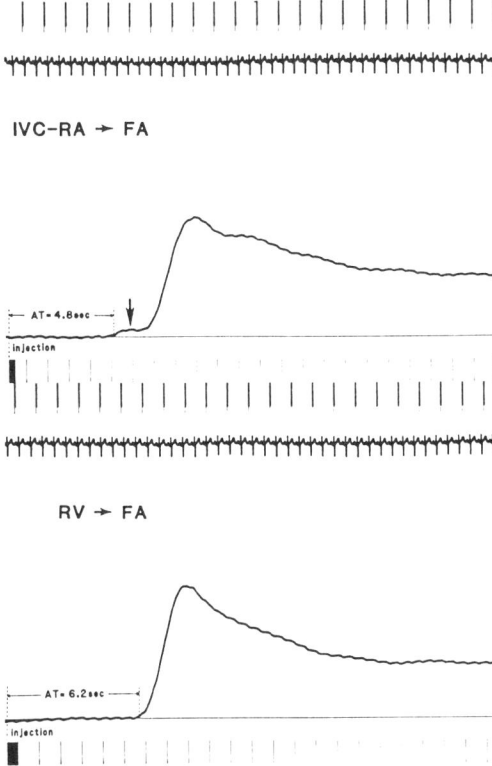

IVC–RA → FA

RV → FA

Figure 5. Dye dilution curve showing mild right to left shunt in patient with no apparent clinical systemic arterial desaturation when the indicator dye was injected into the inferior vena cava-right atrium juncture (top). However, this right to left shunt is not observed with injection of the dye into the right ventricle (bottom). AT = Appearance time; FA = Femoral artery; IVC = Inferior vena cava; RA = Right atrium.

Actual balloon (atrial defect) size is:
Measured balloon size × Magnification Factor

Where:

Magnification factor

$$= \frac{\text{Actual grid dimension}}{\text{Measured grid dimension}}$$

The reliability of this technique has been well documented by Park et al. (1975) and King et al. (1978). However, certain pitfalls should be recognized. When there are multiple atrial defects, an irregular or oval defect, a fibrous band, or a sieve-like network across a large atrial defect, the balloon measurement may underestimate the size of the defect. In contrast, overestimation of the defect size by this technique is not likely unless too much traction is exerted during the pull back or unless the balloon was not actually in the left atrium. Confirmation of the balloon position by lateral fluoroscopy will obviate the latter problem.

A balloon catheter also may be used temporarily to occlude an atrial defect. Hemodynamic evaluation during occlusion of the defect with a balloon is particularly helpful in patients with a right to left shunt through the atrial defect. The maximum balloon diameter that is currently commercially available is 18 mm (a 4 mL Miller septostomy catheter). King et al. (1978) used a custom made balloon catheter which could be inflated to 43 mm in diameter.

Angiocardiography

In patients with an atrial septal defect, angiography is useful in localizing the defect and ruling out associated anomalies, particularly anomalous pulmonary venous return. The atrial septal defect itself usually is best demonstrated in the four-chamber view. The catheter tip is placed just within the right upper pulmonary vein near its junction with the left atrium. (If the catheter tip is placed too far into the pulmonary vein there may be infiltration of contrast material into the

size of the defect. The balloon catheter is gently withdrawn until the balloon is engaged against the interatrial septum. The balloon is then gradually deflated while maintaining gentle traction, until it suddenly passes into the right atrium. This maneuver can be recorded on videotape or cineangiogram (30 frames per second is sufficient). Simultaneous or subsequent recording of a calibrated grid at the level of the heart provides the magnification factor for calculating actual balloon size according to the following formula.

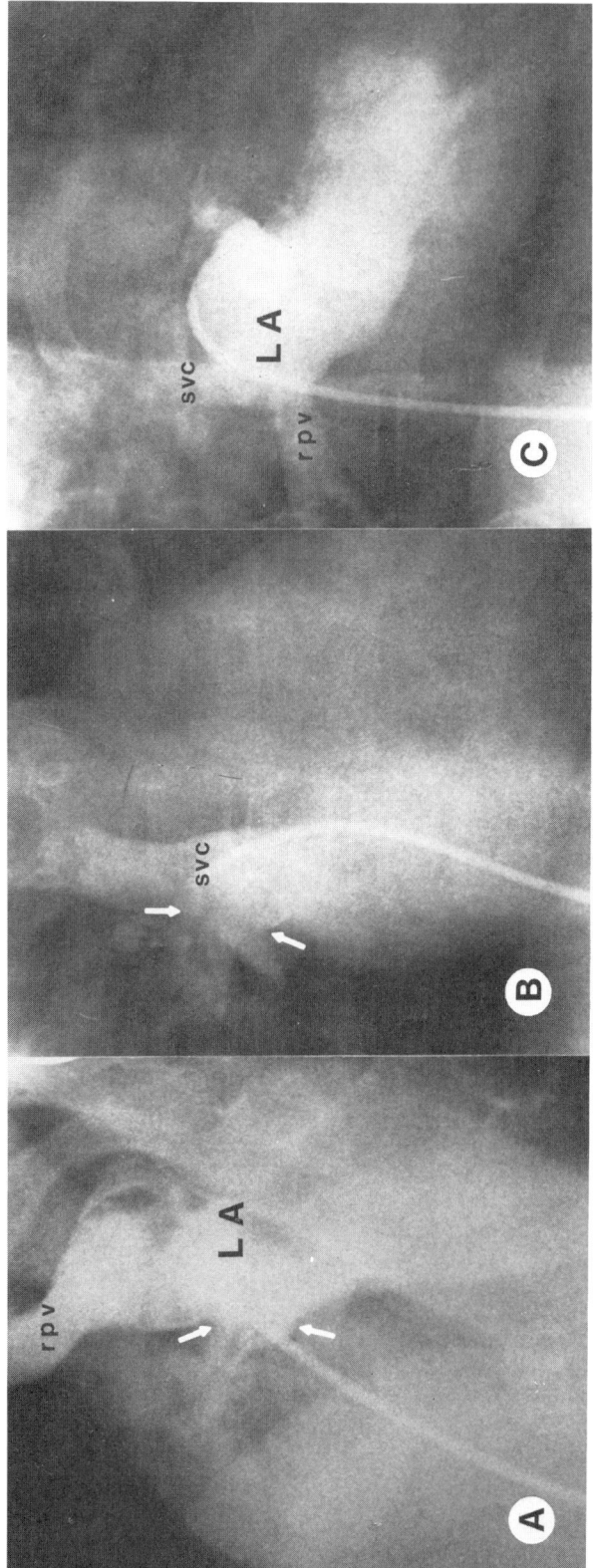

Figure 6. Angiocardiograms of various atrial defects (arrows indicate the limit of the defect). A: Injection in the right upper pulmonary vein (RPV) in a secundum defect. (LA = Left atrium) B: Sinus venosus type (SVC = Superior vena cava) C: Injection in the left atrium (LA) in the same patient as in "B" showing filling of the right lower pulmonary vein and some reflux into the superior vena cava (SVC).

pulmonary parenchyma and paroxysmal coughing). Approximately 0.5 to 1 mL/kg of contrast material is used. This angiogram will usually demonstrate the location of the atrial defect and the site of pulmonary venous drainage (Fig. 6). A sinus venosus defect is located very high in the atrial septum and the right upper pulmonary vein almost invariably drains directly into the superior vena cava. Occasionally, a fossa ovalis type of atrial defect may coexist with a sinus venosus defect and selective angiocardiography of the left atrium in the four-chamber view is helpful.

A selective pulmonary arteriogram in the anteroposterior view is performed to assess pulmonary venous return (Fig. 7). If there is an unusually large pressure gradient across the pulmonic valve (greater than 20 mm Hg) a selective right ventricular angiogram in the anteroposterior and lateral views is preferred. The anteroposterior view demonstrates pulmonary venous return while the lateral view demonstrates the right

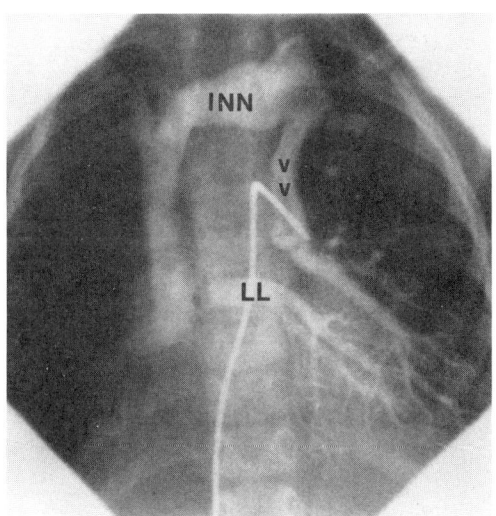

Figure 7. Selective left pulmonary artery angiogram in the anteroposterior view demonstrating partial anomalous pulmonary venous return of the left upper lobe to the innominate vein (INN) via the vertical vein (VV). The left lower lobe pulmonary vein (LL) drains normally to the left atrium.

ventricular outflow obstruction. If an abnormality of the tricuspid valve or of the right ventricle itself is suspected, selective right ventriculography is again essential. Occasionally selective pulmonary arterial angiograms are necessary to define the site of pulmonary venous return.

Other special studies may be useful. For example, a patient with a left upper pulmonary vein draining into a persistent left superior vena cava that connected both to the left innominate vein and to the left atrium was to have surgical correction. To evaluate the adequacy of the communication between the left upper pulmonary vein and left atrium, a Swan Ganz catheter was placed in the persistent left superior vena cava via the left innominate vein and the balloon was inflated. Although angiographically the communication between the left atrium and the pulmonary vein was small, pressure in the pulmonary vein did not increase and therefore the left superior vena cava could be ligated safely at the time of surgical closure of the atrial defect.

Patients with anomalous drainage of the right lower lobe into the right atrial-inferior vena caval junction should have an aortogram or equivalent left-sided angiogram to rule out abnormal systemic arterial supply to the lung (Fig. 8). This anomaly may be associated with hypoplasia of the right lung and dextrocardia and then constitutes a "scimitar" syndrome.

Lastly, a selective left ventricular angiogram is routinely done in both oblique views to rule out clinically unrecognized left heart disease, especially prolapse of the mitral valve.

Associated Cardiac Lesions

While in two-thirds of patients with an atrial septal defect the anomaly is isolated, in the remaining one-third there is an associated anomaly. The most common are valvar pulmonic stenosis, ventricular septal defect, partial anomalous pulmonary venous

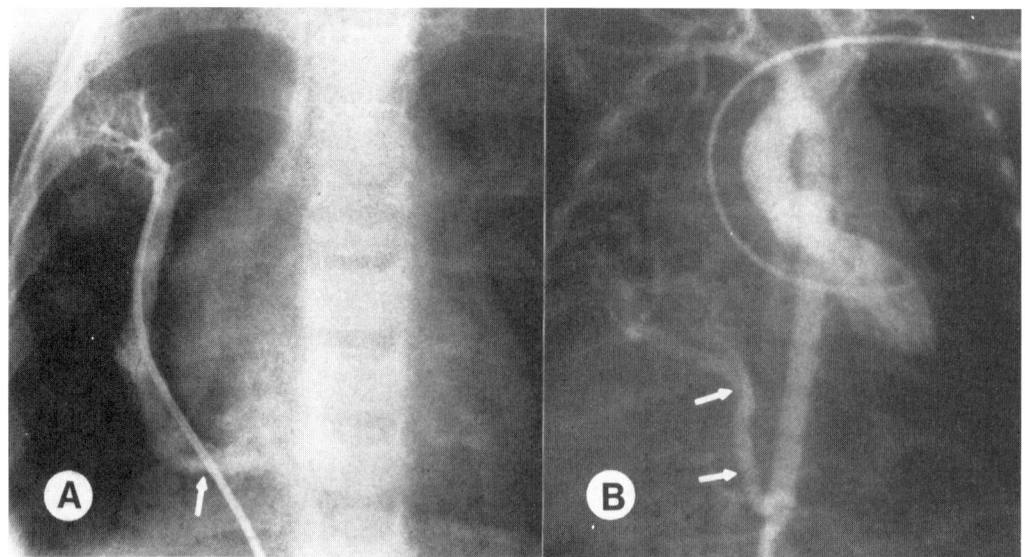

Figure 8. A case of Scimitar syndrome. A: Partial anomalous pulmonary venous return of the right upper lobe pulmonary vein into the right atrial-inferior vena caval juncture (arrow). B: Systemic arterial supply (arrows) from the descending aorta to the right lower lobe.

return, patent ductus arteriosus and coarctation of the aorta. All can be readily recognized clinically and/or echocardiographically.

In the patient with an unusually large left to right atrial shunt, particularly if the defect appears relatively small, the possibility of an additional left to right shunt or a left heart problem should be suspected. Prolapse of the mitral valve occurs in an occasional patient with an atrial septal defect but is rarely important hemodynamically.

Cautions or Precautions

In patients with an atrial septal defect cardiac catheterization is usually technically simple and complications are uncommon. Status of the pulmonary venous return must be carefully evaluated.

References and Suggested Reading

Dimich I, Steinfeld L, Park SC. Symptomatic isolated atrial septal defect. Am Heart J 1983; 85:601-604.

King TD, Thompson SL, Mills NL. Measurement of atrial septal defect during cardiac catheterization: Experimental and clinical results. Am J Cardiol 1978;41:537–542.

Neches WH, Park SC, Lenox CC, et al. Pulmonary artery wedge pressures in congenital heart disease. Catheterization Cardiovasc Diagn 1977;3:11–19.

Park SC, Zuberbuhler JR, Neches WH, et al. A new atrial septostomy technique. Catheterization Cardiovasc Diagn 1975;1:195–201.

Raghib G, Ruttenburg HD, Anderson RC, et al. Termination of left superior vena cava in left atrium, atrial septal defect and absence of coronary sinus. Developmental Complex. Circulation 1965;31:906–918.

18

Ventricular Septal Defect

Sang C. Park, M.D.

Anatomy

Ventricular septal defect is the most common congenital cardiac malformation. As an isolated anomaly it makes up over 20% of all congenital heart disease. Ventricular septal defects are often associated with other cardiac lesions such as atrial septal defect, pulmonic stenosis, coarctation of the aorta, etc. A ventricular septal defect is an integral part of many complex cardiac malformations, including persistent truncus arteriosus, tetralogy of Fallot, double outlet right ventricle, tricuspid atresia, and interrupted aortic arch.

Classification of Ventricular Septal Defect

Many different classifications have been proposed in the past. One commonly used classification is based upon the location of the ventricular septal defect in relation to the crista supraventricularis ("supracristal" and "infracristal") (Becu et al. 1956). Another classification, a numerical one, also refers to position: type I (supracristal); type II (membranous); type III (atrioventricular canal); and type IV (muscular). In 1980, Soto et al. proposed an elegant and comprehensive classification. The ventricular septum is composed of membranous and muscular portions and the muscular portion can be subdivided into inlet (adjacent to the atrioventricular valves), trabecular (apical) and outlet (below the semilunar valves) por-

tions. In this classification defects are grouped into three basic types (Fig. 1). The most common defect is "perimembranous"; in other words it borders the membranous septum. There is usually some deficiency of muscular septum in a perimembranous defect, and the muscular defect may extend into the inlet, trabecular, or outlet portions of the septum. The second most common type of defect is "muscular", or bordered entirely by muscular septum. Muscular defects may be located in the inlet, trabecular, or outlet portion of the septum and may be multiple (so called "swiss cheese" septum). The third type borders both aortic and pulmonic valves and it is called a "doubly committed subarterial defect" (supracristal or subpulmonic ventricular septal defect). This variety results from deficiency of the infundibular septum.

Hemodynamic Considerations

The major hemodynamic effect of a ventricular septal defect is a left to right shunt through the defect with resultant increased pulmonary blood flow. If the defect is sufficiently large, pressures will be equal in the two ventricles and congestive heart failure may occur. If uncorrected, pulmonary vascular disease will eventually occur. The magnitude of the left to right shunt is largely determined by the size of the defect but other factors such as pulmonary vascular resistance and associated cardiac lesions also

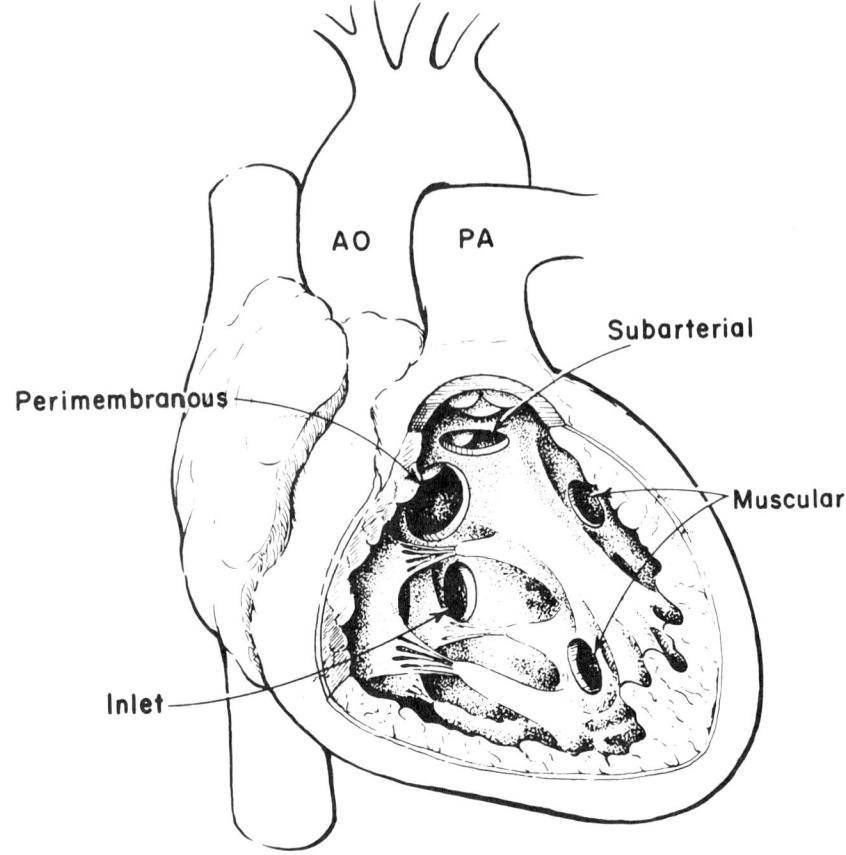

Figure 1. Diagram of the ventricular septum from the right ventricular side with location of various types of ventricular septal defects. AO = aorta; PA = pulmonary artery.

influence the shunt. Age is an important factor because the full-term newborn infant has high pulmonary vascular resistance and as a consequence, the left to right shunt is small. As the pulmonary vascular resistance declines over the first few weeks of life, the left to right shunt becomes larger. Associated cardiac malformations such as patent ductus arteriosus or atrial septal defect, or left-sided obstructive anomalies such as aortic stenosis or coarctation of the aorta, enhance the magnitude of the shunt. In contrast, right ventricular outflow obstruction such as valvar or infundibular pulmonary stenosis or peripheral pulmonary artery stenosis increase the right ventricular pressure

and reduce or eliminate the left to right shunt.

Indications for Cardiac Catheterization

Preoperative Indications

The clinical spectrum of ventricular septal defect is quite wide. A patient with an obviously small ventricular septal defect on clinical or noninvasive evaluation does not require cardiac catheterization. In many patients, a ventricular septal defect can be adequately defined by echocardiography and preoperative cardiac catheterization may not be necessary. However, any patient, particularly an infant, with unusual findings or associated cardiac anomalies should have a diagnostic cardiac catheterization to confirm the diagnosis and obtain hemodynamic data in preparation for possible surgical intervention. If surgical repair is delayed, some patients may require a repeat hemodynamic study, particularly if there is severe pulmonary hypertension. Patients over 6 months of age who have never been in congestive heart failure but have clinical evidence of a large left to right shunt and pulmonary hypertension also require catheterization. Rarely, patients present with predominant findings of pulmonary hypertension without evidence of a large left to right or with no history of congestive heart failure. Such patients are likely to be inoperable but the diagnosis and hemodynamics should be confirmed by cardiac catheterization.

Postoperative Indications

Following surgical correction of ventricular septal defect, repeat cardiac catheterization is not indicated routinely if there is no clinical evidence of residual pulmonary hypertension or left to right shunt. However, if there is persistent cardiomegaly or findings suggestive of pulmonary hypertension or a significant residual defect, postoperative cardiac catheterization is advised.

Catheterization Technique

Cardiac catheterization is usually done via the femoral vessels using percutaneous technique. Initially an end-hole catheter is used and pressures and blood samples are obtained from each right heart position including the pulmonary arterial wedge. An attempt should always be made to traverse the atrial septum and if the left atrium can be entered the pulmonary veins should be explored, particularly if pulmonary artery wedge pressures are high. If there is arterial unsaturation, pulmonary venous saturation should be determined to differentiate an intracardiac shunt from a pulmonary abnormality. For angiography the end-hole catheter is replaced with an NIH catheter. In addition to ventriculography, an aortogram is also valuable to rule out an associated patent ductus arteriosus. To enter the aorta, the catheter is passed into the right ventricular inflow area, then turned clockwise to rotate the tip medially and posteriorly through the ventricular septal defect into the ascending aorta. The success of this maneuver depends upon the size and location of the defect. A large defect is obviously more easily crossed but the location of the defect is even more important. Perimembranous defects extending into the trabecular or infundibular muscular septum are easier to cross than inlet perimembranous or muscular defects. When the ascending aorta cannot be entered by this approach there are two alternative approaches. If there is an interatrial communication, a balloon catheter (Berman or Swan Ganz) is passed into the left atrium and into the left ventricle through the mitral valve. The catheter is looped in the left ventricle, the balloon is inflated and then, hopefully, floats into the ascending aorta (see Chapter 5). However, if there is a large left to right shunt through the defect the balloon catheter tends to pass across the defect into the right ventricle and pulmonary artery rather than into the aorta. If the aorta cannot be entered either by passage of the catheter through the defect or by balloon catheter via the left ventricle, retrograde arterial catheterization is indicated. A percutaneous femoral approach is usual, but if severe coarctation of the aorta is suspected in a small infant, a right axillary artery cutdown is preferable unless there is an aberrant right subclavian artery by clinical examination (absence of the right brachial pulses) or barium esophagram. The left axillary artery is unsatisfactory in a patient with a coarctation of the aorta, since it is difficult to pass the catheter into the ascending aorta. In a small infant, retrograde arterial catheterization carries a significant risk of an arterial complication and a small Long Dwell needle or Intracath (21 gauge) may be used to perform an aortogram to rule out coarctation of the aorta, other aortic arch anomalies or patent ductus arteriosus. When there is clinical evidence of aortic stenosis retrograde arterial catheterization is always indicated.

Hemodynamic Evaluation

Measurements of pressure and oxygen saturations from the various cardiac chambers and vessels are routinely done. The magnitude of the shunt is determined by estimating the pulmonary to systemic flow ratio (Qp/Qs) and the pulmonary vascular bed is assessed by calculating pulmonary vascular resistance (see Chapter 6 and 7).

Pressure Measurement

The pressures in the right ventricle and pulmonary artery are directly related to the size of the defect. With a small defect, pressures are usually normal. If the defect is very large, it is "unrestrictive" and right ventricular systolic pressure is usually the same as left ventricular pressure. Systolic pulmonary arterial pressure also will be equal to aortic systolic pressure although pulmonary artery diastolic pressure may be much lower than aortic diastolic pressure.

Because pressures and saturations can vary during the cardiac catheterization, especially in a small infant, the data should be gathered in rapid sequence. The pulmonary artery wedge pressure is usually somewhat elevated in patients with a large shunt and mean pressure of 10 or 12 mm Hg are usual. The elevation is due both to relative mitral

stenosis related to high flow and to elevated left ventricular end-diastolic pressure. If the pulmonary artery wedge pressure is higher than a simultaneously recorded left ventricular end-diastolic pressure, such anomalies as pathological mitral stenosis, pulmonary vein stenosis or cor triatriatum should be considered. Selective exploration of each pulmonary vein is indicated, if necessary by transseptal puncture technique, particularly when pulmonary vein stenosis is suspected.

Oxygen Saturation Data

In patients with ventricular septal defect and more than a trivial left to right shunt, a step-up in oxygen saturation will be present at right ventricular level. However, in patients with a subarterial defect (supracristal, subpulmonic), shunted blood is preferentially directed into the pulmonary artery and an oxygen step-up may be apparent only in the pulmonary artery or in the right ventricular outflow tract immediately below the pulmonic valve. In general, however, a further increase in oxygen saturation in the pulmonary artery suggests an associated patent ductus arteriosus. In a patient with clinical or catheterization evidence of a ventricular septal defect, an oxygen step-up in the right atrium can be due to an atrial septal defect or partial anomalous pulmonary venous return. A left ventricle to right atrial shunt could theoretically be due to a defect in the atrioventricular portion of the membranous septum but is actually almost always due to flow through a ventricular septal defect and then through a tricuspid valve commissure or cleft.

A low pulmonary arteriovenous oxygen difference indicates large pulmonary blood flow and therefore relatively low pulmonary vascular resistance, even if pulmonary artery pressure is higher than normal. Conversely, a high pulmonary arteriovenous difference indicates low pulmonary blood flow and, if pulmonary artery pressure is high, elevated pulmonary vascular resistance.

Patients who have pulmonary disease or who are heavily sedated may have abnormally low oxygen saturation in pulmonary veins and systemic arteries. Therefore the calculated pulmonary flow and resistance may not reflect accurately the status of the pulmonary vascular bed.

Other Diagnostic Procedures

Pharmacologic Intervention

If systolic pulmonary arterial pressure exceeds 75% of systemic pressure in patients over 6 months of age, the status of the pulmonary arterioles is of concern. Either oxygen or pharmacological manipulation can be used to evaluate the reactivity of the pulmonary vascular bed in such patients. In

general, the use of vasodilators such as tolazoline has not been of value and oxygen is used routinely. The use of oxygen is essential if there is hypoxemia, manifested by a systemic arterial oxygen saturation less than 92%. While the patient receives oxygen by face mask or hood, aortic and pulmonary arterial pressures are recorded and oxygen saturation and preferably also blood gases are obtained from the superior vena cava, aorta (or systemic artery), pulmonary artery and pulmonary vein (or pulmonary arterial wedge position). Oxygen is a potent pulmonary vasodilator and if the pulmonary vascular bed is reactive, calculated pulmonary vascular resistance will decrease and pulmonary flow will increase, or pulmonary artery pressure will decrease (Fig. 2). Systemic arterial pressure response is variable, but a slight increase is common.

When the patient breathes oxygen, the saturation of pulmonary arterial blood can approach systemic arterial saturation, and

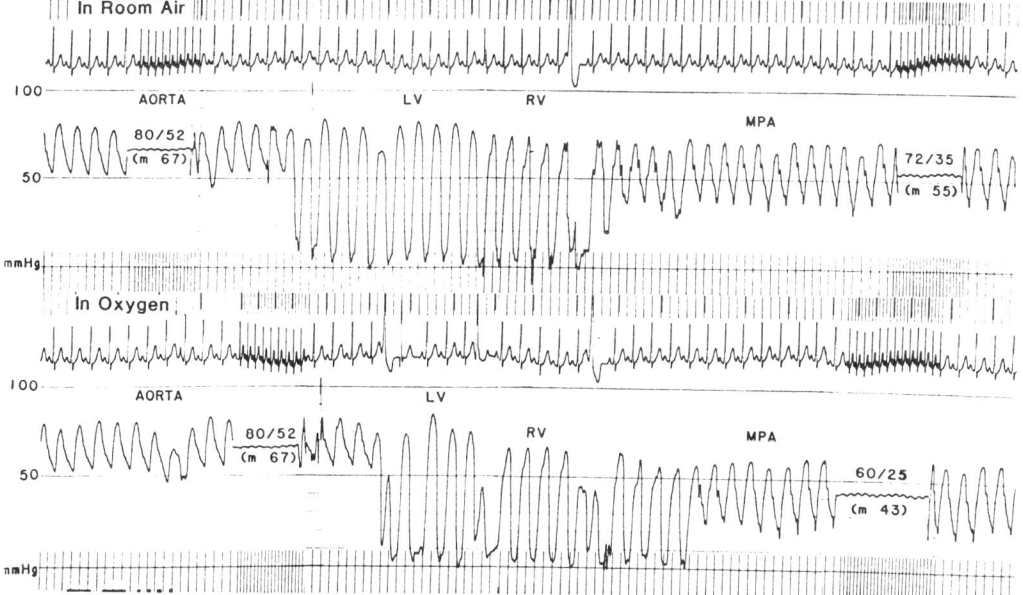

Figure 2. Continuous withdrawal pressure tracings from the aorta to the left ventricle (LV); then to the right ventricle (RV) through ventricular septal defect, and then passed into the main pulmonary artery (MPA). Top: showing high pulmonary artery pressure in room air. Bottom: showing reduction of pulmonary artery pressure in l00% oxygen.

the calculation of pulmonary blood flow from oxygen saturations alone is unreliable. Therefore the PO_2 (partial pressure of oxygen) should also be measured to correct for dissolved oxygen (refer to Chapter 6).

If a pharmacological agent such as Priscoline (tolazoline hydrochloride) is used as a test of pulmonary arteriolar reactivity, 0.1 to 0.2 mg/kg is given intravenously. Unfortunately the systemic arterioles are also affected and a decrease in both pulmonary and systemic arterial pressures commonly occurs.

In general a significant reduction in pulmonary artery pressure with oxygen administration makes irreversible pulmonary vascular disease unlikely. The absence of a fall in pulmonary artery pressure does not exclude reversibility of pulmonary vascular disease after surgical closure of the defect. Unfortunately, even a large calculated rise in pulmonary flow or the pulmonary to systemic flow ratio does not rule out severe pulmonary arteriolar disease.

Balloon Occlusion of the Patient Ductus Arteriosus in Association with the Ventricular Septal Defect

If an infant has an associated patent ductus arteriosus, the contribution of the ductus to the overall hemodynamics is difficult to assess. If the ductus is small on angiocardiography it can be regarded as relatively insignificant, but if it is large its contribution may be less clear. A balloon catheter with a proximal lumen for pressure measurement (e.g., a Berman angiographic catheter) can be used to temporarily occlude the ductus. The catheter tip is passed from the main pulmonary artery to the descending aorta through the ductus and the balloon is inflated and withdrawn against the aortic wall (ductal orifice). If the ductus is large and more hemodynamically significant than the ventricular septal defect, a reduction of pulmonary arterial pressure and con-

comitant rise in systemic pressure is observed (refer to Figure 2 in Chapter 20). In such cases surgical ligation of the ductus alone may be sufficient and closure of the ventricular septal defect may be obviated or at least delayed.

Angiocardiography

The introduction of axial views by Bargeron et al. (1977) enhanced the angiographic diagnosis of many cardiac defects. The technique is particularly helpful in localizing and sizing ventricular septal defects. For optimal visualization of a defect in the ventricular septum the x-ray beam should be parallel to the septum in the region of the defect. It should be noted that the ventricular septum is a curved rather than a flat structure and that the ideal projection varies with the location of the defect.

Left ventriculography in the four-chamber view is usually preferred for defects located relatively posterior in the septum, including perimembranous inlet (Fig. 3A), inlet muscular (Fig. 3B), and trabecular muscular defects (Fig. 3C and 3D). The four-chamber view is less suitable for defects more anterior in the septum.

The long axial view is steeper than the four-chamber view and is therefore more parallel to the anterior portion of the septum. It is the preferred view for subarterial (supracristal), perimembranous outlet, or outlet muscular varieties. On occasion a subarterial defect is better visualized in the lateral projection. The subarterial defect is located just below the aortic and pulmonic valves and contrast usually opacifies the pulmonary artery without opacification of inlet and trabecular portions of the right ventricle (Fig. 4).

A selective aortogram is routinely recommended to evaluate the status of the aortic valve since herniation of the aortic leaflet

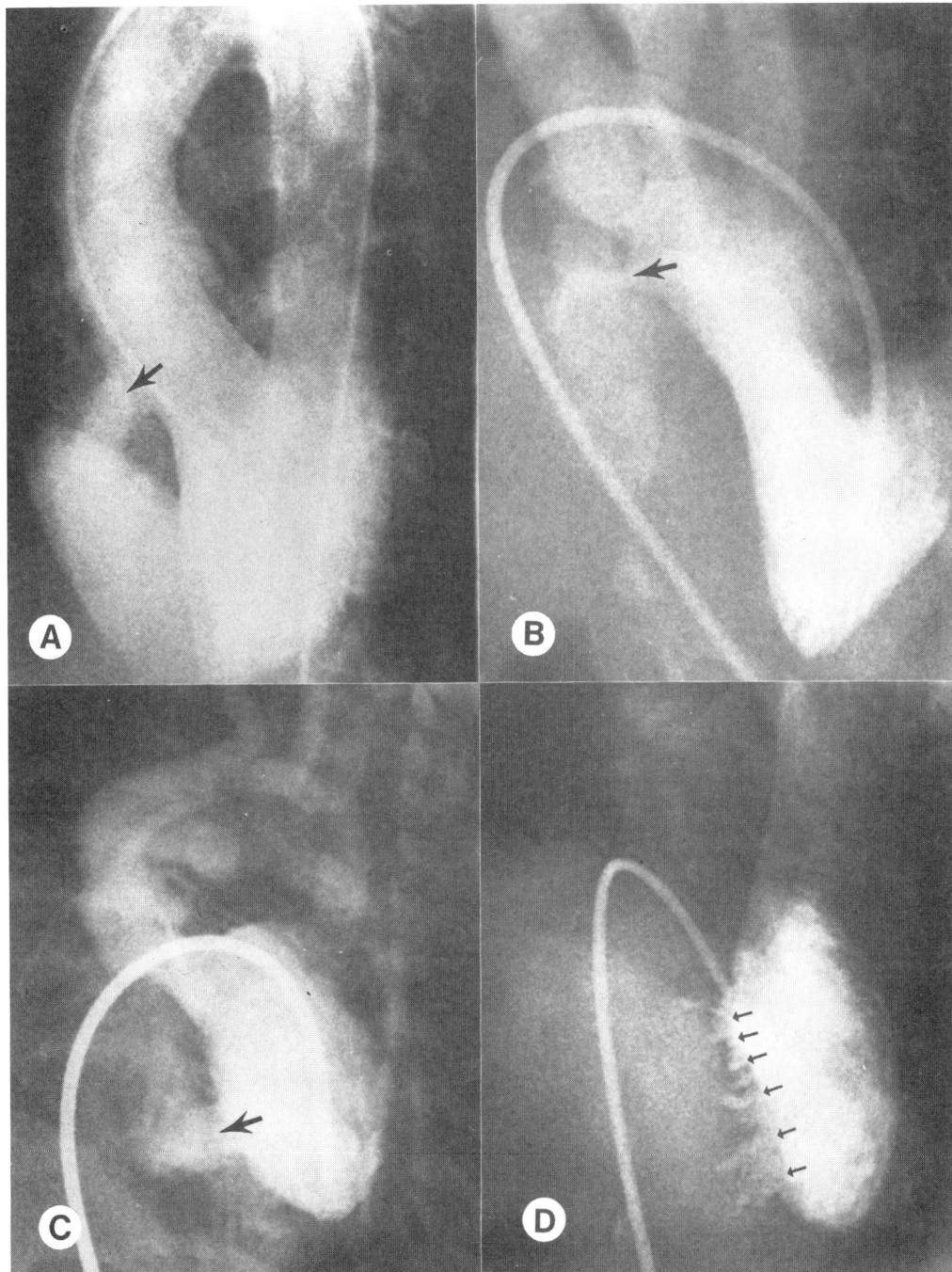

Figure 3. Selective left ventricular angiograms in the four-chamber view demonstrating ventricular septal defects (arrows). A: Perimembranous inlet defect. B: Inlet muscular defect. C: Single trabecular muscular defect. D: Multiple muscular defects.

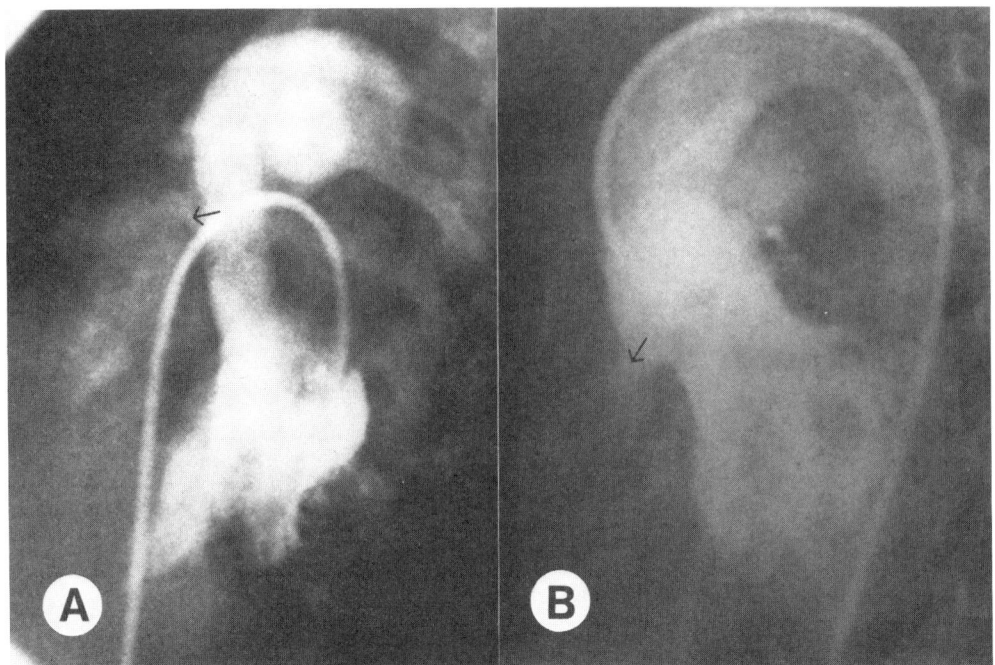

Figure 4. Selective left ventricular angiocardiogram in a patient with a subarterial ventricular septal defect (supracristal defect) (arrows). A: Long axial view. B: Left anterior oblique view.

may be associated with a ventricular septal defect, particularly with the doubly committed subarterial type. The appropriate projection of the angiogram is helpful to identify which leaflet is involved. Generally, combined anteroposterior and lateral views are usually sufficient (Fig. 5) and often oblique views may obscure the presence of herniation. Enlargement of the right sinus of Valsalva and herniation of the right aortic leaflet are rather commonly associated with this defect and are best visualized on the lateral view of an aortogram (Fig. 6A). Involvement of the noncoronary leaflet, which is more common in patients with a perimembranous defect, is best seen in anteroposterior view (Fig. 6B) but also may be well seen in the lateral view (Fig. 6C). The ventricular septal defect occasionally may appear to be small because the herniated right coronary leaflet partially occludes it.

In infants, particularly when there is congestive heart failure, an aortogram should be performed to rule out associated anomalies such as patent ductus arteriosus and coarctation of the aorta, especially when echocardiography is unable to exclude these lesions conclusively.

If there is any question as to the site of pulmonary venous return, a pulmonary arteriogram is indicated. If there is a significant right ventricular outflow gradient or if tricuspid valve disease is suspected, selective right ventricular angiography in the long axial view is indicated.

"Aneurysm of the membranous septum" is a misnomer, because the aneurysm is usually made up of tricuspid valve tissue that partially or completely occludes a perimembranous defect (Beerman et al. 1985). The aneurysm may be small or large and may be smooth walled or "cauliflower"

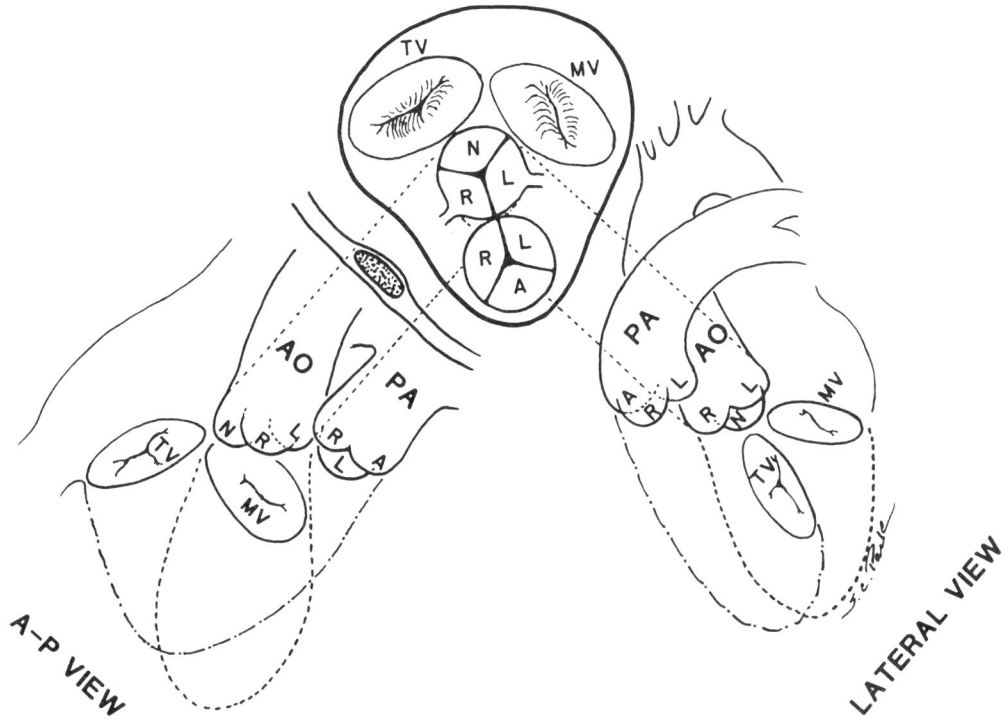

Figure 5. Diagram of the aortic valve showing the relationship of the aortic leaflets in various projections. AO = Aorta; MV = Mitral valve; PA = Pulmonary artery; TV = Tricuspid valve. Valve leaflets: A = Anterior; L = Left; N = Noncoronary; R = Right.

shaped. The ventricular septal defect may be in the apex or along the margin of the aneurysm. The aneurysm is usually best seen in the four-chamber view (Fig. 7).

Associated Lesions

Ventricular septal defect is often associated with other cardiac lesions. Infants in congestive heart failure not infrequently have an associated patent ductus arteriosus, atrial septal defect or coarctation of the aorta. Right ventricular outflow tract obstruction frequently accompanies a ventricular septal defect. Rarely, subaortic stenosis, pulmonary vein stenosis, or anomalous origin of the left coronary artery are associated with ventricular septal defect.

Left Ventricle-Right Atrial Shunt

A left ventricle-right atrial shunt is a rather uncommon condition that causes a direct shunt from the left ventricle to right atrium. Normally, there is an offset arrangement between the mitral and tricuspid valves, forming the atrioventricular septum (Fig. 8). A true left ventricle-right atrial shunt should have a defect in this septal area alone, but the occurrence of this is extremely rare. More commonly, the shunt results from a combination of a perimembranous ventricular septal defect and an abnormality of the tricuspid valve, such as a fenestration, a cleft of the valve or an unusually widened commissure (Fig. 9). Some partial forms of atrioventricular septal defect with atrioventricular valve regurgitation may mimic the left ventricle-right atrial

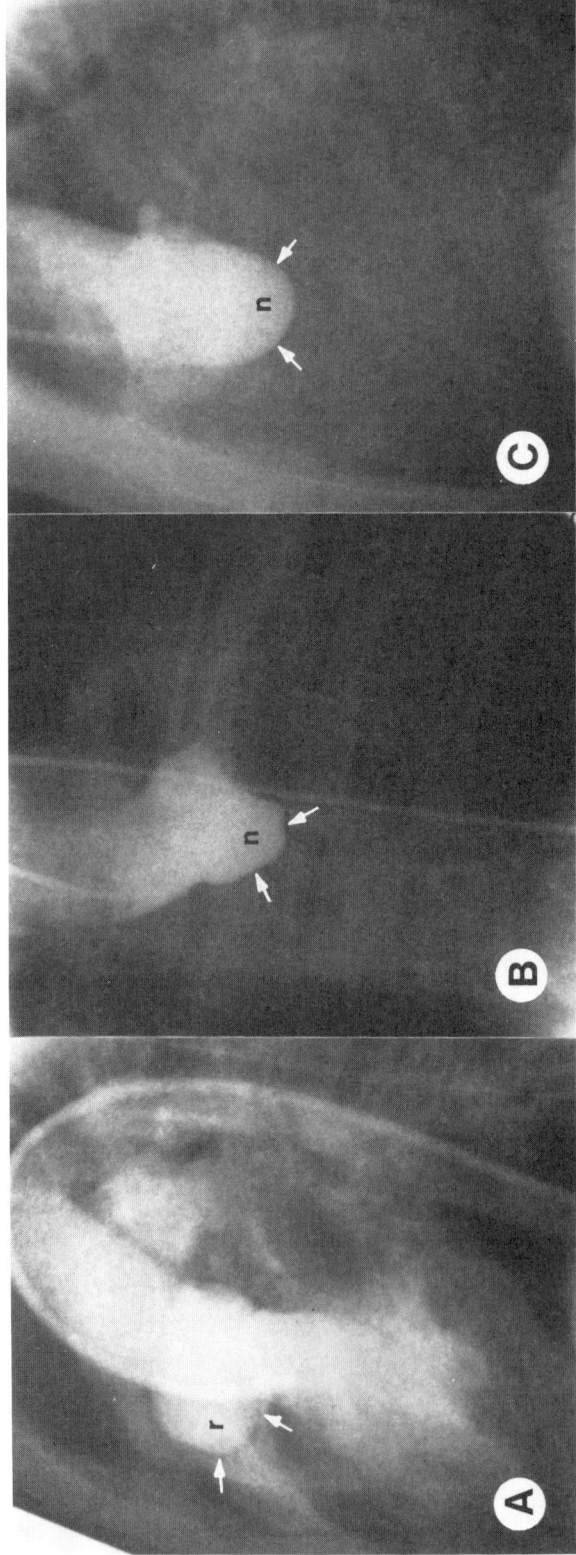

Figure 6. Aortogram in patients with herniation of an aortic valve leaflet (arrows). A: Herniation of the right coronary sinus (r) in a patient with a subarterial defect (lateral view). B: Herniation of the noncoronary sinus (n) in a patient with a perimembranous defect (Antero-posterior view). C: Lateral view of aortogram in the same patient with the perimembranous defect.

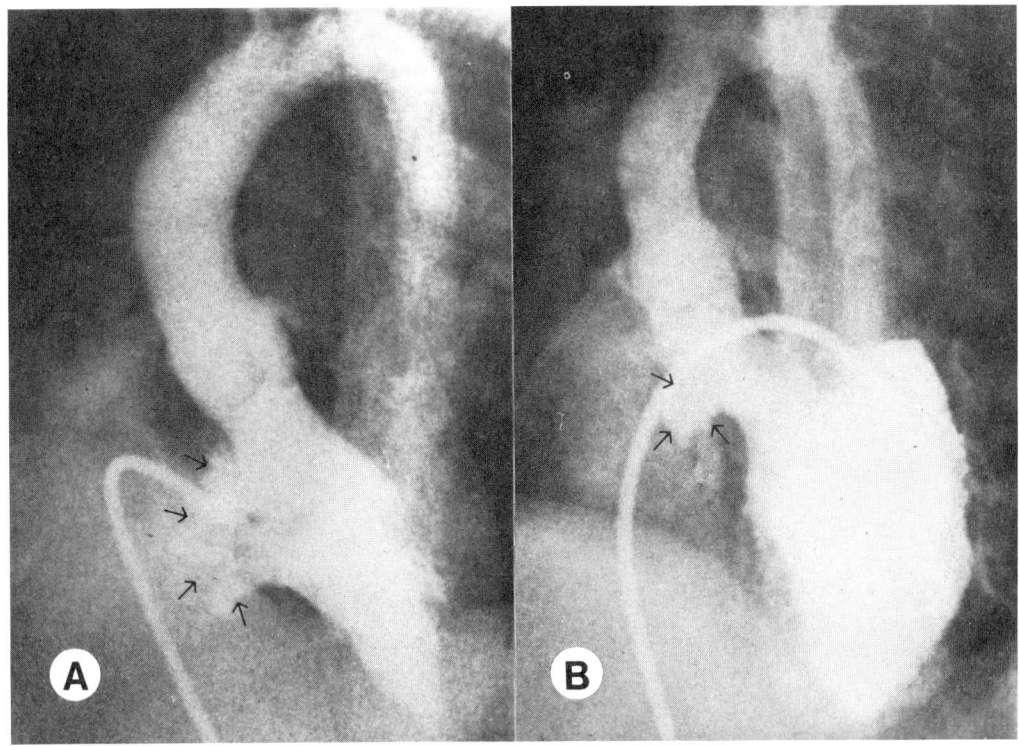

Figure 7. Left ventricular angiocardiograms in the four-chamber view showing a membranous defect and an "aneurysm" of the membranous septum (arrows). A: Catheter through the ventricular defect. B: Catheter passed across the atrial septum.

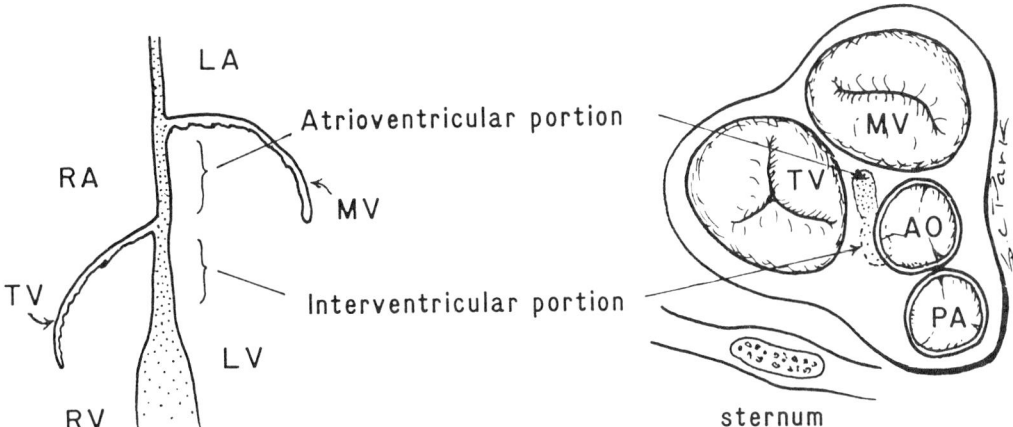

Figure 8. Diagram, illustrating the normal anatomy of the atrioventricular septum. AO = Aorta; LA = Left atrium; LV = Left ventricle; MV = Mitral valve; PA = Pulmonary artery; RA = Right atrium; RV = Right ventricle; TV = Tricuspid valve.

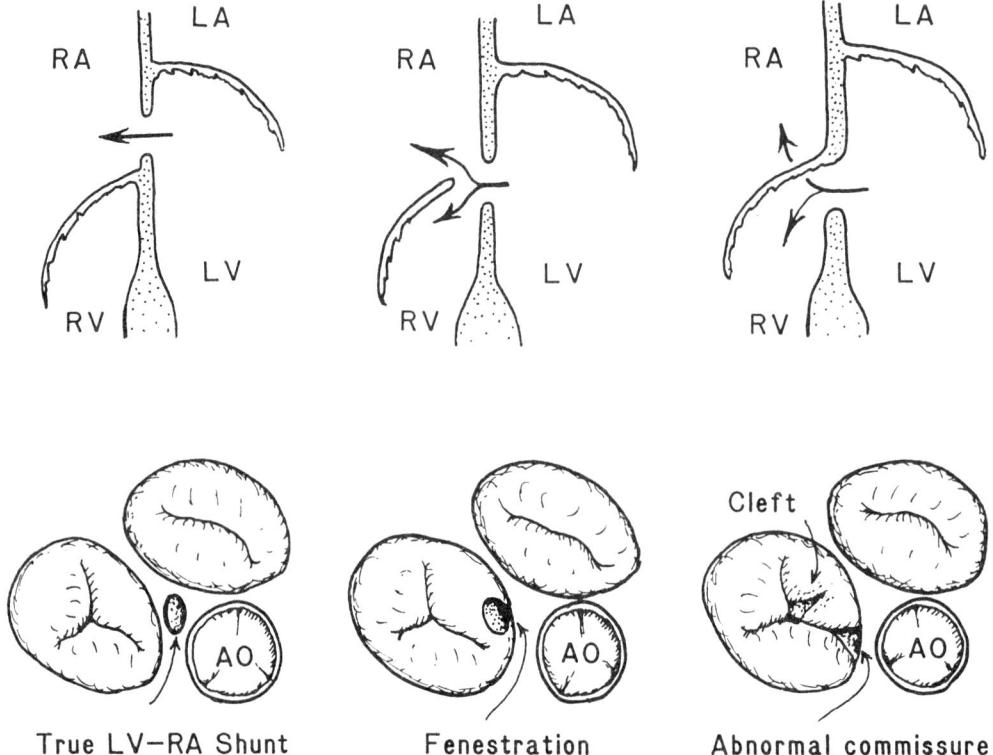

Figure 9. Diagram illustrating the various types of left ventricle-right atrial shunts. (Abbreviations are the same as in Figure 8.)

shunt due to a direct jet of regurgitation to the right atrium via the atrial defect. Cross-sectional echocardiography with color flow mapping may provide useful information regarding the location of the defect and atrioventricular valve status. On hemodynamic evaluation, an oxygen step-up is distinctly noticeable at the right atrial level. Pulmonary blood flow is often increased considerably. Right ventricle and pulmonary artery pressures commonly are elevated and this is dependent upon the size of ventricular septal defect component. A selective left ventricular angiogram in a combination of four-chamber and right anterior oblique views is helpful to localize the defect (Fig. 10A and 10B). A selective right ventricular angiogram is recommended to determine the competence of the tricuspid valve (Fig.

10C). The absence of tricuspid valve regurgitation supports the diagnosis.

Cautions or Precautions

Patients who undergo cardiac catheterization in early infancy are usually symptomatic and may be in frank congestive heart failure. Therefore fluid overload from flushing solution or large quantities of contrast material can lead to deterioration of the clinical status. Thus cautious administration of fluid and contrast material is important. Arterial catheterization in the sick infant also carries a significant risk of a vascular complication.

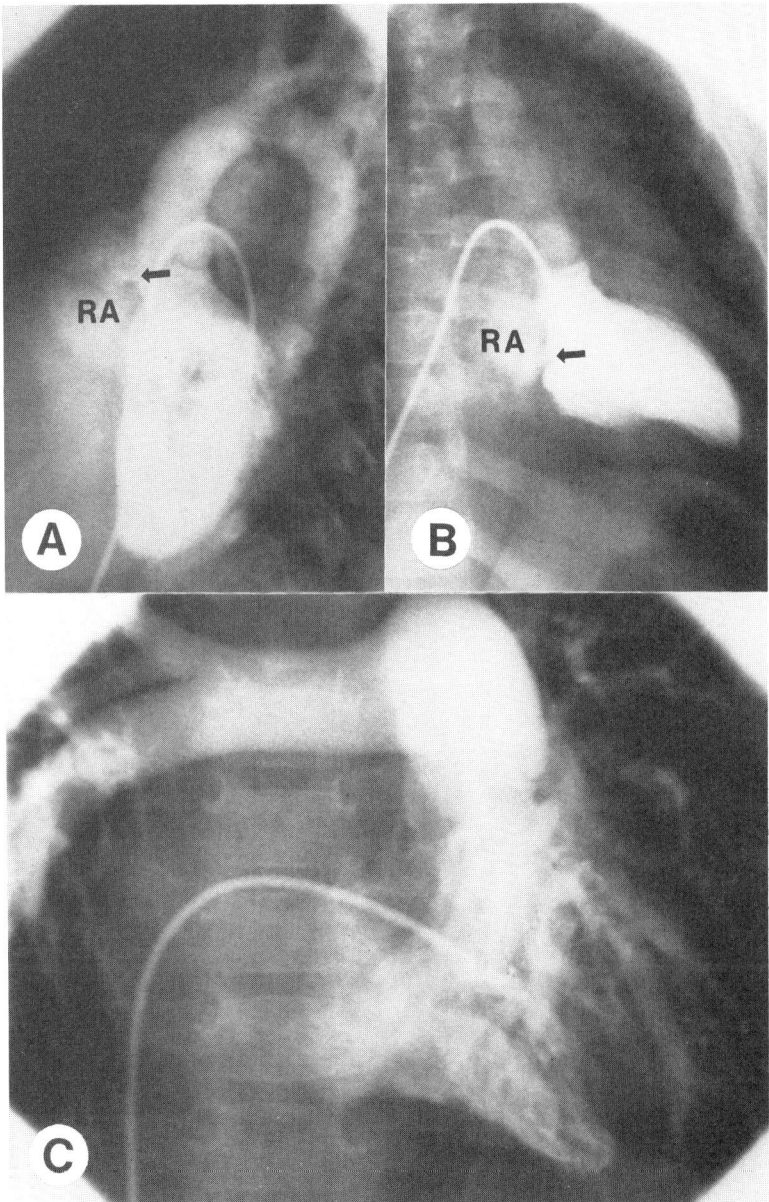

Figure 10. Selective angiograms in left ventricle-right atrial shunt. A & B: Left ventricle in the four-chamber view (A) and right anterior oblique view (B) demonstrating a jet (arrow) filling the right atrium (RA). C: Right ventricle in the anteroposterior view demonstrating absence of tricuispid regurgitation.

References and Suggested Reading

Bargeron LM, Jr., Elliott LP, Soto B, et al. Axial cineangiography in congenital heart disease. Section I Concept, Technical and Anatomic Considerations. Circulation 1977;56:1075–1083.

Becker AE, Anderson RH. Pathology of Congenital Heart Disease. London, Butterworths. 1981;93–117.

Becu LM, Fontana RS, DuShane JW, et al. Anatomic and pathologic studies in ventricular septal defect. Circulation 1957;14:349–364.

Beerman LB, Park SC, Fischer DR, et al. Ventricular septal defect associated with aneurysm of the membranous septum. J Am Coll Cardiol 1985;5:118–123.

Neufeld HN, Titus JL, DuShane JW, et al. Isolated ventricular septal defect of the persistent common atrioventricular type. Circulation 1961;23:685.

Riemenschneider TA, Moss AJ. Left ventricular-right atrial communication. Am J Cardiol 1967;19:710–718.

Soto B, Becker AE, Moulaert AH, et al. Classification of ventricular septal defect. Br Heart J. 1980;43:332–343.

19

Atrioventricular Septal Defect (Endocardial Cushion Defect)

Sang C. Park, M.D.

Anatomy

Atrioventricular septal defect (endocardial cushion defect, atrioventricular canal defect) comprise a group of congenital cardiac anomalies with rather wide spectra of morphology, hemodynamics, and clinical course. The cardinal abnormality is a deficiency of the ventricular septum; the atrioventricular portion of the septum is always absent and the crest of the muscular septum is variably deficient, resulting in a "scooped out" appearance. In most atrioventricular (A-V) septal defects there is an interatrial communication located in the portion of the atrial septum immediately adjacent to the atrioventricular valves. These ostium primum defects may well be secondary to absence of the atrioventricular septum, the lower portion of the developing atrial septum having nothing to which to anchor. The atrioventricular valves are always abnormal. There may be two separate valve orifices, or there may be only a single atrioventricular orifice. These two patterns are really variants of the basic valve morphology of an atrioventricular septal defect, anterior and posterior bridging leaflets, and lateral leaflets. If the anterior and posterior bridging leaflets are not attached to each other a single atrioventricular orifice results and there is usually a large interventricular communication beneath the common atrioventricular valve. Such hearts are called "complete" atrioventricular septal defects

(complete endocardial cushion defect, complete atrioventricular canal, atrioventricularis communis) (Fig. 1). In other hearts the anterior and posterior bridging leaflets join over the ventricular septum and two atrioventricular valve orifices result. With this arrangement, the joined anterior and posterior bridging leaflets are usually attached to the ventricular septum and although there is still deficiency of the crest of the septum there is no interventricular communication. Such hearts are termed "partial" atrioventricular septal defects (partial endocardial cushion defect or incomplete atrioventricular canal) or may be referred to as an ostium primum atrial septal defect (Fig 1). The mitral valve is usually described as being "cleft", the cleft extending to the septum. The cleft is actually just the space between the anterior and posterior bridging leaflets while the apex of the cleft is the point of fusion of these leaflets over the interventricular septum (Anderson et al. 1985; Penkoske et al. 1985)

If the attachment of the leaflets to the septum is incomplete a small interventricular communication results. Such hearts have been termed "transitional forms of atrioventricular canal" or "incomplete" endocardial cushion defect.

The classification described above is imperfect, since not all atrioventricular septal defects can be neatly categorized as "complete", with a single atrioventricular orifice and large interventricular commu-

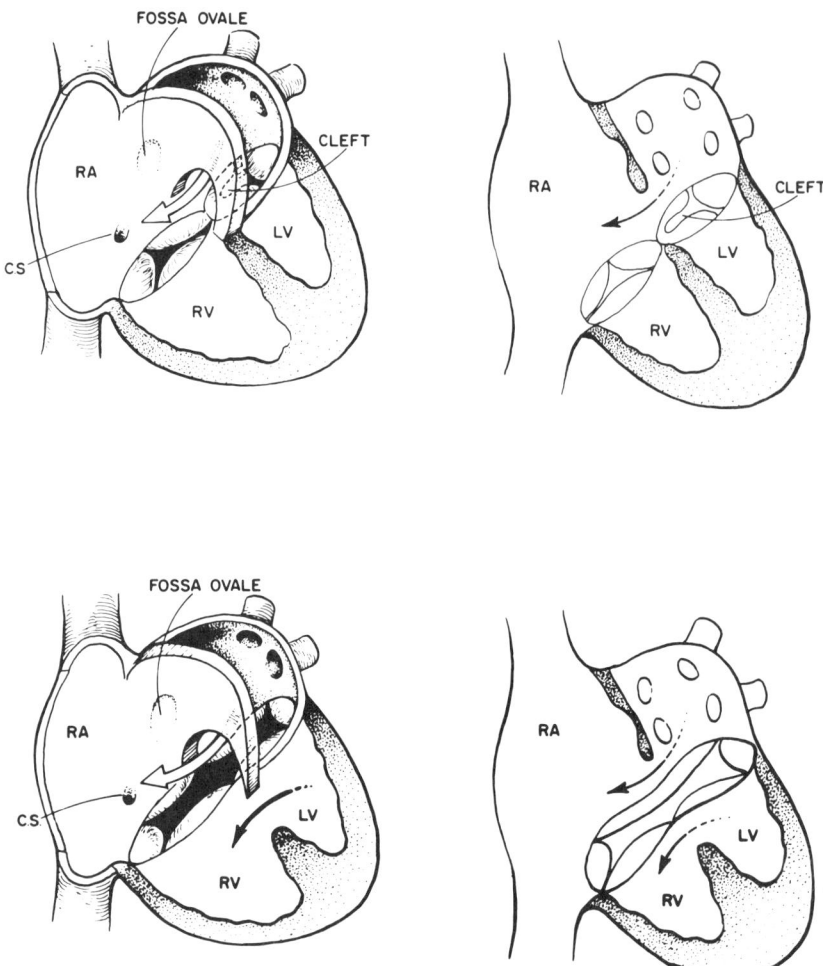

Figure 1. Diagrams of atrioventricular septal defects. Top: Partial form. Bottom: Complete form.

nication; "partial", with two atrioventricular orifices and no interventricular communication; or as transitional forms. The two variables, that is the number of atrioventricular orifices and the presence of an interventricular communication, are to a degree independent. Thus, hearts are occasionally seen where there are two orifices and a large ventricular septal defect (anterior and posterior bridging leaflets joined to each other but not attached to the septum), or anterior and posterior leaflets may not be joined, yet the leaflets are at-

tached to the crest of the septum (single atrioventricular orifice but only a small interventricular communication). Also, some cases of complete atrioventricular septal defect have been seen with spontaneous closure of the ventricular competent "tricuspid pouch" (Pahl et al. 1987). In "common" or "single" atrium, there is complete absence of atrial septal tissue. Although some believe that this anomaly can exist as an isolated lesion, a true "common" atrium, with complete absence of both superior and inferior portions of the atrial septum, is always associated with an atrioventricular septal defect, particularly in the presence of atrial isomerism.

Hemodynamic Considerations

Although the basic anatomic abnormality is remarkably similar in atrioventricular septal defects, the atrioventricular valve morphology is quite variable and is primarily responsible for the wide spectrum of hemodynamic and clinical findings. If the anterior and/or posterior bridging leaflets are not attached to the septum, there is a large interventricular communication, which results in a substantial left to right shunt and high pulmonary artery pressure. Congestive heart failure commonly occurs in early infancy and pulmonary vascular disease has a relatively early onset and may be advanced by a year or two of age. On the other hand, complete attachment of the leaflets to the septum eliminates the interventricular communication, leaving only the ostium primum atrial septal defect. An isolated left to right shunt at atrial level is well tolerated in infancy, whether the shunt be through a secundum or primum type defect. Pulmonary hypertension and pulmonary vascular disease are not expected during childhood. If mitral regurgitation is present, the magnitude of the left to right shunt may be augmented and congestive heart failure may occur early in life.

Thus, the magnitude of pulmonary blood flow, the level of pulmonary artery pressure and resistance, and the presence and severity of mitral regurgitation are important hemodynamic variables that must accurately be assessed at cardiac catheterization.

Indications for Cardiac Catheterization

Cardiac catheterization is usually carried out as part of the preoperative evaluation of atrioventricular septal defects. Some of the morphology of an atrioventricular septal defect can be assessed as well or better by echocardiography than by cineangiocardiography. In addition, the presence of pulmonary hypertension can be inferred from the presence of a large ventricular septal defect on echocardiography, right ventricular hypertrophy on the electrocardiogram, or from a left parasternal lift and a loud pulmonic closure sound on physical examination. The magnitude of the left to right shunt can also be judged from the chest roentgenogram, echocardiogram, and physical examination. Nonetheless, cardiac catheterization is still the "gold standard" for determining pulmonary artery pressure, pulmonary vascular resistance, and magnitude of the left to right shunt. It is also the most reliable way of determining the severity of atrioventricular valve regurgitation. With a partial atrioventricular septal defect, cardiac catheterization is usually not necessary in infancy and is done when surgery is contemplated, often at preschool age. With a complete atrioventricular septal defect, symptoms are usual in infancy. Congestive heart failure and/or poor weight gain may not be controlled with medical therapy and surgery then becomes necessary. Pulmonary artery pressure is always elevated in patients with a complete defect, and pulmonary vascular disease is a feared complication, sometimes developing during the first year of life unless there is associated pulmonic stenosis. Cardiac catheterization and surgical repair therefore should be carried out by 6 months of age in any patient suspected of having pulmonary hypertension. The absence of large pulmonary blood flow (cardiac enlargement, congestive heart failure) indicates a more urgent need for study because of concern that pulmonary vascular resistance is already elevated. Cardiac catheterization is indicated following surgical repair for a variety of reasons: significant residual left to right shunt, atrioventricular valve dysfunction (stenosis or regurgitation) and/or left ventricular outflow obstruction.

Catheterization Technique

The approach to hemodynamic evaluation in patients with atrioventricular septal defect is similar to that in patients with atrial and/or ventricular septal defects (see Chapters 17 and 18). The major difference is in the technique of catheter manipulation. The venous catheter can easily be passed from the right atrium to the left ventricle, either directly or through the left atrium. Because the defect is in the lower portion of the atrial septum the catheter passage across it is substantially lower than the pass with a secundum atrial defect.

Entering the right ventricle from a femoral approach can be difficult and the catheter tends to preferentially pass into the left atrium or left ventricle. In this situation the catheter should initially be hooked against the lateral wall of the right atrium to form a sharp curve. The catheter tip is then rotated clockwise (anteriorly) to enter the right ventricle. In patients with a complete atrioventricular septal defect passage of the catheter into the right ventricle and pulmonary arteries can be especially difficult. In the usual right ventricle to pulmonary artery pass the catheter is rotated clockwise, the tip then pointing posteriorly and sliding up the septum into the pulmonary artery. If this approach is used in the patient with a complete defect, the catheter tip almost invariably enters the left atrium or occasionally left ventricle. Instead, in an atrioventricular septal defect, the catheter should be rotated counterclockwise in the ventricle to keep the tip anteriorly against the right ventricular wall. The pulmonary artery can usually be entered easily with this modification. *A word of caution*: the catheter may also pass across the atrioventricular valve into the left atrium. Thus, a catheter that appears to be in the pulmonary artery may actually be in the left atrial appendage. Therefore, careful monitoring of the pressure tracing is essential during this critical catheter maneuver.

The catheter pass from the right ventricle through the ventricular septal defect to the aorta is usually more difficult with a complete atrioventricular septal defect than with an isolated perimembranous ventricular septal defect. This maneuver is accomplished by passing the tip of the catheter into the right ventricle, rotating it clockwise to position the tip posteriorly and then advancing the catheter directly into aorta. Unfortunately, the tip may encounter the left ventricular free wall and produce ventricular arrhythmia. Also, during the attempt, the catheter tip often flips out of the ventricle into an atrial pressure zone. A balloon catheter may occasionally be useful in entering the aorta or pulmonary artery.

Hemodynamic Evaluation

As with other anomalies with a left to right shunt, oxygen saturations and pressures are obtained from the cardiac chambers and great arteries and veins and shunt magnitude and pulmonary vascular resistance are calculated.

Pressure Evaluation

Pulmonary artery pressure depends both on the volume of pulmonary blood flow and the level of total pulmonary resistance. Pulmonary artery pressure is usually normal or only slightly elevated in a partial atrioventricular septal defect. Even though pulmonary blood flow may be quite large, pulmonary vascular resistance is almost always normal during childhood. There is often a small gradient between the right ventricle and pulmonary artery, which is related to the large flow. Patients with single atrium more frequently have some degree of pulmonary hypertension. Patients with a complete atrioventricular septal defect always have levels of pulmonary artery pressure at or near systemic level unless there is associated pulmonic stenosis. Diastolic pressure in the pulmonary artery is usually lower than in the aorta, unless pulmonary vascular resistance is high or there is an associated pulmonary venous obstructive lesion. A prominent "v" wave may be seen in the atrial pressure tracing when there is significant atrioventricular valve regurgitation.

Oxygen Saturation Data

Arterial blood is usually fully saturated in patients with partial atrioventricular septal defect, but with a single atrium or with complete defect there is often slight systemic arterial desaturation. A significant step-up in oxygen saturation occurs at the right atrial level in both partial and complete forms of atrioventricular septal defect. With a complete defect there may or may not be a further oxygen step-up in the right ventricle. When there is systemic arterial desaturation, sampling should be carried out from both right and left pulmonary veins to look for a pulmonary component of the desaturation.

Other Diagnostic Procedures

In patients with pulmonary artery pressure greater than two-thirds of systemic pressure, oxygen should be administered by hood or face mask and saturations and pressures should be remeasured. (see Chapters 6, 7 and 18).

Angiocardiography

With either a partial or complete atrioventricular septal defect, selective left ventriculography is carried out to evaluate the ventricular septum and left atrioventricular valve function. Some cases with the partial form of atrioventricular septal defect may have a pouch of atrioventricular valve tissue (Fig. 2A) and/or a small interventricular defect between the crest of the ventricular septum and the atrioventricular valve (Fig. 2B). The left ventricular outflow tract characteristically is elongated and narrowed, producing a "scooped out" appearance that is customarily referred to as a "goose-neck deformity". The ventricular septal defect is generally best seen in the four-chamber view and the goose-neck deformity is often readily demonstrated in the anteroposterior projection (Fig. 3A). The concavity of the left ventricular outflow tract is related to the degree of deficiency in the crest of the ventricular septum and may be just as marked in the partial as in the complete form of the anomaly. The basic difference in the two forms lies in the morphology of the atrioventricular valves and not in the extent of the septal deficiency (see section on Anatomy). The concave medial edge of the left ventricular outflow tract is frequently scalloped and often has a nonopacified notch in its midportion. This radiolucent indentation is produced by the coapted free margins of thickened atrioventricular valve tissue and is a marker for a "cleft" between the anterior and posterior bridging leaflets (Fig. 3B). Mitral regurgitation usually occurs through this area and appears as a jet into the left atrium or directly into the right atrium. Mitral regurgitation may be seen with either partial or complete atrioventricular septal defect but is not necessarily present, even with the "free floating" valves of a complete defect. Mitral regurgitation may be induced iatrogenically by ventricular arrhythmia or even by catheter pass across the valve. Thus, angiocardiographic mitral regurgitation in the absence of auscultatory or color flow mapping findings of mitral regurgitation should generally be discounted. The catheter should be properly positioned near the

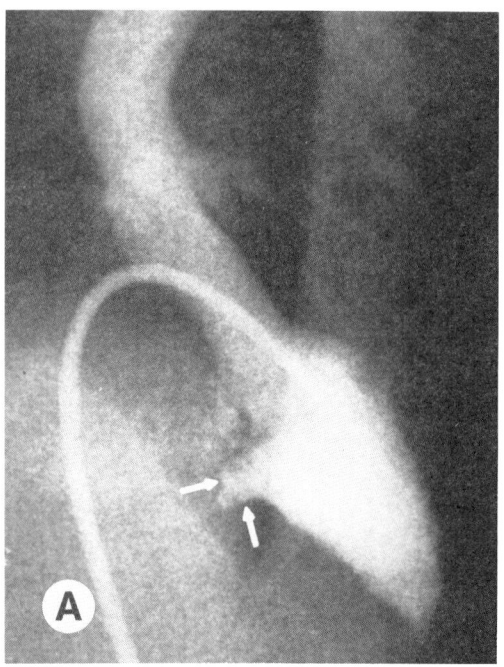

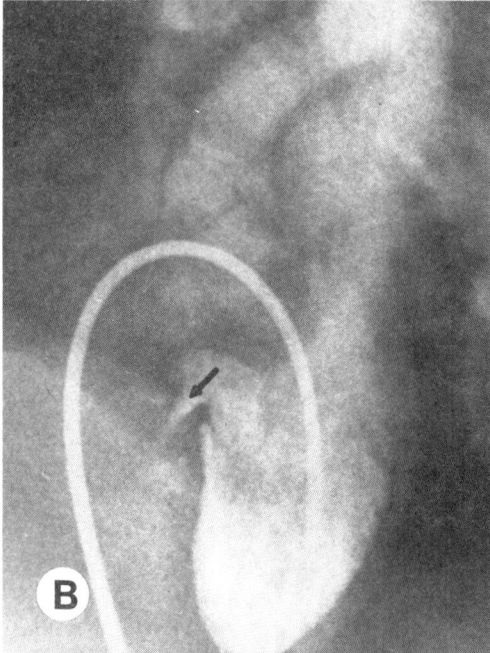

left ventricular apex and the catheter intra-luminal diameter should be sufficiently large to minimize catheter whip during injection. In patients with a large ventricular shunt, contrast medium should be given in a sufficient amount, usually 1.5 mL/kg. Selective right ventriculography is also indicated to evaluate atrioventricular valve function, right ventricular outflow tract, and pulmonary artery anatomy. Determination of the size of each ventricular chamber is important. Usually, the two ventricles are comparable in size, the balanced form (Fig. 4A). At times, however, one of the ventricles is substantially underdeveloped, the asymmetric type. This may occur in either the right ventricle (Fig. 4B) or the left ventricle (Fig. 4C).

Selective right upper pulmonary vein angiography in the four-chamber view provides the best view of the interatrial septum and the defect is usually well visualized (Fig. 5). Selective pulmonary arteriography may be performed in the anteroposterior view if there is a question as to the site of pulmonary venous return. An aortogram is mandatory in infants with complete atrioventricular septal defect and severe pulmonary hypertension particularly when coarctation of the aorta and/or a patent ductus arteriosus are not ruled out by echocardiography.

Figure 2. Selective left ventricular angiograms on the four-chamber view in partial forms of atrioventricular septal defect. A: The ventricular septum is intact. There is a pouch of atrioventricular valve tissue (arrows). B: There is a small interventricular communication (arrow) above the crest of the ventricular septum.

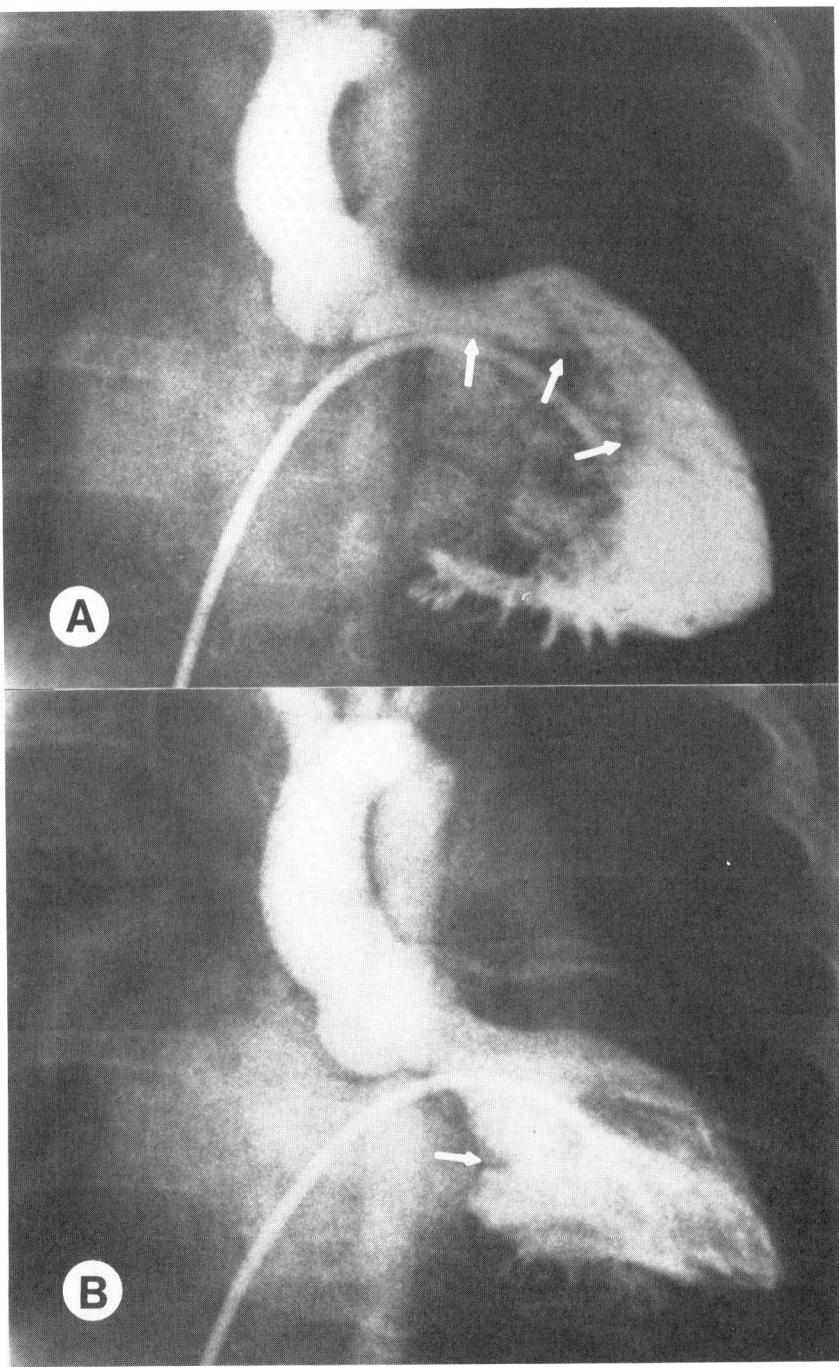

Figure 3. Left ventricular cineangiogram in the anteroposterior view. Arrows indicate the limits of the atrioventricular valve giving the "goose-neck" appearance of the left ventricular outflow. A: Diastole. B: Systole (arrow indicates the "cleft"). Note: Atrioventricular valve insufficiency is present.

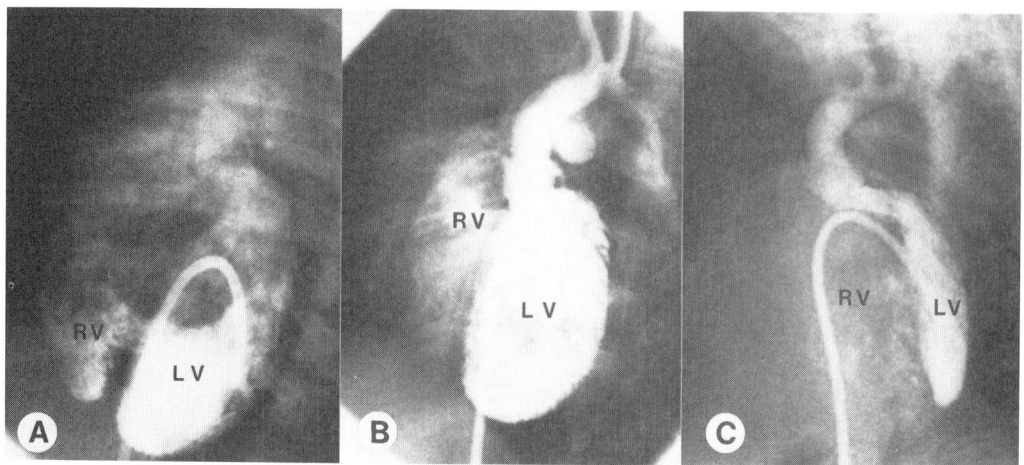

Figure 4. Left ventricular angiocardiograms demonstrating the variable size of the ventricles. LV = left ventricle; RV = right ventricle. A: Balanced. B: Hypoplastic right ventricle. C: Hypoplastic left ventricle.

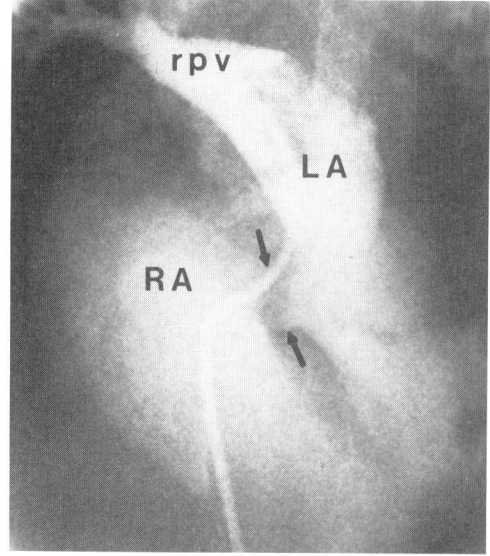

Figure 5. Selective injection of contrast in the right upper pulmonary vein (RPV) in the four-chamber view showing a low lying atrial defect (arrows). LA = Left atrium; RA = Right atrium.

Associated Lesions

Patients with atrioventricular septal defects frequently have associated cardiac anomalies. If there is right or left atrial isomerism (asplenia or polysplenia complexes) anomalies of systemic or pulmonary venous return are common and ventriculoarterial connection may also be abnormal. Associated patent ductus arteriosus and/or coarctation of the aorta should be ruled out in infants with congestive heart failure. Pulmonic stenosis may also be associated and if sufficiently severe, produces cyanosis. Subaortic stenosis occasionally is seen in patients following complete repair of an atrioventricular septal defect, particularly with the partial form (Fig. 6).

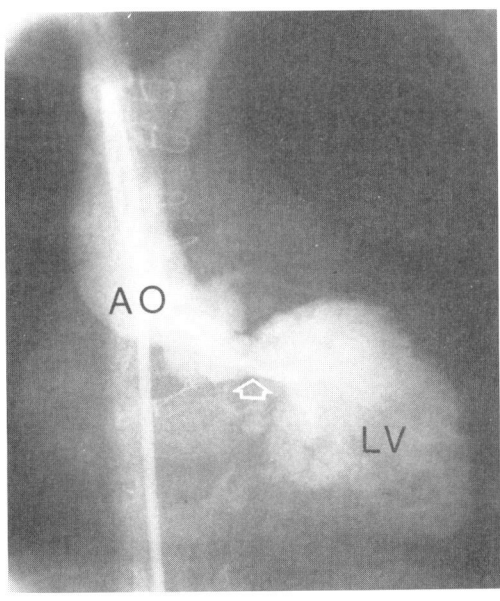

Figure 6. Selective left ventricular angiogram in the anteroposterior view demonstrating subaortic stenosis (arrow) in a postoperative patient.

Cautions or Precautions

Care should be taken to avoid excessive fluid infusion or excessive blood loss in small infants with congestive heart failure. As indicated in the catheter manipulation section it may be difficult to enter the pulmonary artery or aorta from the right ventricle. The catheter tends to enter the left atrium and thus careful monitoring of the pressure tracing is essential during this catheter maneuver. Very forceful manipulation of the catheter may result in serious arrhythmias or myocardial perforation. Many patients with atrioventricular septal defect have Down's syndrome and frequently also have upper airway abnormalities. During cardiac catheterization, aggravation of their airway compromise leads to difficulty in accurate hemodynamic evaluation. It is important to take appropriate precautions to secure an adequate airway during the study. Occasionally, endotracheal intubation may be indicated, particularly when the airway problem is suspected of being the cause of pulmonary hypertension.

References and Suggested Reading

Anderson RH, Zuberbuhler JR, Penkoske PA, et al. Of clefts, commissures, and things. J Thor Cardiovasc Surg 1985;90:605–610.

Baron MG, Wolf BS, Steinfeld L, et al. Endocardial cushion defects. Specific diagnosis by angiocardiography. Am J Cardiol 1964;13:162–175.

Pahl E, Park SC, Anderson RH. Spontaneous closure of the ventricular component of an atrioventricular septal defect. Am J Cardiol 1987;60:1203–1205.

Penkoske PA, Neches WH, Anderson RH, et al. Further observations on the morphology of atrioventricular septal defects. J Thor Cardiovasc Surg 1985;90:611–622.

Rastelli GC, Kirklin JW, Titus JL. Anatomic observations on complete form of persistent common atrioventricular canal with special reference to atrioventricular valve. Mayo Clinic Proc 1966;41:296–308.

Van Mierop LHS. Pathology and pathogenesis of endocardial cushion defects. Surgical implications. In: Second Henry Ford International Symposium on Cardiac Surgery. Davila JC, ed. New York, NY; Appleton-Century-Crofts. 1977;201–207.

20

Patent Ductus Arteriosus

Donald R. Fischer, M.D.

Anatomy

The ductus arteriosus is derived from the distal portion of the embryologic sixth aortic arch and serves to connect the main pulmonary artery with the descending aorta in fetal life. In utero nearly 60% of the combined ventricular output of the fetus crosses the ductus arteriosus. Persistent patency of the ductus arteriosus may occur in the premature infant in which case the ductus is anatomically and histologically normal but presumed to be physiologically immature (Kitterman et al. 1972). The patent ductus arteriosus that is seen in the term infant may be histologically abnormal and unable to constrict and close in a physiologic manner (Gittenberger-de Groot 1977).

In the presence of a left aortic arch, the ductus arteriosus usually connects the main pulmonary artery with the descending aorta slightly distal to the origin of the left subclavian artery (Fig. 1A). If the aortic arch is right sided, the ductus usually arises from the base of the innominate or left subclavian artery or from a retroesophageal left subclavian artery, and connects to the pulmonary artery (Fig. 1B). In some cases it may arise in a mirror image fashion just distal to the origin of the right subclavian artery and connects to the right pulmonary artery. Bilateral ductus arteriosus is uncommon and is usually associated with complex intracardiac malformations (Lenox et al. 1977; Freedom et al. 1984) (Fig. 1C).

A patent ductus arteriosus is often an isolated malformation, but may be associated with other intracardiac defects. Persistent patency of the ductus arteriosus may be crucial in the immediate newborn period if pulmonary or systemic blood flow are ductus dependent, as in pulmonary atresia or interrupted aortic arch. Patent ductus arteriosus is associated with discrete pulmonary arterial stenoses in the rubella syndrome; in this situation the lesions are probably etiologically related to the prenatal effect of rubella virus on arterial elastic tissue. Other defects may coexist with a patent ductus arteriosus and mask its presence, as in the case of a large ventricular septal defect or atrioventricular septal defect with pulmonary hypertension.

Hemodynamic Considerations

The physiologic effect of a patent ductus arteriosus depends on its size and on the relationship between systemic and pulmonary resistance and pressure. An isolated large patent ductus arteriosus may result in congestive heart failure in infancy. With a large ductus the magnitude of left to right shunt varies with the level of pulmonary vascular resistance. If pulmonary artery pressures are at systemic level, the development of pulmonary vascular disease is likely if the defect remains uncorrected. With the development of pulmonary vascular disease, the net left to right shunt decreases and right to left shunting eventually develops.

If the patent ductus arteriosus is small

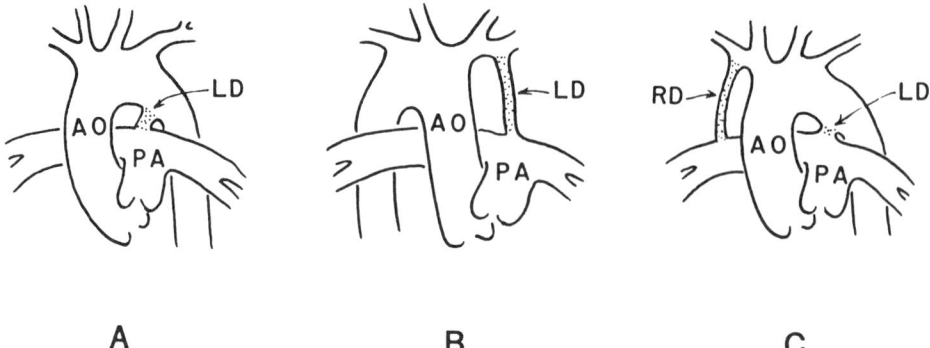

A   B   C

Figure 1. Diagram of patent ductus arteriosus. A: Left aortic arch. B: Right aortic arch. C: Bilateral ductus.

the patient has normal pulmonary artery pressure, only a small left to right shunt and is asymptomatic.

Indications for Cardiac Catheterization

In most institutions the definitive diagnosis of patent ductus arteriosus is made by clinical examination and both cross sectional and Doppler echocardiography. In the case of the premature infant with respiratory distress and a typical course, echocardiographic and physical findings of a ductus, most centers do not perform cardiac catheterization prior to treatment, because the risk of cardiac catheterization and contrast injection in the premature infant with multiple metabolic problems is not warranted.

In patients with a small ductus arteriosus, cardiac catheterization is unnecessary in the presence of classical clinical and echocardiographic features and with an otherwise normal echocardiogram and chest roentgenogram. However, if any unusual findings are present cardiac catheterization prior to surgery identifies the more rare anomalies such as coronary-cardiac fistula, aortopulmonary septal defect, and pulmonary arteriovenous malformation. In a patient with a moderate or large patent duc-

tus arteriosus, cardiac catheterization is again used only if there are unusual clinical findings or when there is a need to determine pulmonary artery pressure or pulmonary vascular resistance. Cardiac catheterization is also used to perform nonoperative (nonthoracotomy) closure of a patent ductus arteriosus with a Rashkind occluder catheter (see Chapter 15).

Catheterization Technique

In most cases of an isolated patent ductus arteriosus, the entire catheterization can be performed from the venous approach. It is usually quite easy to pass a catheter from the main pulmonary artery directly through the patent ductus and into the descending aorta. If the catheter passes into the aorta and then more superiorly into a carotid vessel, an aortopulmonary window is more likely. If the ductus is large, it is often very difficult to pass the catheter from the main to the branch pulmonary arteries. In this situation it is often possible to pass the curved end of a flexible wire into the branch pulmonary artery through the tip of an end-hole catheter positioned in the main pulmonary artery. The catheter can be passed over the wire to the same position. If this effort fails, a balloon-tipped flow directed catheter (e.g., Swan-Ganz) can be used to enter the pulmonary artery branch. If a patent foramen ovale is present, an adequate left heart study can also be performed. If a ductus cannot be traversed from the pulmonary artery, retrograde arterial catheterization with aortic angiography will demonstrate the defect.

Hemodynamic Evaluation

Pressure Data

Pulmonary artery systolic pressure is usually high with a large ductus, but the diastolic pressure usually remains low if there is low resistance. Aortic pulse pressure is wide due to the large diastolic runoff into the pulmonary bed. Accurate calculation of pulmonary resistance is often not possible due to incomplete pulmonary arterial mixing. Pulmonary pressure would be expected to be normal in the case of a small ductus.

Oxygen Saturation Data

Oxygen saturations should be obtained from the descending aorta, pulmonary wedge, branch and main pulmonary arteries, and right ventricle. Venous saturations should also be obtained in a sampling sweep from the superior vena cava to the lower right atrium. An isolated patent ductus arteriosus would be expected to show an oxygen saturation step-up at the level of the main pulmonary artery. Due to streaming of ductal flow into one or the other pulmonary artery branches, it is often impossible to get an accurate mixed pulmonary artery saturation. For this reason it is frequently impossible to determine pulmonary blood flow and a pulmonary to systemic flow ratio reliably. An oxygen saturation step-up in the right ventricular outflow tract is occasionally seen due to mild pulmonic insufficiency, but a coexisting ventricular septal defect must be ruled out.

In an infant with a very large ductus shunt, the left atrium is enlarged and the foramen ovale may stretch to the point of causing interatrial left to right shunting. An oxygen saturation step-up at the level of the right atrium would be noted in association with a mean pressure gradient between the left and right atria. In the presence of a true atrial septal defect, it would be expected that mean pressures in the two atria would be nearly identical.

Other Diagnostic Procedures

If severe pulmonary hypertension is present, 100% oxygen should be administered with repeat measurement of hemodynamics. If pulmonary artery diastolic pressure drops pulmonary vascular resistance is probably labile. If diastolic pressure does not fall it is difficult to be sure that resistance is labile even in the face of a substantial increase in calculated pulmonary flow. If pulmonary artery pressure does not drop, and does not increase with oxygen administration, irreversible pulmonary vascular disease is certain.

It may be worthwhile in certain patients to determine the effect of closure of the ductus arteriosus on pulmonary artery pressure. This can be done by temporarily occluding the ductus with a balloon catheter and then repeating hemodynamic measurements (Fig. 2). This may be particularly useful if there is a coexisting ventricular septal defect; the relative contributions of each to pulmonary flow and pressure can be determined by this technique.

Angiocardiography

Injection of contrast media in the descending aorta with the catheter just beyond the ductus usually visualizes the defect adequately. It can usually best be seen in the lateral or in the left anterior oblique projection. The ductus may be either long or short and usually has a segment of larger diameter

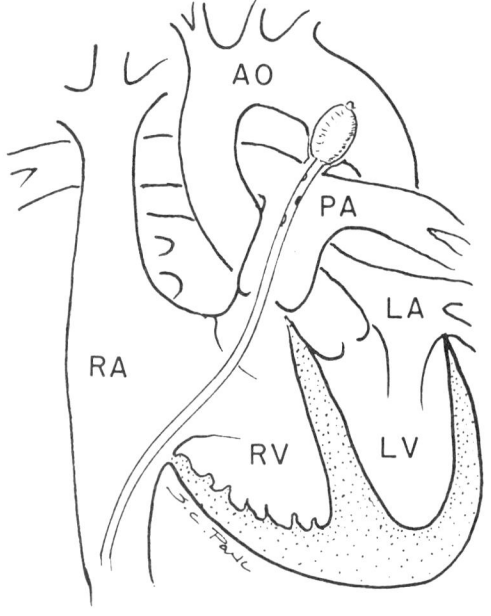

Figure 2. Simultaneous pressure tracing of aorta and pulmonary artery in a patient with a large patent ductus arteriosus and severe pulmonary artery hypertension. Temporary occlusion of the duct (arrow) using an angiographic Swan catheter (with proximal openings) demonstrates a substantial fall of the pulmonary artery pressure and a rise of the aortic pressure. A: Diagram. B: Pressure tracing.

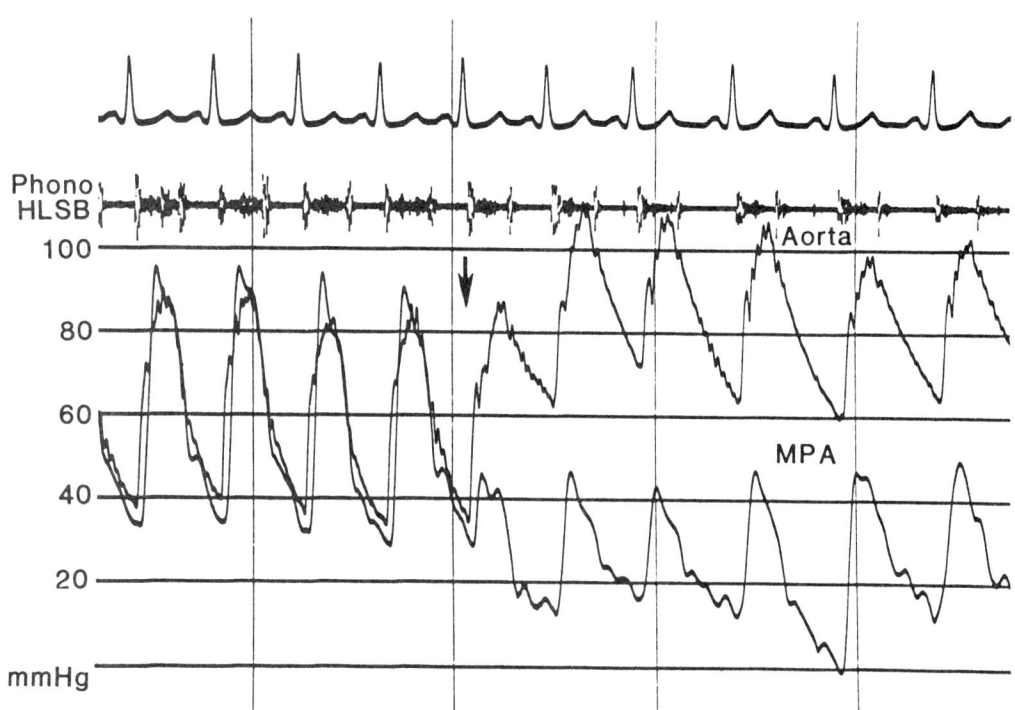

at the aortic origin (Fig. 3). If a small ductus cannot be traversed from the pulmonary arterial side, retrograde arterial catheterization with injection in the descending aorta is necessary. If the ductus fails to visualize with the standard injection, an aortic root injection in the anteroposterior lateral, or oblique views, should adequately visualize the site of origin of the ductus and will also rule out a coronary arteriovenous fistula or

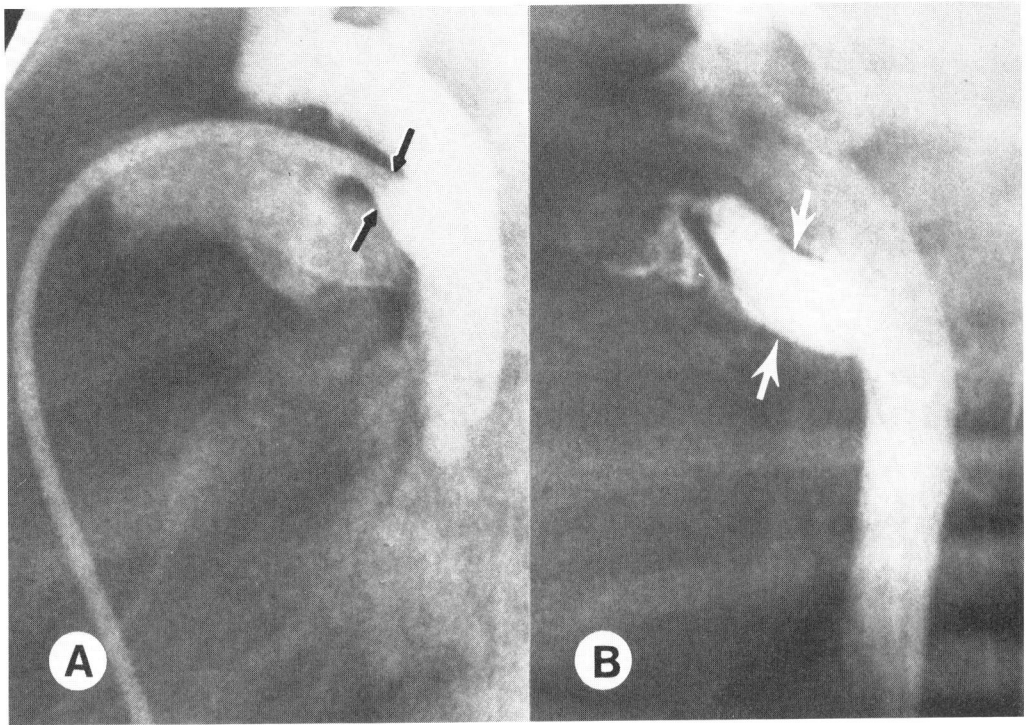

Figure 3. Lateral angiograms showing two types of patent ductus arteriosus (arrows) with a: A: Short segment. B: Long segment.

an unusual aortopulmonary connection. Between 0.5 and 1 mL of contrast media/kg of body weight should be given on the initial injection; the lesser amount should be adequate if there is a small left to right shunt.

A pulmonary arteriogram with follow through levophase may be adequate to screen for associated left to right shunting at atrial or ventricular level.

Cautions or Precautions

Occasionally, other anomalies may be confused with a ductus arteriosus. The presence of two separate semilunar valves by echocardiography rules out a common arterial trunk, as does an intact ventricular septum. A catheter pass from the pulmonary artery to a brachiocephalic vessel is more suggestive of an aortopulmonary window defect. If a ductus is suspected clinically, but not found at catheterization, a coronary cardiac fistula or other systemic or aortopulmonary connection should be considered. The ductus may be in an unusual position if there is a right aortic arch and the possibility of a bilateral ductus should be considered if there is a complex cardiac lesion with pulmonary atresia (Lenox et al. 1977). The origin of the ductus can be in an unusual position; not infrequently from the subclavian artery or from the inferior surface of the transverse aortic arch, particularly in a patient with a complex cardiac lesion and/or in association with right aortic arch (Fig. 4). A specific search for a ductus arteriosus should always be made when performing cardiac catheterization in a patient with a large ventricular septal defect or atrioven-

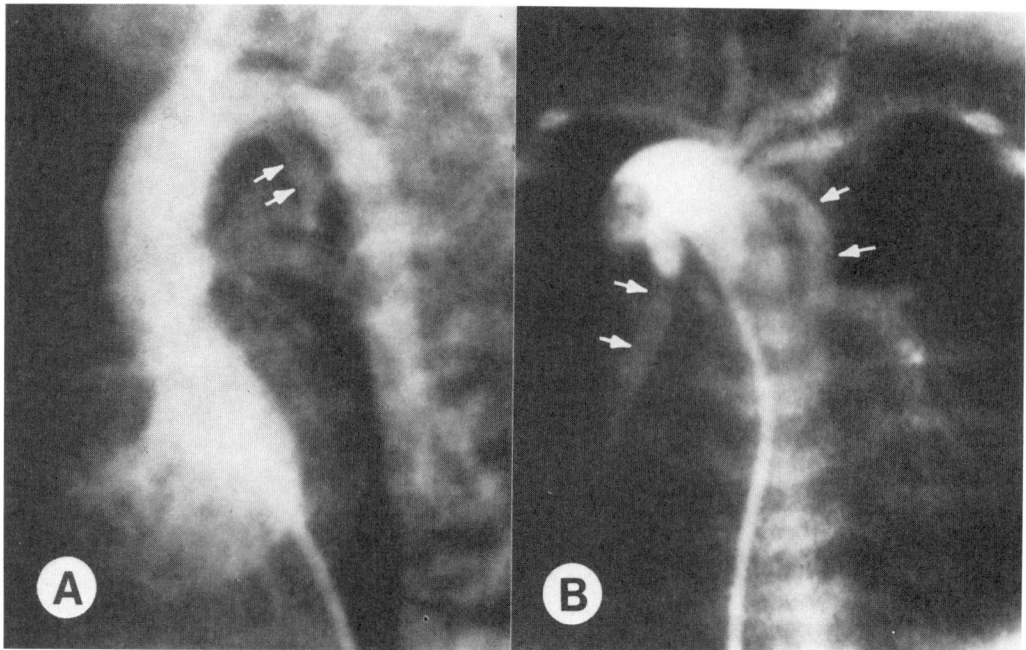

Figure 4. Angiograms demonstrating unusual forms of patent ductus arteriosus in complex congenital heart disease. A: Left anterior oblique view demonstrating a ductus arising from the inferior surface of the transverse arch (arrows) B: Aortogram demonstrating a bilateral ductus in a patient with a right aortic arch. There is a left ductus arteriosus originating from the left innominate artery and a right-sided ductus arteriosus as well (arrows).

tricular septal defect with pulmonary hypertension, as the ductus may not be evident on clinical examination.

References and Suggested Reading

Freedom RM, Moes CAF, Pelech A, et al. Bilateral ductus arteriosus (or remnant): An Analysis of 27 patients. Am J Cardiol 1984;53:884–891.

Gittenberger-de Groot AC. Persistent ductus arteriosus: Most probably a primary congenital malformation. Br Heart J 1977;39:610–618.

Kitterman JA, Edmunds H, Gregory GA, et al. Patent ductus arteriosus in premature infants. Incidence, relation to pulmonary disease and management. N Engl J Med 1972; 287:473–477.

Lenox CC, Neches WH, Zuberbuhler JR, et al. Management of bilateral ductus arteriosus in complex congenital heart disease. J Thorac Cardiovasc Surg 1977;74:607–613.

21

Aortopulmonary Window

Donald R. Fischer, M.D.

Anatomy

Aortopulmonary window (aortopulmonary septal defect, aortopulmonary fenestration) is a rare congenital anomaly consisting of a communication between the ascending aorta and the pulmonary artery. The most common type is located proximally in the ascending aorta just above the sinuses of Valsalva and opens into the main pulmonary artery (Fig. 1). Rarely, the defect extends inferiorly to the semilunar valve level. This variety is thought to result from incomplete septation of the aortopulmonary trunk during embryogenesis. A less common type is more distal in the ascending aorta and connects to the right pulmonary artery (Doty et al. 1981;, Berry et al. 1982). An aortopulmonary window is usually large and most commonly is isolated. Associated defects have been described and include patent ductus arteriosus, ventricular and atrial septal defects, anomalous origin of a coronary artery, tetralogy of Fallot, pulmonary arteriovenous fistula, subaortic stenosis, and aortic arch anomalies including coarctation of the aorta, interrupted aortic arch, and aortic isthmus hypoplasia (Newfeld et al. 1962; Richardson et al. 1979; Blieden and Moller, 1974; Berry et al. 1982).

Hemodynamic Considerations

An isolated aortopulmonary window is usually large and behaves hemodynamically like a large patent ductus arteriosus or ventricular septal defect. There is a large left to right shunt, the magnitude of which varies with the level of pulmonary vascular resistance. Pulmonary artery pressure is at systemic level and the development of pulmonary vascular disease is likely if the defect remains uncorrected. Congestive heart failure often develops early in infancy. In the rare case of a small aortopulmonary window, the patient may manifest no symptoms, have normal pulmonary artery pressure, and only a small left to right shunt.

Indications for Cardiac Catheterization

Although cross-sectional and Doppler echocardiography enable accurate diagnosis of this lesion, cardiac catheterization should be performed for a definitive diagnosis in anticipation of surgical repair. In the majority of cases the setting will be that of an infant who has been in congestive heart failure and has physical findings of pulmonary hypertension. Bounding pulses are usual and suggest the possibility of an aortic runoff. Cardiac catheterization is necessary for hemodynamic measurements to determine the magnitude of the left to right shunt and the level of pulmonary vascular resistance. Angiography will confirm the diagnosis, localize the defect, and rule out other cardiac or vascular anomalies.

In the exceptional case without congestive heart failure or findings of pulmonary

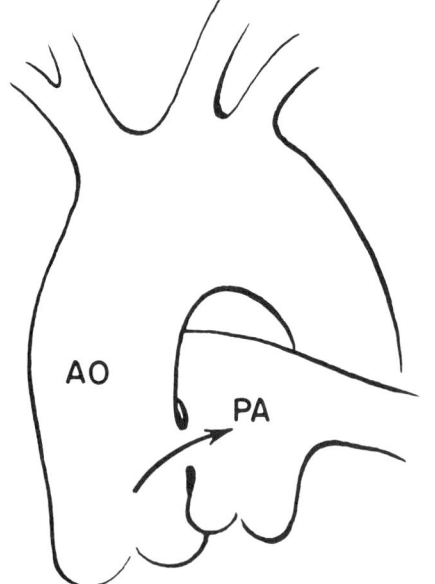

Figure 1. Diagram of aortopulmonary window.

hypertension, catheterization may be deferred until the age at which elective surgery would be performed, but this occurrence is rare.

Catheterization Technique

It is usually possible to traverse the aortopulmonary window from the main pulmonary artery with a standard woven Dacron catheter. The catheter then passes into the innominate or left carotid artery rather than the descending aorta, differentiating this entity from a patent ductus arteriosus. It is more difficult to traverse a more distal defect from the pulmonary artery. In that case, retrograde arterial catheterization is necessary.

Hemodynamic Evaluation

Pressure Data

Pulmonary artery systolic pressure is usually high because the defect is usually large and unrestrictive. Diastolic pressure may be lower than that in the aorta, however aortic pulse pressure is wide due to the diastolic runoff into the pulmonary bed. The hemodynamics are comparable to a large patent ductus arteriosus. Accurate calculation of pulmonary resistance is impossible if there is incomplete mixing in the pulmonary artery.

Oxygen Saturation Data

Oxygen saturations should be obtained from all cardiac chambers, great arteries, and veins. The magnitude of the left to right shunt may be difficult to calculate with the usual proximal defect due to streaming of flow within the pulmonary arterial tree. Accurate determination of the pulmonary to systemic blood flow ratio in a distal defect is often impossible because of the discrepancy in oxygen saturation between the right and left pulmonary arteries. Systemic arterial blood is fully saturated unless pulmonary vascular resistance is at systemic level and there is bidirectional shunting, or if the patient has pulmonary edema. A comparison of pulmonary venous or pulmonary wedge saturation and systemic arterial saturation is important to rule out an intracardiac or interarterial right to left shunt.

Other Diagnostic Procedures

If the patient is noted to have severe pulmonary hypertension (pulmonary artery pressure greater than two thirds of systemic pressure), 100% oxygen should be administered by hood or face mask and hemodynamic measurements repeated (see Chapters 6, 7, and 18) for the evaluation of pulmonary vascular reactivity.

Angiocardiography

Aortic root injection in multiple views is crucial to the diagnosis of this abnormality. An injection of contrast in the ascending aorta will demonstrate filling of the pulmonary artery prior to opacification of the descending aorta. This indicates a communication with the pulmonary artery at the level of the proximal aorta (Fig. 2). The demonstration of two distinct semilunar valves rules out a persistent truncus arteriosus. It is often difficult to profile the defect but the oblique views with cranio-caudal tilt are probably best. At least 1 mL of contrast media per kg of body weight should be given rapidly within the first second on the initial injection. A distal defect shows direct filling of the right pulmonary artery and reflux into the left pulmonary artery, without concomitant filling of the main pulmonary artery.

If the oblique views are inadequate to assess coronary artery anatomy, then additional aortic root injections or selective coronary angiograms need to be performed (Doty et al. 1981). An injection in the distal arch is necessary to rule out a patent ductus arteriosus and coarctation of the aorta. An injection of contrast media into the left ventricle in the hepatoclavicular view is sufficient to assess ventricular function and rule out an associated ventricular septal defect.

Cautions or Precautions

The most important differential diagnoses are common arterial trunk (truncus arteriosus) and a large, short patent ductus arteriosus. The presence of two semilunar valves by angiography or echocardiography rules out a common trunk as does an intact interventricular septum. Unilateral origin of a pulmonary artery from the aorta can be confused easily with this lesion (refer to the following chapter). A catheter pass from the pulmonary artery to a brachiocephalic vessel makes a patent ductus arteriosus most unlikely. Conversely, passage of the catheter into the descending aorta does not rule out

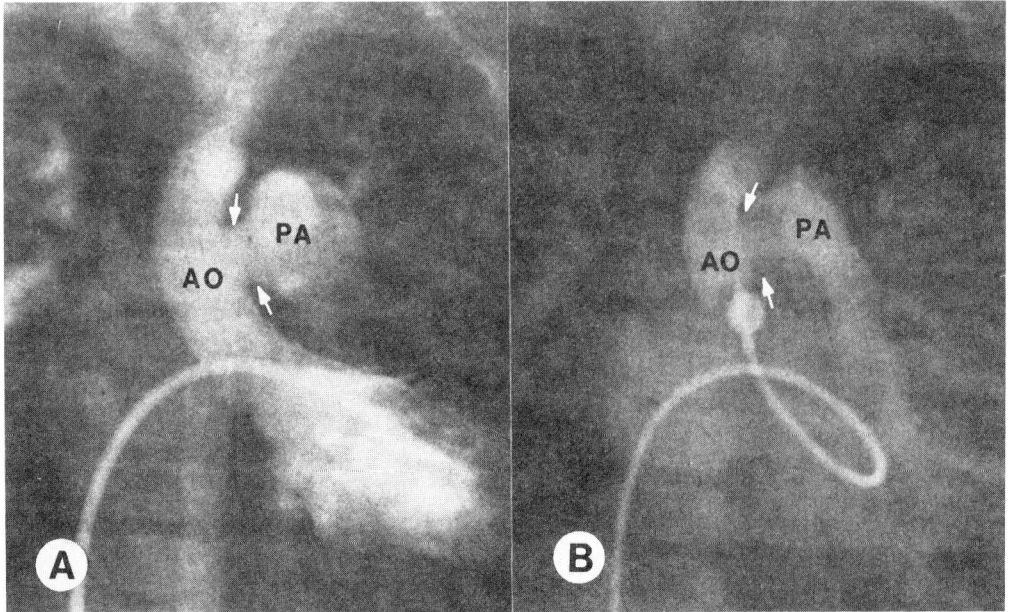

Figure 2. Angiography in aortopulmonary window (arrows). AO = Aorta; PA = pulmonary artery. A: Selective left ventricular angiocardiogram. The site of shunting into the pulmonary artery is not easily determined. B: Selective aortogram. There is opacification of the pulmonary artery before contrast appears in the descending aorta.

an aortopulmonary window since this lesion may coexist with a patent ductus arteriosus. Because other associated lesions are often masked by the dominant primary defect, careful assessment of other potential associated anomalies must be made.

References and Suggested Reading

Berry TE, Bharati S, Muster AJ, et al. Distal aortopulmonary septal defect, aortic origin of the right pulmonary artery, intact ventricular septum, patent ductus arteriosus and hypoplasia of the aortic isthmus: A newly recognized syndrome. Am J Cardiol 1982; 49:108–116.

Blieden LC, Moller JH. Aorticopulmonary septal defect: An experience with 17 patients. Br Heart J 1974;36:630–635.

Doty DB, Richardson JV, Falkovsky GE, et al. Aortopulmonary septal defect: Hemodynamics, angiography, and operation. Ann Thorac Surg 1981;32:244–250.

Kutsche LM, Van Mierop LHS. Anatomy and pathogenesis of aorticopulmonary septal defect. Am J Cardiol 1987;59:443–447.

Newfeld HN, Lester RG, Adams P Jr, et al. Aorticopulmonary septal defect. Am J Cardiol 1979;9:12–25.

Richardson JV, Doty DB, Rossi ND, et al. The spectrum of anomalies of aortopulmonary septation. J Thorac Cardiovasc Surg 1979; 78:21–27.

22

Common Arterial Trunk (Truncus Arteriosus) or Origin of a Single Pulmonary Artery from the Aorta (Hemitruncus)

William H. Neches, M.D.

Anatomy

Common arterial trunk or persistent truncus arteriosus is a congenital cardiovascular anomaly that results from lack of septation of the truncus arteriosus during fetal development. This results in an anomaly that is characterized by the biventricular origin of the single arterial trunk over what is usually a large and unrestrictive ventricular septal defect. In addition to the coronary and brachiocephalic vessels, the common trunk also gives rise to the pulmonary arteries. The classification developed by Collett and Edwards (1949) is still useful although others have been suggested (Calder et al. 1976; Van Praagh 1976; Crupi et al. 1977). In the first three categories of this classification, the pulmonary arteries arise from the ascending aorta either as a single trunk (type I) or as separate vessels from the posterior (type II) or lateral (type III) aspects of the aorta (Fig. 1). In many patients with a common arterial trunk, it is not always possible to differentiate between type I and type II and in fact, the overwhelming majority of patients represent an intermediate form between types I and II where the pulmonary arteries arise separately but have origins that are very close together on the posterior

aspect of the aorta. It is thus extremely difficult to determine the true classification in many patients prior to open heart repair or pathological examination.

In type IV truncus arteriosus, there are no true right and left pulmonary arteries and pulmonary blood flow is via systemic to pulmonary artery collaterals. Although rare examples of this type probably exist, most patients previously thought to have truncus arteriosus type IV can be shown to have tetralogy of Fallot with pulmonary atresia (pulmonary atresia with a ventricular septal defect). In such patients, hypoplastic but distinct pulmonary arteries usually can be found at postmortem examination. Also, it is usually possible to demonstrate true pulmonary arteries during life by selective injection into collateral arteries or by pulmonary venous wedge angiography (see Chapter 9). Thus, most patients with a single great artery arising from the heart who have systemic to pulmonary collaterals arising from the descending aorta should be classified as tetralogy of Fallot with pulmonary atresia.

Origin of a single pulmonary artery from the ascending aorta is a rare condition that will also be considered in this chapter. In patients with this anomaly, one pulmonary artery arises from the lateral or posterola-

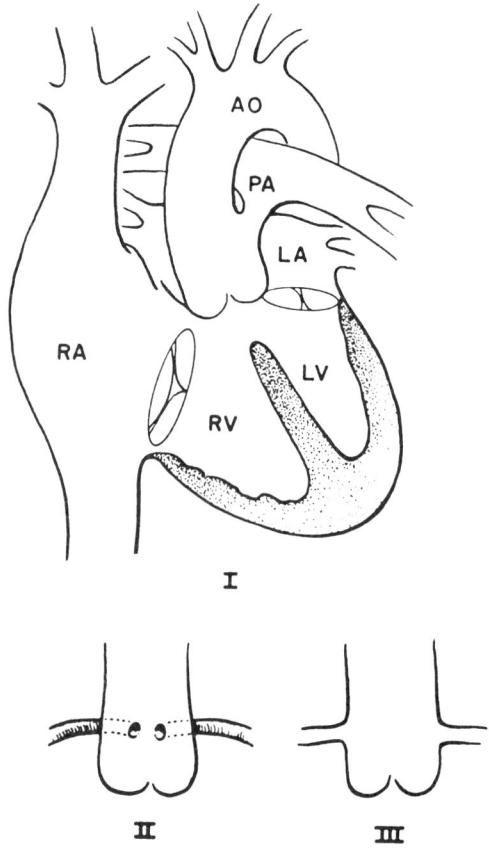

Figure 1. Diagram of truncus arteriosus—types I, II and III.

nitude of pulmonary blood flow. Pulmonary artery stenosis is uncommon and thus presentation is usually with congestive heart failure during the first month or two of life. Congestive failure is uncommon during the first week of life, unless there is associated truncal valve regurgitation, but develops as pulmonary vascular resistance falls and pulmonary blood flow increases. Stenosis of the origin of the pulmonary arteries is occasionally seen in patients with type II and type III lesions and if severe, the patient may present with cyanosis rather than congestive heart failure. In patients with unilateral origin of a pulmonary artery from the aorta, pulmonary artery stenosis is uncommon and thus systemic pressure is usually present in the anomalous pulmonary artery. If pulmonary vascular resistance decreases in a normal manner during early infancy, then pulmonary blood flow will be increased considerably and congestive heart failure will occur. On the other hand, some patients do not experience a fall in pulmonary vascular resistance in this anomalous vessel and thus may present with milder findings such as failure to thrive, or possibly with just a heart murmur.

teral wall of the ascending aorta while the contralateral pulmonary artery arises normally from the pulmonary trunk (Fong et al. 1989). In the past, this lesion has been called hemitruncus and although its origin may be embryologically similar to that of the common arterial trunk, it differs in that there are two great vessels arising from the heart rather than a single trunk. In over 80% of patients with this anomaly, the right-sided pulmonary artery arises anomalously from the aorta while the left is normally connected.

Hemodynamic Considerations

The presentation of patients with common arterial trunk depends upon the mag-

Indications for Cardiac Catheterization

Cross-sectional and Doppler echocardiography can accurately make the diagnosis of a common arterial trunk. However, anomalous origin of a single pulmonary artery from the aorta may be difficult to diagnose by echocardiography. Cardiac catheterization is important to assess the hemodynamic alterations including the degree of pulmonary hypertension and the presence or absence of pulmonary stenosis. Angiography is required to determine pulmonary artery size and to evaluate for the presence of multiple ventricular septal defects or other associated lesions, especially coronary artery anomalies. The competence of a truncal valve and origin of the pulmonary arteries from the truncus are often better demonstrated by echocardiographic techniques.

Catheterization Technique

The ventricular septal defect of a common arterial trunk is almost always large and unrestrictive and right and left ventricular pressures are equal. It is usually possible to enter the trunk from the right ventricle and the catheter often can be manipulated into the pulmonary arteries. A prograde catheter pass into the pulmonary artery is most often accomplished when there is a main pulmonary artery arising from the base of the trunk (type I). In the other types, it is more difficult to enter each pulmonary artery selectively and a retrograde arterial approach may be necessary. If the pulmonary blood flow is quite large, a flow-directed balloon catheter should be tried in the hope that it will float into a pulmonary artery.

Hemodynamic Evaluation

It is essential that the right and left pulmonary arteries be entered selectively for pressure measurements and selective angiography because significant arterial stenoses will protect the pulmonary vascular bed and permit delay of surgery. Truncal valve stenosis is indicated by a significant gradient (greater than 15 mm Hg) between the ventricles and the trunk. A mild pressure gradient across the truncal valve may be found in the absence of truncal valve stenosis particularly when there is large pulmonary blood flow.

Oximetry usually indicates a substantial left to right shunt at or distal to the ventricular level. It would seem that the oxygen saturation in the trunk and pulmonary artery should be the same. Actually, streaming of the blood flow from the two ventricles often causes some variation in the saturation be-

tween these two areas. It is thus important to measure the oxygen saturation in both the trunk and the pulmonary arteries. There is always arterial desaturation but it is mild if the pulmonary blood flow is large.

Angiocardiography

The diagnosis of a common arterial trunk may be apparent following selective angiocardiography in either ventricle. However, the ventricular angiocardiograms must be carefully scrutinized because absence of a true right ventricular outflow tract can be missed because of the rapid appearance of contrast material in the proximal aorta following injection in a ventricle. The selective injection of contrast material into the truncal root in the anteroposterior and lateral or oblique views is diagnostic although it is sometimes difficult to demonstrate clearly the origin of the pulmonary artery (Fig 2). A further selective injection into or near the orifice of each pulmonary artery may delineate the origin and size of the pulmonary arteries. Whenever the assessment of cardiovascular structures is important, a few cine frames of a calibration block or grid should be obtained to enable correction for magnification during later analysis of films.

An aorticopulmonary window may have a somewhat similar angiographic appearance to a common arterial trunk but there is rarely a ventricular septal defect in the former lesion. Also, it should be possible to visualize separate aortic and pulmonary valves. Another lesion that needs to be differentiated from a common arterial trunk is origin of a single pulmonary artery from the aorta (Fig. 3). In this entity, the anomalous pulmonary artery will be seen to arise directly from the ascending aorta following an aortic root injection while the opposite pulmonary artery, which arises normally, will be visualized with a selective injection in the right ventricle (Penkoske et al. 1983; Fong et al. 1989).

The truncal valve is often abnormal and may have two to four or more leaflets. Al-

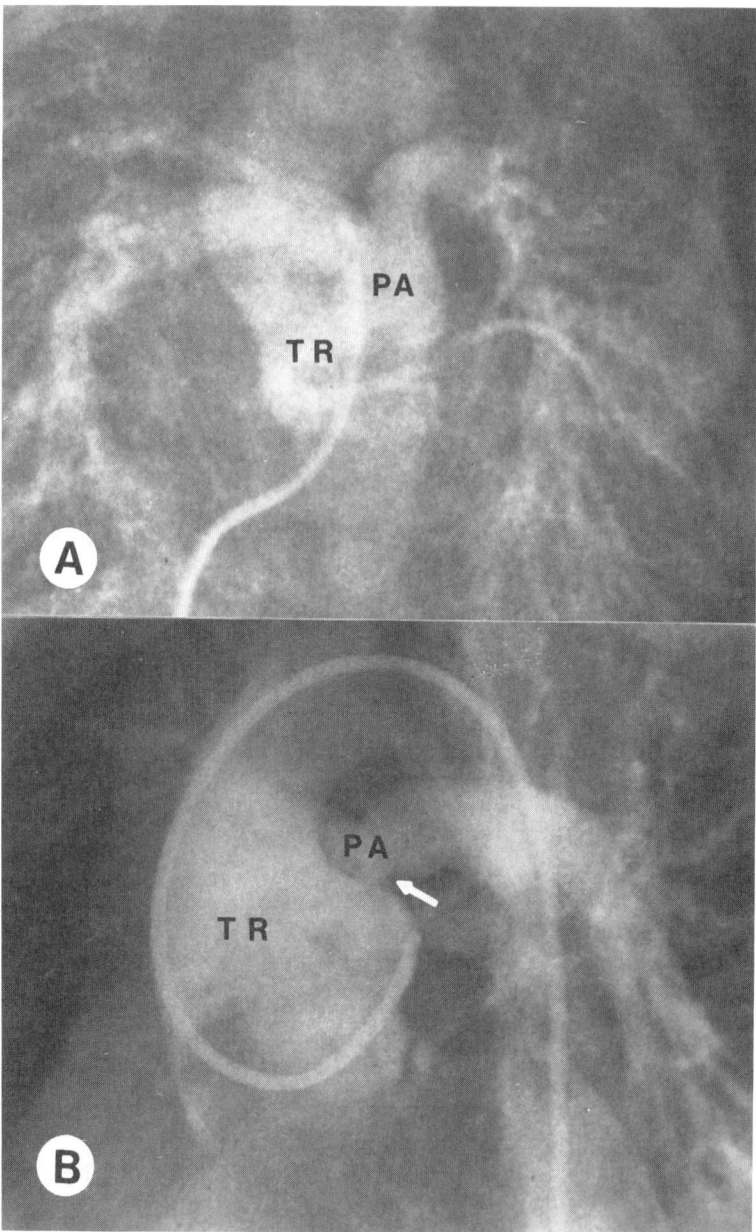

Figure 2. Selective angiograms in truncus arteriosus (TR), type I. A: Injection in the pulmonary artery (PA) demonstrating filling of the aorta and pulmonary artery. The origin of the pulmonary artery is not well seen. B: Injection in the common trunk in the left anterior oblique view demonstrating mild narrowing of the common pulmonary trunk (arrows).

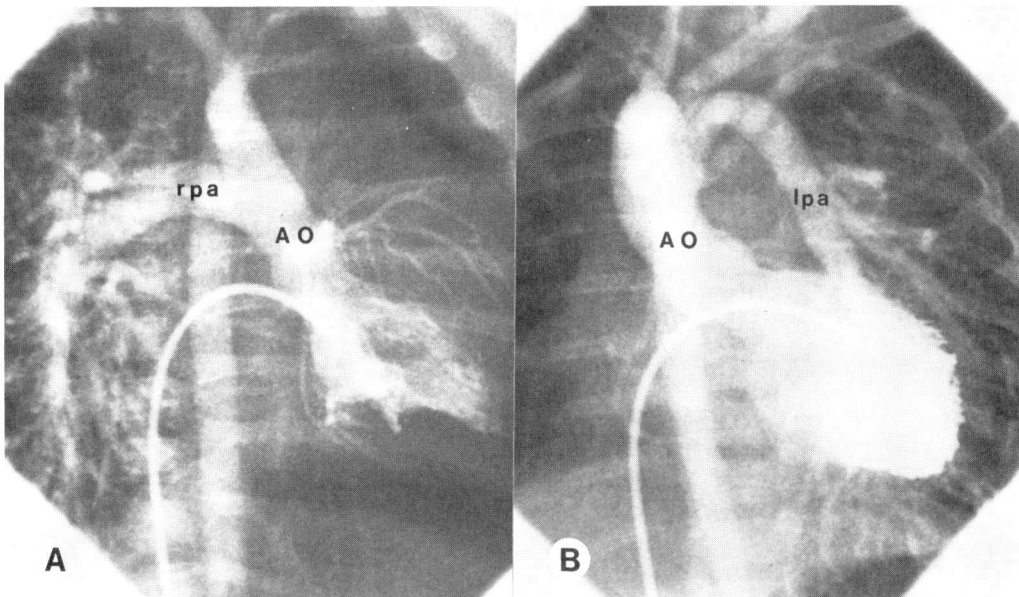

Figure 3. Angiograms of patients with anomalous origin of the pulmonary artery from the aorta showing: A: Right pulmonary artery (rpa) arising from the aorta (AO). B: Left pulmonary artery (lpa) arising from the aorta.

though truncal valve stenosis may occur, truncal insufficiency is more common. The anatomy of the truncal valve is best evaluated with a selective injection in the trunk in the oblique views. The injection must be made close enough to the valve to outline the valve sinuses and to gauge valvar regurgitation, but not so close as to artificially induce regurgitation. The catheter is best positioned approximately one rib space above the level of the truncal valve. A vigorous hand injection of a small amount of contrast material in the left anterior oblique view confirms proper positioning of the catheter. As with other lesions, it is important to correlate the angiographic evaluation of truncal regurgitation with the clinical findings as well as findings on Doppler echocardiography.

The size, location, and number of ventricular septal defects should be evaluated by selective left ventricular cineangiocardiography in the four-chamber or long axial oblique view. A separate muscular ventricular septal defect may occur and should be documented at catheterization.

Associated Anomalies

The importance of identifying truncal valve stenosis and regurgitation and pulmonary artery stenosis has already been discussed. In addition to these abnormalities, an atrial septal defect should be sought not only by catheter pass but by oximetry and by viewing the atrial septum on the recirculation phase of the pulmonary artery injection. A variety of aortic arch anomalies also can occur in conjunction with a common arterial trunk. A right aortic arch is present in about 30% of patients and a double aortic arch, as well as coarctation of the aorta or interrupted arch, have also been reported (Thiene et al. 1976; Crupi et al. 1977). An associated patent ductus arteriosus is rare but should be ruled out by small injection of contrast material into the distal aortic arch. Anomalies of the coronary arteries are also common and if suspected, coronary anatomy should be defined either by aortography or selective coronary angiography (Shrivastava and Edwards 1977; Anderson et al. 1978). Since conotruncal anomalies are commonly associated with the DiGeorge's syndrome, the status of the patient's thymus gland and parathyroid function should be evaluated, especially in sick infants with this anomaly. If DiGeorge's syndrome is found, the patient needs to be carefully monitored for abnormalities of calcium metabolism and, in addition, the patient should receive irradiated blood if transfusion is required.

Cautions and Precautions

Young infants who present with this anomaly are often extremely ill with congestive heart failure. Careful attention needs to be paid to the maintenance of normothermia and an adequate airway if there is any respiratory compromise. In these small sick infants, care must be taken to avoid excessive fluid administration and a limited amount of low or nonionic contrast material should be utilized to minimize the volume load.

References and Suggested Reading

Anderson KR, McGoon DC, Lie JT. Surgical significance of the coronary arterial anatomy in truncus arteriosus communis. Am J Cardiol 1978;41:76–81.

Calder L, Van Praagh R, Van Praagh S, et al. Truncus Arteriosus Communis. Clinical, angiocardiographic and pathologic finidngs in 100 patients. Am Heart J 1976;92:23–38.

Collett RW, Edwards JE. Persistent truncus arteriosus: A classification according to anatomic types. Surg Clin North Am 1949; 29:1245–1270.

Crupi G, Macartney FJ, Anderson RH. Persistent truncus arteriosus. A study of 66 autopsy cases with special references to definition and morphogenesis. Am J Cardiol 1977; 40:569–578.

Fong LV, Anderson RH, Siewers RD, et al. Anomalous origin of one pulmonary artery from the ascending aorta: A review of echocardigraphic, catheter, and morphological features. Br Heart J 1989;62:389–395.

Penkoske PA, Castenada AR, Fyler DC, et al. Origin of pulmonary artery branch from ascending aorta. J Thorac Cardiovasc Surg 1985;85:537–545.

Shrivastava S, Edwards JE. Coronary arterial origin in persistent truncus arteriosus. Circulation 1977;55:551–554.

Thiene G, Bortolotti U, Gallucci V, et al. Anatomical study of truncus arteriosus communis with embryological and surgical consideration. Br Heart J 1976;38:1109–1123.

Van Praagh R. Classification of truncus arteriosus communis. Am Heart J 1976;92:129–132.

23

Pulmonary Stenosis with Intact Ventricular Septum

William H. Neches, M.D.

Anatomy

Obstruction to right ventricular outflow may be at the valvar, subvalvar, and/or supravalvar level (Fig. 1). When valvar stenosis is the predominant lesion, the leaflets are usually thickened with varying degrees of fusion of the commissures. The valve is most commonly bicuspid although tricuspid and unicommissural valves also occur. A dysplastic pulmonary valve is usually trileaflet and is characterized by markedly thickened valve leaflets with a large amount of redundant, poorly differentiated myxomatous tissue. Some degree of subvalvar infundibular stenosis is often found in association with valvar pulmonary stenosis. In general, the more severe the valvar stenosis, the most likely there will be substantial reactive infundibular hypertrophy. However, this is not the primary lesion and is a consequence of the right ventricular hypertrophy secondary to the severe valvar stenosis. In most cases of isolated valvar pulmonary stenosis, the pulmonary valve annulus is normal to slightly below normal in size. Poststenotic dilatation of the main pulmonary artery is commonly seen in patients with valvar pulmonary stenosis and it must be remembered that the degree of poststenotic dilatation has no relationship to the degree or severity of valvar stenosis.

Isolated subvalvar pulmonary stenosis at the infundibular level is uncommon, with obstruction at this level usually accompanying either valvar stenosis or being part of the overall picture of tetralogy of Fallot. More commonly, isolated muscular subpulmonic stenosis occurs within the body of the right ventricle, the so-called "double chamber right ventricle". In patients with this lesion, there are severely hypertrophied anomalous muscle bundles or a moderator band within the body of the right ventricle that result in right ventricular outflow obstruction. These muscle bundles are usually present below the infundibular level and subdivide the right ventricle into a high-pressure inflow region and a low-pressure outflow region. In most cases, this is the only level of obstruction with the pulmonary valve and pulmonary valve annulus being normal in caliber. Lastly, pulmonary stenosis can be limited to the pulmonary artery trunk or the proximal portion of the branches and occasionally in the distal branches, especially when there are multiple stenotic areas.

Hemodynamic Considerations

The clinical presentation ranges from the asymptomatic patient with a heart murmur to the critically ill newborn infant with severe pulmonary stenosis and cyanosis due to right to left shunting at atrial level. However, most patients with pulmonary stenosis and intact ventricular septum are asymp-

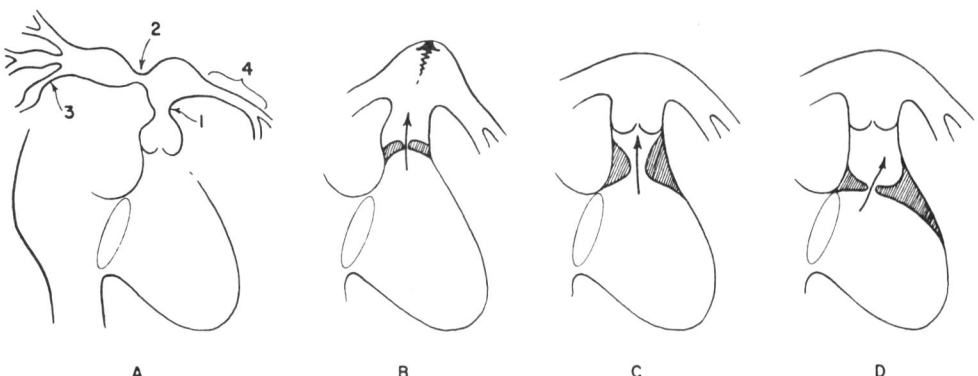

Figure 1. Diagram of various forms of right ventricular outflow obstruction. A: Pulmonary artery stenosis. (1) Supravalvar stenosis; (2) Main branch stenosis; (3) Peripheral stenosis; (4) Diffuse hypoplasia. B: Pulmonary valve stenosis. C: Infundibular pulmonary stenosis. D: Anomalous muscle bundle.

tomatic and cardiomegaly is unusual unless obstruction is very severe and right ventricular failure occurs. As a result of the obstruction to right ventricular outflow, the right ventricular pressure is elevated leading to right ventricular hypertrophy. Outside of the newborn period, right ventricular hypertension is well tolerated and rarely causes hemodynamic compromise even when the right ventricular pressure is suprasystemic. However, if suprasystemic pressure is present for a long time, eventually right ventricular failure will occur. If an atrial communication is also present (patent foramen ovale or atrial septal defect), then right to left shunting will result in systemic hypoxemia. In the absence of an interatrial communication the patient will develop signs of severe right-sided congestive heart failure with systemic venous engorgement, hepatosplenomegaly, and peripheral edema. Tricuspid regurgitation, if present, will be manifest clinically by abnormal hepatic and jugular venous pulsations.

In the newborn with critical pulmonary stenosis, right ventricular pressure may be at systemic level and is often suprasystemic. Right ventricular dysfunction and tricuspid regurgitation are often present and result in elevated right atrial pressure and right to left shunting at atrial level with systemic hypoxemia. This is usually recognized in the first few hours of life because of the presence of cyanosis and a heart murmur.

Indications for Cardiac Catheterization

In most patients with valvar pulmonary stenosis, the diagnosis is easily made on the basis of an ejection click, a systolic murmur, and thrill at the mid- to upper left sternal border, right ventricular hypertrophy on the electrocardiogram and Doppler echocardiographic evidence of a significant transvalvar gradient. In the past, cardiac catheterization was performed in anticipation of possible surgical valvotomy. Today, however, the estimation of severity and the delineation of accompanying abnormalities is made easily by the previously mentioned noninvasive means. Cardiac catheterization therefore usually is undertaken to perform a balloon dilation valvotomy in an attempt to avoid a thoracotomy and cardiac surgery (Rao 1989). For those patients with subvalvar pulmonary stenosis, Doppler estimation of the gradient across the obstruction often is not precise and direct measurement by cardiac catheterization is necessary. Similarly, in patients with pulmonary arterial stenosis, adequate Doppler evaluation of the pulmonary artery branches is not possible. Thus, when the clinical and electrocardiographic findings suggest significant right ventricular hypertension, cardiac catheterization is warranted to assess the severity and to perform balloon dilation angioplasty.

Catheterization Technique

Cardiac catheterization is performed percutaneously via the femoral approach. An end-hole catheter is used to determine oxygen saturations in the various sites and to record pressures in the right heart, particularly to localize the site of right ventricular outflow and/or pulmonary arterial obstruction. When an interatrial communication is present, the catheter can easily be passed into the left atrium and from there to the left ventricle. This enables determination of left ventricular pressure that is valuable for comparison with right ventricular pressure before and after any interventional procedures. The procedures for pressure measurement are described in Chapter 7 while the technique and procedures for balloon valvotomy are described in Chapter 13.

Hemodynamic Evaluation

Pressure Data

The right ventricular pressure curve has a characteristic "isosceles triangle" configuration in patients with valvar pulmonary stenosis and intact interventricular septum (Fig. 2). In patients with right ventricular outflow obstruction it is important to localize the gradient and to rule out additional stenoses at other levels. This is best accomplished by slow withdrawal of an end-hole catheter such as a Lehman or flow directed

Swan-Ganz (with a side-hole catheter the holes may straddle the obstruction and prevent accurate localization). In any patient with right ventricular outflow obstruction, it must be remembered that there may be more than one stenotic site. It is, therefore, extremely important to withdraw the catheter from the distal right and left pulmonary arteries all the way to the right ventricular inflow area while pressure is monitored (see Chapter 7). If this is not done, it is easy to miss an additional obstruction in a pulmonary artery or within the body of the right ventricle. It is also important to compare right ventricular and systemic pressure, either by direct catheter measurement in the left ventricle or aorta or by determining arterial blood pressure by a sphygmomanometer. In patients with valvar pulmonary stenosis, a negative pressure may be recorded on a pressure tracing during the early phase of systole. This phenomenon known as the "Venturi effect" results from negative lateral pressure at the tip of the catheter as a result of the high-velocity jet in the direction of the long axis of the catheter (Chapter 7) (Fig. 3).

Oxygen Saturation Data

Oxygen saturations in the right heart chambers and pulmonary artery are normal in patients with pulmonary stenosis unless there is an associated left to right shunt at atrial level. If pulmonary stenosis is severe, interatrial shunting is more likely to be right to left and systemic oxygen saturation should always be determined. This is especially true if a right to left shunt has been documented prior to cardiac catheterization with the use of noninvasive methods such as contrast or Doppler color flow echocardiography. If arterial desaturation is demonstrated, it may be important to rule out other reasons for desaturation such as intrapulmonary shunting, especially in a newborn. This is accomplished by determining the oxygen saturation in the right and left pulmonary veins because desaturation in

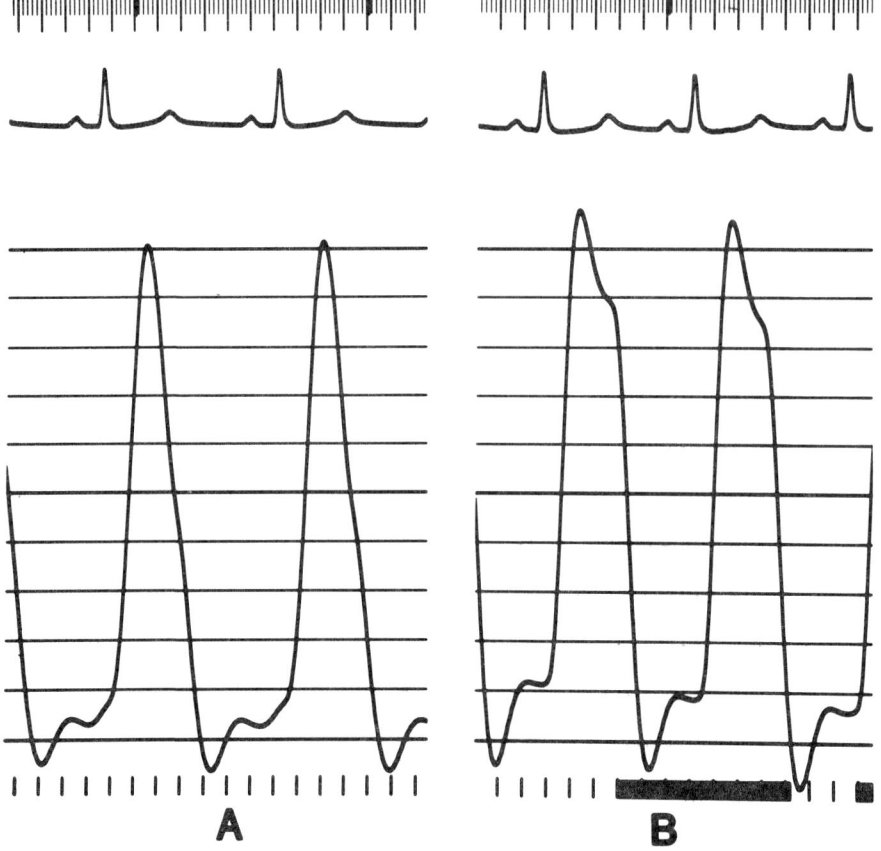

Figure 2. Pressure curve in patients with right ventricular hypertension due to: A: Valvar pulmonary stenosis. B: Pulmonary stenosis with ventricular septal defect.

the pulmonary veins indicates intrapulmonary shunting and the presence of some pulmonary parenchymal abnormality. In addition to noninvasive echocardiographic techniques, right to left shunting at atrial level can be documented by angiography and quantitated by indicator dilution curves. The assessment of cardiac output is helpful in the overall assessment of the severity of pulmonary stenosis since patients with a low cardiac output may have a lowered right ventricular outflow gradient. In most cases with severe pulmonary stenosis, assessment of cardiac output by thermodilution technique is not practical due to difficulty in crossing the stenotic pulmonary valve with a balloon catheter. Determination of cardiac output from the oxygen consumption as measured by a computer using a flow-through hood and from oxygen saturation data, is the preferred method (Chapter 8). Following balloon dilation, cardiac output is again determined to insure that a reduction of right ventricular outflow gradient is as a result of the balloon dilation and not caused solely by reduction in cardiac output.

Other Diagnostic or Therapeutic Procedures

In patients with valvar pulmonary stenosis and an intact ventricular septum balloon dilation valvotomy can successfully reduce the transvalvar gradient and right

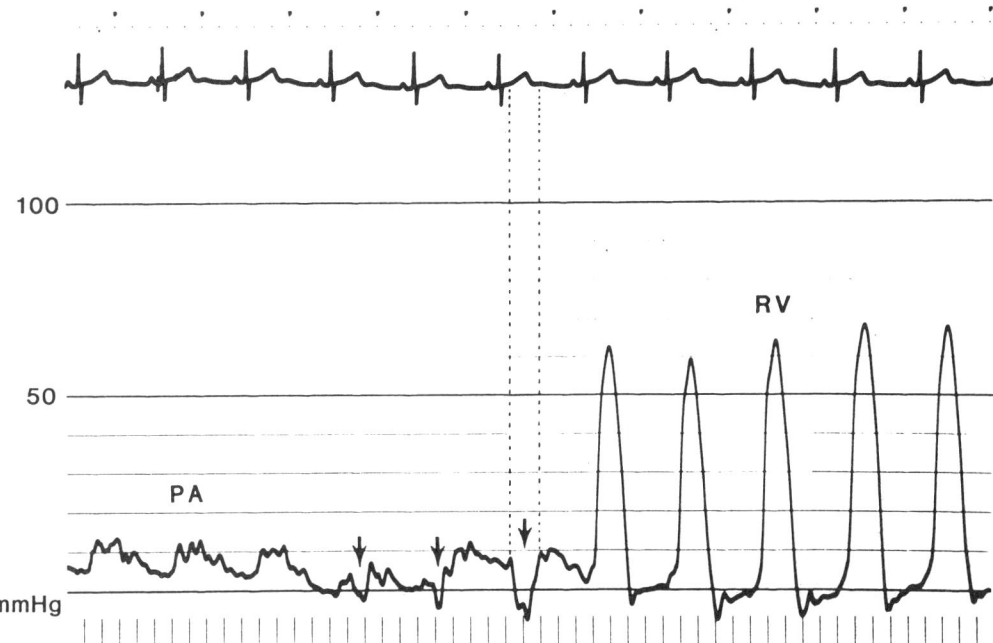

Figure 3. Withdrawal pressure tracing from the pulmonary artery to the right ventricular demonstrating the "Venturi" effect (arrows). Dotted lines indicate the negative pressure recorded during systole.

ventricular pressure to acceptable, if not near normal levels (see Chapter 13). This procedure may not be successful if the pulmonary valve is dysplastic and usually is not indicated for isolated subvalvar muscular stenosis (Rothman 1990). It has met with only limited success in patients with pulmonary arterial stenosis. In neonates with critical pulmonary stenosis, a normal-sized right ventricle and where there is some forward flow across the pulmonary valve, it may be possible to pass a wire across the pulmonary valve and perform balloon dilation valvotomy with progressively larger balloon catheters (see Chapter 13). In some cases, however, even if it is possible to pass a guidewire across the pulmonary valve and into the pulmonary artery, the degree of stenosis of the pulmonary valve may be so severe that it will not be possible to advance a balloon catheter over the wire. In these cases, surgical valvotomy will be management of choice.

Angiocardiography

Selective right ventricular angiocardiography is important in the localization of the site of pulmonary stenosis. Becuase there is no right to left shunting at ventricular level, right ventricular angiocardiography in the elongated right anterior oblique or the anteroposterior and lateral views demonstrates the infundibulum and the pulmonary valve quite well (Fig. 4A). The characteristic angiographic feature of valvar pulmonary stenosis is a somewhat thickened pulmonary valve that domes in systole. A jet of contrast material through a central orifice is usually seen, as is poststenotic dilatation of the main pulmonary artery. In patients with pulmonary stenosis due to a dysplastic pulmonary valve a markedly thickened pulmonary valve is seen (Jeffrey 1972). This often is present in association with Noonan syndrome (Noonan 1968). In contrast to the

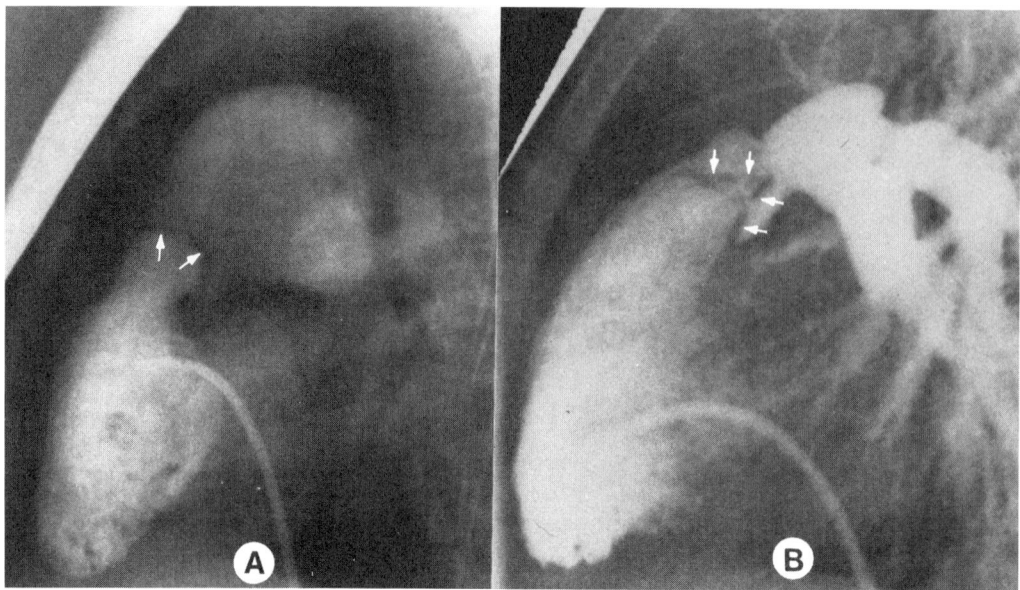

Figure 4. Valvar pulmonary stenosis with intact ventricular septum A: Right ventricular angiogram in the lateral view demonstrating valvar pulmonary stenosis. Note the doming pulmonary valve (arrows). B: Right ventricular angiogram in the lateral view demonstrating a dysplastic pulmonary valve (arrows).

usual form of pulmonary valve stenosis, the dysplastic pulmonary valve does not dome and remains in nearly the same position in systole and diastole (Fig. 4B). Many patients with valvar pulmonary stenosis have an associated dynamic infundibular obstruction. The right ventricular outflow tract narrows in systole but opens widely in diastole. Rarely, patients with valvar pulmonary stenosis may have an associated obstructing anomalous muscle bundle in the body of the right ventricle. It is therefore important to visualize the entire right ventricle on angiocardiography to make certain that intraventricular obstruction is not present. Abnormal muscle bundles are generally best visualized in the elongated right anterior oblique, or in the anteroposterior view, of the right ventricular injection (Fig. 5). It should be emphasized that an injection of contrast material into the right ventricular outflow tract may not visualize the body of the right ventricle and an anomalous muscle bundle may be missed.

Pulmonary artery stenosis rarely accompanies isolated valvar obstruction. If suspected, the pulmonary artery and its branches should be visualized in an anteroposterior projection of a selective injection in the main pulmonary artery or right ventricle. The main pulmonary artery and the area of pulmonary artery bifurcation are readily visualized in the anteroposterior projection with 30° of cranio-caudal angulation (sitting-up view) (Fig. 6). An alternative is a 15° left anterior oblique projection with 30° of cranio-caudal angulation. This view will better visualize the proximal left pulmonary artery while still demonstrating the proximal right pulmonary artery. A simultaneous lateral view is helpful to define the pulmonary valve status as well as supravalvar area.

Associated Lesions

An interatrial communication is the anomaly most commonly associated with

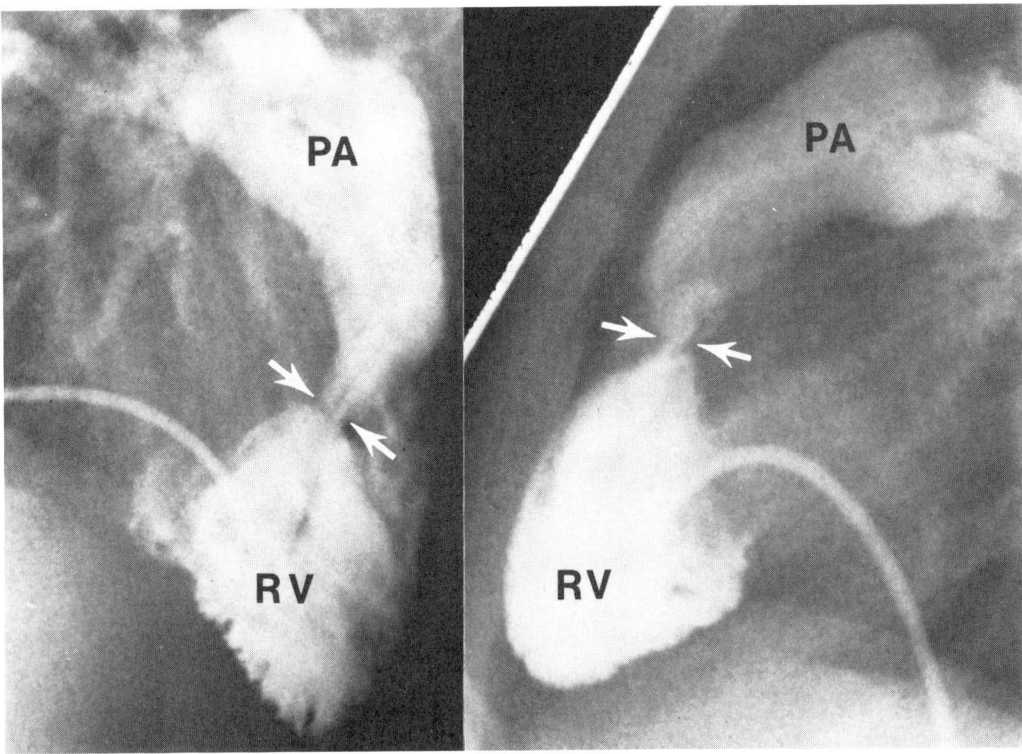

Figure 5. Right ventricular angiogram in pulmonary stenosis due to an anomalous muscle bundle (arrow). A: Elongated right anterior oblique view. B: Lateral view. PA = pulmonary artery; RV = right ventricle.

pulmonary stenosis and an intact ventricular septum. Left to right or right to left shunting should be assessed by oximetry and angiocardiography. With left to right shunting at atrial level, the right atrium opacifies on the recirculation phase of a pulmonary arteriogram. The atrial septum may be visualized with a hand injection of contrast media in the right upper pulmonary vein with the patient in the four-chamber view.

In patients with severe valvar pulmonary stenosis and systemic or suprasystemic right ventricular pressure, a variable degree of tricuspid regurgitation is found. In many cases, though mild, this provides the availability to assess right ventricular pressure using Doppler echocardiography. There is an association between Ebstein's malformation of the tricuspid valve and pulmonary stenosis. In general, when this combination

is present, both the pulmonary stenosis and the Ebstein's malformation are severe. However, it is also possible for a mild degree of Ebstein's anomaly to be present and angiographically this is best seen in either the anteroposterior or right anterior oblique views of a right ventriculogram. Since the attachment of the tricuspid valve and its relationship to the atrioventricular septum are best visualized using cross-sectional echocardiography, it is important to evaluate for tricuspid anomalies with this noninvasive technique prior to cardiac catheterization of patients with pulmonary stenosis. A patent ductus arteriosus is commonly present in the newborn with critical valvar pulmonary stenosis and is the source of pulmonary blood flow. This is also usually visualized echocardiographically and can be demonstrated angiographically with a selective in-

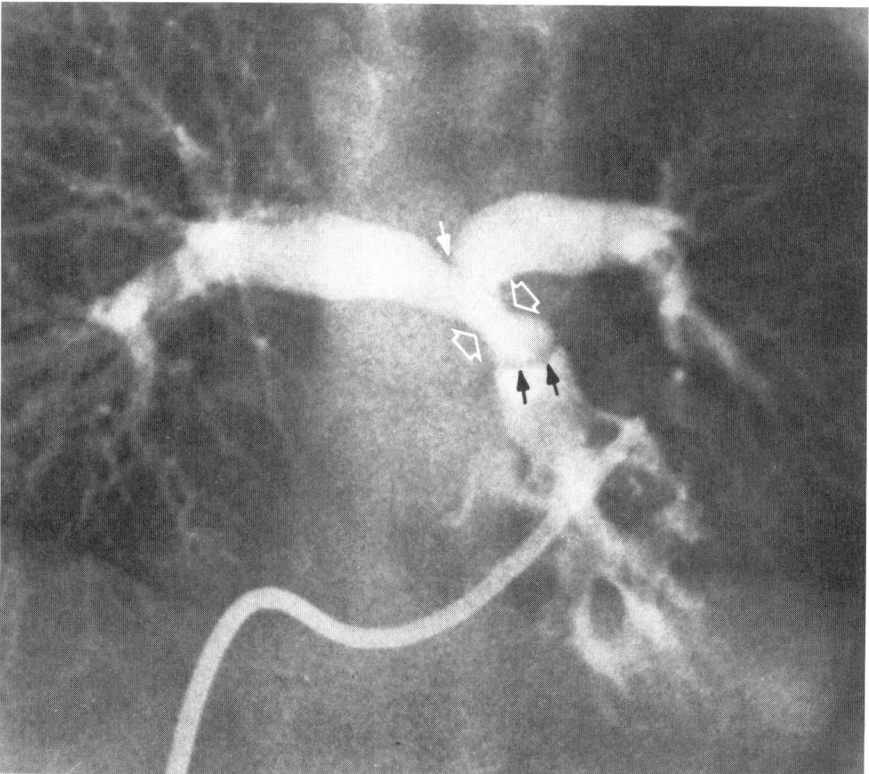

Figure 6. Right ventricular outflow angiogram (anteroposterior view with cranio-caudal angulation = sitting up view) showing a thickened pulmonary valve (black arrows), supravalvar narrowing (open arrows) and mild proximal branch stenosis (solid white arrow).

jection in the left ventricle or with an aortogram.

Pulmonary artery stenosis is often present in association with other anomalies both cardiac and noncardiac. The cardiac association includes tetralogy of Fallot, transposition of the great arteries and more complex congenital heart disease particularly with other pulmonary outflow obstruction. Noncardiac associations include rubella syndrome, Williams syndrome (with or without supravalvar aortic stenosis) and Allagille syndrome (with intrahepatic biliary atresia).

Cautions and Precautions

In patients with a severely stenotic pulmonary valve, especially in the newborn infant, catheter passage into the right ventricular outflow tract and across the pulmonary valve is difficult and hazardous. The right ventricular outflow tract can be quite thin and is easily perforated by the relatively stiff catheter or by the guidewire as attempts are made to pass the wire across the pulmonary valve. In attempts to cross the pulmonary valve in a very small infant, it may be preferable to use a sharply curved woven Dacron catheter (Chapter 5), because the sharp curve will orient the tip of the catheter toward the pulmonary valve rather than cephalad against the right ventricular outflow tract. It is important to remember that as a guidewire is advanced through the end of the catheter, even the soft flexible end of a guidewire is relatively stiff until at least 5 or 6 mm of the wire have advanced beyond the catheter tip. Thus, it is preferable to withdraw the catheter slightly before advancing the guidewire through the catheter tip. This will insure that the distal end of the guidewire is sitting freely within the outflow of the right ventricle just below the pulmonary valve, before attempts are made to pass it across the valve. Passing a catheter across a critically stenotic pulmonary valve may be hazardous beause it can almost completely obstruct the outflow across a very small orifice. In a newborn infant during the first week or so of life, prostaglandin E_1 should be administered during the catheterization to maintain patency of the ductus arteriosus, thereby providing a source for pulmonary blood if the outflow from the right ventricle is obstructed.

References and Suggested Reading

Jeffrey RF, Moller JH, Amplatz K. The dysplastic pulmonary valve: A new roentgenographic entity. With a discussion of the anatomy and radiology of other types of valvular pulmonary stenosis. Am J Roentgen Radium Ther Nucl Med 1972;114:322–339.

Kan JS, White RI, Mitchell SE, et al. Percutaneous balloon valvuloplasty: A new method of treating congenital pulmonary valve stenosis. N Engl J Med 1982;307:540–542.

Noonan JA. Hypertelorism with Turner phenotype: A new syndrome associated with congenital heart disease. Am J Dis Child 1968;116:373–380.

Rothman A, Perry SB, Keane JF, et al. Early results and follow-up of balloon angioplasty for branch pulmonary artery stenoses. J Am Coll Cardiol 1990;15:1109–1117.

Rao PS. Balloon pulmonary valvuloplasty: A review. Clin Cardiol 1989;12:55–74.

24

Pulmonary Atresia with Intact Ventricular Septum

William H. Neches, M.D.

Anatomy

In most cases with this lesion the pulmonary valve annulus, main pulmonary artery and the pulmonary branches appear to be normal structures. The pulmonary valve is usually a membranous structure with three, or sometimes two, formed valve leaflets with fused commissures. In an occasional case, there are no pulmonary valve leaflets. The right ventricular outflow tract is usually patent although in some cases there also may be outflow tract atresia. The right ventricular cavity varies from an extremely small or "cherry pit" cavity to one that is normal or even larger than normal in size. In about two thirds of cases, the right ventricle would be classified as moderately to markedly underdeveloped (Fig. 1) (Zuberbuhler 1979).

The tricuspid valve may be abnormal with thickened and dysplastic leaflets and abnormal chordal attachments or an Ebstein-like malformation with a variable degree of displacement from the site of the annulus. The size of the tricuspid valve annulus is usually proportional to the size of the right ventricular cavity and these, in turn, are related to the degree of tricuspid valve regurgitation (Bull 1982). Thus, when the tricuspid valve is stenotic and/or competent, the right ventricular cavity usually is extremely small with a good portion of the cavity further obliterated by extremely hypertrophied trabecular muscle. An increasing degree of tricuspid incompetence results in a larger right ventricular cavity. The right atrium is usually dilated with the largest atria found in those cases with the most severe degree of tricuspid regurgitation.

Right ventricular myocardial sinusoids with direct connection to the right coronary artery system are common in patients with pulmonary atresia and an intact ventricular septum. These fistulous connections are particularly well developed in small hypoplastic right ventricles with a competent tricuspid valve and suprasystemic right ventricular pressure.

Hemodynamic Considerations

Patients with pulmonary atresia and an intact ventricular septum present in the newborn period with severe cyanosis and most have a murmur of tricuspid regurgitation. Pulmonary blood flow is almost always via a patent ductus arteriosus but rarely, systemic to pulmonary collateral circulation may be present. Newborns with critical pulmonary stenosis present similarly in the newborn period. During fetal life, the systemic venous return cannot exit from the right heart and thus passes across the foramen ovale and is handled by the left ventricle. The left side of the heart thus is usually larger than normal in these patients. The flow to the pulmonary artery branches is normal in volume but occurs in a reverse

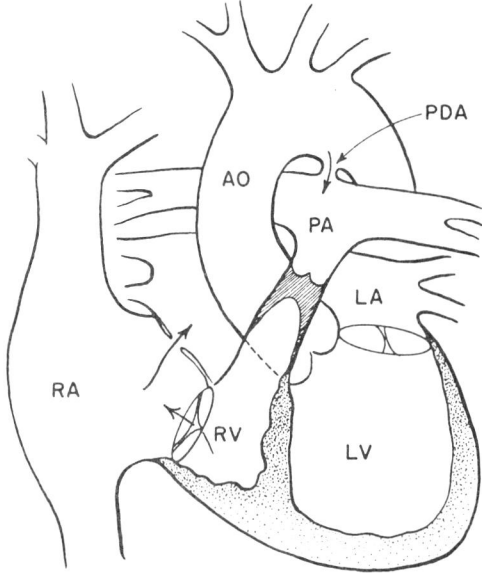

Figure 1. Diagram of pulmonary atresia with intact ventricular septum.

Indications for Cardiac Catheterization

The diagnosis of pulmonary atresia with intact ventricular septum is often obvious on the basis of the clinical examination and the radiographic findings of an increased heart size with an extremely large right atrium and normal or reduced pulmonary vascular markings. Cross-sectional and color Doppler echocardiography are valuable tools to demonstrate the anatomic abnormality and the relative sizes of the ventricles, atria, and great vessels. Color Doppler echocardiography will document the presence of tricuspid regurgitation and both color flow and contrast echocardiography are helpful in demonstrating the right to left shunt at atrial level. These noninvasive tools provide a very accurate delineation of the basic anatomic abnormality and many of the associated features. However, cardiac catheterization and angiocardiography remain extremely important for measuring pressures, precise definition of additional anatomic abnormalities such as the myocardial sinusoidal connections between the right ventricle and the coronary arteries, and to perform atrial septostomy since this is required in the majority of patients.

Catheterization Technique

Because almost all patients with this lesion present on the first day or two of life, the ductus venosus is usually patent and cardiac catheterization as well as balloon atrial septostomy can be performed easily from the umbilical venous route (see Chapters 4 and 5). If the ductus venosus is not patent, the procedure can be performed either by percutaneous or cutdown technique using the femoral vessels. An umbilical arterial line is useful for monitoring systemic arterial pressure, systemic oxygen saturation, and blood gases throughout the procedure. If an umbilical arterial line has not been

direction from the aorta through the patent ductus arteriosus rather than from the main pulmonary artery. The pulmonary blood flow, as well as the systemic blood flow to the lower half of the body and the placenta, traverse the aortic isthmus. This results in this structure being quite large in comparison to the normal fetus and newborn infant where the aortic isthmus is small in relationship to the adjacent proximal and distal aorta.

Postnatally, there is still no forward flow from the right ventricle into the pulmonary artery and thus the fetal circulatory pattern described above is maintained. Once the umbilical cord is clamped and the placental circulation is interrupted, there is total admixture of the systemic and pulmonary venous return and the patient's systemic oxygen saturation will then depend upon the degree of pulmonary blood flow. Because this in turn is totally provided by flow from the aorta through the patent ductus arteriosus, severe systemic hypoxemia becomes apparent as soon as the patent ductus arteriosus begins to close, as it does normally in the first day or so of life.

placed previously, this can be inserted at the time of cardiac catheterization. Continuous monitoring of systemic arterial oxygen saturation by means of pulse oximeter is extremely valuable throughout the procedure. In almost all cases, the patency of the ductus arteriosus is maintained by continuous intravenous infusion of prostaglandin E_1 at a rate of 0.05 to 0.1 $\mu g/kg/min$.

It is quite easy to pass a catheter from right atrium into the left side of the heart from either the umbilical or femoral venous routes, with entry into the left ventricle through the use of a guidewire or with a flow-directed balloon catheter (see Chapter 5). Entry into the right ventricle, which is often quite small, may be extremely difficult in these patients and it is usually not possible to accomplish this with a flow-directed balloon catheter. The use of an NIH angiographic catheter with a closed end and multiple side holes is not recommended because the cavity of the right ventricle is often extremely small and will not have enough depth to accommodate all of the holes of the catheter. This will result in the distal holes being within the cavity of the right ventricle while the proximal holes are still within the right atrium. Thus, it would not be possible to measure the right ventricular pressure accurately with this catheter and angiography might result in a false impression as to the degree of tricuspid regurgitation. A Goodale-Lubin catheter, which has an end-hole and two distal side holes, is quite useful in this situation. A preformed catheter with a sharp curve at the distal end may enter the right ventricular cavity easily and if this is not successful, then the J shaped curve on the stiff end of a guidewire can be used to shape the catheter within the heart and direct the tip into the right ventricular cavity (see Chapter 5). If this technique is utilized, it is important to remember that the stiff end of the guidewire be inserted only up to the tip of the catheter, but must not be advanced passed the distal end of the catheter. Proper positioning of the catheter tip within the right

ventricle is suggested by its position in the anteroposterior and lateral views fluoroscopically and if some ventricular ectopic beats are elicited by the catheter when it reaches what appears to be an appropriate position. If the catheter is advanced without the need for a guidewire, then pressure measurement will confirm the catheter's position in the right ventricle.

Hemodynamic Evaluation

Pressure Data

Systemic pressure is usually normal with systolic pressures in the left ventricle and aorta of approximately 60–80 mm Hg. Right ventricular pressure is commonly suprasystemic and it is not unusual to record systolic pressures of well over 100 mm Hg. Right atrial pressure may be normal or elevated with mean pressure similar to, or higher than, left atrial pressure. In patients with moderate or a large degree of tricuspid regurgitation, a large "v" wave may be present in the right atrium. It must be remembered that the right atrium is quite distensible and has a higher capacitance. Thus, although the patent foramen ovale may be small and restrictive, there may be either no or a small pressure gradient between the right and left atrium.

Oxygen Saturation Data

Oximetry demonstrates marked desaturation of the left atrium, left ventricle and aorta. Mixed venous saturation is usually quite low and often extremely variable during the procedure. We usually obtain a single mixed venous sample in the superior vena cava. Since incomplete mixing of systemic and pulmonary venous return is often present in the left atrium as well as the left ventricle, the true level of systemic oxygenation is best determined by blood gases drawn from an umbilical arterial line. Since there is total admixture of the systemic and pulmonary venous return, the patient's systemic oxygen saturation depends on the magnitude of the pulmonary blood flow which in turn, is dependent upon adequate flow through the patent ductus arteriosus. If it is noted that the patient's systemic oxygen saturation is falling during the procedure, it is important to check the prostaglandin E_1 infusion. If the infusion is running adequately it may be necessary only to increase the rate of administration to a higher level.

Other Diagnostic or Therapeutic Procedures

Because all the systemic venous return must traverse the atrial septum, an interatrial communication, usually a patent foramen ovale, is present in patients with this abnormality. In many centers, when a small right ventricular cavity is present, balloon atrial septostomy is performed at cardiac catheterization, followed by a systemic to pulmonary artery anastomosis. If the right ventricle is of moderate to large size, a pulmonary valvotomy with or without outflow tract reconstruction, or in combination with a systemic-pulmonary artery anastomosis, is performed (deLeval 1985). If a systemic to pulmonary artery anastomosis is contemplated for management of a patient, it is advisable to perform a balloon atrial septostomy even if there is no pressure gradient between the right and left atrium and the interatrial communication seems adequate. If balloon atrial septostomy is not contemplated, at least the adequacy of the size of the interatrial communication should be es-timated by balloon catheter withdrawal and, if possible, by angiocardiography (see Chapter 12). If right ventricular size is considered adequate to enable primary right ventricular to pulmonary artery reconstruction, balloon atrial septostomy should not be performed. Clearly, in patients with pulmonary atresia, regardless of the size of the right ventricle, the pulmonary valve is not patent and thus balloon dilation valvotomy is not possible unless some technique is used first to make an opening in the pulmonary valve.

Angiocardiography

Selective right ventricular angiocardiography will demonstrate the presence of pulmonary atresia as well as assess the proximal level of obstruction and determine the size of the right ventricular cavity. Both of these anatomic features are important in the management of patients with this disorder. Angiography can be performed in the anteroposterior and lateral views by a hand injection of a small amount of contrast material (0.5 mL/kg). A calibration block or grid should also be recorded to enable subsequent measurement of the magnification factor. In the past, right ventricular size has been described using nonspecific terms such as "large" or "small", or "cherry pit" or "peach pit" in most series (Fig. 2). Unfortunately, these terms do not allow comparison of surgical results on the basis of preoperative right ventricular size. Techniques for measuring tricuspid valve and right ventricular dimensions and for determining right ventricular volume have been reported (Fricker 1987; Patel 1980; deLeval 1985). Although these angiographic studies

Figure 2. Pulmonary atresia with intact ventricular septum and right ventricles of various sizes. (Top: Anteroposterior views. Bottom: Lateral views). A: Severe hypoplasia ("cherry pit") showing coronary cardiac fistulae with reversed flow into the ascending aorta. B: Moderate hypoplasia. C: Normal size.

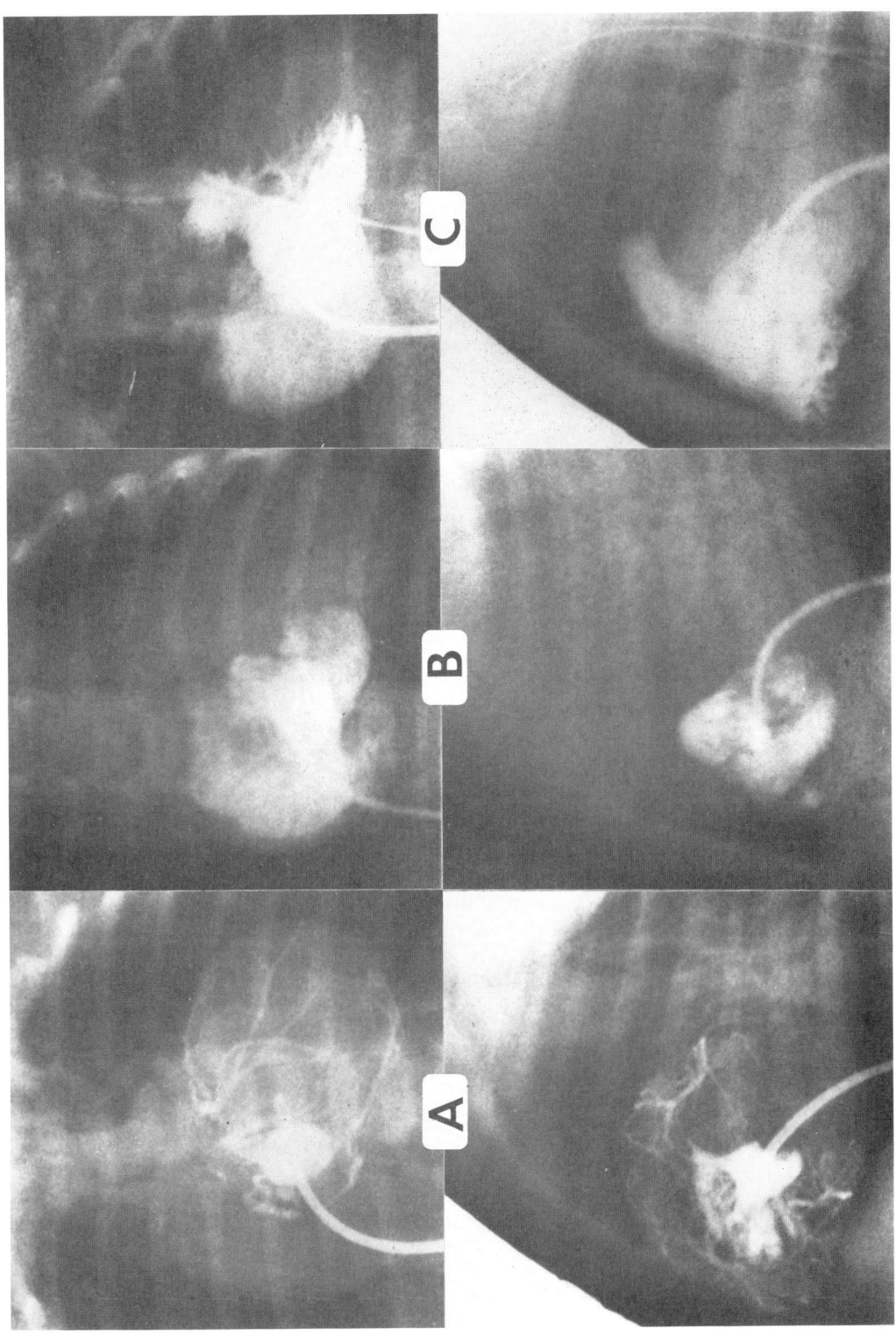

generally have shown good correlation with the anatomic findings in postmortem specimens, they may underestimate right ventricular cavity size due to cavity obliteration caused by the presence of severely hypertrophied trabecular muscle (Bull 1982).

The proximal level of atresia is also an important consideration in determining whether or not it is possible simply to open the atretic pulmonary valve or whether there is atresia or severe stenosis of the infundibulum as well. Sequential injections in the right ventricle and aorta may visualize this area adequately. Otherwise, a simultaneous double injection with one catheter in the right ventricle and the other in the aorta at the site of the ductus arteriosus or in the pulmonary artery shows both the right ventricular outflow tract and main pulmonary artery and demonstrates the extent of the obstruction (Fig. 3). In patients with pul-

monary atresia and intact ventricular septum, there may be some natural decompression of the right ventricle either by tricuspid regurgitation or by fistulous connections between the right ventricle and coronary arteries. Tricuspid regurgitation is best demonstrated during catheterization by a right ventricular angiogram in the anteroposterior or right anterior oblique projection. As was indicated earlier in this chapter, it may be worthwhile to use a Goodale-Lubin catheter (end-hole and two distal side holes) for angiography in these patients. Mild tricuspid regurgitation may be induced by the catheter position or by dysrhythmia, but dense opacification of the right atrium following right ventricular injection indicates significant regurgitation. In general, right ventricular cavity size correlates well with the presence and severity of tricuspid regurgitation. A very large right ventricle is almost always

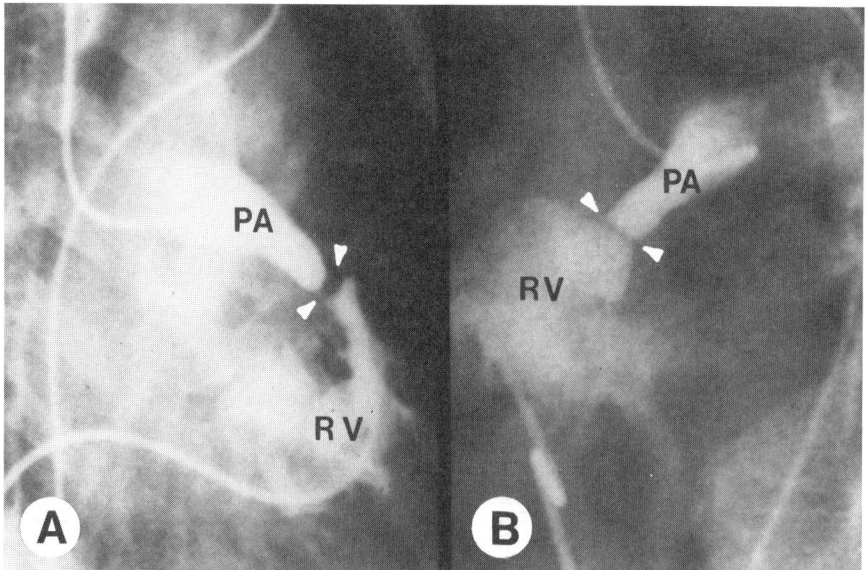

Figure 3. Right anterior oblique (A) and shallow left anterior oblique (B) views of a simultaneous injection in right ventricle and pulmonary artery in pulmonary atresia with intact ventricular septum (see text). The venous catheter is in the right ventricular outflow tract while the arterial catheter has been passed through a systemic to pulmonary shunt into the main pulmonary artery. (Arrows indicate the atretic valve). PA = pulmonary artery. RV = right ventricle.

associated with severe tricuspid regurgitation while a tiny right ventricle usually has no accompanying regurgitation.

Right ventricle to coronary artery fistulae also correlate, but inversely, with right ventricular cavity size being found most commonly in patients with a tiny right ventricular cavity and suprasystemic right ventricular pressure. The fistulae are demonstrated on right ventricular angiography, usually in the anteroposterior and lateral projections. Bidirectional coronary flow is often present, with flow from aorta to coronary arteries in diastole and from right ventricle to coronary arteries in systole. In some cases retrograde systolic flow passes all the way from the right ventricle through the length of the coronary artery and into the aorta. It is important to evaluate this bidirectional flow carefully to be certain that there are no segments of the coronary artery that are supplied solely by flow from the right ventricle (Burrows 1990). This is especially true at the time of a subsequent catheterization in a patient with a very small right ventricle and coronary fistulae who is being considered for a procedure to occlude right ventricular inflow. Clearly, this might be disastrous if a portion of coronary blood flow is supplied only from the right ventricle. Thus, if additional operative procedures are contemplated and the coronary artery patterns have not been identified adequately, selective coronary angiography should be performed.

Lastly, selective left ventricular angiocardiography should be performed to evaluate size and function of the left ventricle. This should be done routinely, even if no left ventricular problem is suspected because left ventricular function may be abnormal (Sideris 1982). It permits estimation of "relative" right and left ventricular sizes and screens for unanticipated left heart abnormalities. Since the foramen ovale is always patent in patients with this abnormality, access to the left ventricle is easy. The selective left ventricular angiocardiogram will also demonstrate the pulmonary artery anatomy via the patent ductus arteriosus. If the anatomy of the pulmonary artery is not well visualized, then a selective aortogram with the umbilical artery line is essential.

Associated Lesions

Pulmonary atresia with an intact ventricular septum usually occurs as an isolated lesion and not in the context of other congenital cardiac anomalies. As was mentioned previously, there is often an associated Ebstein's malformation of the tricuspid valve that may cause tricuspid regurgitation or, less commonly, tricuspid stenosis. The left side of the heart and aortic arch and its branches are usually normal although left ventricular function may be depressed especially if systemic hypoxemia has been prolonged or particularly severe. Lastly, although abnormalities of the pulmonary veins are not usually associated with this condition, it is important to be certain that there is full saturation in the pulmonary veins and that they drain normally to the left atrium.

Cautions or Precautions

In patients with pulmonary atresia and intact ventricular septum, the size of the tricuspid orifice correlates strongly with the size of the right ventricular cavity. It may be quite difficult, therefore, to enter a very small right ventricle.

Because patients with this lesion have ductal dependent pulmonary blood flow, a continuous infusion of prostaglandin E_1 is necessary to maintain adequate oxygenation. Inadequate delivery of prostaglandin E_1 because of too low a dose, or failure of a peripheral venous line into which it is being infused, may result in a sudden rapid fall in systemic oxygen saturation. The adequacy of the peripheral infusion site should be ascertained prior to cardiac catheterization and if there is any question during the procedure, immediate transfer of the infusion line to the cardiac catheter will result in immediate patient improvement and confirm the source of the problem. It is important to remember that a number of undesirable side effects of prostaglandin such as a rash, fever, or seizures can occur. Apnea is also a particular problem at high infusion rates or if a bolus of prostaglandin is inadvertently administered during an attempt to purge or flush a venous line. Because this can occur at any time, advance preparation should also be made to provide assisted ventilation by means of an Ambu bag and mask, or intubation, of any patient who is receiving intravenous Prostaglandin infusion. Lastly, careful attention must be paid to the patient's blood gas status upon arrival in the catheterization laboratory and periodically during the procedure. If the patient has had a prolonged period of systemic hypoxemia, a considerable degree of metabolic acidosis may be present at the start of the procedure and require treatment with sodium bicarbonate. If there is any doubt as to the stability of the patient before catheterization, it may be preferable to perform an elective intubation prior to the procedure rather than attempting to do this on an emergency basis during the catheterization.

References and Suggested Reading

Bull C, deLeval MR, Mercanti C, et al. Pulmonary atresia and intact ventricular septum: A revised classification. Circulation 1982;66: 266–272.

Burrows PE, Freedom RM, Benson LN, et al. Coronary angiography of pulmonary atresia, hypoplastic right ventricle, and ventriculocoronary communications. Am J Roentgen 1990;154:789–795.

deLeval M, Bull C, Hopkins R, et al. Decision making in the definitive repair of the heart with a small right ventricle. Circulation 1985; 72(Suppl II):II-52-II-60.

Fricker FJ, Zuberbuhler JR. Pulmonary atresia with intact ventricular septum. In: Paediatric Cardiology. Anderson RH, Macartney FJ, Shinebourne EA, et al. eds. Edinburgh; Churchill Livingstone, 1987:771–720.

Patel RG, Freedom RM, Moes CAF, et al. Right ventricular volume determinations in 18 patients with pulmonary atresia and intact ventricular septum. Analysis of factors influencing right ventricular growth. Circulation 1980;61:428–440.

Sideris EB, Olley PM, Spooner E, et al. Left ventricular function and compliance in pulmonary atresia with intact ventricular septum. J Thorac Cardiovasc Surg 1982;84:192–199.

Zuberbuhler JR, Anderson RH. Morphological variations in pulmonary atresia with intact ventricular septum. Br Heart J 1979;41:281–288.

25

Tetralogy of Fallot with Pulmonary Stenosis or Atresia

William H. Neches, M.D.

Anatomy

The term tetralogy of Fallot refers to a spectrum of anatomic abnormalities that have a large and unrestrictive ventricular septal defect and right ventricular outflow tract obstruction. The anatomic hallmark of the tetralogy of Fallot is the anterocephalad deviation of the outlet septum. This deviation significantly narrows the right ventricular outflow tract and is responsible for most of the infundibular pulmonary stenosis and also accounts for the ventricular septal defect and the aortic override (Fig. 1). The severity of infundibular obstruction ranges from mild to severe pulmonary stenosis, to pulmonary atresia. Further obstruction to pulmonary blood flow often occurs at other levels including the pulmonary valve and annulus, supravalvar region and branch pulmonary arteries. Pulmonary valve stenosis is common and can be due to a stenotic three leaflet valve, a bicuspid or unicuspid valve.

In about 80% of patients, there is a large unrestrictive membranous ventricular septal defect, while in 20% of patients this defect has a muscular posteroinferior rim separating the tricuspid valve from the aortic valve. An additional ventricular septal defect, or multiple defects, may also be present in the trabecular portion of the interventricular septum.

Hemodynamic Considerations

The hemodynamic features produced by the anatomic abnormalities in tetralogy of Fallot are: (1) equalization of right and left ventricular pressure, and (2) normal or reduced pulmonary artery pressure. Because the ventricular septal defect is large and unrestrictive, and the right and left ventricles contract simultaneously, the end result is in effect a "common" ventricular chamber ejecting into the systemic and pulmonary circulations. Therefore, the pulmonary and systemic blood flows are dependent upon the relative relationship between the pulmonary and systemic outflow resistances. In tetralogy of Fallot, the pulmonary vascular "arteriolar" resistance is usually normal or less than normal and the total outflow resistance to right ventricular ejection into the pulmonary vascular bed is instead related to relatively fixed anatomic obstruction. These potential areas for anatomic obstruction include right ventricular outflow tract at the subvalvar, annular, or valvar levels and supravalvar or distal arterial stenoses as well. Thus, the resistance to systemic outflow depends solely upon the arteriolar resistance of the distal vascular bed, while the resistance to pulmonary outflow is the cumulative effect of the various levels of anatomic obstruction. If the right ventricular outflow obstruction is less than the systemic resis-

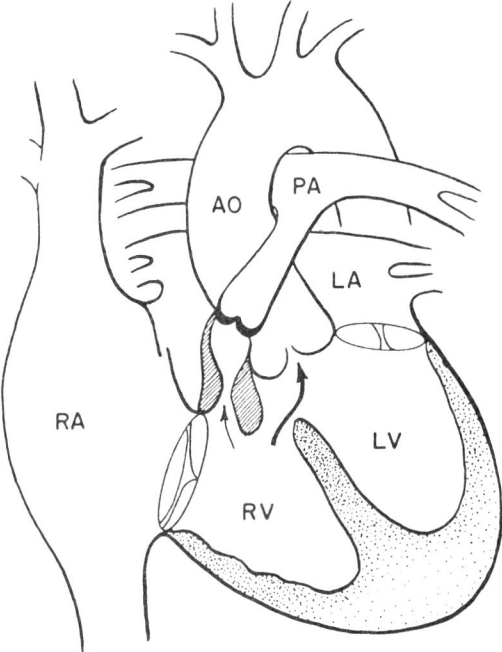

Figure 1. Diagram of tetralogy of Fallot.

the right ventricular outflow tract, the distribution and size of the pulmonary arteries and hopefully to predict accurately whether the repair is likely to be successfully accomplished. It is extremely important to demonstrate other associated lesions such as multiple ventricular septal defects or coronary artery anomalies that may have an adverse affect on the success of surgical repair. An anomalous coronary artery is found in as many as 5%–10% of patients with tetralogy of Fallot and an accurate assessment of this anomaly is not possible by echocardiography. The assessment of the hemodynamic result, ventricular function, residual anatomic abnormalities, and electrophysiologic studies are important in the postoperative evaluation and follow-up of patients.

Catheterization Technique

A standard protocol is followed for hemodynamics and oximetry while the sites of injection and views for angiocardiography are selected to define the anatomy and associated anomalies in tetralogy of Fallot. Catheters are usually inserted into the femoral vessels and entry into the pulmonary artery can be difficult from this position. Because crossing the right ventricular tract with the catheter is sometimes associated with hypoxemic spells, we recommend measurement of oxygen consumption and assessment of hemodynamics and oximetry at all other sites prior to attempts at crossing the right ventricular outflow tract with a catheter. In this way, even if a hypoxemic spells is induced, baseline measurements will have been obtained before hand. In many laboratories, flow directed balloon catheters are used for right heart procedures. In patients with tetralogy of Fallot with moderate to severe pulmonary stenosis, the right to left shunt will result in a flow-directed balloon catheter passing from the right ventricle into the aorta. In these patients, entry into the pulmonary artery, if de-

tance, there will be a net left to right shunt and the clinical manifestations will be similar to those of patients with a small to moderate-sized ventricular septal defect. On the other hand, if the right ventricular outflow obstruction and systemic resistances are similar, there will be a balanced shunt with nearly equal pulmonary and systemic blood flows at rest. Lastly, when the right ventricular outflow obstruction exceeds systemic resistance, there will be a net right to left shunt and the patient will be cyanotic.

Indications for Cardiac Catheterization

The anatomic features of tetralogy of Fallot can be accurately identified by cross-sectional echocardiography. Cardiac catheterization and angiocardiography are important both preoperatively and postoperatively. In the preoperative patient it is important to define the levels of stenosis in sired, may be accomplished only with a woven Dacron or some other type of non-flow-directed catheter. It is usually possible to enter the left heart and aorta with a venous catheter in patients with tetralogy of Fallot. Because an atrial communication, either a patent foramen ovale or atrial septal defect is commonly present, the venous catheter can be advanced across the atrial septal communication into the left atrium and from there to the left ventricle. Also, the venous catheter often can be passed from the right ventricle out into the aorta. Even if the atrial septum is intact, it may be possible to manipulate a catheter that has been advanced into the aorta into the left ventricle across the ventricular septal defect. This is accomplished by maintaining a counter-clockwise twist on the catheter as it is withdrawn from the ascending aorta into the ventricle. This counterclockwise twist will result in the catheter tip flipping into the left ventricle rather than into the right ventricle as it is withdrawn from the aorta (see Chapter 5).

Hemodynamic Evaluation

Pressure Data

The ventricular septal defect is unrestrictive in patients with tetralogy of Fallot and thus the systolic pressures are the same in both ventricles and the aorta. If it is possible to pass a catheter into the pulmonary artery, the slow withdrawal of an end-hole catheter from the distal pulmonary arteries to the right ventricle may demonstrate additional sites of stenosis in the distal pulmonary artery, in the supravalvar region, or at the valvar level. However, the proximal infundibular stenosis and right to left shunt at ventricular level will make the pressure gradient across most distal areas of stenosis an unreliable measure of severity. This is best assessed by angiocardiography. It is important to measure the pulmonary artery pressure in patients who are being considered for corrective surgery and who previously have undergone a systemic to pulmonary artery anastomosis. This is especially true if the patient has had a Waterston, Potts, or other central shunt. Pulmonary hypertension may occur in patients who have undergone these palliative procedures and if present, may be a serious complicating factor at the time of complete repair. In patients with a Waterston or Potts anastomosis, there may be severe acquired pulmonary artery stenosis proximal to the shunt with resultant unilateral pulmonary hypertension only on the same side as the anastomosis.

Oxygen Saturation Data

Oxygen saturations are determined from various sites within the cardiovascular system and the data used for calculation of pulmonary and systemic flow. If oxygen consumption is measured, then actual pulmonary and systemic blood flows can be calculated. Otherwise, the pulmonary to systemic flow ratio can be used. Although some patients have a balanced shunt or net left to right shunt, most patients with tetralogy of Fallot have a net right to left shunt and at least some degree of systemic arterial desaturation. The degree of right to left shunting can be quantified either by oximetry or by means of indicator dilution curves (see Chapter 6).

Other Diagnostic or Therapeutic Procedures

Electrophysiology

Most centers do not routinely perform intracardiac electrophysiologic studies postoperatively despite the fact that a significant incidence of atrioventricular conduction abnormalities have been reported following complete repair of this anomaly.

We have found that approximately 25% of postoperative patients show abnormalities of atrioventricular conduction that were not present preoperatively (Neches 1977). If a postoperative cardiac catheterization is indicated for another reason, additional electrophysiologic screening procedures are easily performed with a single catheter. If abnormalities are found, further, more sophisticated evaluation is warranted. The studies performed with a single catheter include obtaining a His bundle electrogram, measurement of resting AH and HV intervals, and incremental atrial pacing to determine AV node refractoriness and sinus node recovery time. Although the significance of the abnormalities that have been found in these patients is still unknown, the high incidence of abnormalities found in this group and not present in other groups of postoperative patients is bothersome and indicates that this subgroup that may be at greater risk for problems in the future.

Ventricular arrhythmias may be found following repair of tetralogy of Fallot. It has been suggested that the finding of premature ventricular beats on resting or exercise electrocardiography may be a marker for those patients who may develop serious ventricular arrhythmias and sudden death. An intracardiac electrophysiologic study would be indicated for those postoperative patients in a high-risk category such as those with previous episodes of syncope or suspected arrhythmia, or to facilitate the selection of pharmacologic therapy in patients with serious and life threatening arrhythmias.

Interventional Catheterization Procedures

Percutaneous balloon dilation angioplasty has been used in a few preoperative patients with tetralogy of Fallot (Wright 1986) and successful balloon dilation of a stenotic Blalock-Taussig systemic to pulmonary artery anastomosis has also been reported (Fischer 1985). In addition, balloon dilation of residual pulmonary artery stenosis in patients who have undergone complete repair of tetralogy of Fallot may be important in the future. In the past, balloon dilation of pulmonary artery stenosis usually has not been successful due to the inability to maintain the area of pulmonary artery stenosis in its dilated state. A potentially valuable technique that is currently under investigation involves the use of the wire mesh stent that surrounds the surface of a deflated balloon dilation catheter (Mullins 1988). When this device is inserted into a stenotic area of the pulmonary artery and the balloon inflated, the stent assumes a new and larger diameter. When the balloon is deflated, the metal stent retains the enlarged diameter and thus prevents the surrounding stenotic area of pulmonary artery from returning to its previous size.

Some patients have multiple systemic to pulmonary artery collaterals that provide pulmonary blood flow preoperatively and are difficult to approach at the time of surgical repair. These vessels can be occluded either preoperatively or postoperatively by coil or other embolization techniques or by the use of a Rashkind patent ductus arteriosus occluder (see Chapter 15).

Angiocardiography

The angiocardiographic evaluation of the patient with tetralogy of Fallot is designed to provide information regarding a number of anatomic and functional features. The number, size, and location of ventricular septal defects must be ascertained. It is also important to determine the level and severity of the right ventricular outflow tract obstruction and whether or not additional sites of obstruction are present proximal or distal to the major area of stenosis. It is also important to determine the presence of associated abnormalities such as an atrial septal defect, pulmonary artery stenosis, coronary artery abnormalities, or anomalies of the aortic arch and its branches (Soto 1982).

Selective left ventricular angiocardiography is best performed in multiple views. If only one left ventricular injection is possible, this should be done in the four-chamber view, which adequately visualizes the ventricular septum in the area of the usual ventricular septal defect. The anteroposterior and lateral or oblique views of the left ventricular angiogram can be used to assess quantitatively left ventricular volume and function if a reference grid is recorded before or after the angiogram. Selective right ventricular angiocardiography is useful to evaluate right ventricular function, the presence of tricuspid regurgitation and most importantly, the site of the right ventricular outflow tract obstruction (Fig. 2). This injection should be in the body of the right ventricle rather than in the right ventricular

outflow tract, so that subinfundibular obstruction due to an anomalous muscle bundle is not missed. The elongated right anterior oblique view is probably the best for demonstrating the entire right ventricular outflow tract, as well as pulmonary artery. In the simultaneously recorded four-chamber view, right to left shunting at ventricular level opacifies the aorta. If the right ventricular outflow tract has not been visualized adequately by right ventricular angiocardiography due to a very severe pulmonary stenosis, a small injection of contrast (safest by hand) in the right ventricular outflow tract is helpful.

There are often multiple sites of obstruction in patients with tetralogy of Fallot, including infundibular, valvar and pulmonary arterial stenosis (Fig. 3). The pulmonary valve annulus and main pulmonary artery, as well as the bifurcation of the main

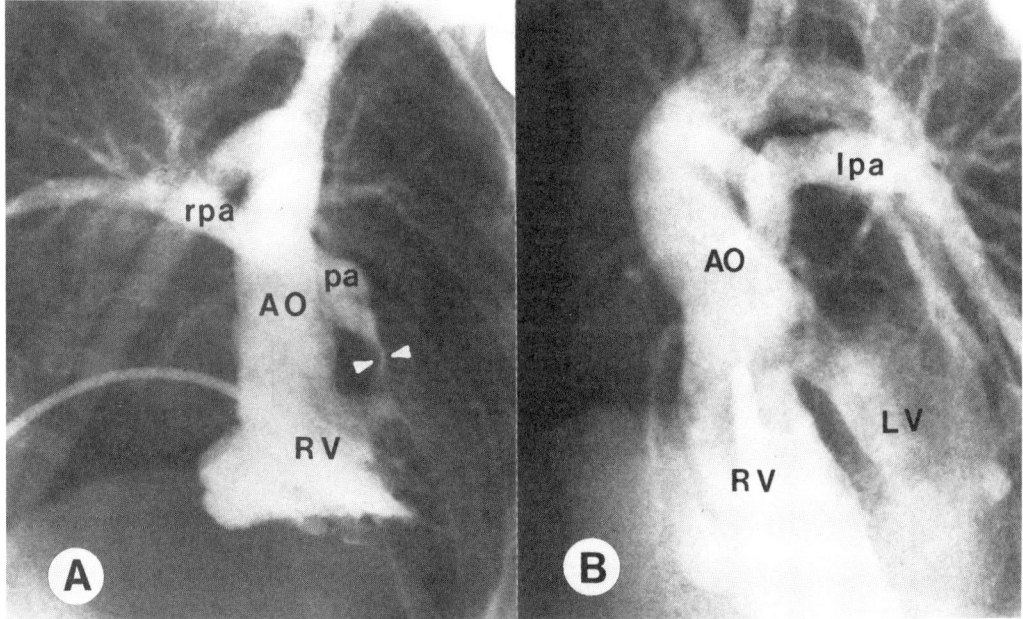

Figure 2. Right ventricular injection in tetralogy of Fallot demonstrating marked infundibular stenosis (arrows). Note substantial right to left shunting has opacified the aorta. AO = Aorta; PA = pulmonary artery; RV = right ventricle. A: Elongated right anterior oblique view. Right pulmonary artery (RPA) is visualized best in this view. B: Four-chamber view that also demonstrates marked override of the aorta. The left pulmonary artery (LPA) is visualized in this view.

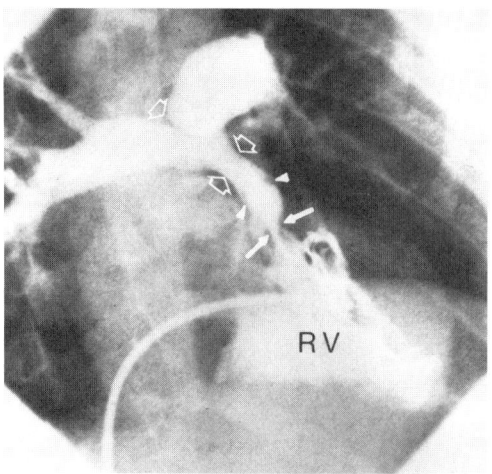

Figure 3. Selective injection in the right ventricle (RV) in the elongated right anterior oblique view demonstrating multiple levels of obstruction. Solid arrows = infundibular stenosis. Arrow points = valvar stenosis. Open arrows = pulmonary artery stenosis.

pulmonary artery, must be well visualized, especially if these areas have not been traversed with the catheter. Stenosis in these areas has significant bearing on both the method of surgical repair and the surgical risk. If these areas of the pulmonary artery have not been visualized adequately with the preceding injections, a pulmonary arteriogram in the anteroposterior or shallow left anterior oblique projection with 25°–40° of cranio-caudal angulation is advisable (Fig. 4).

It has been suggested that inadequate relief of distal obstruction in the pulmonary vascular bed will result in an increase in the postoperative right to left ventricular pressure ratio ($P_{RV/LV}$). A number of methods have been developed to predict the success of surgical repair based upon a preoperative cineangiographic measurement of the pul-

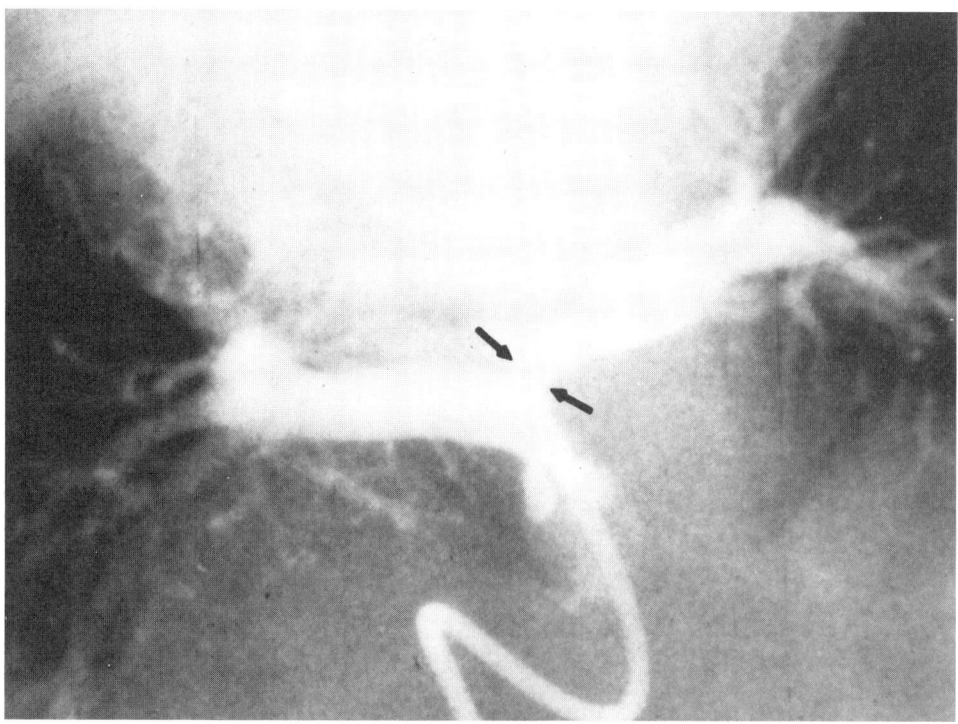

Figure 4. Selective pulmonary artery injection in the shallow left anterior oblique projection with 40° of cranio-caudal angulation demonstrating proximal left pulmonary artery stenosis (arrows).

monary arteries. Blackstone et al. (1979) developed a formula to predict postrepair $P_{RV/LV}$ related to the diameter of the right and left pulmonary arteries and the pulmonary valve annulus as measured from preoperative cineangiograms and normalized to the patient's descending aorta.

$$P_{RV/LV} = \frac{0.4840}{\dfrac{D_{RPA} + D_{LPA}}{D_{DAo}}} + 0.2007$$

Where: D = Diameter of vessel
RPA = Right pulmonary artery
LPA = Left pulmonary artery
DAo = Descending thoracic aorta

These measurements are the maximal systolic diameter of the right and left pulmonary arteries measured just before the take-off of the first branch and the descending aorta just above the level of the diaphragm (Fig. 5). To insure the accuracy of these calculations, a calibration grid must be recorded following angiography to enable correction for the magnification factor. The angiographic catheters can be used to calculate this factor, but this method is often inaccurate due to the small size of the catheter. The pressure ratio predicted by this formula assumes complete relief of all areas of obstruction proximal to the point of measurement including the right ventricular outflow tract, pulmonary valve, annulus, main pulmonary artery, and proximal branches.

Another approach was taken by Nakata et al. (1984) who calculated the pulmonary artery area index by measurement of right and left pulmonary arteries from preoperative cineangiograms.

PA_{index}

$$= \frac{RPA\ area\ (mm^2) + LPA\ area\ (mm^2)}{BSA\ (m^2)}$$

$$PA\ area\ (mm^2) = \pi \left(\frac{D}{2}\right)^2$$

BSA = Body surface area (m^2)
PA = Pulmonary artery
RPA, LPA = Right or left pulmonary artery

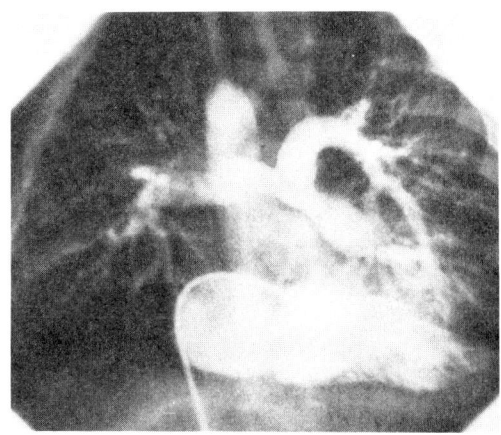
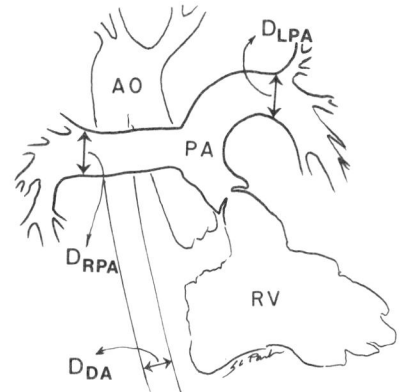

Figure 5. Diagram and angiogram demonstrating the measurements to predict the postoperative right ventricular pressure (see text). D = Diameter of vessel. LPA = Left pulmonary artery. RPA = Right pulmonary artery.

As in the Blackstone formula, the pulmonary arteries are measured just proximal to the first branch. Normal value for PA_{index} was 330 ± 30 mm²/BSA. Although their index was not used to predict postoperative right ventricular pressure, those patients with a pulmonary artery area index of less than 55% of normal either had severe problems with low cardiac output and congestive heart failure, or died in the postoperative period.

Coronary artery abnormalities often are present in patients with tetralogy of Fallot and may have significant bearing on the operative risk and overall results. The most common serious abnormality is an anomalous anterior descending coronary artery which arises from the right coronary artery rather than from the left (Fig. 6). A variant is an accessory anterior descending coronary artery arising from the right and paralleling the normal left anterior descending vessel. In either case, a substantial portion of myocardium is supplied by a vessel that crosses the right ventricular outflow tract. In the presence of severe tetralogy of Fallot, especially in the small infant, it is often necessary to patch the right ventricular outflow and to carry the patch across the pulmonary annulus and out onto the pulmonary artery. Thus, the presence of the anomalous coronary artery precludes the placement of this patch since division of the artery may result in ventricular dysfunction, or a myocardial infarction that may be fatal. It is therefore mandatory to visualize the major branches

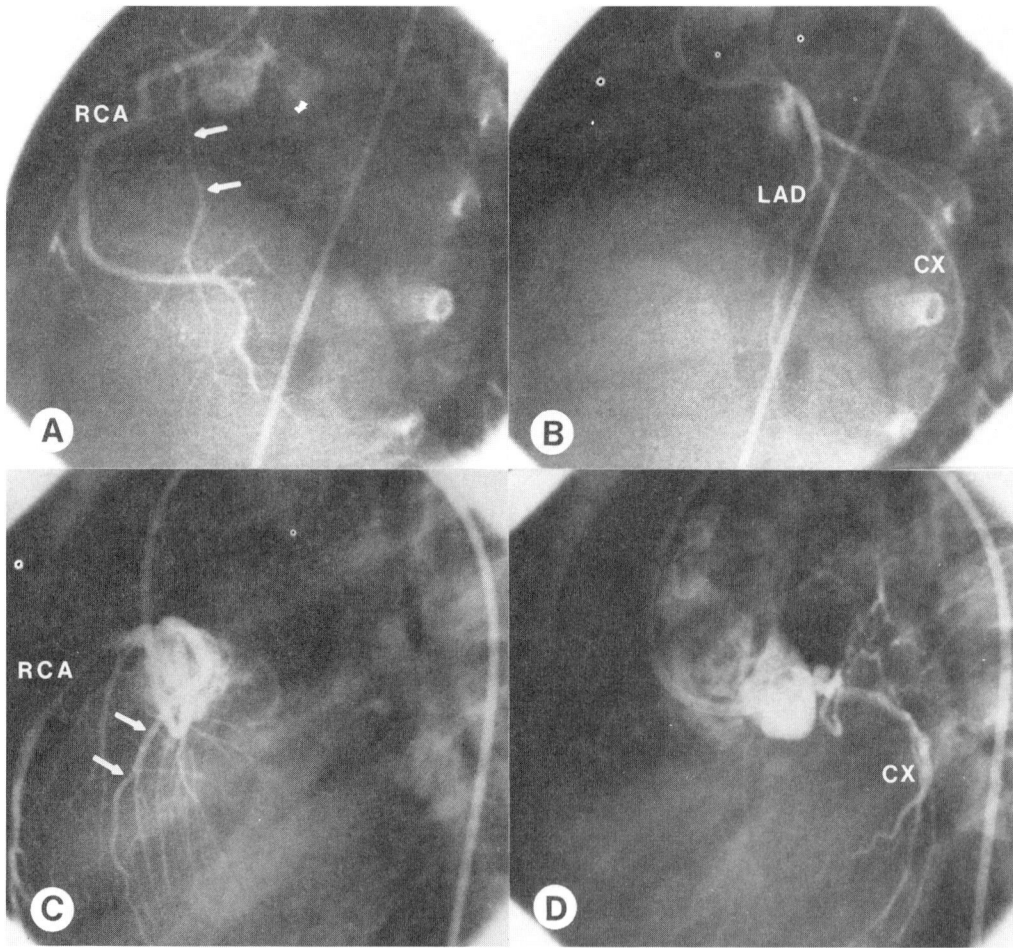

Figure 6. Selective coronary angiograms demonstrating anomalous anterior descending coronary arteries Top = Accessory anterior descending (arrows) from the coronary artery. Selective injection in the right coronary artery (RCA) (A) and the left coronary artery (B) in the four-chamber view. Bottom = Anterior descending coronary artery (arrows) from the right coronary artery. Selective injection in the right coronary artery (C) and the left coronary artery (D) in the left anterior oblique view. Note absence of the anterior descending from the left coronary trunk. CX = circumflex coronary artery. LAD = left anterior descending artery.

of both coronary arteries in any patient with tetralogy of Fallot prior to corrective surgery. In general, the coronary arteries are well visualized following an aortic root injection in right and left anterior oblique views. In a small patient, aortography can be performed with a venous catheter passed from the right ventricle out into the aorta, avoiding arterial catheterization. In an older child it can be done safely by a retrograde arterial catheterization toward the end of the catheterization procedure. Since ventriculography will have been performed using the prograde catheter, the retrograde arterial catheter can be relatively small and is in place in the artery for only a short time. If the coronary arteries are not visualized adequately with aortography, selective coronary arteriography must be considered.

Associated Lesions

The presence of an associated atrial septal defect (so called "pentalogy of Fallot") should be determined at the time of cardiac catheterization. It is also mandatory that the ventricular septum be visualized adequately so that additional muscular ventricular septal defects or an associated atrioventricular septal defect can be identified. As was stated previously, it is essential to determine the coronary artery anatomy and to rule out the presence of double outlet right ventricle, especially if the patient is to undergo corrective surgery. Lastly, a right-sided aortic arch is a common associated abnormality. Although the presence of a right-sided aortic arch has no physiologic significance, there may also be an associated anomalous retroesophageal subclavian artery. This assumes great significance if the patient is to undergo a subclavian to pulmonary artery anastomosis.

Absent pulmonary valve syndrome is considered to be part of tetralogy of Fallot complex. However, the features of this syndrome that are different from the usual patient with tetralogy of Fallot are: marked hypoplasia or absence of pulmonary valve tissue with narrowing of the pulmonary annulus and concomitant severe dilation of the pulmonary arteries (Fig. 7). These patients rarely present with cyanosis. Instead, many

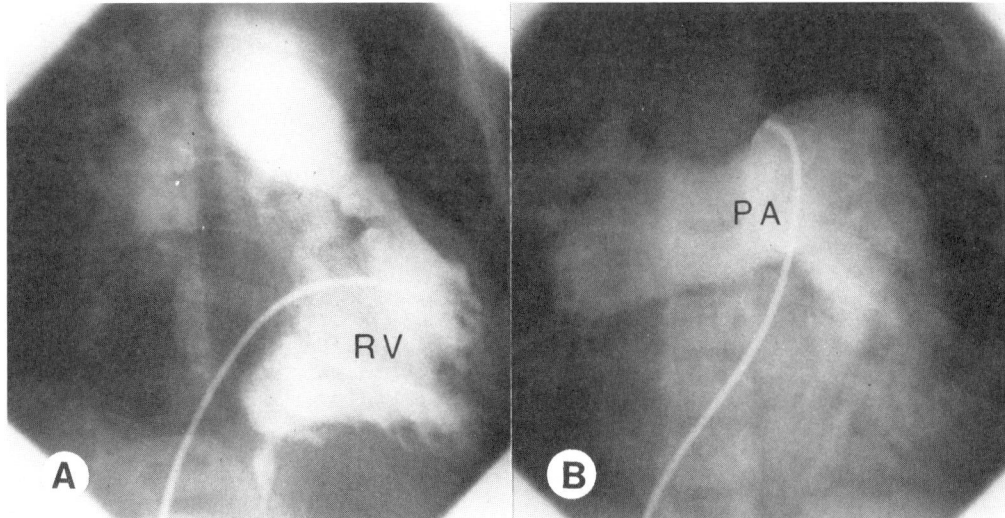

Figure 7. Tetralogy of Fallot with absent pulmonary valve A: Right ventricular angiogram in an elongated right anterior oblique view demonstrating marked narrowing of the pulmonary annulus. B: Pulmonary arteriogram in the anteroposterior view showing marked dilation of the pulmonary arteries. PA = Pulmonary artery. RV = Right ventricle.

present during infancy with respiratory distress due to compression of the tracheobronchial tree by the aneurysmally dilated pulmonary arteries.

Cautions or Precautions

Patients with tetralogy of Fallot, especially those with severe pulmonary stenosis, or with a history of previous hypoxemia episodes, may be predisposed to have a hypoxemic spell during cardiac catheterization. Thorazine should not be used as part of the premedication since it tends to lower peripheral resistance and may precipitate a spell. Morphine sulfate alone is a good alternative for premedication in these patients. If there is considerable potential for a hypoxemic spell during a cardiac catheterization, then general anesthesia rather than only sedation might be used for the procedure. In some cases, the presence of a catheter in the right ventricular outflow tract may precipitate a hypoxemic episode. Continuous monitoring of the systemic arterial oxygen saturation by pulse oximetry during cardiac catheterization, especially in infants and small children with tetralogy of Fallot, will enable immediate recognition of a decrease in systemic oxygenation. If a hypoxemic spell occurs, oxygen should be administered by face mask as soon as possible and the use of morphine sulfate 0.1 mg/kg, administered intravenously, should be considered. If the hypoxemic spell persists despite two or three doses of morphine sulfate 20–30 minutes apart, intravenous propranolol (0.01–0.05 mg/kg) may be used. It should be emphasized that the myocardium of the right ventricular outflow tract is relatively thin, even in patients with tetralogy of Fallot. This area is easily traumatized or perforated by intense attempts to traverse a stenotic right ventricular outflow tract or pulmonary valve with the catheter or guidewire. Care must be taken during these manipulations to be certain that the catheter tip or guidewire are directed posteriorly toward the

pulmonary valve and pulmonary artery rather in a cephalad direction against the right ventricular outflow tract myocardium.

Tetralogy of Fallot with Pulmonary Atresia (Pulmonary Atresia with Ventricular Septal Defect)

Patients with tetralogy of Fallot and pulmonary atresia (also called pulmonary atresia and ventricular septal defect) generally present with cyanosis in early infancy. Pulmonary blood flow is via a patent ductus arteriosus and/or systemic-pulmonary artery collateral vessels (Fig. 8). The intensity of the cyanosis depends on the volume of pulmonary blood flow. If only a patent ductus is present, flow is usually low and cyanosis often severe. With systemic-pulmonary collaterals, flow may be greater and cyanosis less marked or even inapparent. If systemic to pulmonary collateral vessels are large and pulmonary blood flow is excessive, patients may present with congestive heart failure. The diagnosis is usually established

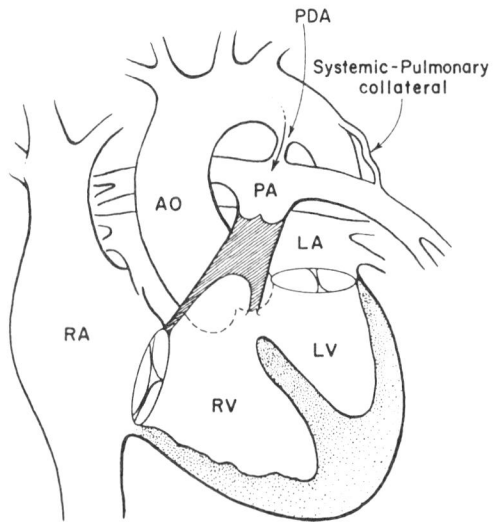

Figure 8. Diagram of tetralogy of Fallot with pulmonary atresia.

echocardiographically and cardiac catheterization is indicated to confirm the diagnosis and to evaluate the status of the pulmonary blood flow. This should be done promptly in a newborn since pulmonary blood flow may depend solely upon patency of the ductus arteriosus. If this diagnosis is suspected and significant hypoxemia is present, the intravenous infusion of prostaglandin E_1 is important to maintain patency of the ductus arteriosus, thereby improving oxygenation and relieving acidosis.

Hemodynamic Evaluation

Pressure Data

Pulmonary hypertension is a serious complication that may be seen in patients with tetralogy of Fallot and pulmonary atresia who have had a systemic to pulmonary artery anastomosis or who have large systemic to pulmonary collateral arteries. Thus, it is important to measure pressure in the collaterals, or in the pulmonary artery in the patient who has had palliative surgery. Considerable effort must thus be made to catheterize selectively all collateral vessels and to manipulate the catheter into the pulmonary artery through a systemic to pulmonary artery anastomosis.

Oxygen Saturation Data

The findings in patients with this anomaly are similar to those in patients with tetralogy of Fallot. The exception, of course, is that the catheter cannot be passed into the pulmonary artery across the right ventricular outflow tract. There is usually no oxygen step-up in the right atrium or right ventricle unless an associated atrial septal defect is present. Pulmonary venous and left atrial saturations are usually normal. The systemic arterial oxygen saturation is decreased and is dependent upon the volume of pulmonary blood flow. It is important to

note that the level of systemic oxygenation also varies with the systemic cardiac output. Because the volume of pulmonary blood flow is generally fixed, any increase in cardiac output results in a larger volume of desaturated systemic venous blood. The net result is the decrease in systemic arterial oxygen saturation that occurs with activity, crying, etc.

Angiocardiography

Angiocardiographic features of tetralogy of Fallot with pulmonary atresia are similar to those of tetralogy of Fallot and pulmonary stenosis. Left ventricular function and the location and size of the ventricular septal defect are best evaluated using the four-chamber view. As in tetralogy of Fallot, an injection of contrast media into the body of the right ventricle is necessary to judge right ventricular and tricuspid valve function. The right anterior oblique view is probably best. If the outflow tract is not well seen, a hand injection directly into the area should be done. With this selective injection the right ventricular out flow tract can be nicely visualized in almost any view.

The pulmonary artery anatomy must be demonstrated adequately angiocardiographically. Because all pulmonary blood flow is from the aorta, via either a patent ductus arteriosus, systemic-pulmonary artery collaterals or a surgical anastomosis, the pulmonary circulation should be defined initially by an aortogram (Fig. 9). An injection into the distal arch in the anteroposterior and lateral projections should visualize both a patent ductus (lateral view) and collateral arteries (anteroposterior view). If only a ductus is present and only the ipsilateral pulmonary artery fills, discontinuity of the right and left pulmonary arteries should be suspected. The contralateral artery may then connect to another ductus on that side, which may or may not be patent at the time of the study. One should also be certain that a pulmonary arterial supply is

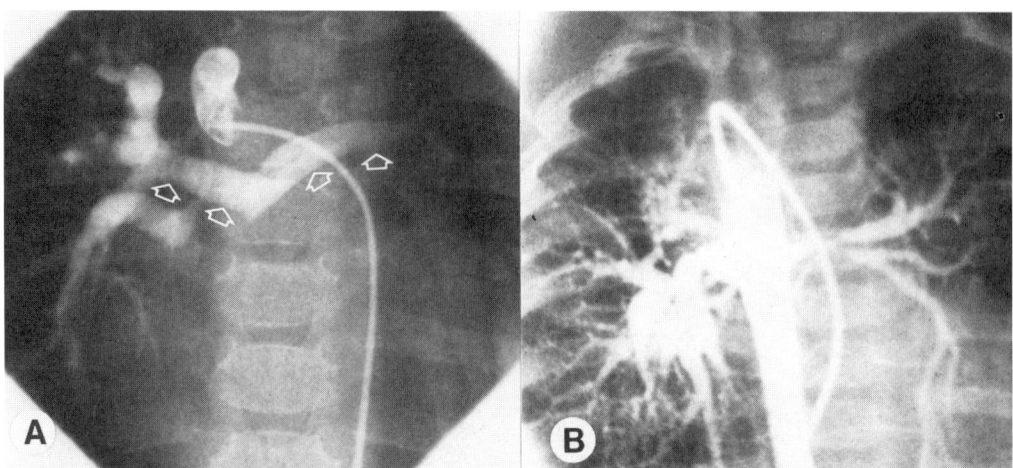

Figure 9. Tetralogy of Fallot with pulmonary atresia A: Selective injection in a systemic to pulmonary artery collateral demonstrating true pulmonary arteries (arrows) which have a "sea gull" appearance. B: Aortogram demonstrating multiple systemic to pulmonary collaterals.

present to all parts of both lungs. With this entity it is possible to have systemic collateral arteries supplying part or all of the flow to a lobe or lung (Liao 1985). If large collateral arteries are seen on the aortogram, selective injection into each artery is advisable, again, in the anteroposterior and lateral views. The collateral arteries may connect to small true pulmonary arteries, which opacify later after the selective collateral injection (Fig. 10). Occasionally, competitive flow from two different ipsilateral collateral arteries may prevent adequate delineation of the connections to true pulmonary arteries. Balloon occlusion of one collateral with selective injection in the other may be helpful in this situation (Hruda 1989).

If distinct pulmonary arteries are not seen with aortography or selective injection in the systemic to pulmonary artery collaterals, it is often possible to demonstrate these vessels using pulmonary vein wedge angiography (Fig. 11) (Nihill 1978). This technique is easily performed if an interatrial communication is present and if the

atrial septum is intact, the transseptal technique may be used (Fig. 12).

The demonstration of the degree of separation between the right ventricular outflow tract and the main pulmonary artery is also an important part of the angiocardiographic evaluation of patients with tetralogy of Fallot and pulmonary atresia. This is done by comparing the position of the most distal portion of the right ventricular outflow tract on the hand injection in this area, with the most proximal position of the main pulmonary artery as seen in other studies. An even better evaluation of this atretic segment can be obtained by simultaneous injection of a small amount of contrast material in the right ventricular outflow tract and a large injection at whatever site best opacifies the main pulmonary artery. Although this technique is of little importance in patients with extremely hypoplastic pulmonary arteries, it may have considerable value in the occasional patient with a large main pulmonary artery and a short atretic segment in whom reconstruction of the right ventricular outflow tract is possible.

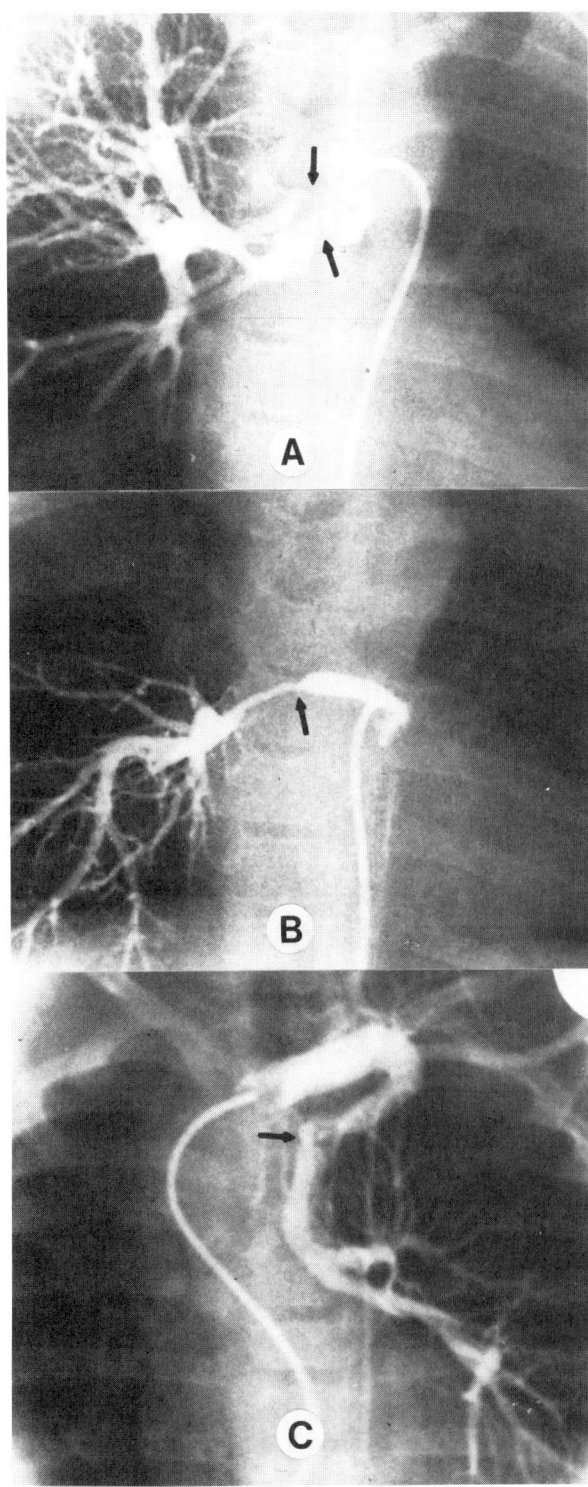

Figure 10. Selective injections in multiple systemic to pulmonary collaterals in a patient with tetralogy of Fallot and pulmonary atresia. Note area of stenosis in the collaterals (arrows).

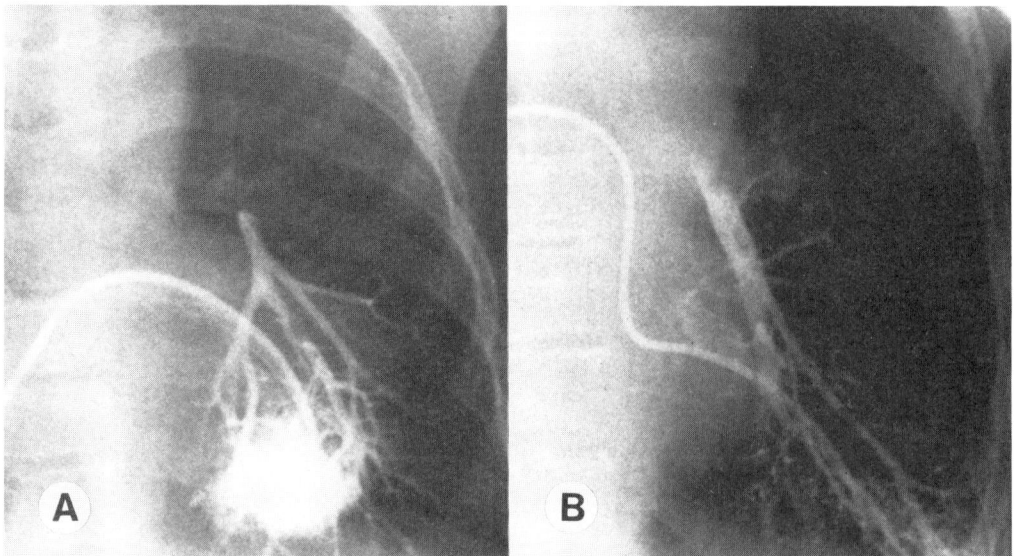

Figure 11. Pulmonary vein wedge angiogram in tetralogy of Fallot and pulmonary atresia demonstrating left lower lobe pulmonary artery.

Associated Lesions

The associated abnormalities seen in these patients are similar to those found in

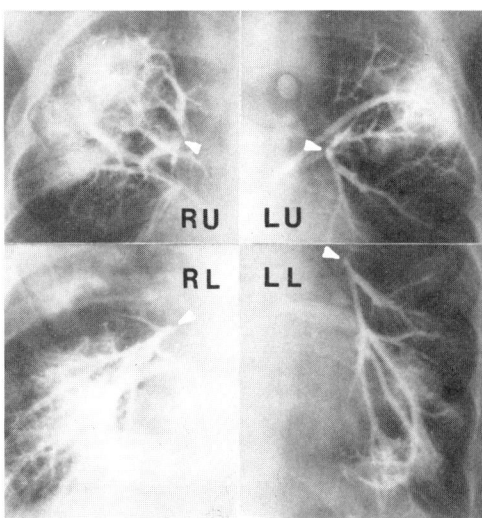

Figure 12. Transseptal pulmonary vein wedge angiograms in tetralogy of Fallot and pulmonary atresia demonstrating the the true pulmonary arteries (arrows). LL = Left lower. LU = Left upper. RL = Right lower. RU = Right upper.

patients with tetralogy of Fallot. Aortography should be performed to determine the presence or absence of aortic regurgitation and to evaluate the coronary artery anatomy. An abnormality of the origin of the left anterior descending coronary artery is not as serious an impediment to the surgical repair in these patients as in tetralogy of Fallot with pulmonary stenosis, because most patients with associated pulmonary atresia will require a right ventricle to pulmonary artery conduit. An interatrial communication should be sought. The importance of pulmonary artery abnormalities has already been emphasized. Lastly, abnormalities of pulmonary venous drainage are extremely unusual but it is still a good idea to make certain that these vessels drain normally.

References and Suggested Reading

Blackstone EH, Kirklin JW, Bertranou EG, et al. Preoperative prediction from cineangiograms of postrepair right ventricular pressure in tetralogy of Fallot. J Thorac Cardiovasc Surg 1979;78:542–552.

Fischer DR, Park SC, Neches WH, et al. Successful dilatation of a stenotic Blalock-Taussig anastomosis by percutaneous transluminal balloon angioplasty. Am J Cardiol 1985;56:861–862.

Hruda J, Julsrud PR. Diagnostic selective balloon occlusion technique in pulmonary valve atresia and ventricular septal defect. Am J Cardiol 1989;63:1408–1409.

Liao P, Edwards WD, Julsrud PR, et al. Pulmonary blood supply in patients with pulmonary atresia and ventricular septal defect. J Am Coll Cardiol 1985;6:1343–1350.

Mullins CE, O'Laughlin MP, Vick GW, et al. Implantation of balloon-expandable intravascular grafts by catheterization in pulmonary arteries and systemic veins. Circulation 1988;77:188–189.

Nakata S, Imai Y, Takanashi Y, et al. A new method for the quantitative standardization of cross-sectional areas of the pulmonary arteries in congenital heart disease with decreased pulmonary blood flow. J Thorac Cardiovasc Surg 1984;88:610–619.

Neches WH, Park SC, Mathews RA, et al. Tetralogy of Fallot. Postoperative electrophyisologic studies. Circulation 1977;56:713–719.

Nihill MR, Mullins CE, McNamara DG. Visualization of the pulmonary arteries in pseudotruncus by pulmonary vein wedge angiography. Circulation 1978;58:140–147.

Soto B, Pacifico AD, Ceballos R, et al. Tetralogy of Fallot: An angiographic-pathologic correlative study. Circulation 1981;64:558–566.

Wright JGC, Arnold R, Bini RM, et al. Percutaneous balloon dilation of right ventricular outflow tract and pulmonary valve in patient with tetralogy of Fallot. Br Heart J 1986;55:516–517.

26

Double Outlet Right Ventricle

Elfriede Pahl, M.D.

The term double outlet right ventricle represents a wide spectrum of anatomic abnormalities, and disagreement regarding classification and definition of this malformation persists. Some believe that double outlet right ventricle should be diagnosed only when there is mitral-great artery discontinuity (i.e., a bilateral infundibulum), and that substantial separation between the mitral valve and a semilunar valve must exist (Baron 1971). Others define double outlet right ventricle solely as a specific ventriculoarterial connection in that both great arteries have more than 50% of their origin from the right ventricle (50% rule), regardless of the presence or absence of mitral-aortic discontinuity (Leu 1972; Tynan 1977). Nevertheless, this entity refers to a diverse group of defects with common origin of both great arteries primarily from the right ventricle.

If the ventriculoarterial connection view is applied, a tetralogy of Fallot with moderate aortic override can be regarded as a double outlet connection, while remaining a tetralogy morphologically. Consequently, this definition has the inherent problem of being dependent on a precise determination of the extent of override of the aorta or pulmonary artery by echocardiography or angiocardiography. In many situations, this is difficult even by inspection of the pathological specimen. In spite of these difficulties, an attempt will be made to describe the broad categories of variation that are found in patients with this anomaly, defined from the morphologic and physiologic perspective rather than from the connection point of view.

Anatomy

Morphologically, double outlet right ventricle consists of a continuum of defects, depending upon the anatomic variables associated with the common origin of both great arteries from the right ventricle. The most important variables are the location of the ventricular septal defect, the spatial relationships of the great arteries, and the presence of pulmonary or aortic outflow obstruction. The ventricular septal defect may be related predominantly to the aorta (subaortic), to the pulmonary artery (subpulmonic), to both great arteries (doubly committed subarterial), or to neither (noncommitted) (Fig. 1). The ventricular septal defect is commonly large and unrestrictive although a small restrictive defect may be found in the subaortic variety.

In the normal heart, the pulmonary valve is anterior, superior, and to the left, of the aortic valve. In double outlet right ventricle, the spacial arrangement of the great arteries is variable, although the classic description is for side-by-side vessels with their respective semilunar valves at the same height. This elevation of the aortic valve in relationship to the pulmonary valve is a result of the subaortic infundibulum. However, in many cases of double outlet right ventricle, the great arteries are not side-by-side and may have a normal (pul-

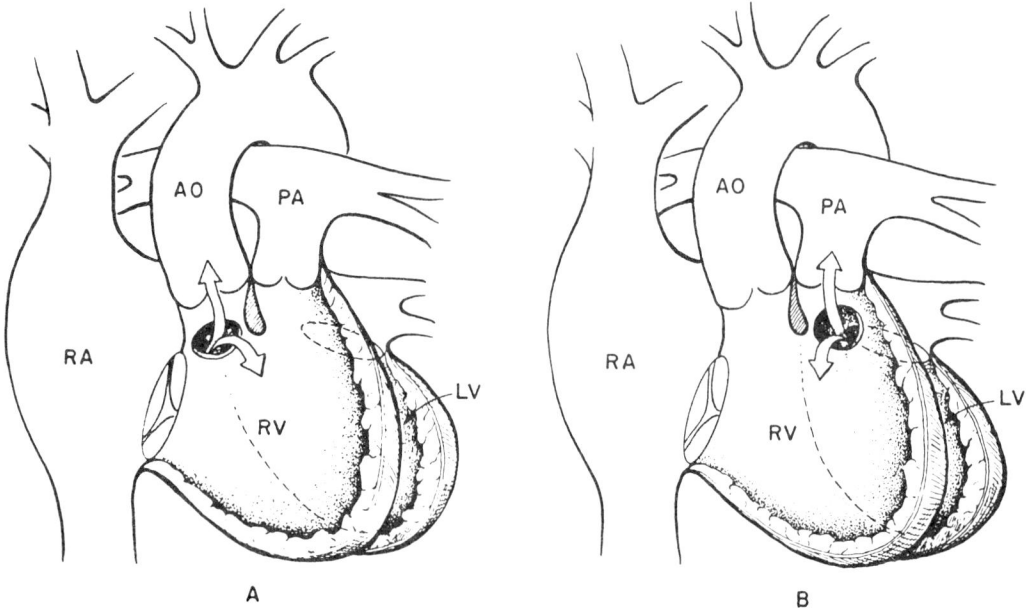

Figure 1. Diagram of double outlet right ventricle. A: With a subaortic ventricular septal defect (VSD). B: With a subpulmonary VSD (Taussig-Bing anomaly). Ao = aorta; LV = left ventricle; PA = pulmonary artery; RA = right atrium; RV = right ventricle.

monary valve anterior and to the left) or a spatial relationship similar to transposition of the great arteries (aortic valve anterior).

Outflow obstruction may be found bilaterally. In the pulmonary outflow, this may be valvar or infundibular and is common in association with a subaortic ventricular septal defect. Aortic outflow obstruction, if present, is usually subvalvar and is caused by the bilateral infundibulum.

Hemodynamic Considerations

In most cases of double outlet right ventricle the ventricular septal defect is large and the ventricular pressures are equal. A gradient between the left and right ventricle of more than 5 mm Hg confirms the presence of a restrictive defect. Furthermore, a gradient between either ventricle and the aorta suggests subaortic obstruction, due to either the subaortic infundibulum or to a restrictive ventricular septal defect as the sole outlet of the left ventricle. When the ventricular septal defect is subaortic, subpulmonic obstruction is common and patients will clinically appear to have tetralogy of Fallot, with the presence or absence of cyanosis dependent upon the degree of obstruction. However, if no pulmonary stenosis exists and the ventricular septal defect is large and subaortic, the pulmonary artery pressure will be elevated and pulmonary vascular resistance may be increased.

On the other hand, if the defect is subpulmonic, the clinical presentation is that of transposition of the great arteries with a large ventricular septal defect. Despite having considerably increased pulmonary blood flow, these patients are usually quite cyanotic because left ventricular outflow is directed to the pulmonary artery and systemic venous inflow is directed to the aorta. Some would call this group the "Taussig-Bing" anomaly (Taussig 1949). Left ventricular outflow tract obstruction, or mitral valve or aortic arch abnormalities are associated with this subgroup.

Indications for Cardiac Catheterization

Cardiac catheterization should be performed preoperatively in all patients with double outlet right ventricle. Although the majority, if not all, anatomic features may be identified accurately by cross-sectional echocardiography, hemodynamic information is essential before deciding the ideal timing and best approach for surgery. In addition, ventricular angiography will confirm the location, size, and number of ventricular septal defects, as well as define the spatial relationship of the great arteries, and identify the degree of subaortic or subpulmonic stenosis.

Cardiac catheterization should be performed in infants with subaortic ventricular septal defects and congestive heart failure unresponsive to medical therapy, in anticipation of corrective surgery or palliation with pulmonary banding. Hemodynamic investigation is indicated if pulmonary hypertension is suspected in an asymptomatic patient before 6 months of age. If significant pulmonic obstruction is suggested by echo/Doppler study, catheterization is recommended electively at 12 months of age in anticipation of repair, or sooner if cyanosis is moderately severe and surgical intervention is contemplated. All infants with cyanosis, a subpulmonic ventricular septal defect, and transposition physiology should undergo cardiac catheterization once an echocardiographic diagnosis is made. Balloon atrial septostomy is indicated if the interatrial communication is restrictive and surgical repair is to be delayed.

Postoperatively, cardiac catheterization may be helpful in determining the extent or development of subaortic or subpulmonic obstruction, or in defining any residual ventricular defect. If pulmonary artery banding was performed for palliation, catheterization is also indicated before corrective surgery is undertaken.

Catheterization Technique

A standard protocol is followed to obtain access, generally from a femoral approach. The complete study can often be performed solely from the venous approach. Blood samples for oxygen saturation are obtained from all sites. Usually, an end-hole catheter is used initially to enter the pulmonary artery and obtain pressures and saturations. If pulmonary hypertension is present, pulmonary artery wedge pressures should be obtained to rule out pulmonary vein stenosis or other left heart inflow obstructive lesions, such as mitral valve stenosis. Hemodynamic and oximetric data also should be obtained in 100% oxygen if pulmonary hypertension is present.

In most cases, the aorta is right of the pulmonary artery and usually can be entered from the right ventricle. After an arterial blood sample is obtained, a withdrawal pressure is recorded from aorta to right ventricle. We prefer to use a woven Dacron catheter for these initial studies, although in many centers a flow-directed balloon catheter is used. A flow-directed catheter may be useful to enter the aorta if a Dacron catheter pass is unsuccessful, particularly when an aortic arch anomaly such as a coarctation of the aorta is suspected. In this case, the catheter should be advanced from the ascending aorta to the descending aorta to measure the gradient.

If an interatrial communication exists, the catheter can be passed from left atrium to left ventricle with the aid of a guidewire (see Chapter 5). If this is not feasible, it may be possible to enter the left ventricle by passing the prograde catheter across the ventricular septal defect when it is being withdrawn from the aorta to the right ventricle. This is accomplished by maintaining counterclockwise torque on the catheter while it is withdrawn (see Chapter 5). From the retrograde arterial approach, a catheter passed across the aortic valve usually enters the right, rather than the left ventricle. However, a retrograde catheter that enters the right ventricle can be manipulated through the ventricular defect into the left ventricle by maneuvering the curved catheter tip in a posterior and leftward direction against the ventricular septum as the catheter is withdrawn to the aortic root. Lastly, transseptal puncture of an intact atrial septum also can be used to obtain left atrial and ventricular access.

Hemodynamic Evaluation

Pressure Data

Since the ventricular septal defect is usually large and unrestrictive, right and left ventricular pressures are equal. Pulmonary stenosis may be present to any degree and if significant, the pulmonary artery pressure will be low and the pulmonary vascular bed protected. Conversely, in the absence of pulmonary stenosis, pulmonary hypertension is present and pulmonary vascular disease will occur eventually. Occasionally, there may be a restrictive interventricular communication, with resultant left ventricular outflow obstruction (Fig. 2). In this situation, the left ventricular pressure exceeds right ventricular, aortic, or pulmonary artery pressure. Thus, in the setting of double outlet right ventricle, with equal right ventricular and aortic pressures, it is always crucial to measure the left ventricular pressure to rule out a restrictive interventricular communication (Marin-Garcia 1978). An unusual situation with a tunnel-like structure may produce restrictive communications between the tunnel, the aorta, and both ventricles (Neches 1976). In the Taussig-Bing type anomaly with a subpulmonic ventricular septal defect, systolic pressures are usually equal in both ventricles and great vessels, unless subaortic stenosis exists.

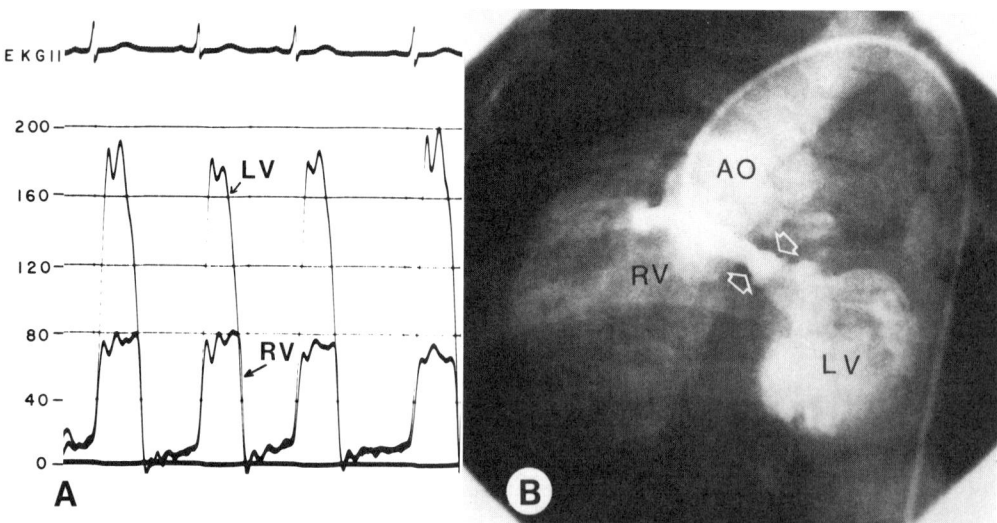

Figure 2. Double outlet right ventricle with a restrictive ventricular septal defect (VSD). A: Pressure tracing showing a left ventricular pressure B: Selective left ventricular angiocardiogram in the four-chamber view demonstrating a tunnel-like, long, restrictive ventricular septal defect (arrows). AO = aorta. LV = left ventricle; RV = right ventricle.

Oxygen Saturation Data

Oxygen saturations are obtained in all cardiac chambers, great vessels and the superior vena cava. An increase in oxygen saturation in the right atrium suggests an atrial septal defect, while an increase in the right ventricle is from the ventricular septal defect. Without subpulmonic obstruction, a further step-up may be evident in the pulmonary artery. Patients with tetralogy of Fallot physiology manifest aortic desaturation consistent with a net right to left shunt. In patients with double outlet right ventricle and a subpulmonary ventricular septal defect (the so-called Taussig-Bing anomaly), the pulmonary artery receives the left ventricular blood, as it does in complete transposition of the great arteries (Fig. 1). In these anomalies with transposition physiology, pulmonary artery saturation substantially exceeds aortic saturation by greater than 10%. Pulmonary stenosis rarely accompanies the Taussig-Bing anomaly, and pulmonary hypertension is the rule.

Angiocardiography

Ventricular angiography is crucial in defining the anatomy, and 1 to 1.5 mL/kg of contrast is used for each angiogram. The most important distinguishing features of double outlet right ventricle are visualized on right ventricular angiogram and are related to the presence of bilateral infundibula supporting both the aorta and pulmonary artery, and origin of both vessels primarily from the right ventricle. If the infundibula are of nearly equal length, the aortic and pulmonic valves are at the same horizontal level, which is best shown in the anteroposterior view. This view also shows the abnormal orientation of the infundibular outlet septum, which is at a nearly right angle to the rest of the septum and appears as a "tear drop" separating the aorta and pulmonary artery (Fig. 3A). This orientation of the infundibular septum also results in a side-by-side relationship of the great arteries in the anteroposterior view. Because the arteries

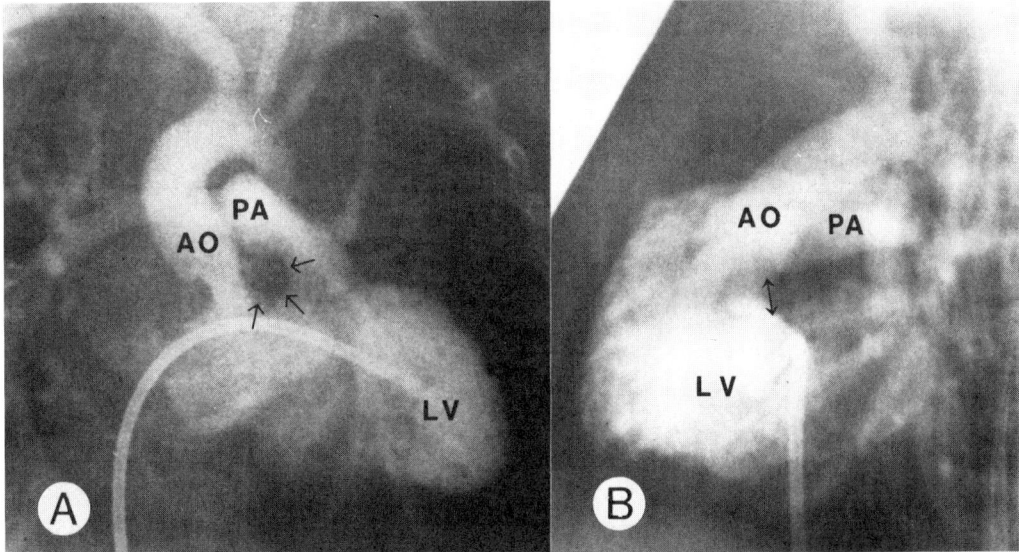

Figure 3. Selective left ventricular angiocardiogram in double outlet right ventricle. A: Anteroposterior view showing the "teardrop" of the bilateral infundibulum (arrows). B: Lateral view showing discontinuity between the mitral valve and the aortic valve (arrow). AO = aorta; LV = left ventricle; PA = pulmonary artery.

do not spiral, and are parallel as they ascend from the heart, they are often superimposed in the lateral view of the ventricular angiogram.

The bilateral infundibula also result in discontinuity between the mitral and semilunar valves. This is best seen in the lateral or long axial oblique projection of a left ventricular angiogram (Fig. 3B), but may also be evident in the anteroposterior view. A short infundibulum may not be apparent angiographically.

The location of the ventricular defect with respect to the aorta and pulmonary artery is an important variable, but may be difficult to define angiographically. Left ventricular angiograms in multiple views are usually required, including standard anteroposterior and lateral, oblique and craniocaudal views. A membranous defect is usually subaortic but may be subpulmonic (Fig. 4). A defect in the inlet septum is usually noncommitted, and will be present with an atrioventricular septal defect. An outlet defect is usually subpulmonic but may be doubly committed. Aortic root angiography

should be performed to delineate coronary arterial anatomy, and the aortic arch should be imaged to exclude coarctation of the aorta or brachiocephalic vessel abnormalities.

Associated Lesions

Aortic and pulmonic stenosis (valvar and subvalvar) may be associated with this lesion and already have been mentioned. Patients with infundibular pulmonary stenosis may have an anomalous coronary artery branch crossing the right ventricular outflow tract as is also seen in tetralogy of Fallot. Interrupted aortic arch and coarctation of the aorta are found in association with double outlet right ventricle, particularly when there is a subpulmonic ventricular septal defect ("Taussig-Bing" complex). Mitral valve abnormalities and subaortic obstruction also occur in this group. Other defects such as a patent ductus arteriosus, atrial septal defect, atrioventricular septal defect, and total anomalous pulmonary ve-

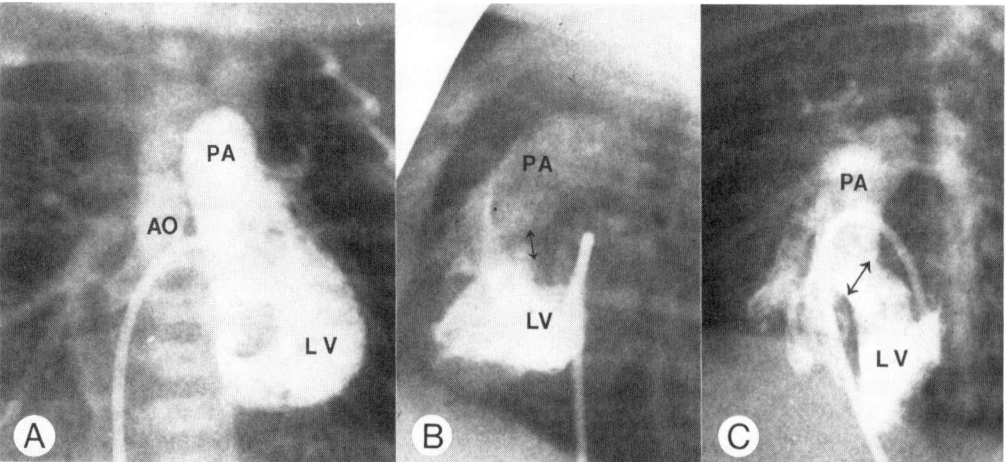

Figure 4. Selective left ventricular angiogram demonstrating the Taussig-Bing anomaly. A: Anteroposterior view demonstrating side by side great arteries with predominant flow from the left ventricle into the pulmonary arteries. B: Lateral view demonstrating mitral-pulmonary discontinuity (arrow). C: Four-chamber view demonstrating right ventricular origin of the pulmonary artery and a large ventricular septal defect (arrow). AO = aorta. LV = left ventricle. PA = pulmonary artery.

nous return also may be seen in association with double outlet right ventricle. Careful cross-sectional and Doppler echocardiographic study should be performed to rule out these anomalies prior to catheterization.

Cautions and Precautions

Catheter manipulations may be intense or difficult and may result in atrioventricular block or arrhythmia. If a catheter pass is difficult, the use of a flow-directed balloon catheter is important to minimize potential myocardial trauma. Hemodynamically significant or surgically important associated lesions such as a restrictive ventricular septal defect, coarctation of the aorta, coronary anomalies, or mitral stenosis are common in patients with double outlet right ventricle. Each of these anomalies must be specifically eliminated by appropriate hemodynamic measurements or angiographic delineation.

If a large left to right shunt through a ventricular septal defect is present, high doses of contrast, as much as 1.5 to 2.0 mL/kg, may be needed and nonionic contrast may be preferable. Because a number of angiograms will be required it is important to watch for volume overload, especially in small sick infants.

Patients with severe pulmonary stenosis may react in a similar fashion to those with tetralogy of Fallot when a catheter is passed across the area of subpulmonary stenosis. This may precipitate a hypoxemic spell and one should be prepared to treat this with oxygen, morphine, volume infusion, or propranolol.

If a subpulmonary ventricular defect (Taussig-Bing anomaly) is found and immediate operation is not contemplated, a balloon septostomy should be performed to facilitate atrial mixing and reduce cyanosis.

References and Suggested Reading

Baron MG. Radiologic notes in cardiology—angiographic differentiation between tetralogy of Fallot and double outlet right ventricle. Relationship of the mitral and aortic valve. Circulation 1971;43:451–455.

Leu M, Bharati S, Meng CCL, et al. A concept of double outlet right ventricle. J Thorac Cardiovasc Surg 1972;64:271–281.

Marin-Garcia J, Neches WH, Park SC, et al. Double outlet right ventricle with restrictive ventricular septal defect. J Thorac Cardiovasc Surg 1978;76:853–858.

Neches WH, Dankner E, Park SC, et al. Double outlet right ventricle with tunnel from left ventricle to aorta. J Thorac Cardiovasc Surg 1976;71:685–690.

Taussig HB, Bing RJ. Complete transposition of the aorta and a levoposition of the pulmonary artery. Am Heart J 1949;37:551–559.

Tynan MJ, Anderson RH, Macartney FJ, et al. The ventricular origin of the great arteries. In: Pediatric Cardiology. Edinburgh, Churchill Livingstone. 1987;36–42.

27

Transposition of the Great Arteries

Lee B. Beerman, M.D.

Transposition of the great arteries (or complete transposition) is a serious anomaly whose devastating natural history has been transformed by aggressive diagnostic and therapeutic interventions. The noninvasive techniques now available to the pediatric cardiologist complement cardiac catheterization in the management of these patients, and in many cases may be the only studies performed prior to an arterial switch operation in a newborn. However, a number of catheterizations are often still required in early childhood. The clinical settings in which these studies are indicated include: the acutely ill cyanotic newborn who needs a balloon atrial septostomy; preoperative evaluation of an infant awaiting an elective atrial baffle procedure or a delayed arterial switch operation; and postoperative assessment of residual hemodynamic, anatomic and electrophysiologic abnormalities.

Anatomy

Transposition of the great arteries is characterized by ventriculoarterial discordance, the right ventricle giving rise to the aorta and the left ventricle to the pulmonary artery (Figs. 1 and 2). The aorta usually lies directly in front of or slightly to the right of the pulmonary artery, but rarely it may be to the left. The most common associated intracardiac anomaly is a ventricular septal defect, which is present in 40% of patients. These are usually perimembranous in location, but muscular and doubly committed

subarterial defects also occur. Left ventricular outflow tract obstruction is present in one third of cases and often coexists with a ventricular septal defect. This obstruction is subvalvar in the great majority of cases. When the ventricular septum is intact, the most common cause of left ventricular outflow obstruction is a dynamic bulging of the upper portion of the septum into the outflow tract, resulting in close apposition between the septum and the anterior leaflet of the mitral valve. When a ventricular defect is present, this same mechanism may occur.

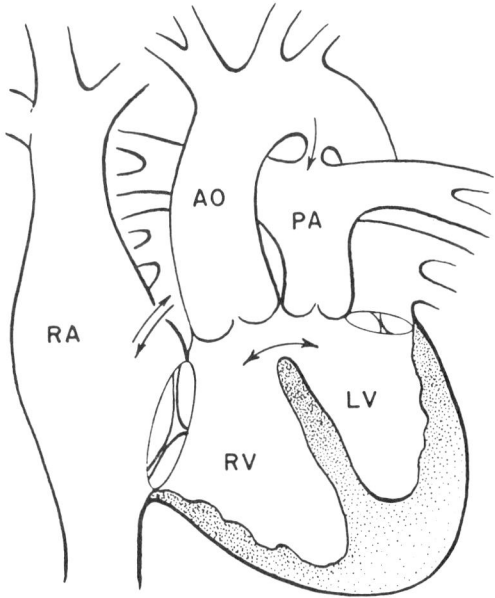

Figure 1. Diagram of transposition of the great arteries with sites of potential mixing: atrial, ventricular, and ductal communications.

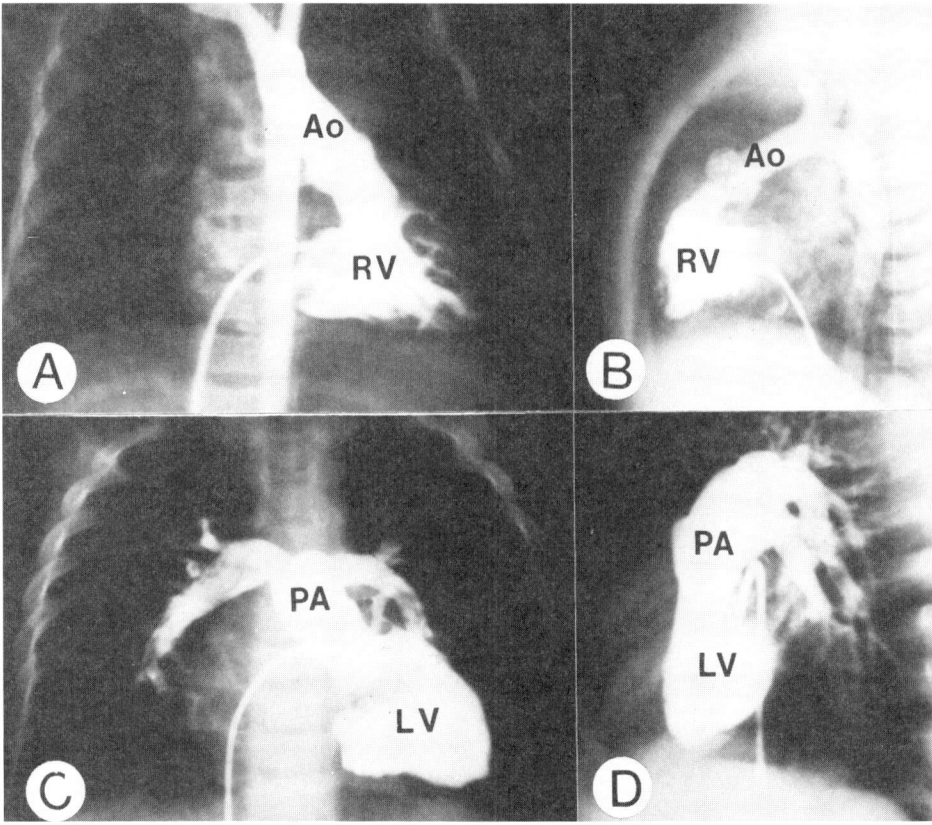

Figure 2. Selective ventricular angiocardiograms in transposition of the great arteries. Top: Right ventricular injection in the anteroposterior (A) and lateral (B) views demonstrating filling of the anteriorly positioned aorta. Bottom: Left ventricular injection in the anteroposterior (C) and lateral (D) views demonstrating filling of the posteriorly positioned pulmonary artery. AO = aorta; LV = left ventricle; PA = pulmonary artery; RV = right ventricle.

However, other causes should be considered and include a discrete subvalvar membrane, a posterior deviation of the outlet septum creating a subpulmonic tunnel, "aneurysmal tissue" arising from the environs of the membranous septum, and valvar pulmonic stenosis. A patent ductus arteriosus is usually present in a newborn, but persistent patency is uncommon. Other less common associated abnormalities include right aortic arch, coarctation of the aorta, varying degrees of hypoplasia of the right ventricle, mitral valve anomalies, and an overriding tricuspid valve when an inlet ventricular septal defect is present. Variations in coronary ar-

tery anatomy have become extremely important in the current era of the arterial switch approach to operative repair.

Hemodynamic Considerations

Transposition of the great arteries results in the systemic and pulmonary circulations being parallel rather than in series. This leads to profound hypoxemia shortly after birth and is incompatible with life unless there is some mixing of the circulations.

This mixing can take place at the atrial, ventricular, or great arterial level. Because newborns usually have a degree of incompetence of the flap of the foramen ovale, a variable amount of highly saturated left atrial blood crosses to the right atrium and enters the systemic circulation. In general, the degree of aortic hypoxemia is inversely related to the size of the interatrial communication. Defects of the ventricular septum, or aorta to pulmonary artery communications such as a patent ductus arteriosus or systemic to pulmonary collateral arteries, result in better systemic saturation.

In the usual patient with transposition, superior vena caval saturation is very low and there is a variable oxygen step-up in the right atrium, depending on the degree of interatrial mixing. There may be a further oxygen step-up in the right ventricle if a large ventricular septal defect is present. Left atrial and left ventricular oxygen saturations are usually quite high, sometimes approaching 100% in a very sick newborn. Pulmonary artery oxygen saturation is always higher than aortic oxygen saturation and this finding is strongly suggestive of transposition of the greater arteries, although it may also occur with other lesions such as the Taussig-Bing complex (double outlet right ventricle with subpulmonic ventricular septal defect) or total anomalous pulmonary venous return.

Pressure data are variable and depend upon factors such as left ventricular outflow tract obstruction, the size of an associated ventricular septal defect or patent ductus arteriosus, and the level of pulmonary vascular resistance. In a patient with uncomplicated transposition, the left ventricular pressure is less than the aortic pressure and this finding is diagnostic. Left and right atrial mean pressures are nearly identical in the presence of a large atrial defect, while elevation of the left atrial pressure with a significant gradient between the two atrial chambers indicates a restrictive interatrial communication.

Pulmonary and systemic flows and re-

sistances may be calculated as in any catheterization study. In patients with transposition of the great arteries, however, there are several potential sources of error in these calculations that limit their usefulness (Rudolph 1974). If oxygen consumption is not measured, a significant error may be introduced by using an assumed oxygen consumption, because the actual consumption may be reduced in a severely hypoxemic infant. Also, because both systemic and pulmonary arteriovenous oxygen content differences are quite small, minor errors in determining saturations produce large errors in calculated flows. Still another error is introduced if systemic-pulmonary collateral circulation is large, because relatively unsaturated systemic arterial blood enters the pulmonary circuit distal to the sampling sites in the pulmonary arteries. This leads to an underestimation of pulmonary blood flow by over estimating the pulmonary arteriovenous difference. A final factor peculiar to transposition of the great arteries is uneven pulmonary perfusion, with the right pulmonary artery flow usually being greater than the left. Keeping the above limitations in mind, pulmonary and systemic flows and pulmonary and systemic resistances can be calculated by standard techniques.

The terms "anatomic" and "physiologic" shunt were introduced by Rudolph (1974) to facilitate understanding of the hemodynamics of TGA. The "anatomic" left to right shunt is the actual volume of blood which passes from the left to the right heart, and can also be referred to as "effective systemic flow" (i.e., volume of pulmonary capillary blood perfusing the systemic circulation). The "anatomic" right to left shunt is the volume of blood flowing from the right to the left heart, and is the "effective pulmonary flow" (i.e., volume of systemic venous blood perfusing the pulmonary circulation). Necessarily, in a steady state, anatomic left to right and right to left shunts (and effective pulmonary and systemic flows) must be equal. The "physiologic" left to right shunt is the volume of pulmonary venous return that recirculates through the pulmonary bed without an intervening course through the systemic circuit. Similarly, the "physiologic" right to left shunt is the volume of systemic venous return that goes directly back out the aorta. Thus, from the above, pulmonary blood flow equals effective pulmonary blood flow plus the physiologic left to right shunt, and systemic blood flow equals effective systemic blood flow plus the physiologic right to left shunt. The chief value of these calculations is in aiding understanding that, in transposition, the larger the anatomic shunt the higher the systemic saturation.

Indications for Cardiac Catheterization

Any newborn with cyanosis should have an accurate diagnosis expeditiously established by echocardiography. Usually, definitive anatomic and hemodynamic data can be obtained by a combination of imaging and Doppler studies. Once the diagnosis of transposition of the great arteries is made by these noninvasive studies, the infant should be started on a prostaglandin E$_1$ infusion. This is because even an infant with transposition who appears to be well compensated with only mild cyanosis, may experience sudden deterioration with progressive hypoxemia and acidosis as a closing ductus arteriosus and/or foramen ovale lead to inadequate mixing. The decision to perform a catheterization in the newborn period is dependent on several factors including response of the infant to the prostaglandin infusion, institutional preference for operative approach (i.e., early arterial switch versus delayed atrial baffle procedure), and the surgeon's comfort with the Doppler and cross-sectional echocardiographic diagnostic data.

Although most infants respond well to prostaglandin with a significant increase in arterial oxygenation, some will not respond adequately and occasionally an infant will actually deteriorate. This poor response is due to an extremely restrictive interatrial communication and demands urgent catheterization in order to perform a balloon septostomy. If the infant is stable with an adequate systemic saturation and an arterial switch operation is planned within the first week of life, cardiac catheterization may not be necessary. However, some institutions prefer to proceed with a balloon septostomy despite clinical stability in order to be able to discontinue prostaglandins prior to surgery. Furthermore, catheterization allows angiographic delineation of coronary artery anatomy that may be desired by some surgeons.

If early surgical repair is not performed, neonatal catheterization and balloon septostomy are performed. Repeat catheterization prior to an atrial baffle procedure or a delayed arterial switch may be indicated. The purpose of this study would be to redefine associated defects and measure pulmonary arterial and left ventricular pressure. The presence of left ventricular outflow tract obstruction, which usually develops after the newborn period, needs to be assessed. If an arterial switch procedure is being considered, pulmonary artery and left ventricular pressures must be determined.

Routine postoperative catheterization is performed within 1 or 2 years of the operation. This recommendation is made even if the child is clinically well, because significant hemodynamic abnormalities (e.g., pulmonary or systemic venous obstruction following an atrial baffle procedure, or pulmonary arterial stenosis or coronary artery anomalies after an arterial switch operation) may be present without clinical signs or symptoms (Hagler et al. 1978; Park et al. 1983, Wernovsky, 1988). If the patient is not doing well postoperatively, catheterization should be performed as soon as it is evident that improvement is not occurring.

Cardiac Catheterization Technique

Newborn Catheterization

Essential supportive care for these often critically ill neonates involves the recognition and management of the following problems:

1. Hypothermia—The infant should be placed on a heating pad during the procedure and rectal temperatures should be continuously monitored.
2. Metabolic acidosis—Blood gases should be monitored by an umbilical artery line with administration of bicarbonate as needed.
3. Severe hypoxemia—Umbilical artery line monitoring may indicate severe and progressive hypoxemia demanding urgent balloon septostomy. Prostaglandin infusion is important in this situation. Continuous transcutaneous pulse oximetry monitoring should be utilized allowing early recognition of a deteriorating clinical status.
4. Congestive heart failure—This is unusual within the first week of life, but requires digoxin and diuretic therapy when it occurs. Intravenous inotropic support may be required.
5. Respiratory insufficiency—Sedation should be avoided and ventilatory support should be provided as needed. Hypoventilation or apnea are common side effects of a prostaglandin infusion.
6. Hypovolemia and blood loss— This may be related to perinatal complications or iatrogenic blood loss during the procedure. Furthermore, prostaglandin may

cause relative hypovolemia and hypotension due to systemic vasodilation. A type and cross match should always be done so that packed red cells are available if needed. Blood pressure, central venous or right atrial pressure and hemoglobin level should be monitored during the catheterization.

Initially, a #5 French feeding tube or umbilical artery catheter is inserted into the umbilical artery and advanced into the descending aorta to monitor arterial blood gases and systemic pressure throughout the procedure. It also may be useful for aortography if the venous catheter does not pass easily from the right ventricle to the aorta. The umbilical vein can be used for both diagnostic studies and balloon atrial septostomy (Porter et al. 1978). This technique has the advantage of preserving the inguinal region for future catheterizations and eliminating the risk of ileofemoral thrombosis, a common complication in this setting (Mathews et al. 1979). Disadvantages of this approach include a high likelihood of nonpatency of the ductus venosus after 48 hours and a frequently difficult pass into the right ventricle from the right atrium.

If the umbilical venous route is not used, a catheter is inserted into the right femoral venous system, either percutaneously, or by a cutdown exposing the saphenous bulb and common femoral vein. Care must be taken to select a site for venous entry large enough to accommodate a septostomy catheter. The percutaneous technique requires the use of a #6 or #7 French sheath to accommodate the septostomy catheter.

Because there is rarely uncertainty regarding the diagnosis of transposition of the great arteries following an adequate echocardiographic examination, limited hemodynamic and angiographic data are required. In general, balloon septostomy should be performed before the other studies.

Although several catheters are available for performing balloon atrial septostomy, we prefer a #5 French Fogarty balloon septostomy catheter (Edwards Laboratories). If a cutdown is required, the catheter usually can be inserted into the proximal saphenous bulb, but it may be necessary to extend the venotomy into the common femoral vein. Once inserted, the catheter is advanced into the right atrium and then across the atrial septum to the left atrium. The proper location of the catheter can be confirmed by entering a pulmonary vein or, preferably, by using the lateral camera to show a posterior position of the catheter tip. Echocardiography can also be used to localize the position of the balloon catheter. In fact, in some centers echocardiography alone has been used to perform the entire balloon septostomy procedure at the bedside rather than in the cardiac catheterization laboratory. In performing balloon septostomy, whether by fluoroscopy or echocardiographic guidance, the first pullback is the most critical one in producing an adequate interatrial opening. If the balloon is not inflated sufficiently or if the pullback is too slow, the flap of the foramen ovale may be stretched rather than torn and this may preclude successful septostomy on subsequent attempts. It is important to establish a defect of at least 10 to 12 mm in diameter. A measuring pullback should be performed by slowly withdrawing the catheter from the left atrium while gradually deflating the balloon. Most of the early complications of balloon septostomy were due to balloon failure (e.g., rupture, deflation failure), and these have been essentially eliminated by technical improvements in the septostomy catheters. Other unusual complications include injury to the tricuspid or mitral valves and rupture of a pulmonary vein or the inferior vena cava. (For detailed description of balloon septostomy see Chapter 12).

After the performance of the septos-

tomy, this catheter is replaced with an NIH or angiographic flow-directed balloon catheter. If the infant is stable and no difficulties are encountered, it may be useful to obtain pressure and oximetry data from all cardiac chambers, the aorta and at least one pulmonary vein. Of particular importance are the following: aortic blood gases and saturation, right ventricular and left ventricular pressures recorded in rapid succession, and left atrial to right atrial pullback pressures. Entering the pulmonary artery is not essential in a newborn catheterization, particularly if the cross-sectional and Doppler echocardiographic studies show no left ventricular outflow tract obstruction. However, an effort should be made to enter the pulmonary artery if a left ventricular outflow tract gradient is suspected. A flow-directed catheter (e.g., Swan-Ganz) (American Edwards Labs, Irvine, CA, USA) is used (See Chapter 5). Saturation from the pulmonary artery and a pressure pullback from this vessel to the left ventricle should be recorded. In a patient with a patent ductus arteriosus, the umbilical artery catheter can sometimes be passed retrogradely across the ductus and into the main pulmonary artery. Only limited angiography is required during the newborn catheterization, with the most valuable injection being in the aortic root, to visualize and define coronary artery anatomy being the most valuable when an arterial switch procedure is anticipated. This will be discussed later in the **Angiography** section.

If a cutdown is performed and the saphenous vein or bulb is used, it is simply ligated after the catheter is removed. If the femoral vein itself is used by cutdown, repair of this vessel is optional but preferred. It is often helpful to leave the umbilical artery catheter in place for 24 hours to follow arterial blood gases in the critical hours after the catheterization.

Preoperative Catheterization

After the newborn period, the femoral vein can usually be approached by the per-

cutaneous technique. If ileofemoral thrombosis is documented, venous access may
need to be via cutdown on the brachial or
axillary vein or, as preferred at our institution, a percutaneous approach to the internal jugular vein (Chapter 4). An end-hole
flow-directed balloon catheter is used initially so that the pulmonary artery can be
entered. Pressure and oximetry data are obtained from the usual sites and the atrial defect may be measured using the technique
described in Chapter 12. After completion of
the collection of hemodynamic data, baseline preoperative electrophysiologic data
are obtained, including a His bundle recording, rapid atrial pacing and sinus node recovery time (see Chapter 10). The final step
in this catheterization is angiocardiography.
If the infant is severely hypoxemic secondary to inadequate atrial mixing, a blade atrial
septostomy should be considered at this
catheterization. (This procedure is described in detail in Chapter 12). If venous
access proves to be difficult, adequate information may be obtained from an arterial
approach and even the pulmonary artery
can be entered (Fig. 3). A deflated flow-directed balloon catheter is introduced into
the femoral artery and passed around the
aortic arch, across the aortic valve and retrogradely across the tricuspid valve (Fig.
3A). The catheter is then advanced from the
right to the left atrium and after inflating the
balloon, the left ventricle (Fig. 3B) and subsequently the pulmonary artery can be entered (Fig. 3C). If a ventricular septal defect
is present, this complex maneuver can be
simplified (Fig. 3D).

Postoperative (Atrial-Baffle) Catheterization

The route of venous entry is the same
as described in the previous section. In addition, the femoral artery should be entered
percutaneously. The procedure is begun
with insertion of an end-hole flow-directed
balloon catheter into the femoral vein and

pressure and oximetry data are obtained
from each chamber and great vessel as it is
entered. The catheter is advanced to the inferior vena cava and then into the systemic
venous atrium. From this chamber, the superior vena cava can be entered by passing
the catheter medially and then superiorly to
the right. If this soft catheter cannot be maneuvered into the superior vena cava, use of
a stiffer NIH catheter facilitates this maneuver unless caval obstruction is severe or virtually atretic. With the balloon inflated, the
flow-directed catheter passes easily from
the systemic venous atrium across the mitral valve into the left ventricle. The pulmonary artery is entered by forming a loop
in the left ventricle and orienting the balloon
superiorly and medially.

Once the catheter passes into the main
pulmonary artery, an attempt should be
made to enter both right and left branches
and obtain bilateral wedge pressures. At this
point a catheter (either an NIH or end-hole
catheter is acceptable) is inserted into the
femoral artery and advanced retrogradely
across the aortic valve into the right ventricle (see Chapter 5). Simultaneous pulmonary artery wedge and right ventricular
end-diastolic pressures should be obtained.
If no gradient is present, pulmonary venous
obstruction is ruled out and it is not necessary to enter the pulmonary venous
atrium. However, if a significant gradient exists it is useful to enter this chamber to determine the site of obstruction (see Chapter
5). The arterial catheter can be manipulated
into the proximal portion of the pulmonary
venous atrium or pulmonary veins by a passage retrogradely across the tricuspid valve.
Pressures are obtained in both portions of
the pulmonary venous atrium and an injection of contrast in the proximal chamber in
the anteroposterior and lateral views is performed.

Postoperative hemodynamic data
should include withdrawal pressure measurements from the pulmonary artery to left
ventricle, superior vena cava to systemic venous atrium, systemic venous atrium to in-

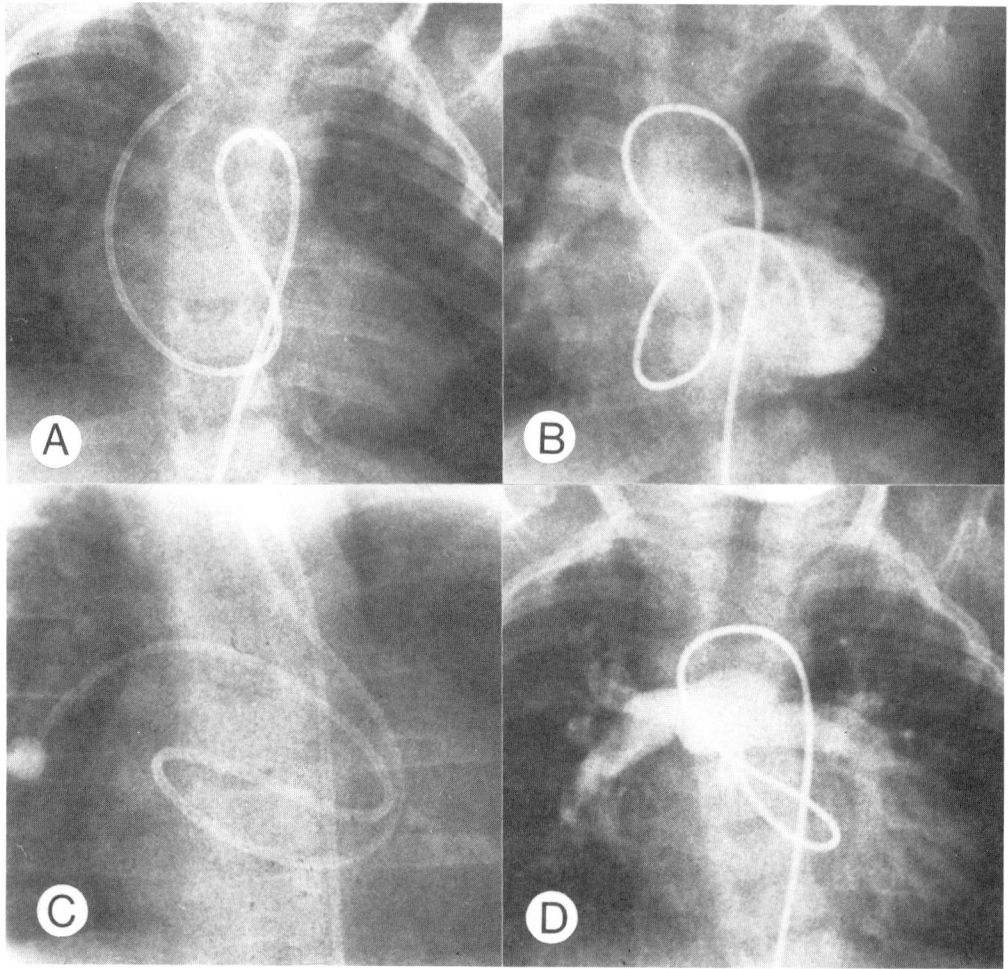

Figure 3. Retrograde arterial catheterization in transposition of the great arteries for access to the left ventricle and pulmonary artery (anteroposterior views). A: Retrograde catheter passed from the aorta to the right ventricle to right atrium to superior vena cava. B: Catheter in "A" passed across the atrial communication to left atrium and then to left ventricle. C: The same balloon catheter can then be floated into the pulmonary artery. D: When a ventricular septal defect is present, the retrograde catheter can be advanced from the right ventricle to the left ventricle and then into the pulmonary artery.

ferior vena cava, proximal pulmonary venous atrium to distal pulmonary venous atrium, and right ventricle to aorta. A simultaneous right ventricular end-diastolic and wedge pressure may be substituted for the direct pulmonary venous atrial pressures.

Cardiac output should be measured by the Fick technique measuring oxygen con-

sumption, or by thermodilution studies with an appropriate catheter in the pulmonary artery. Alternatively, indicator dilution (e.g., indocyanine green dye) studies may be utilized. Sampling is from a catheter in the aorta or femoral artery and injections are into the pulmonary artery (to determine cardiac output and to rule out a left to right shunt) and the superior and inferior vena cavae (to rule out right to left shunting across the baffle).

In our laboratory, an electrophysiologic study is done routinely at this catheterization. A #5 or #6 French multipolar catheter is inserted into the femoral artery and advanced across the aortic valve into the right ventricle. A His bundle recording can usually be obtained near the tricuspid valve (Fig. 4A). At times it may be necessary to loop the catheter and pass it into the pulmonary venous atrium as described in Chapter 5. The His bundle can often be recorded as the catheter is slowly withdrawn across the tricuspid valve. Following the His bundle study, a quadripolar catheter is inserted into the femoral vein and advanced into the systemic venous atrium. The tip of the catheter is positioned in the superior rightward portion of this chamber (Fig. 4B). The two distal electrodes can be used for atrial pacing, while the two proximal electrodes record an atrial electrogram (See Chapter 10). Resting intervals including high right atrium to low septal right atrium, AH and HV intervals are obtained. Rapid atrial pacing and single premature atrial beats introduced into a paced atrial rhythm are performed to assess AV conduction, sinus node recovery times, sinoatrial conduction time, and atrial and AV node refractory periods. These data may prove to have prognostic value, especially if a preoperative study is available for comparison. Further atrial or ventricular extrastimulus studies may be indicated in selected patients with clinically important tachyarrhythmias. Angiography should be performed following the hemodynamic and electrophysiologic studies. Specific injection sites will be discussed subsequently.

In summary, in a patient who has had an interatrial baffle procedure, the postoperative catheterization should rule out systemic and pulmonary venous obstruction, assess right ventricular and tricuspid valve function, identify residual abnormalities such as a ventricular defect, baffle leak, or left ventricular outflow tract obstruction, and document any electrophysiologic aberrations.

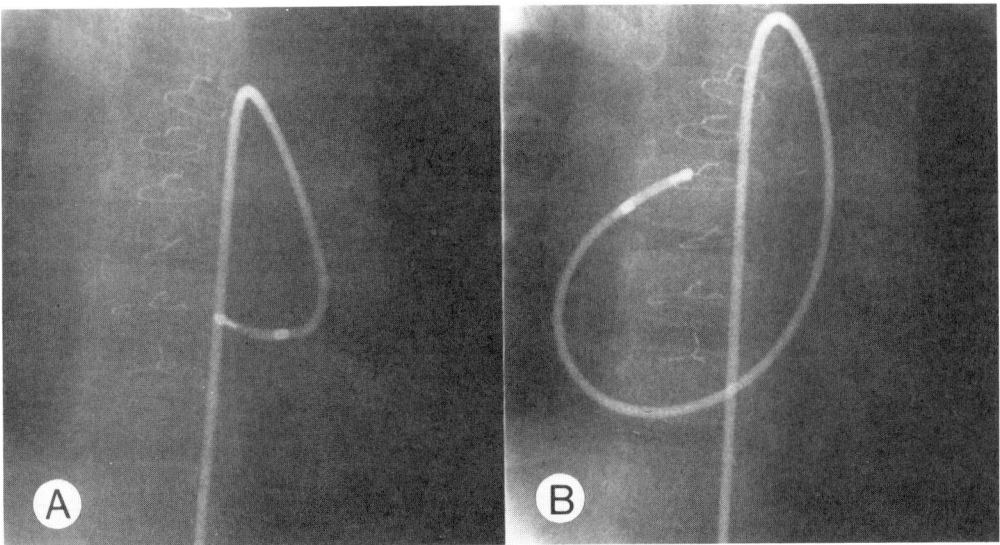

Figure 4. Catheter position for electrophysiologic studies following atrial baffle surgery. A: Retrograde catheter passed across the aortic valve and positioned near the tricuspid valve to record this His bundle. B: The catheter advanced across the tricuspid valve and positioned in the right atrium for an atrial pacing study.

Postoperative (Arterial Switch) Operation

If a patient has had an arterial switch procedure, the areas of postoperative concern are the reimplanted coronary arteries, aortic and pulmonary artery anastomoses, aortic and pulmonic valve function, and ventricular function (Wernovsky 1988). Cross-sectional and Doppler echocardiographic studies are invaluable in the assessment of these concerns. However, the possibility of coronary artery stenosis or kinking can only be adequately evaluated by aortography, or by selective coronary arteriography in selected cases.

Hemodynamic Evaluation

Newborn

In the newborn with transposition of the great arteries, superior vena caval saturation is quite low before balloon septostomy. A large step-up at atrial level suggests a sizable interatrial communication and an increase at the ventricular level suggests a ventricular septal defect. Left atrial and left ventricular saturations are usually quite high and pulmonary artery saturation is always higher than aortic saturation. Very low aortic saturation indicates inadequate mixing at any levels. Following adequate enlargement of the atrial defect by septostomy, the aortic, right ventricular and superior vena caval saturations rise and the left atrial left ventricular and pulmonary artery values decrease.

In the newborn, pressures are often similar in the right and left ventricles before balloon septostomy. This is due to the presence of pulmonary hypertension, regardless of whether a ventricular septal defect or left ventricular outflow tract obstruction are present. A left ventricular pressure lower than aortic pressure is diagnostic of transposition. If the interatrial communication is small, left atrial pressure is generally higher than right atrial, although this is not uniformly the case in the newborn period. If septostomy is successful, mean left and right atrial pressure usually equalize. "Fixed" pulmonic or subpulmonic stenosis may be present in a newborn with transposition but is rare if the ventricular septum is intact. Even "dynamic" subpulmonic stenosis in association with an intact ventricular septum is rarely seen in this age group.

Preoperative

The hemodynamic data obtained at the elective preoperative catheterization outside of the neonatal period have the same implications as in the newborn. Aortic oxygen saturation and a step-up in saturation in the right atrium and/or right ventricle reflect the adequacy of intracardiac mixing. Pulmonary artery and left ventricular pressures are critically important data because they allow evaluation of pulmonary vascular resistance and the presence and degree of left ventricular outflow obstruction. Both of these factors are extremely important in planning surgical intervention.

Postoperative

Hemodynamic data obtained at the postoperative catheterization following an atrial baffle repair should reflect normal circulatory physiology unless there are significant residual abnormalities. Mixed venous saturation in the superior vena cava is generally in the normal range. A step-up in oxygen saturation in the systemic venous atrium or left ventricle indicates trans-baffle shunting or a residual ventricular septal defect, respectively. Oxygen saturations in the pulmonary venous atrium, right ventricular, and aorta should be greater than 94%, even with drainage of the coronary sinus into the pulmonary venous atrium, unless there is right to left baffle shunting.

Left ventricular peak systolic pressure

is usually in the range of 25 to 40 mm Hg. The presence of a systolic gradient between the left ventricle and pulmonary artery indicates left ventricular outflow obstruction. Small gradients, up to 20 mm Hg, are frequently found even in the absence of anatomic pulmonic stenosis, probably due to the more acute angulation of the left ventricular outflow tract in transposition combined with mild bulging of the ventricular septum into the outflow tract. Elevation of right ventricular end-diastolic pressure suggests right ventricular dysfunction. Pressure gradients between the superior and inferior vena cavae and the systemic venous atrium indicate systemic venous obstruction from the baffle (Fig. 5). Similarly, obstruction within the pulmonary venous return pathway is reflected by a pulmonary artery wedge pressure higher than the right ventricular end-diastolic pressure. If the pulmonary artery wedge pressure is elevated, the pressure within the pulmonary venous atrium should be measured with the arterial catheter passed retrogradely across the tricuspid valve as was described earlier in this chapter (Fig. 6).

Hemodynamic data following an arterial switch procedure should be normal if there are no residual intracardiac defects or great vessel anastomotic stenoses. Since supravalvar pulmonic artery stenosis is the most common hemodynamic abnormality, a careful measurement of pressure in both distal pulmonary arteries with withdrawal into the main pulmonary artery and right ventricle is important. Elevation of end-diastolic pressure in the right or left ventricle reflects abnormal function of that chamber.

Angiocardiography

Preoperative

In the past, selective ventricular angiography was required to establish a diagnosis of transposition of the great arteries (Fig. 2). Today, in view of the usually precise anatomic information that can be obtained by cross-sectional and Doppler echocardiography, angiography should be limited to defining abnormalities or structures that are not visualized adequately by noninvasive techniques.

In a patient in whom an arterial switch procedure is anticipated, it is very useful to

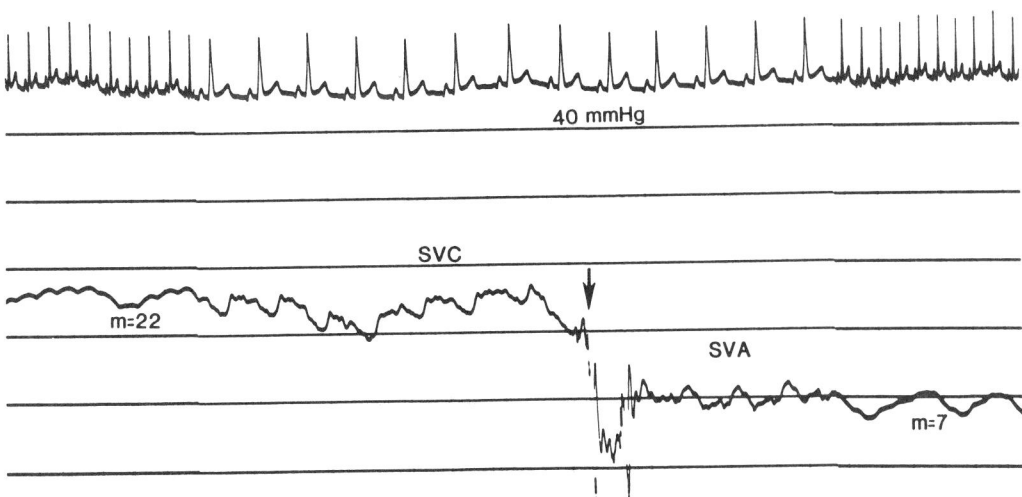

Figure 5. Withdrawal pressure tracing from the superior vena cava (SVC) to the systemic venous atrium (SVA) demonstrating severe superior vena caval obstruction.

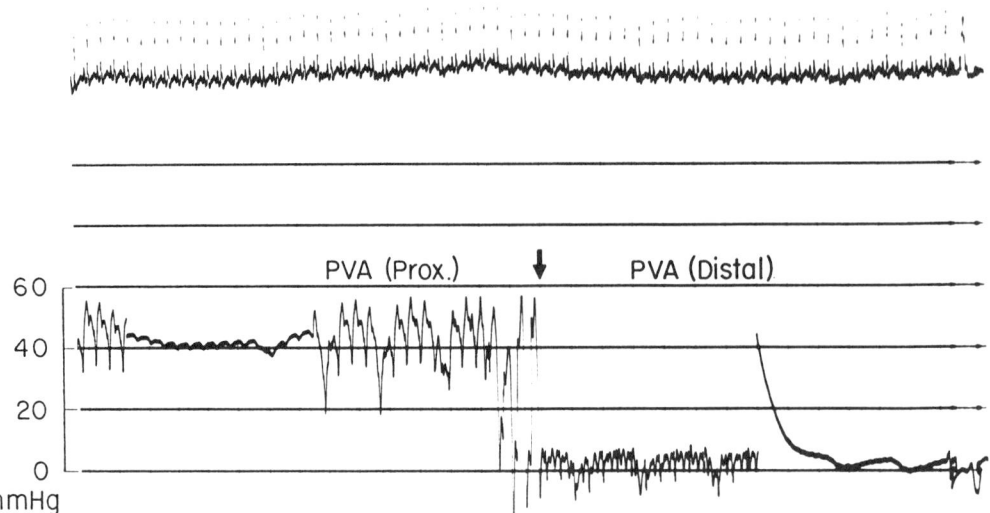

Figure 6. Withdrawal pressure tracing using the retrograde catheter from the proximal pulmonary venous atrium (PVA) near the pulmonary vein to the distal pulmonary venous atrium just above the tricuspid valve. The marked elevation of pressure in the proximal pulmonary venous atrium indicates severe pulmonary venous obstruction.

establish the coronary artery pattern by an aortic root injection. This may be done by advancing the umbilical artery catheter into the aortic root, or alternately by maneuvering an NIH or angiographic balloon tipped catheter prograde from the right ventricle to the aorta. A technique for selective coronary angiography using a venous catheter also has been described (Day 1989). In a newborn, temporary inflation of the balloon to occlude the ascending aorta briefly during the injection may be done to facilitate visualization of the coronary arteries (Mandrell 1990). The best view to identify the coronary origin is a shallow left anterior oblique with caudocranial angulation (Fig. 7). However, other views may be needed because of the numerous variations in the position of the "facing" coronary sinuses. The usual coronary artery pattern in transposition of the great arteries is for the noncoronary sinus to be anterior with the right and left "facing" sinuses (as viewed from the noncoronary sinus facing the pulmonary artery) giving rise to the left and right coronary arteries respectively. Many variations are possible,

with the most common one being the circumflex artery arising from the right coronary.

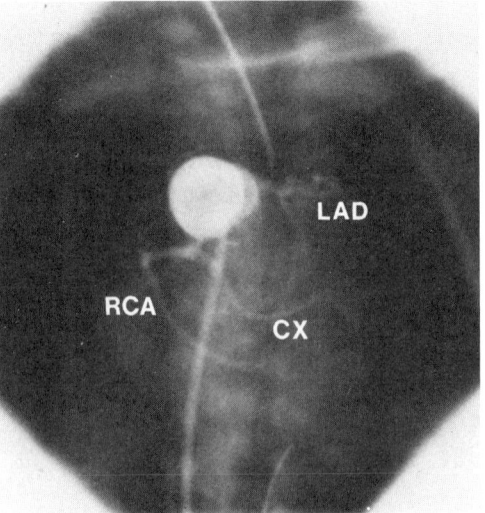

Figure 7. Selective balloon-occlusion aortogram in the shallow left anterior oblique view with caudocranial angulation. The circumflex coronary artery (CX) arises from the right coronary artery (RCA). LAD = Left anterior descending coronary artery.

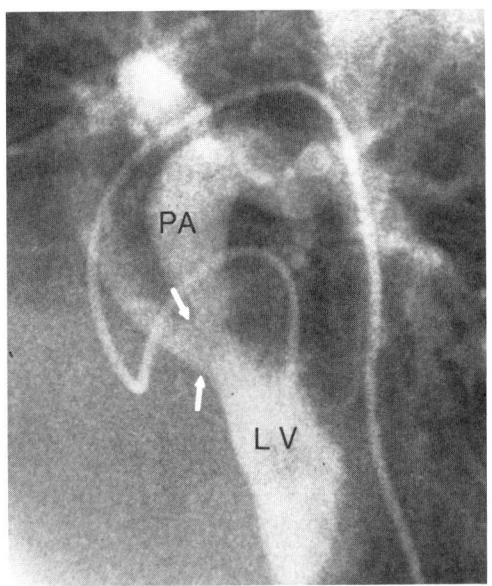

Figure 8. Selective left ventricular angiogram in the four-chamber view demonstrating a membranous ventricular septal defect (arrows). LV = left ventricle; PA = pulmonary artery.

Some associated anomalies that may also require angiographic studies include ventricular septal defects, left ventricular outflow tract obstruction, branch pulmonary artery stenosis, and aortic isthmus hypoplasia or coarctation. Defects in the ventricular septum are profiled best by a right ventricular angiogram in a steep left anterior oblique or lateral view with cranio-caudal angulation, or a left ventricular angiogram in the four-chamber view (Fig. 8). The pulmonary arteries will be shown by left ventricular angiography in the anteroposterior and four-chamber views. Abnormalities of the aortic arch are clearly demonstrated by an injection in the region of the aortic isthmus.

Postoperative

At the postoperative catheterization the purpose of angiography is to evaluate residual defects, ventricular function and specific hemodynamic abnormalities resulting from an atrial baffle repair or an arterial switch procedure. In the patient who has had an atrial baffle procedure, injections should be made in the superior and inferior vena cavae in the anteroposterior and lateral views to rule out obstruction at the junction of these vessels with the systemic venous atrium. (Enough contrast may reflux into the inferior vena cava from the superior vena caval injection to make a direct injection in this vessel unnecessary) (Fig. 9). Superior vena caval obstruction is much more frequent than inferior vena caval narrowing. If the superior vena caval obstruction is severe or completely atretic, collateral flow or drainage via the azygos system into the inferior vena cava is often present (Fig. 10). A right ventricular angiogram in the anteroposterior and lateral views is usually performed to determine right ventricular size, function, and tricuspid valve competency. A relatively slow injection (a total of 1 mL/kg over 1.5 to 2 seconds) minimizes arrhythmia. If a ventricular septal defect is present, a four-chamber view is desirable.

A left ventricular angiogram should be done in the four-chamber or long axial projection if there is left ventricular outflow tract obstruction (Fig. 11). An injection in the proximal pulmonary venous atrium should be made in the anteroposterior and lateral views if an elevated wedge pressure suggests pulmonary venous obstruction. With baffle induced pulmonary venous obstruction, a constriction in the midportion of the pulmonary venous atrium in the lateral view gives a "dumbell" or hour glass appearance (Fig. 12). An aortogram in the anteroposterior and lateral or the oblique views is useful in evaluating aortic valve competence, coronary artery anatomy and systemic to pulmonary collateral circulation.

In a patient who has had an arterial switch procedure, the great artery anastomoses and the coronary arteries need to be evaluated. Semilunar valve incompetence may occur and can be evaluated by selective

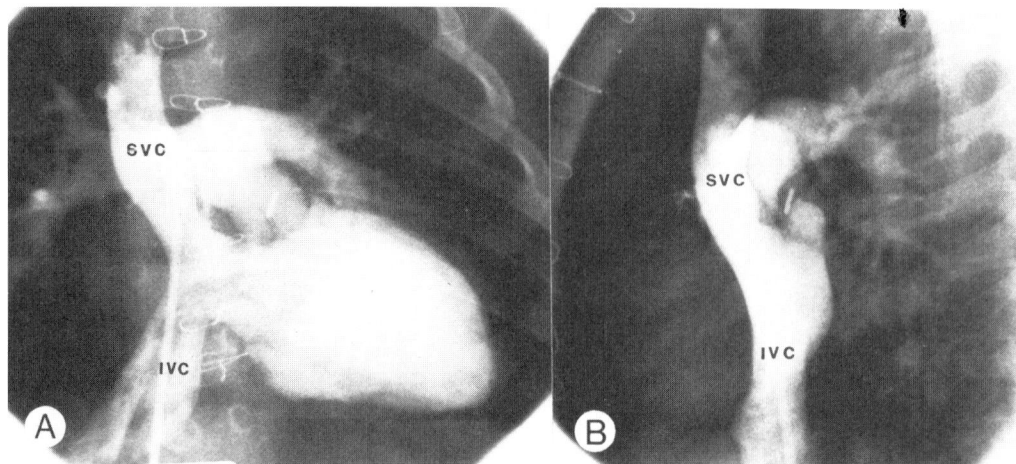

Figure 9. Selective injection in the superior vena cava (SVC) following an atrial baffle procedure. There is no evidence of obstruction and reflux of contrast into the inferior vena cava (IVC) is adequate to visualize this area. A = Anteroposterior view B = Lateral view.

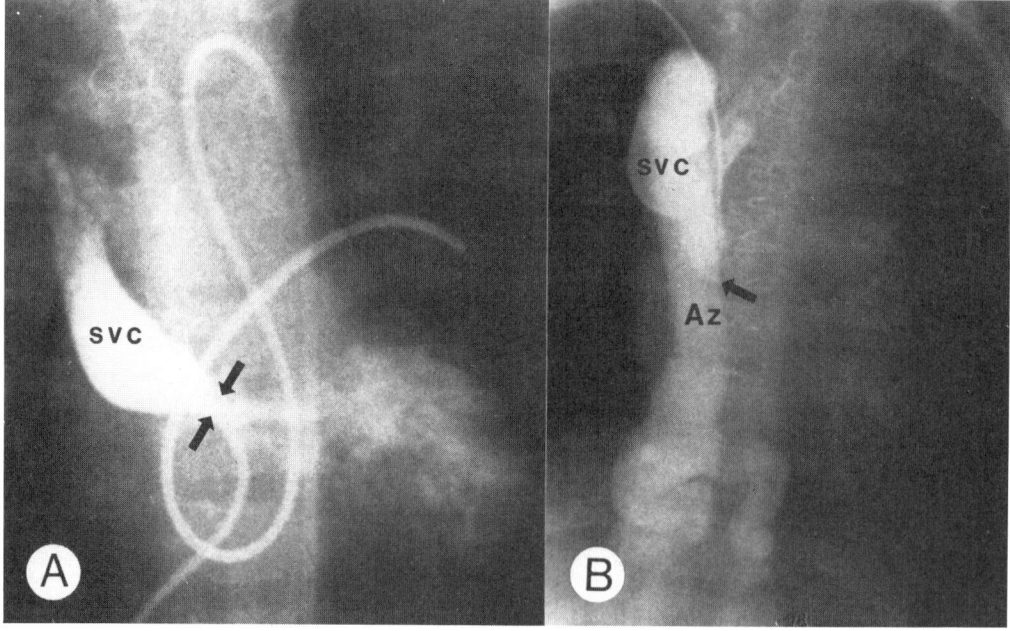

Figure 10. Selective injection in the superior vena cava (SVC) demonstrating obstruction following an atrial baffle procedure A: Severe obstruction (arrows). B: Complete obstruction (arrows) with retrograde filling of the azygos vein (AZ) and subsequent drainage into the inferior vena cava.

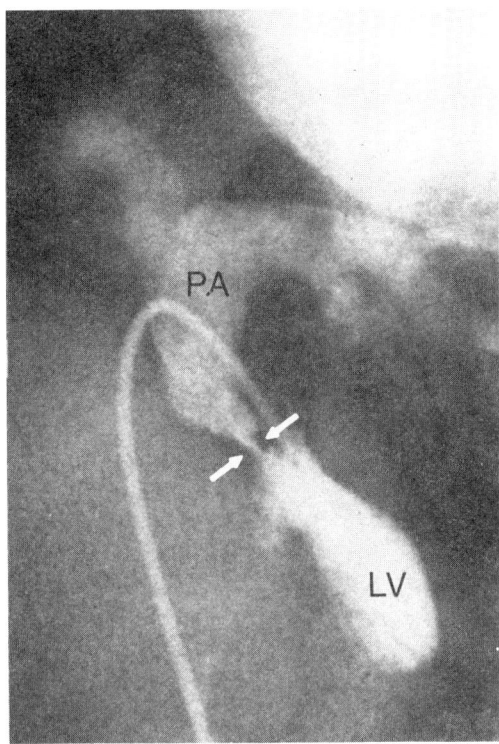

Figure 11. Selective left ventricular angiogram in the four-chamber view demonstrating severe left ventricular outflow obstruction (arrows). LV = Left ventricle; PA = Pulmonary artery.

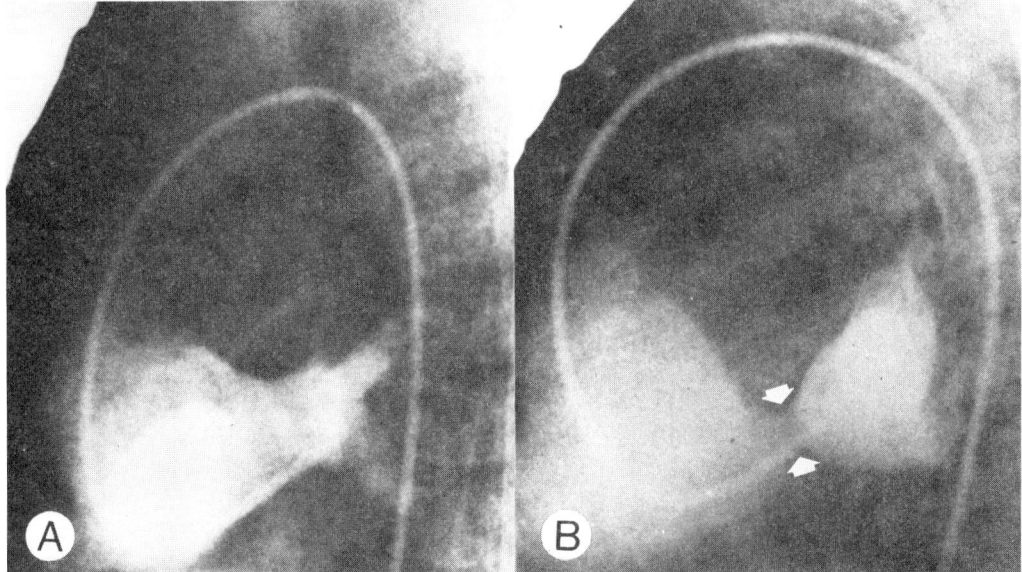

Figure 12. Selective injection in the proximal pulmonary venous atrium in the lateral view following an atrial baffle procedure. A: There is no evidence of obstruction. B: There is severe obstruction (arrows) with a "dumbbell" or "hour glass" appearance.

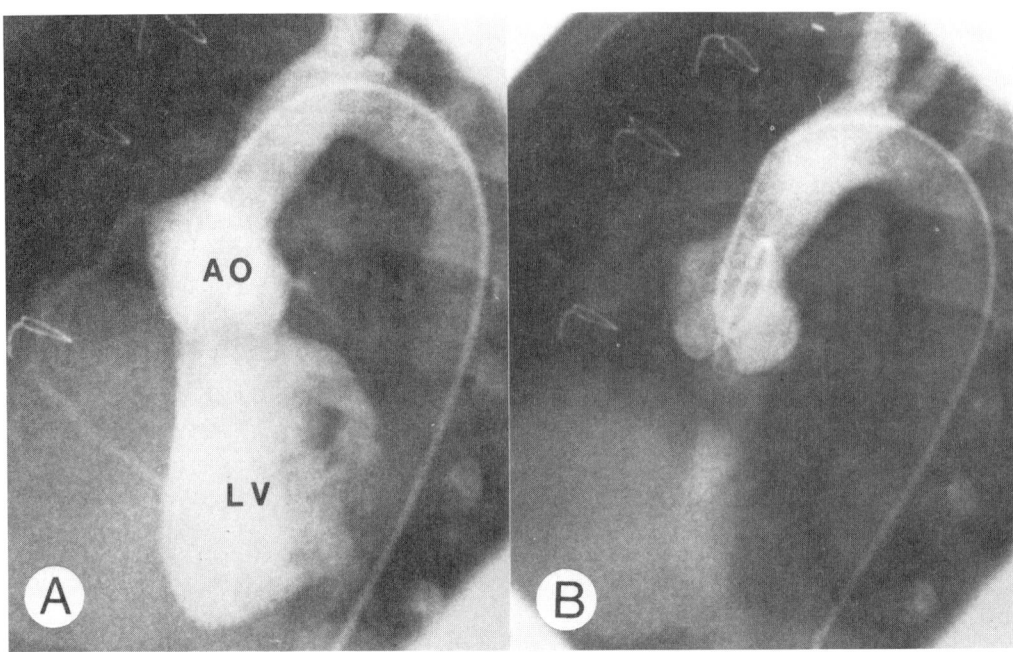

Figure 13. Selective angiography following an arterial switch operation. A: Left ventricular injection. B: Aortic root injection demonstrating mild aortic regurgitation and patency of the coronary arteries. AO = aorta; LV = Left ventricle.

aorta and pulmonary artery injections. An aortic root injection in oblique views with caudocranial angulation is usually sufficient to delineate the coronary artery anatomy. On occasion, selective coronary arteriography may be indicated to better visualize kinking, stenosis, or ostial abnormalities of the coronary vessels. Either a left ventricular or aortic root injection is useful for evaluating the aortic anastomosis and distortion or dilation of the proximal neo-aortic root, while a selective aortic root injection is necessary to assess aortic valve competency (Fig. 13). A right ventricular or main pulmonary artery injection is important to evaluate the pulmonary artery anastomotic site and bifurcation, as supravalvular pulmonary artery narrowing is the most common residual hemodynamic abnormality following the arterial switch procedure (Fig. 14). The optimal views for this injection are an anteroposterior or a very shallow left an-

terior oblique projection with as much cranio-caudal angulation as possible, in addition to the lateral view (Fig. 13).

Associated Anomalies and Anatomic Variants

Pulmonary atresia may accompany transposition of the great arteries, when there is an associated ventricular septal defect. Pulmonary blood supply is usually via a patent ductus arteriosus. As in any ductus dependent anomaly, continuity between right and left pulmonary arteries should be demonstrated, because bilateral patent ducts may provide a separate blood supply to each lung. Transposition may also occur in the setting of other complex cardiac malformations, including double inlet ventricle and atrioventricular septal defect. The Taus-

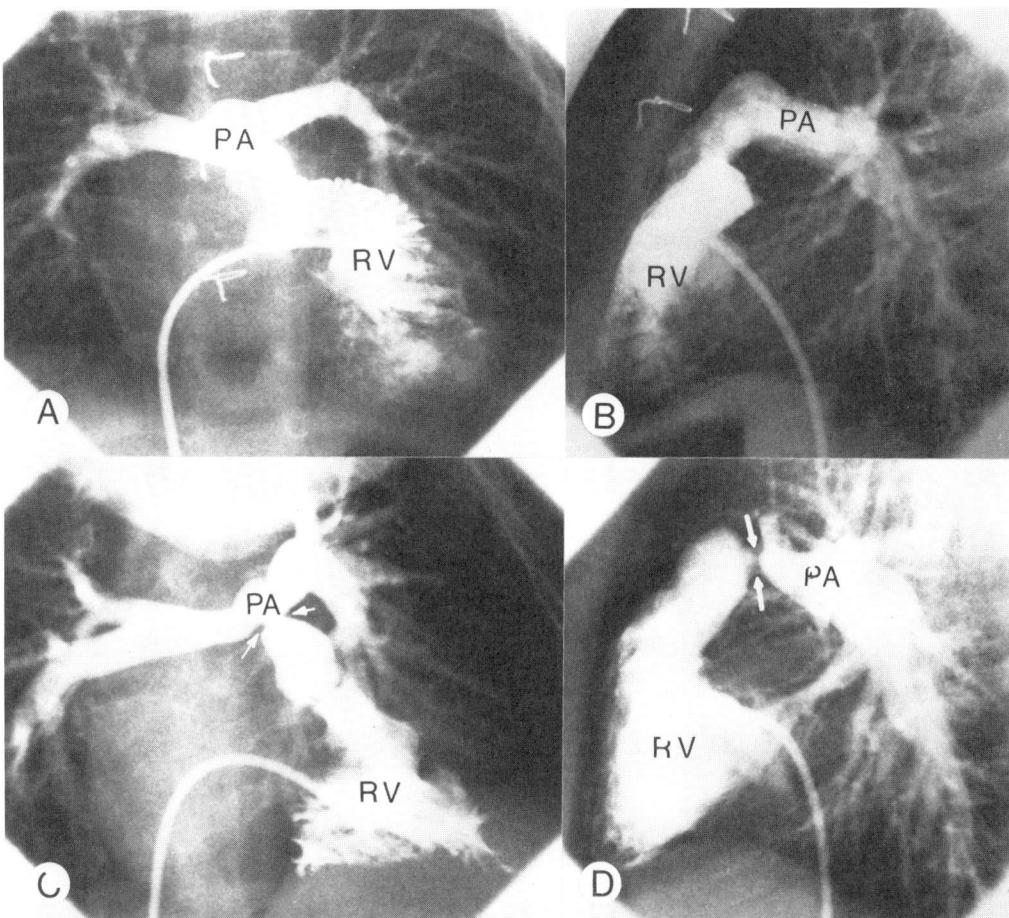

Figure 14. Selective right ventricular angiography following an arterial switch operation. Top: Anteroposterior (A) and lateral view (B) demonstrating the marked angulation normally seen without stenosis at the anastomotic site in the pulmonary artery. Bottom: Right anterior oblique view with cranio-caudal angulation (C) and lateral view (D) demonstrating stenosis in the main pulmonary artery at the anastomotic site (arrows).

sig-Bing complex, while morphologically a double outlet right ventricle, is physiologically similar to transposition. The aorta arises from the right ventricle as does the pulmonary artery. However, the latter great vessel may override the subpulmonic defect to a varying degree and thus have a biventricular origin. Infants with Taussig-Bing complex are intensely cyanotic and require balloon septostomy. As in other patients with transposition of the great arteries and a ventricular septal defect, pulmonary hy-

pertension leads to early pulmonary vascular disease. Unlike other forms of transposition, pulmonary stenosis is almost never present, but aortic outflow tract narrowing or, more commonly, coarctation may occur.

In the Taussig-Bing complex the great arteries are nearly side by side, with the pulmonary artery to the left of the aorta (see Chapter 26). During cardiac catheterization the pass from the right ventricle to the pulmonary artery is usually easy and resembles the pass in the patient with normally connected great arteries. The pass to the aorta is more medial. The hemodynamics are indistinguishable from the patient with transposition and a large ventricular septal defect. The distinguishing features angiographically, include side-by-side great vessels, and either a bilateral infundibulum or marked overriding of the pulmonary artery over a subpulmonic ventricular septal defect. A subpulmonary infundibulum results in mitral-pulmonary discontinuity, usually best seen in the lateral projection of a left ventricular angiogram. In this anomaly an aortogram is essential, since coarctation of the aorta is common.

Cautions and Precautions

Two potential complications of preoperative catheterization in the infant with transposition of the great arteries deserve special mention. Hypovolemia may occur due to a combination of factors including perinatal blood loss, a period of no oral intake prior to the procedure and significant blood loss during the catheterization. Hypovolemic infants with transposition are prone to develop severe and progressive hypoxemia, presumably because of a lowering of left atrial pressure and a consequent decrease in interatrial mixing. This pathophysiologic process can be successfully reversed with volume or blood replacement if recognized early enough. Thromboembolic complications are also relatively common in this group of very cyanotic and polycythemic patients who have such large "physiologic right to left" shunts prior to operative repair.

References and Suggested Reading

Day RW, Isabel-Jones JB, Wetzel GT, et al. Description of a venous technique for selective coronary arteriography in newborns with d-transposition of the great arteries. J Am Coll Cardiol 1989;14:1308–1311.

Hagler DJ, Ritter DG, Mair DD, et al. Clinical, angiographic and hemodynamic assessment of late results after Mustard operation. Circulation 1978;57:1214–1220.

Keith JD, Rowe RD, Vlad P. (eds) Heart Disease in Infancy and Childhood, 3rd ed., New York, NY; MacMillan.

Mathews RA, Park SC, Neches WH, et al. Iliac venous thrombosis in infants and children after cardiac catheterization. Catheterization Cardiovasc Diagn 1979;5:67–74.

Mandrell VS, Lock JE, Mayer JE, et al. The "laidback" aortogram: An improved angiographic view for demonstration of coronary arteries in transposition of the great arteries. Am J Cardiol 1990;65:1379–1383.

Mullins CE, Neches WH, McNamara DG. The infant with transposition of the great arteries. I. Cardiac Catheterization Protocol. Am Heart J 1972;84:597–602.

Park SC, Neches WH, Mathews RA, et al. Hemodynamic function after the Mustard operation for transposition of the great arteries. Am J Cardiol 1983;51:1514–1519.

Porter CJ, Gillette PC, Mullins CE, et al. Cardiac catheterization in the neonate. A comparison of three techniques. J Pediatr 1978;93:97–101.

Rudolph, AM. Congenital Diseases of the Heart. Chicago, IL; Year Book Medical Publishers, 1974.

Wernovsky G, Hougen TJ, Walsh EP, et al. Mid term results after the arterial switch operation for transposition of the great arteries with intact ventricular septum: Clinical, hemodynamic, echocardiographic, and electrophysiologic data. Circulation 1988;77:1333–1344.

Corrected Transposition of the Great Arteries

Lee B. Beerman, M.D.

Anatomy

Atrioventricular discordance associated with ventriculoarterial discordance has many appellations, but the most widely accepted is corrected transposition of the great arteries (or just corrected transposition). In this chapter, this entity and its commonly associated defects will be discussed. In uncomplicated corrected transposition, the systemic veins drain normally into the right atrium, which connects via a mitral valve to a right-sided but morphologic left ventricle, which then gives rise to the pulmonary artery (Fig. 1). Pulmonary venous drainage is into the left atrium, which empties through a tricuspid valve into a left-sided but morphologic right ventricle, that supports the aorta. There is usually atrial and visceral situs solitus, a left-sided cardiac apex, and thus the morphologic left ventricle lies to the right of the morphologic right ventricle. The aorta is to the left of the pulmonary artery and usually slightly anterior, although it may be side by side or even somewhat posterior to the pulmonary artery.

It is unusual for corrected transposition to exist without associated intracardiac defects. The most common associated anomalies are ventricular septal defect, an abnormal tricuspid (left atrioventricular) valve and pulmonic stenosis. Cardiac malposition, including meso- or dextrocardia with situs solitus or situs inversus may be seen. Ap-

proximately 30% of patients have first, second, or third degree atrioventricular block and the block is frequently progressive. An extensive morphologic study (Allwork et al. 1976) demonstrated that a tricuspid (left atrioventricular) valve abnormality occurred in 91% of cases, ventricular septal defects in 78% and pulmonic stenosis in 44%. The most frequent abnormality of the left atrioventricular valve was Ebstein's anomaly (76% of the patients had this defect). In most of these cases the extent of the displacement of valve tissue into the ventricle was not great, but other dysplastic features such as short and thickened chordae or nodular excrescences on the free edges of the leaflets were common. Non-Ebstein's deformities of this valve also occur; usually deficient leaflet tissue, dilatation of the annulus, or abnormalities of the papillary muscles and chordae. In spite of the high incidence of anatomic abnormalities, left atrioventricular valve regurgitation is clinically detectable in only about one third of the cases and stenosis occurs very rarely. However, in patients with corrected transposition, abnormalities of the tricuspid, left atrioventricular valve may have more serious long-term implications because this valve is the systemic atrioventricular valve.

Most ventricular septal defects are perimembranous (84%). These defects are usually large and often extend well into the posterior inlet septum, allowing continuity between the mitral and tricuspid valves. So

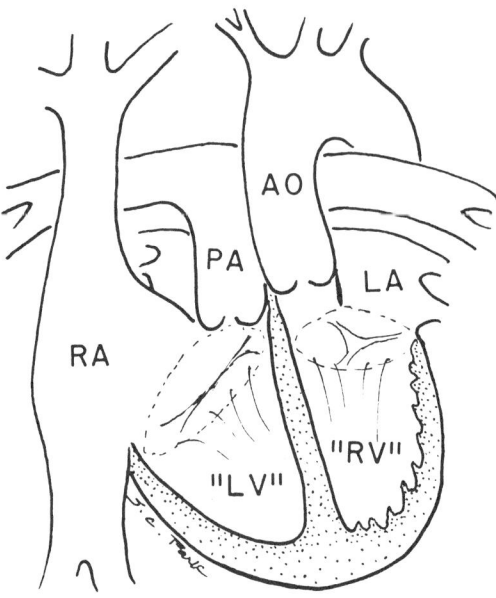

Figure 1. Diagram of corrected transposition of the great arteries. AO = Aorta; LA = Left atrium; "LV" = Morphologic left ventricle; PA = Pulmonary artery; RA = Right atrium; "RV" = Morphologic right ventricle.

called "aneurysms of the membranous septum" are sometimes associated with perimembranous defects and are usually comprised of left atrioventricular valve tissue. Defects of the infundibular or muscular trabecular septum also occur. Left ventricular (pulmonary) outflow tract obstruction is common, usually associated with a ventricular septal defect, and is most often both valvar and subvalvar. The subvalvar pulmonic stenosis may be muscular or related to tissue arising from the membranous septum ("aneurysm of the septum") or a left atrioventricular valve leaflet prolapsing through a ventricular septal defect.

Hemodynamic Considerations

The hemodynamic findings reflect the associated defects. If a large ventricular septal defect is present, the pressure in the pul-

monary (right-sided, morphologic left) ventricle is elevated. The ventricular and pulmonary artery pressures are also affected by the presence and degree of pulmonic stenosis. In a patient with a ventricular septal defect, oximetry may show left to right, bidirectional, or right to left shunting, depending upon the pulmonary vascular resistance and the presence and severity of pulmonic stenosis. Left atrioventricular valve regurgitation may result in elevation of the left atrial or pulmonary artery wedge pressure and a prominent "V" wave. (The intermittent "cannon" venous waves of third degree atrioventricular block must be differentiated from the "V" waves of severe atrioventricular regurgitation.) When pulmonary artery hypertension is present because of either a large ventricular septal defect or left atrial hypertension, pulmonary vascular resistance should be carefully evaluated, including its response to oxygen (See Chapter 7).

Indications for Cardiac Catheterization

Preoperative

Cardiac catheterization may be indicated because of the severity of associated defects or because of a conduction disturbance. Cross-sectional and Doppler echocardiographic studies can accurately diagnose corrected transposition, define associated defects, and assess their hemodynamic consequences. Pulmonary hypertension, excessive or insufficient pulmonary blood flow, and severe regurgitation of the systemic atrioventricular valve (i.e., tricuspid valve) are the usual indications for catheterization. The timing of the investigation is similar to that in isolated ventricular septal defect, pulmonic stenosis, or left-sided atrioventricular valve regurgitation. In patients with ventricular septal defect and suspected pulmonary hypertension, catheterization should be done within the first 6 months of life to accurately assess pulmonary vascular resistance. When severe pulmonic stenosis is associated with a ventricular defect, cyanosis may be apparent as early as the newborn period. This may warrant catheterization at that time if echocardiographic data are not sufficient for planning an aortic to pulmonary artery shunt.

Because of the high incidence of associated atrioventricular conduction abnormalities, electrophysiologic studies are indicated at the time of catheterization. Gillette et al. (1979) have shown that the site of the atrioventricular block in corrected transposition can be determined in approximately 80% of cases. In a newborn with symptomatic third degree atrioventricular block, cardiac catheterization may be helpful to determine the site of the block and to assess hemodynamics before a decision is made with regard to permanent pacing. In an older child with second or third degree atrioventricular block and questionable symptoms or marked bradycardia, establishing whether the block is above, below, or within the bundle of His is very helpful, because pacemaker implantation is almost always indicated with infra- or intra-His block. Documented episodes of syncope or near syncope associated with high-grade atrioventricular block are absolute indications for pacemaker insertion and an electrophysiologic study is not unnecessary, unless a hemodynamic study is planned for other reasons. Wolff-Parkinson-White syndrome occurs with corrected transposition and may lead to recurrent supraventricular tachycardia. If this arrhythmia is refractory to treatment or associated with severe hemodynamic embarrassment, electrophysiologic testing may be helpful in management.

Postoperative

Routine postoperative catheterization is not usually necessary but should be considered if the echo-Doppler studies suggest significant residual hemodynamic abnormalities. This is particularly true following complex procedures such as use of a conduit to bypass pulmonic stenosis.

Cardiac Catheterization Technique

When the percutaneous femoral approach is used, the catheter pass from the right atrium across the right atrioventricular (mitral) valve into the right-sided (morphologic left) ventricle is much more difficult than usual. The plane of the mitral valve orifice is oblique rather than vertical (as is the normal, right-sided tricuspid valve) and requires a sharper bend on the catheter. Furthermore, with the posteriorly positioned pulmonary artery and the acute angulation of the inflow and outflow tracts of the right-sided morphologic left ventricle, the pass from the left ventricle to the pulmonary artery is often quite difficult with standard catheters. In addition to this, the conduction system (His bundle) is more vulnerable in corrected transposition than in a normal heart because of its anterosuperior position and traumatic injury secondary to catheter manipulation is more likely. Therefore a balloon-tipped flow-directed catheter (e.g., Swan-Ganz) is preferred for the right-sided hemodynamic study. If an approach from the arm is used, the pass across the mitral valve is easier but entering the pulmonary artery is still difficult without a balloon-tipped catheter. If the left-sided chambers cannot be entered via a foramen ovale or an atrial or ventricular septal defect, retrograde arterial catheterization may be necessary. The systemic (morphologic right) ventricle can be easily entered by passing the catheter across the aortic valve, and frequently the left atrioventricular valve can be retrogradely traversed. This is accomplished by backing a loop of catheter across the aortic valve and then by directing the catheter tip posteriorly and rightward in the inflow portion of the systemic ventricle (See Chapter 5). In corrected transposition, the His bundle electrogram can sometimes be obtained by passing an electrode catheter across the right-sided atrioventricular (mitral) valve, rotating the tip clockwise and observing the intracardiac electrogram as the catheter is withdrawn from the ventricle.

Hemodynamic Evaluation

As has already been stated, the hemodynamics of isolated corrected transposition should be normal; however, associated defects are almost always present and lead to predictable hemodynamic alterations. When a large ventricular septal defect is present, pulmonary hypertension and a large left to right shunt generally occur during early life and pulmonary vascular disease may develop if there is no surgical intervention. When severe pulmonic stenosis occurs in association with a large ventricular septal defect, physiology identical to that of tetralogy of Fallot is present. Less commonly, pulmonic stenosis may occur as an isolated abnormality and lead to markedly elevated pressure in the pulmonary (morphologic left) ventricle. Even with "isolated" corrected transposition, dysfunction of the systemic (morphologic right) ventricle may occur, with elevated diastolic pressure in that chamber. Wedge and pulmonary artery pressures are increased if the dysfunction is severe. Estimation of pulmonary vascular resistance is important when pulmonary hypertension is present. In addition to the calculation of pulmonary and systemic blood flows and resistances, the response of the pulmonary vascular bed to vasodilators such as oxygen can provide useful information. Cardiac output should be determined by indicator dilution, thermodilution, or the Fick method to assess the significance of the measured gradient and allow calculation of absolute pulmonary and systemic vascular resistances.

In the presence of a large ventricular septal defect, the systemic (morphologic right) ventricle is occasionally relatively hypoplastic. Ventricular hypoplasia is often associated with varying degrees of overriding of the left-sided atrioventricular valve that may occur with an inlet ventricular septal defect. Ventricular volume studies may help to assess the functional potential of this chamber when open heart repair is contemplated.

Angiography

Cross-sectional and Doppler echocardiography are usually sufficient to diagnose the anatomic malformation of corrected transposition and to accurately define the associated defects. However, angiography often provides valuable complementary information. To establish a diagnosis of atrioventricular discordance, it is necessary to determine visceral situs, identify the atrial positions and define ventricular anatomy. Situs can be determined by echocardiography, by abdominal and overpenetrated chest radiographs and during catheterization by outlining the course of the systemic veins (particularly the inferior vena cava) as they enter the atrium. (This latter information can be also obtained by catheter pass and rarely requires selective venous injections.) The right atrium can be identified by its appendage, which is pyramidal in shape with a broad base attaching to the body of the atrium, and the left atrium by its appendage, which is finger-like with a narrow waist at the site of its attachment. If atrial identity can not be inferred by other means (e.g., echocardiographic visualization of appendages, site of pulmonary or systemic venous return, etc.), angiographic imaging of the appendages may be useful. Analysis of ventricular anatomy in the presence of corrected transposition can be done reliably by selective ventricular angiography. The morphologic left ventricle (which is right-sided with situs solitus) is finely trabeculated, oval in shape and, in the usual situation with a left-sided apex, has its right superior border formed by the mitral (right atrioventricular) valve (anteroposterior projection). This valve is slightly oblique to the sagittal plane and mitral-pulmonary valve continuity can be seen on both the anteroposterior and lateral views (Fig. 2A and 2B). Another characteristic finding in the lateral view is the anterior recess that results from the posterior take-off of the pulmonary artery from this ventricle. The morphologic right ventricle is left-sided and slightly superior. The tricuspid valve is vertically oriented and in the anteroposterior view forms the right border of the coarsely trabeculated, triangular shaped right ventricular chamber (Fig. 2C

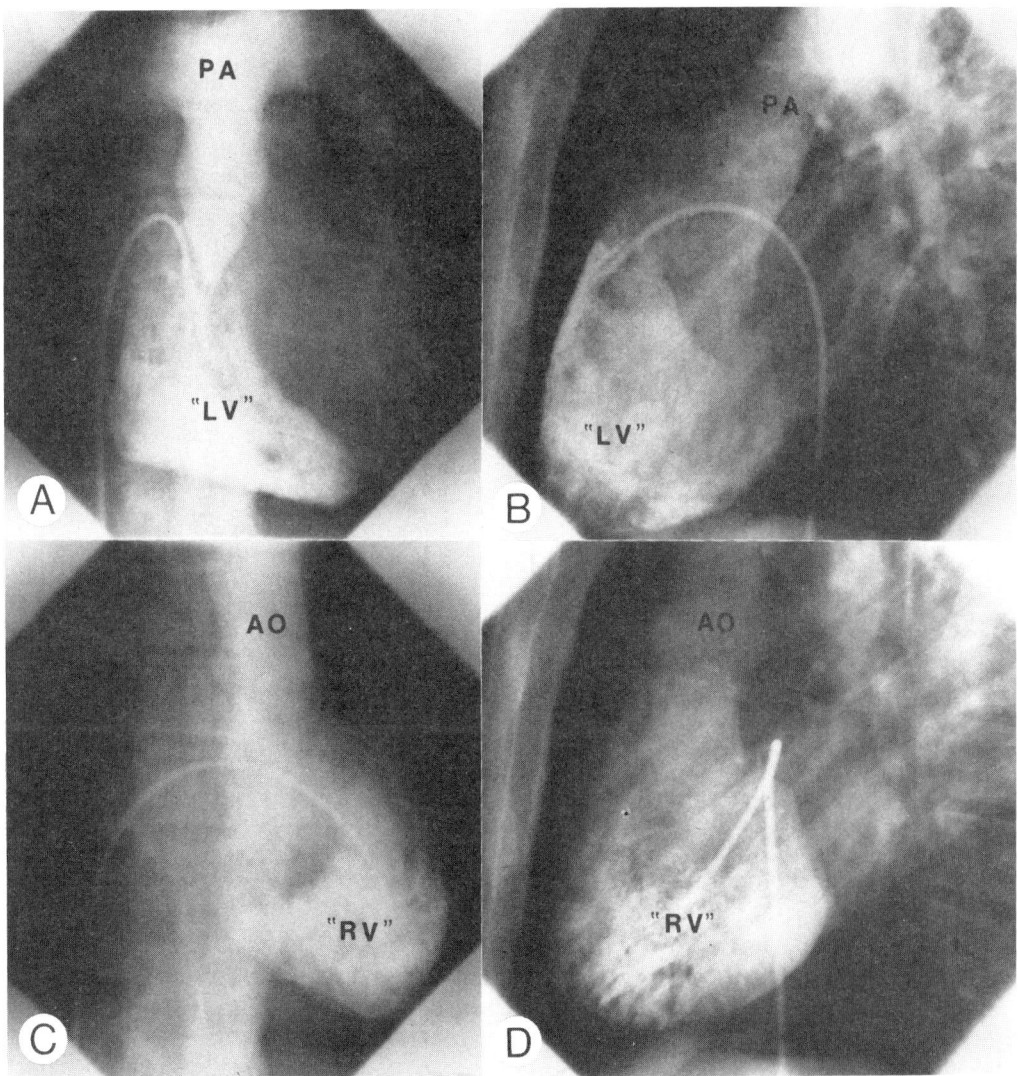

Figure 2. Selective ventricular angiocardiograms in corrected transposition. Top: Injection in the right-sided morphologic left ventricle ("LV") that gives rise to a posterior pulmonary artery (PA). Bottom: Injection in the left-sided morphologic right ventricle ("RV") that gives rise to an anterior aorta (AO). A and C: Anteroposterior view; B and D = Lateral view.

and 2D). A distinguishing feature of this ventricle is the presence of an infundibulum that separates the tricuspid valve from an anterior aorta. The pulmonary artery usually lies rightward, inferior, and slightly posterior to the aorta, although in rare cases the pulmonary artery may be directly behind or to the left of the aorta.

In corrected transposition, the ventricular septum is nearly in the sagittal plane and is well profiled in the anteroposterior view, slanting from right superior to left inferior. The coronary artery pattern is "inverted" in this entity, with the right-sided sinus giving rise to an artery that corresponds to a morphologic left coronary artery that bifurcates into a circumflex (following the right-sided atrioventricular groove) and an anterior descending artery. The other coronary artery, corresponding to a morphologic right coronary artery arises from the left-sided sinus and runs in the left atrioventricular groove. The anterior sinus is the noncoronary one in corrected transposition. Other abnormalities of the coronary arteries occur, but are not common.

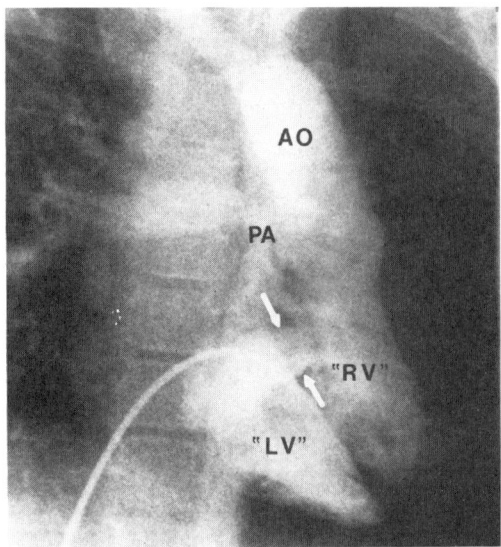

Figure 3. Anteroposterior view of a selective injection in the right-sided morphologic left ventricle in a patient with corrected transposition, pulmonary stenosis, and a muscular inlet ventricular septal defect (arrows) AO = Aorta; "LV" = Morphologic left ventricle; PA = Pulmonary artery; "RV" = Morphologic right ventricle.

Associated Lesions

Due to their relative frequency in corrected transposition, the accurate definition of associated abnormalities is especially important. Defects in the ventricular septum are present in the majority of cases and are usually of the perimembranous type. They usually can be profiled best in the anteroposterior view, particularly with craniocaudal angulation, because of the unusual septal orientation. An injection in the morphologic left (pulmonary) ventricle may define the defect more clearly as compared to a right (systemic) ventricular angiogram if there is right to left shunting due to pulmonary stenosis (Fig. 3). Axial views (e.g., four-chamber and long-axial) also may be helpful in outlining ventricular septal defects, particularly when they extend into the posterior (inlet) septum (Soto et al. 1978).

Pulmonic stenosis may be an isolated finding but more often occurs with a ventricular septal defect. Usually there is a combination of valvar and subvalvar obstruction, and the anteroposterior and shallow left anterior oblique (normal cardiac position) or right anterior oblique (dextrocardia) views with cranio-caudal angulation are best for visualizing the left ventricular outflow tract. As with noninverted ventricles, the lateral view is best for assessment of valvar pulmonic stenosis. Other discrete causes of obstruction, such as an aneurysm of the membranous septum or prolapse of left atrioventricular valve tissue through a ventricular septal defect, may be present and are best visualized in the anteroposterior or axial views (Fig. 4). Because left atrioventricular valve abnormalities are very common, the morphology and function of this valve should be evaluated with a selective systemic ventricular injection. The anteropos-

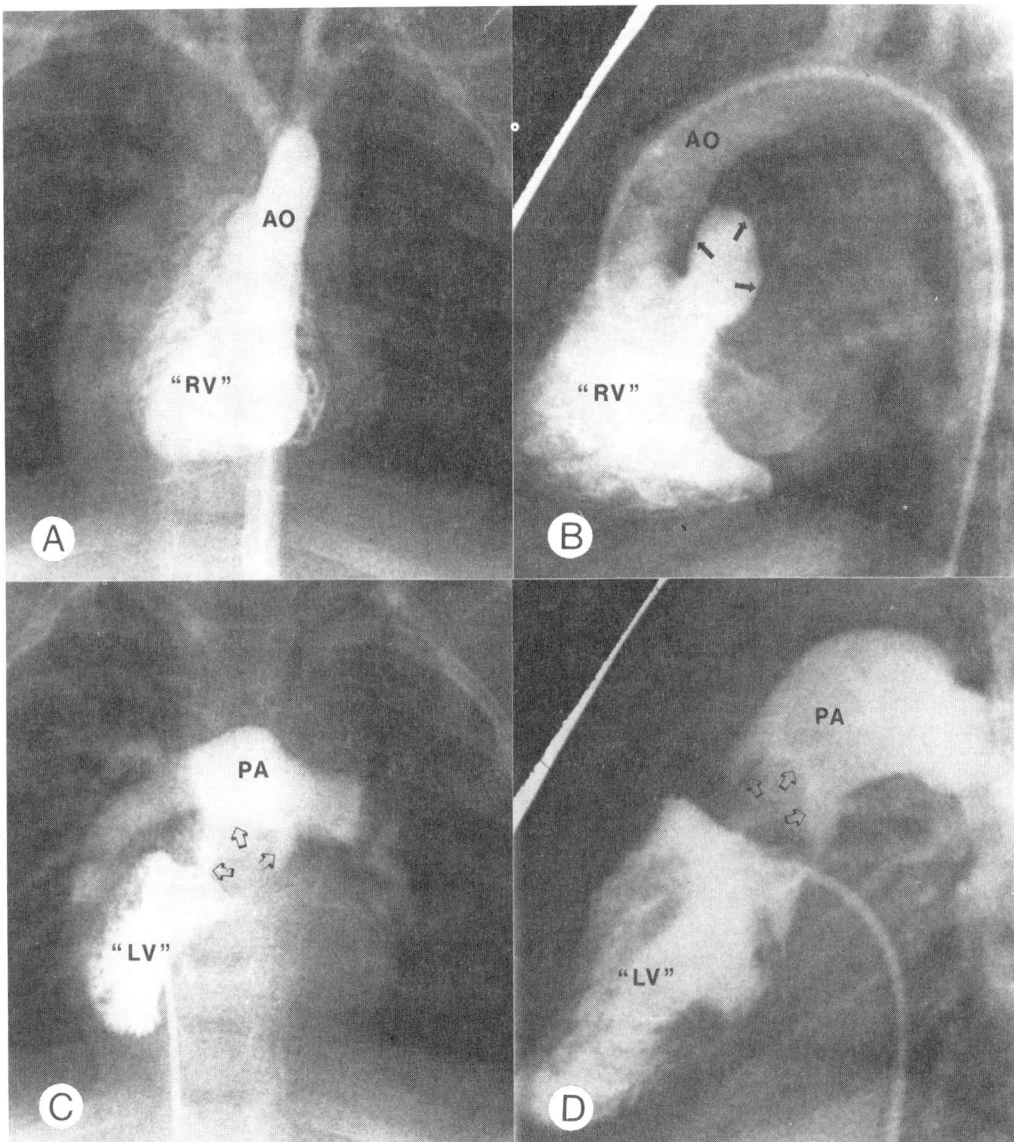

Figure 4. Selective ventricular angiocardiograms in corrected transposition and pulmonary stenosis due to accessory left atrioventricular valve tissue prolapsing through a ventricular septal defect. Note the cardiac apex is toward the right. Top: Injection in the left-sided, morphologic right (systemic) ventricle demonstrating the large aneurysmal pouch (arrows) protruding into the subpulmonic area. Bottom: Injection in the right-sided, morphologic left (pulmonary) ventricle demonstrating the radiolucent filling defect (arrows) in the outflow area due to the aneurysmal pouch. A and C: Anteroposterior view. B and D: Lateral view. AO = Aorta; "LV" = Morphologic left ventricle; PA = Pulmonary artery; "RV" = Morphologic right ventricle.

terior view is best for detecting prolapse or displacement of the septal or inferior leaflets from the atrioventricular groove (Ebstein's anomaly). (A good marker for the site of the annulus is the left coronary artery as it courses in the left atrioventricular groove). When Ebstein's anomaly is present, the hinge point of the septal or inferior leaflet is displaced inferiorly and toward the left lateral cardiac border. The "atrialized" portion of the ventricle has a very smooth appearance.

Cardiac malposition is common in corrected transposition and the presence of mesocardia or dextrocardia with situs solitus will somewhat alter the angiographic landmarks. When malposition is present, the morphologic left ventricle is not so oval shape, does not have the tail-like projection in the anteroposterior view and its major

axis is nearly vertical. The septum is *en face* in the anteroposterior view and is extremely well profiled by ventriculograms in this plane. Cranio-caudal tilt in the anteroposterior position further enhances septal imaging and is particularly useful in visualizing the left ventricular outflow tract when subpulmonic stenosis is present.

It is very important to distinguish corrected transposition angiographically from double inlet (single) ventricle with rudimentary outlet chamber. In the latter entity there is usually transposition, with the aorta arising from the outlet chamber and lying to the left of the pulmonary artery (see Chapter 31). The orientation of the great arteries is therefore very much like that in corrected transposition and if the outlet chamber is unusually large, the similarity to corrected transposition may be striking. The crucial

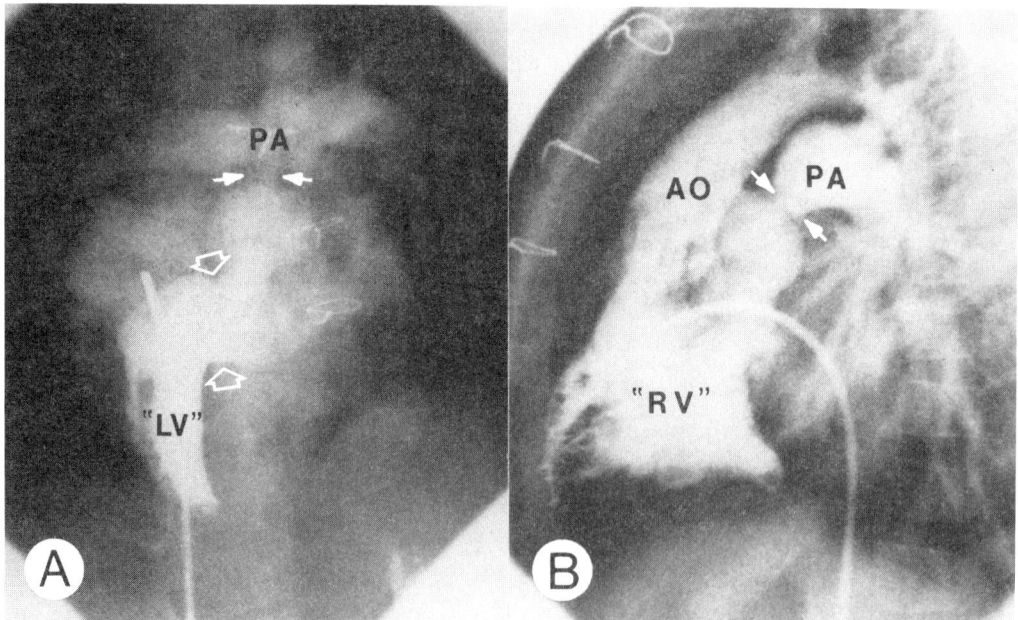

Figure 5. Angiocardiograms in corrected transposition of the great arteries with double outlet of the right (systemic) ventricle and a hypoplastic morphologic left ventricle. A: Selective injection in the morphologic left ventricle ("LV") demonstrating a large ventricular septal defect (open arrows) and a pulmonary artery (PA) band (solid arrows). B: Selective injection in the morphologic right (systemic) ventricle("RV") in the lateral view demonstrating both the aorta (AO) and pulmonary artery (PA) arising from the ventricle. Arrows indicate the pulmonary artery band.

difference is in the atrioventricular connection. With double inlet left ventricle, both atrioventricular valves enter the large right-sided, morphologic left ventricle. The left atrial blood flow first enters the main left ventricular chamber, then the outlet chamber, and then the aorta. In corrected transposition, left atrial exit is to the left-sided morphologic right ventricle and then directly to the aorta. In both of these groups of anomalies, cross-sectional and Doppler echocardiographic evaluation is invaluable in determining atrioventricular relationships.

Double outlet of the morphologic right (systemic) ventricle also may occur, but rarely. This is best evaluated by angiography (Fig. 5).

Cautions and Precautions

Special attention must be paid to catheter manipulation in patients with corrected transposition, particularly in traversing the right-sided, mitral, atrioventricular valve and attempting to enter the pulmonary artery. The atrioventricular conduction system is particularly vulnerable to traumatic injury because of its course in the morphologic left ventricular side of the septum. The rather abruptly angled pass from the inflow

to outflow region of the morphologic left ventricle can be performed more easily and safely with the use of a balloon-tipped flow-directed catheter. Patients with corrected transposition and the Wolff-Parkinson-White syndrome may also be prone to the inadvertent induction of supraventricular tachycardia.

References and Suggested Reading

Allwork SP, Bentall HH, Becker AE, et al. Congenitally corrected transposition of the great arteries: Morphologic study of 32 cases. Am J Cardiol 1976;38:910–923.

Attie F, Soni J, Ovseyevitz J, et al. Angiographic studies of atrioventricular discordance. Circulation 1980;62:407–415.

Gillette PC, Busch U, Mullins CE, et al. Electrophysiologic studies in patients with ventricular inversion and "corrected transposition". Circulation 1979;60:939–945.

Jaffe RB. Systemic atrioventricular valve regurgitation in corrected transposition of the great vessels. Angiographic differentiation of operable and non-operable valve deformities. Am J Cardiol 1976;37:395–402.

Soto B, Bargeron LM Jr, Bream PR, et al. Conditions with atrioventricular discordance-Angiographic study. In: Paediatric Cardiology. Anderson RH, MaCartney FJ, Shinebourne EA, et al., eds. Edinburgh; Churchill Livingston, 1987:207–223.

29

Ebstein's Anomaly of the Tricuspid Valve

J.R. Zuberbuhler, M.D.

Anatomy

In Ebstein's anomaly, the origin of one or more leaflets of the tricuspid valve is displaced into the right ventricle from the tricuspid annulus (Fig. 1). The septal and inferior (posterior) leaflets may display this feature, but the anterior superior leaflet always arises at the annulus. The leaflets are usually dysplastic to a degree, and sometimes severely so. The septal leaflet may consist of a clumpy mass of dysplastic valve tissue attached to the septum at a distance from the annulus, while the anterior superior leaflet may be large and "sail-like" with numerous fenestrations, The abnormal origin of the septal and inferior leaflets results in a shift of the tricuspid orifice from the annulus into the body of the right ventricle. This divides the right ventricle into an inlet, or atrialized portion proximal to the tricuspid orifice, and an outlet portion distal to it.

The distal attachments of the tricuspid valve leaflets are also often abnormal. In the normal heart, the tricuspid support apparatus has focal attachments to the right ventricular myocardium. Some examples of Ebstein's anomaly have relatively normal chordae tendineae and papillary muscles. In others, the distal attachment of the leaflets is not focal and to papillary muscles but is more or less linear and to a muscular ridge located laterally in the right ventricle. This linear attachment emphasizes the division of the right ventricle into inlet and outlet portions and may compromise the effective tricuspid orifice. There is a spectrum of the resultant obstruction ranging from mild through severe stenosis, to an imperforate membrane or muscular partition completely subdividing the right ventricle (Zuberbuhler et al. 1979). The relative size of the inlet and outlet portions of the right ventricle is variable, depending on the degree of displacement of the tricuspid valve attachments. If the origin of the inferior leaflet is displaced well into the right ventricle, the portion of the right ventricle proximal to the origin of the leaflet is "atrialized" physiologically, because it is part of an atrial pressure zone.

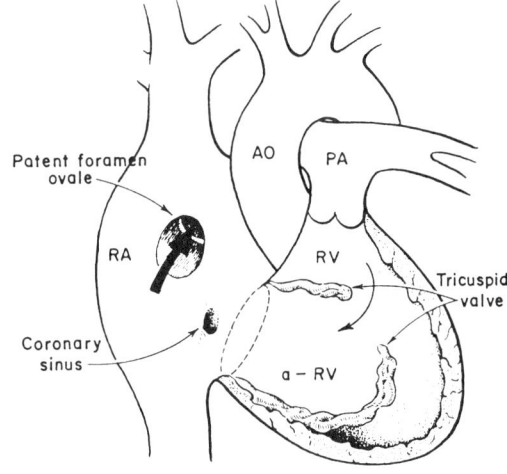

Figure 1. Ebstein's anomaly diagram. AO = Aorta; a-RV = Atrialized right ventricle; PA — Pulmonary artery; RA = Right atrium; RV = Right ventricle.

The inferior wall of the right ventricle is often atrialized anatomically as well, being thin and stretched. With Ebstein's anomaly, the left ventricle is often also abnormal and may be misshapen and have an abnormal contraction pattern (Monibi et al. 1978).

Hemodynamics Considerations

The morphology of the tricuspid valve in Ebstein's anomaly may result in valvar and right ventricular dysfunction. The tricuspid regurgitation that is so often present results both from the dysplasia of the leaflets which prevents good coaptation, and sometimes from fenestrations in the anterosuperior leaflet. Tricuspid stenosis, when it occurs, is a consequence of a relatively linear distal attachment of the leaflets, which restricts egress of blood from the atrialized portion of the right ventricle. In the rare "imperforate" variety of Ebstein's there is functional tricuspid atresia. If the "ventricular" portion of the right ventricle (the portion distal to the tricuspid orifice) is small, an element of ventricular restriction is introduced. Each of these hemodynamic abnormalities, the tricuspid regurgitation, tricuspid stenosis, and the restriction tends to compromise right ventricular forward output. If there is an interatrial communication, a right to left shunt will result if the tricuspid valve and/or ventricular dysfunction is even moderately severe. Right ventricular outflow obstruction is present in some hearts displaying Ebstein's anomaly and may consist of valvar pulmonic stenosis or may result from tricuspid valve tissue protruding into the right ventricular outflow tract. Such obstruction tends to accentuate right to left shunting across the atrial septum. It is important to note that the hemodynamic abnormalities associated with Ebstein's anomaly are most severe in the newborn period, because the elevated pulmonary vascular resistance characteristic of this age group further impedes right ventricular outflow and increases right to left atrial shunting. After the newborn period there is usually clinical improvement and older infants and children with Ebstein's anomaly may be asymptomatic.

Indications for Cardiac Catheterization

Cardiac catheterization is rarely necessary to establish a firm diagnosis of Ebstein's anomaly. In most cases the clinical picture is distinctive and the diagnosis is often strongly suggested by typical auscultatory findings, including a loud early systolic "sail-sound" (tricuspid valve closure), S3 and/or S4 gallops, and soft systolic and diastolic murmurs at the low left sternal border. A chest x-ray is also often highly suggestive with cardiomegaly and a "box-shaped" heart. This peculiar contour of the heart is usually due to right atrial enlargement and to prominence of the high left cardiac border due to the displaced right ventricular outflow tract. The cross-sectional echocardiogram is diagnostic and shows the displacement of the origin of the tricuspid valve leaflets. Cardiac catheterization with angiography may be valuable in preoperative evaluation. The echocardiographic description of the tricuspid valve abnormality can be supplemented by angiography, and the size of the functional right ventricle can be defined. The severity of the tricuspid regurgitation can be evaluated angiographically as well as by Doppler color flow mapping, and the associated anomalies, especially right ventricular outflow tract obstruction, can be identified and quantitated. Postoperatively, cardiac catheterization is indicated if there is clinical evidence of an important residual abnormality of tricuspid valve or right ventricular function.

Catheterization Techniques

The usual approach is via the femoral vein. Hemodynamic data are best gathered with an end-hole catheter, because the site of transition from atrial to ventricular pressure within the right ventricle can best be determined if there are no side-holes or if the side-holes are very near the tip. If there is marked tricuspid leaflet displacement, the physiologic right ventricle will be at the high left cardiac border and the pass to the pulmonary artery may be difficult. The pass is safer using an end-hole catheter because tip entrapment is more obvious. A flow-directed balloon catheter can be used, but the dilated right atrium, right ventricle, and tricuspid regurgitation may make it difficult to manipulate such a catheter into pulmonary artery. There is usually a patent foramen ovale and thus the left ventricle can be entered with the venous catheter. Otherwise, a retrograde arterial approach is used to obtain left ventricular pressure or if a left ventriculogram is needed. Any of the standard angiographic catheters can be used for contrast injection.

Hemodynamic Evaluation

Pressure Data

If the anomaly is a severe one, the transition from atrial to ventricular pressure will be well to the left of the usual site, and in extreme cases the right ventricular pressure zone is confined to the left upper cardiac border. It should be noted that the plane of the tricuspid orifice is usually oblique, with the superior pole of the orifice being nearly normally positioned and the inferior pole being more leftward displaced. Thus, a high catheter pass will show a relatively small "atrialized" portion of right ventricle, or may miss it entirely, while a lower pass shows a larger atrialized area. A withdrawal pressure tracing from pulmonary artery to right ventricle demonstrates any right ventricular outflow tract gradient and identifies pulmonic stenosis. However, tricuspid valve hemodynamics are harder to define. Even with

severe tricuspid regurgitation the right atrial pressure contour may not show an abnormally large V wave, since right ventricular pressure is usually low and the right atrium is large with resultant damping of pressure. Similarly, even with severe tricuspid stenosis, there is rarely more than a few mmHg pressure gradient from right atrium to right ventricle during diastole. The gradient will be even less or be absent if there is an interatrial communication which permits right to left atrial shunting. In this circumstance, flow across the tricuspid orifice is decreased and the gradient small.

Oxygen Saturation Data

Unless there is an associated ventricular septal defect (rare) no right heart oxygen step-up is expected. If there is a patent foramen ovale or atrial septal defect, the potential for right to left shunting is present and will be realized if there is sufficient tricuspid stenosis or tricuspid regurgitation or if the right ventricular pressure zone is small. Such a shunt is documented by finding left atrial oxygen saturation to be lower than pulmonary venous saturation. Left ventricular and systemic arterial saturation will be similarly decreased.

Other Diagnostic or Therapeutic Procedures

The use of an end-hole electrode catheter has been recommended for the diagnosis of Ebstein's anomaly. The characteristic finding is an atrial pressure zone with ventricular electrical characteristics. False negative results are common and the procedure is no longer indicated since echocardiography and angiocardiography are far more reliable diagnostic methods.

Angiocardiography

Ebstein's anomaly is diagnosed angiographically by demonstrating that the tricuspid orifice is displaced into the right ventricle away from the tricuspid annulus (Leung 1988). With injection into the proximal "atrialized" portion of right ventricle the site of the tricuspid annulus is indicated by a notch along the inferior border of the heart near the spine. The site of the tricuspid orifice is usually evident during diastole and there is usually filling of the outflow portion of the right ventricle before the trabecular zone opacifies. Flow from the atrialized right ventricle to the atrium does not indicate tricuspid regurgitation. The functional right ventricle can better be defined and tricuspid regurgitation quantitated with a selective direct injection into the ventricular pressure zone, also in the anteroposterior or right anterior oblique projection (Fig. 2). Tricuspid stenosis may be seen with injection into either proximal or distal right ventricle. A thin, vertical radiolucency is often seen within the right ventricle and represents a more or less linear attachment of the anter-

osuperior leaflet to the lateral septum. This structure defines the extent of the atrialized right ventricle. With injection into the functional right ventricle, contrast medium first appears distal to the structure but is eventually seen proximally as well if there is tricuspid regurgitation. The septal and inferior leaflets are often dysplastic and/or diminutive and are often not well defined angiographically. A left ventricular angiogram should be obtained in the oblique or elongated projections, because dyskinesia of the left ventricle and mitral valve prolapse are common (Fig. 3).

In the newborn period severe Ebstein's anomaly may mimic pulmonary atresia, and a right ventricular angiogram may show massive tricuspid regurgitation but no forward flow into the pulmonary artery (functional pulmonary atresia) (Fig. 4). Because Ebstein's anomaly occurs with true pulmonary atresia the distinction can be very difficult. An aortic injection will show pulmo-

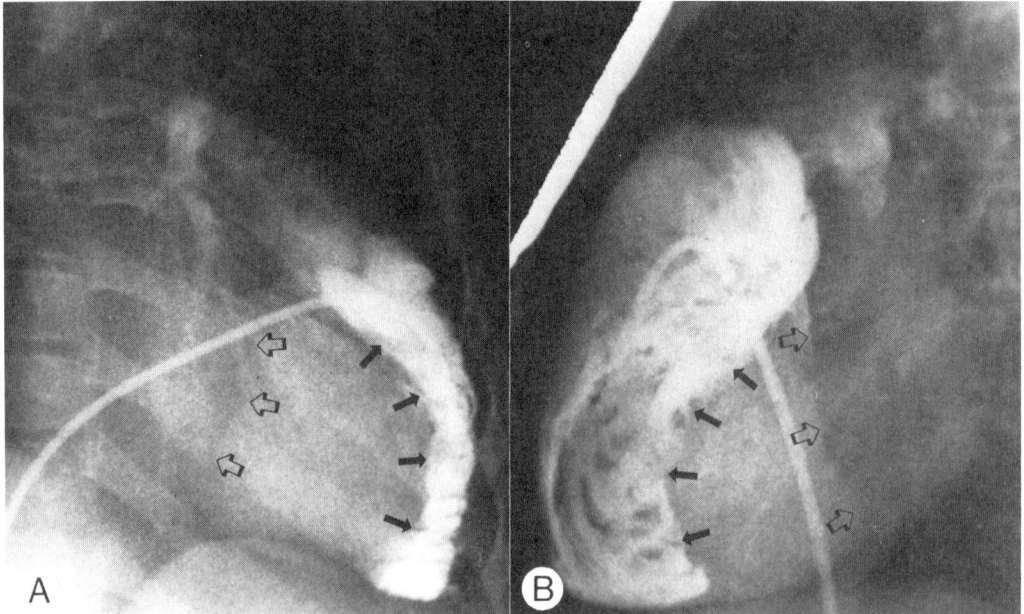

Figure 2. Selective injection into the right ventricular pressure zone. Open arrows indicate the tricuspid valve annulus. Solid arrows indicate the plane of the displaced tricuspid valve orifice. A: Shallow right anterior oblique. B: Lateral view.

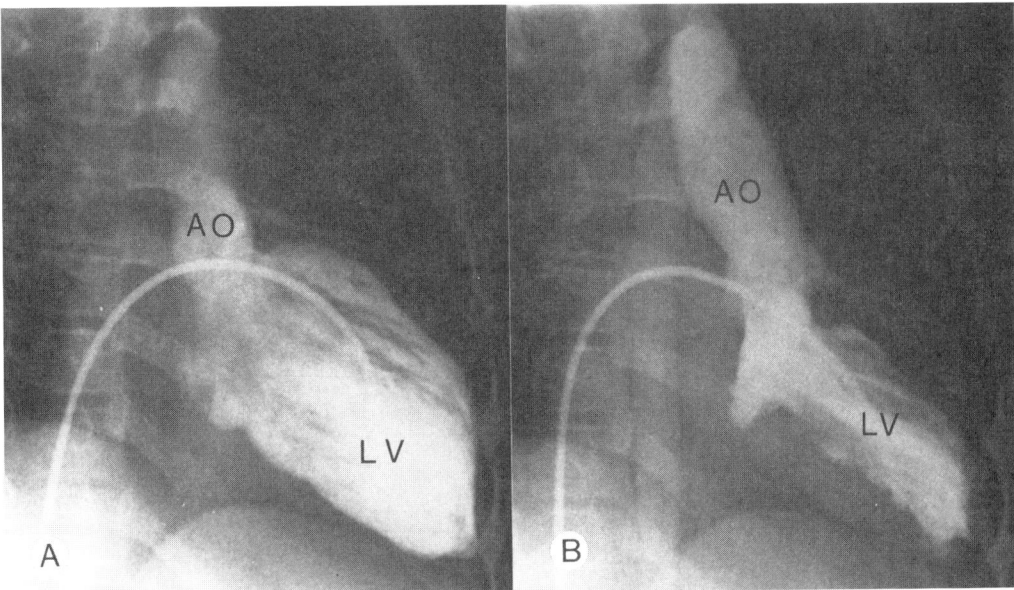

Figure 3. Left ventricular angiogram in Ebstein's anomaly in the right anterior oblique view. An abnormal contraction pattern is seen. A: Diastolic frame. B: Systolic frame. AO = Aorta; LV = left ventricle.

nary artery filling via the patent ductus in either case, but with Ebstein's anomaly there may be pulmonic regurgitation, ruling out morphologic pulmonary atresia.

Imperforate Ebstein's Anomaly

There is a spectrum of tricuspid valve obstruction ranging from a widely patent tricuspid orifice through varying degrees of tricuspid stenosis to complete subdivision of the right ventricle by a fibrous, fibromuscular, or muscular partition (Zuberbuhler et al. 1979). The sometimes linear attachment of the anterior leaflet of the tricuspid valve has been mentioned, and imperforate Ebstein's can be thought of as an unbroken linear attachment of the anterior leaflet to the septum and walls of the right ventricle. There is usually a ventricular septal defect connecting the left ventricle to the distal right ventricle and functionally this anomaly is identical to tricuspid atresia. The distinction is angiographic (Zuberbuhler et al.

1984). With injection into the proximal right ventricle there is reflux to the right atrium but no antegrade flow to the distal right ventricle (Fig. 5A). The left ventricular angiogram shows normal filling of the aorta and also visualizes the distal right ventricle and pulmonary artery (Fig. 5B).

Associated Lesions

Pulmonic Stenosis

Right ventricular outflow obstruction is identified and quantitated by pressure measurements in the right ventricle and pulmonary artery, and the site of the obstruction is determined angiographically.

Ventricular Septal Defect

A ventricular septal defect is a rare accompaniment of Ebstein's anomaly and is best demonstrated by left ventricular injec-

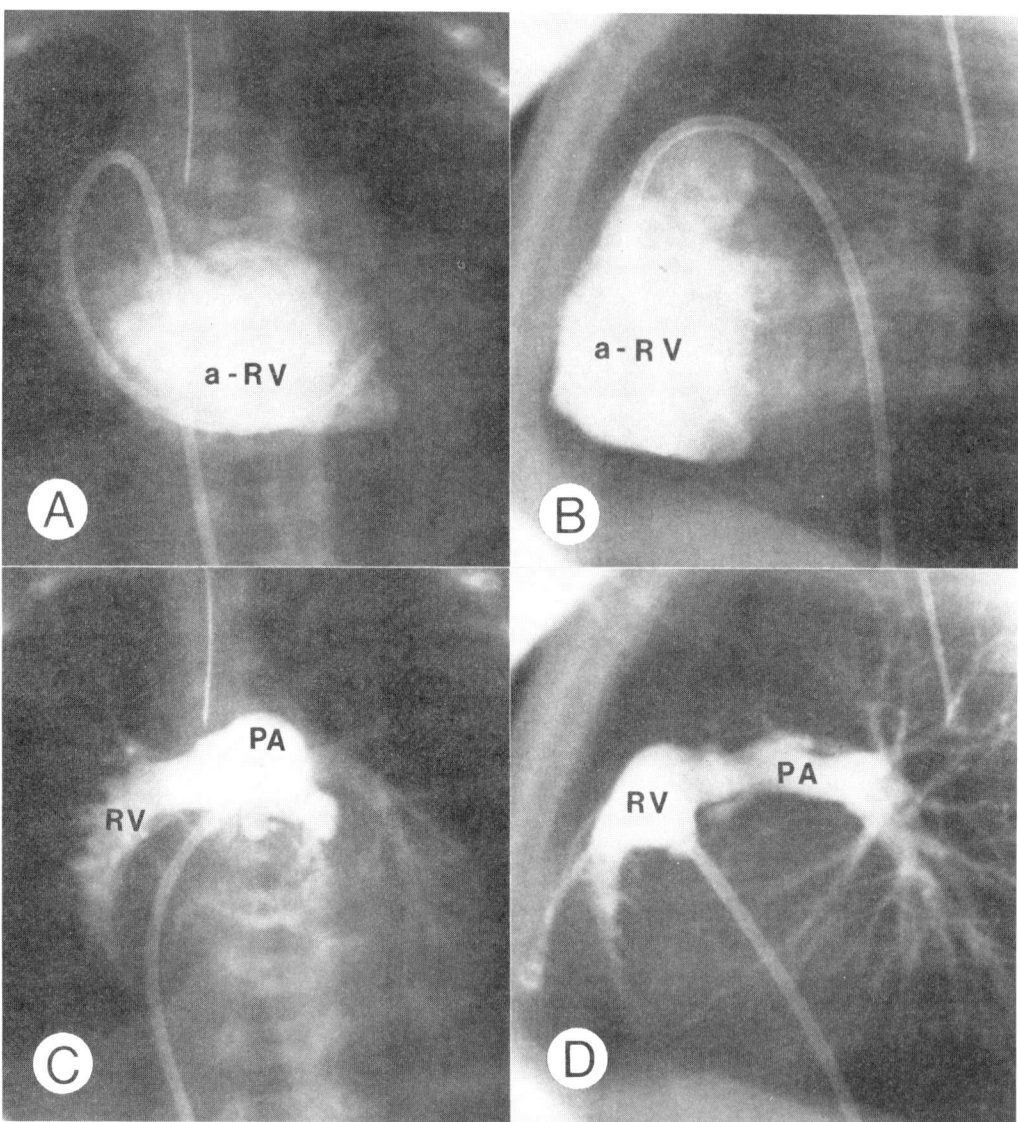

Figure 4. Functional pulmonary atresia in Ebstein's anomaly Top: Right ventricular injection demonstrating massive tricuspid regurgitation and absence of forward flow. Bottom: Passage of catheter into the right ventricular outflow area and demonstration of patency of the pulmonary valve. A and C = Anteroposterior views. B and D = Lateral view. a-RV = Atrialized right ventricle; PA = Pulmonary artery; RV = Right ventricle.

tion in the left anterior oblique or four-chamber view.

Pulmonary Atresia with Intact Ventricular Septum

Ebstein's anomaly accompanies pulmonary atresia with intact ventricular sep-tum in approximately 25% of cases (Zuber-buhler and Anderson, 1979). The anomaly ranges from slight displacement of a dys-plastic septal leaflet into a small right ven-tricle to extensive displacement with a very large fenestrated anterior leaflet. In the lat-ter variant the right ventricle is usually quite large. The differential diagnosis of Ebstein's

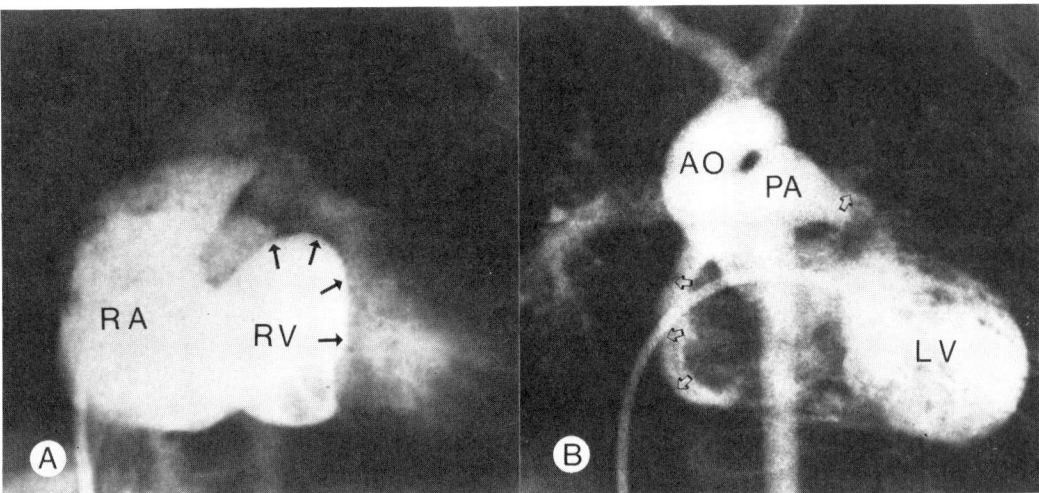

Figure 5. Imperforate Ebstein's anomaly (anteroposterior view) A: An injection into the atrialized ventricle shows filling of the right atrium and no forward flow through the tricuspid valve (arrows). B: Distal right ventricle (open arrows) and pulmonary artery fill via a patent ductus arteriosus following a left ventricular injection. AO = aorta. LV = left ventricle. PA = pulmonary artery. RA = right atrium. RV = right ventricle.

anomaly and pulmonary atresia is discussed above (also see Chapter 24).

Corrected Transposition of the Great Arteries

Ebstein's anomaly may also accompany corrected transposition of the great arteries (atrioventricular discordance with ventriculoarterial concordance) (Jaffe 1976), and is discussed in the chapter dealing with corrected transposition (see Chapter 28).

Cautions or Precautions

Cardiac catheterization was once considered to be quite dangerous in patients with Ebstein's anomaly. The chief hazard is the induction of supraventricular dysrhythmias and supraventricular tachycardia or atrial fibrillation are poorly tolerated in some individuals. With reasonable care in catheter manipulation, most patients can be catheterized successfully without inducing sustained tachycardia. Electrical conversion

is occasionally necessary if an induced dysrhythmia is not well tolerated hemodynamically.

References and Suggested Readings

Jaffe RB. Systemic atrioventricular valve regurgitation in corrected transposition of the great arteries. Am J Cardiol 1976;37:395–402.

Leung MP, Baker E, Anderson RH, et al. Cineangiographic spectrum of Ebstein's malformation: Its relevance to clinical presentation and outcome. J Am Coll Cardiol 1988;11:154–161.

Monibi AA, Neches WH, Lenox CC, et al. Left ventricular anomalies associated with Ebstein's malformation of the tricuspid valve. Circulation 1978;, 57:303–306.

Zuberbuhler JR, Allwork SP, Anderson RH. The spectrum of Ebstein's anomaly of the tricuspid valve. J Thorac Cardiovasc Surg 1979;77:202–211.

Zuberbuhler JR, Anderson RH. Morphologic variations in pulmonary atresia with intact ventricular septum. Br Heart J 1979;41:281–288.

Zuberbuhler JR, Becker AE, Anderson RH, et al. Ebstein's malformation and the embryological development of the tricuspid valve. Ped Cardiol 1984;5:289–295.

30

Atrioventricular Valve Atresia

Robert A. Mathews, M.D.

Tricuspid and mitral atresia can also be referred to as right and left atrioventricular valve atresia, respectively (Tynan et al. 1979). The latter terms are particularly useful in complex varieties of congenital heart disease where it is not entirely clear that atrioventricular valve is the "tricuspid" or the "mitral". The terms "absent right" and "absent left atrioventricular connection" also must be defined. They indicate not only lack of a patent communication between the respective atrium and ventricle, but also a lack of contiguity between the expected site of the atrioventricular valve and the ventricular musculature. Thus, with absent connection the atrioventricular groove extends well beyond the usual atrioventricular connection. Rarely, an atrioventricular valve can be "atretic" in the sense that there is no patent orifice but still be contiguous to the ventricular mass. In such cases the atrioventricular connection is "imperforate" rather than absent.

Right or left atrioventricular valve atresia inevitably produce severe hemodynamic alterations and these alterations usually become evident early in life. Arterial unsaturation is always present, but is usually more severe with absence of the right connection. Conversely, congestive heart failure is more common with left than with right atrioventricular valve atresia. Associated anomalies are the rule. Because there is no direct communication between an atrium and a ventricle the atrium must have another outlet, almost always an interatrial communication. Rarely, with left atrioventricular valve atresia, the atrial septum is anatomically or functionally intact and the left atrium empties via an ascending vertical vein into the left innominate vein, hemodynamically simulating total anomalous pulmonary venous connection. Other associated anomalies are common and will be discussed under absent right and left atrioventricular atresia headings.

Right Atrioventricular Valve (Tricuspid) Atresia

Anatomy

With right atrioventricular valve atresia (tricuspid atresia), the right ventricle is hypoplastic but normally related to the left ventricle (anterior and to the right). The ventriculoarterial connection is usually concordant but may be discordant (tricuspid atresia with transposition) (Fig. 1). Pulmonic stenosis is common and is most often infundibular, although obstruction may be at the valve level or may be due to a restrictive interventricular communication. With absent right connection there is always a ventricular septal defect unless there is associated pulmonary atresia.

Hemodynamic Considerations

With right atrioventricular valve atresia, the entire systemic venous return must pass from right to left atrium through either

345

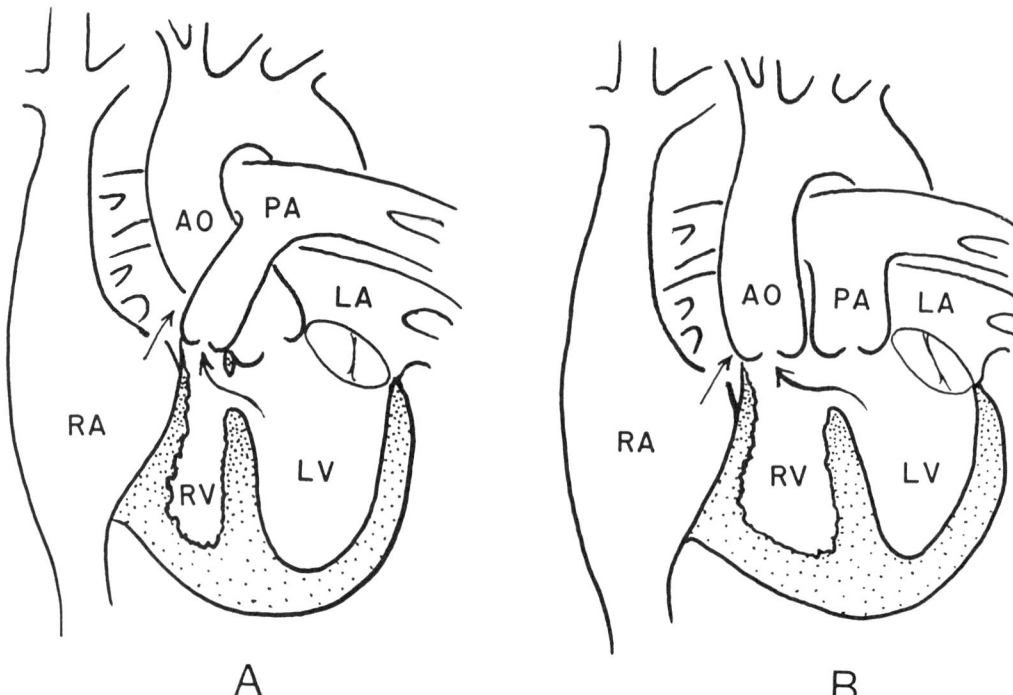

Figure 1. Diagram tricuspid atresia with (A) Concordant (normally connected) or (B) discordant (transposition) ventriculoarterial connection.

a patent foramen ovale or a true atrial septal defect. Systemic venous blood mixes with pulmonary venous return in the left atrium and then enters the left sided ventricular chamber. In hearts with two ventricles, the course of blood flow to the aorta and pulmonary artery depends on the variety of ventriculoarterial connection. Because there is complete mixing of systemic and pulmonary venous returns, the degree of arterial unsaturation (and hence of cyanosis) is inversely related to the magnitude of pulmonary blood flow, which in turn depends upon whether or not there is pulmonic stenosis or pulmonary vascular disease.

When ventriculoarterial discordance accompanies right atrioventricular valve atresia, associated pulmonic stenosis is unusual. The most obvious hemodynamic abnormality is a torrential pulmonary blood flow, and pulmonary artery pressure is usually elevated as well. Most such patients present in early infancy with congestive heart failure, and although a diagnosis usu-

ally is made echocardiographically, cardiac catheterization is indicated before pulmonary artery banding. In this variety of right atrioventricular valve atresia, a restrictive ventricular septal defect constitutes subaortic stenosis, because the aorta arises from the diminutive right ventricle. The appearance of myocardial ischemia, evidenced by ST-T wave shifts on the electrocardiogram or a clinical picture suggestive of angina, are indications for catheterization, even in a patient who has a previously proven diagnosis of tricuspid atresia with transposition of the great arteries. (Neches et al. 1973).

Indications for Cardiac Catheterization

Preoperative

The diagnosis of absent right atrioventricular connection is made by cross-sectional echocardiography. Nevertheless, cardiac catheterization is required in most patients before surgical intervention. If a systemic to pulmonary shunt or pulmonary artery banding is contemplated, the size of the interatrial communication should be assessed and the opening enlarged by balloon or blade septostomy if it is restrictive. Cardiac catheterization is also required to ascertain pulmonary artery size and pulmonary artery pressure. This information is vital in the patient who is to undergo a Fontan operation, and may be needed in some patients being considered for pulmonary banding, especially if the banding is primarily intended to prevent pulmonary vascular disease rather than to treat congestive heart failure. Although pulmonary artery anatomy can be assessed to some degree by cross sectional and Doppler echocardiography, the consequences of overlooking discontinuity of the right and left pulmonary arteries, or of significant stenosis or hypoplasia of the pulmonary arteries, can be disastrous in the patient undergoing a systemic-pulmonary artery shunt or a Fontan procedure. For that reason, in our laboratory, the pulmonary arterial tree is always visualized cineangiographically in patients who are to undergo surgery.

Postoperative

Cardiac catheterization is advisable in most patients who have undergone palliative surgical procedures. A catheterization should be done to measure pulmonary artery pressure following a systemic-pulmonary artery shunt, in particular if there is evidence of excessive pulmonary blood flow and especially if a subsequent Fontan operation is planned. Another specific indication is a discrepancy in right and left lung vascular markings on chest radiograph that would suggest kinking of a pulmonary artery by the shunt, native pulmonary artery stenosis or discontinuity between the right and left pulmonary arteries. Catheterization should also be carried out following pul-

monary artery banding to determine the adequacy of the band and insure that there is normal distal pulmonary artery pressure. In a patient who has undergone a Fontan operation, cardiac catheterization provides a hemodynamic and angiographic assessment of the results of the operation that compliments the information obtained by echocardiography.

Cardiac Catheterization Technique

By definition, the right ventricle cannot be entered from the right atrium. If the catheterization is done from the femoral approach, the catheter preferentially crosses the atrial septum into the left atrium. In patients with a concordant ventriculoarterial connection, it is then easy to enter the pulmonary veins and the left ventricle, and it is usually possible to float a balloon catheter from the left ventricle into the ascending aorta. If there is no pulmonic stenosis, particularly in the small infant, the balloon often preferentially crosses the ventricular septal defect into the right ventricular outflow tract and then into the pulmonary artery. If there is pulmonic stenosis, the pulmonary artery usually can be entered only by a retrograde arterial approach. The catheter can usually be passed into the pulmonary artery from the aorta if a systemic to pulmonary artery shunt has been performed (Fig. 2). If not, then it is still possible to enter the right ventricle from the left ventricle across the ventricular septal defect. To do this, a sharply curved catheter is used, either an end-hole or multiple side-hole variety, depending on whether angiography or precise localization of the pressure gradient is most important. The catheter is positioned above the aortic valve with fluoroscopy in the left anterior oblique projection. The catheter is passed across the aortic valve into the left ventricle and the tip rotated anteriorly and rightward against the interventricular septum (Fig. 3). By probing this area the ventricular septal

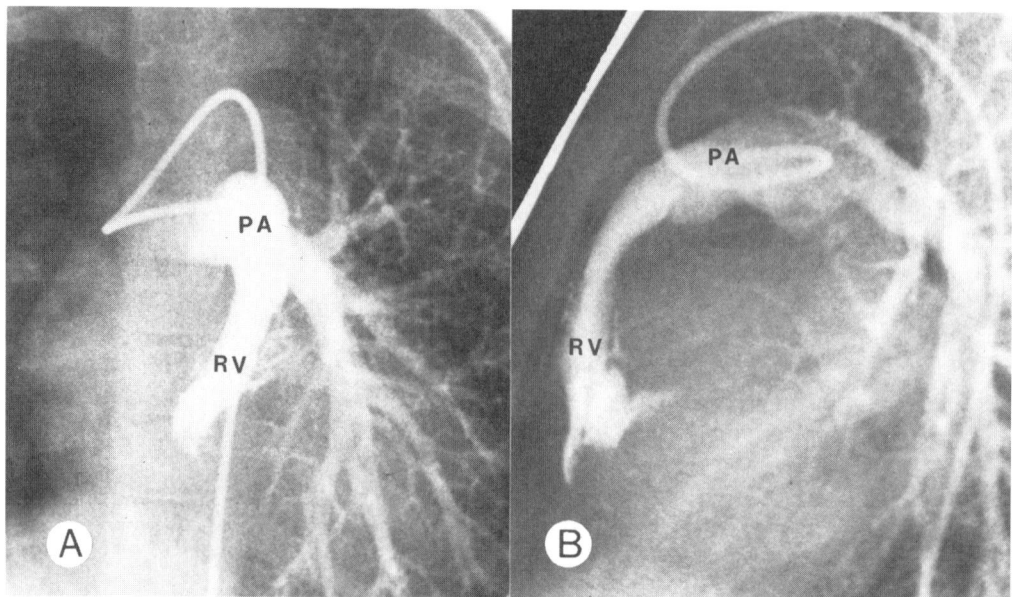

Figure 2. Selective injection in the right ventricular outflow area in tricuspid atresia. The arterial catheter has been passed through a systemic to pulmonary artery shunt. Note the hypoplastic right ventricle (RV). Left = Anteroposterior; Right = lateral; PA = Pulmonary artery.

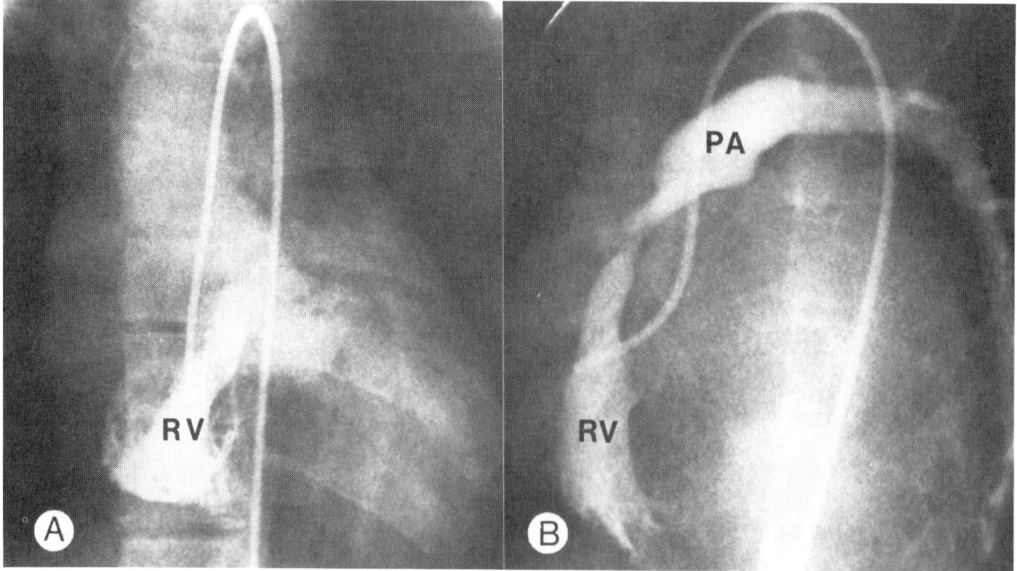

Figure 3. Selective right ventricular injection in tricuspid atresia. The arterial catheter has been passed across the ventricular septal defect. Left = Anteroposterior; Right = Lateral view; PA = Pulmonary artery; RV = Right ventricle.

defect usually can be crossed. If the tip of the catheter is sufficiently curved, it may be advanced into the right ventricular outflow tract and across the pulmonic valve into the pulmonary artery. A curved guidewire facilitates the above pass, especially if an end-hole catheter is used. A withdrawal pressure measurement from the pulmonary artery localizes the site(s) of obstruction. In our experience, obstruction is usually at infundibular level but is occasionally valvar. The interventricular communication is usually not restrictive in infants and young children and pressures are similar in the left ventricle and in the hypoplastic right ventricle. In patients with discordant ventriculoarterial connection (tricuspid atresia and transposition), in the first few months of life, it is especially important to measure pulmonary artery pressure and to visualize adequately the main and proximal right and left pulmonary arteries, because pulmonary artery banding is the usual surgical approach to this anomaly at that age. The pulmonary artery usually can be entered with a flow-directed balloon catheter via the right atrium, left atrium, and left ventricle. Because pulmonary blood flow usually far exceeds systemic flow, there is little tendency for the balloon to cross the ventricular septal defect into the small right ventricle and enter the aorta instead of entering the pulmonary artery. If an angiographic balloon catheter is used, the pulmonary arteries can be visualized directly, preferably in the anteroposterior view with cranio-caudal angulation (sitting-up view). Alternatively, a left ventricular angiogram can be done in the same view. It is also important to look for evidence of a restrictive ventricular septal defect, both by recording a pressure during a withdrawal of the catheter across the ventricular septal defect from the right to the left ventricle and by visualizing the ventricular septal defect angiographically. Although it may be possible to enter the right ventricle antegrade (via the right atrium, left atrium, left ventricle and ventricular septal defect), it is usually necessary to use a retrograde arterial approach. The ventricular septal defect is best seen on a left ventricular angiogram done in the four-chamber view. As in the more common tricuspid atresia with normally connected great arteries, the adequacy of the interatrial communication should be assessed, both with withdrawal pressure recording and by balloon measurement (see Chapter 12).

Hemodynamic Evaluation

Pressure Data

"A" waves are often large in the right atrial pressure tracing, occasionally reaching 30 or even 40 mm Hg. Markedly exaggerated "A" waves usually indicate a restrictive interatrial opening and this can be confirmed by a withdrawal pressure recording from left to right atrium showing a mean gradient between the two chambers. Right atrial "A" waves may be large in the absence of a small interatrial opening and then usually are related to an elevation of left ventricular end diastolic pressure. Left ventricular dysfunction, as evidenced by high end diastolic pressure, is common in this entity but its genesis is not completely understood. There is volume overload of the left ventricle if there is only mild pulmonic stenosis and large pulmonary flow, and there is marked arterial (including coronary arterial) unsaturation if pulmonic stenosis is severe. The left ventricular dysfunction often seems out of proportion to either volume overload or arterial unsaturation, however.

In patients who are being considered for any type of atrial-pulmonary connection or variant of the Fontan operation, systemic venous pressure is the only, or at least the most important, factor in propelling blood through the pulmonary circuit. Clearly, an elevation of pulmonary vascular resistance precludes a successful result. Therefore, in any patient being considered for this operation, it is mandatory carefully to assess pulmonary vascular resistance. The pulmonary artery must be entered and pressure recorded. In general, a mean pressure of less than 12 mm Hg is a prerequisite for a successful procedure. Pulmonary blood flow influences pressure, however, and a mean pressure of 20 mm Hg in the presence of high flow is less worrisome than a mean pressure of 12 mm Hg with very restricted flow. If the pulmonary to systemic flow ratio is less than 1, we would insist on a mean pressure of 12 mm Hg or less before recommending a Fontan procedure. If the flow ratio is equal to or greater than 2, a mean pressure of up to 20 mm Hg is probably acceptable.

Oxygen Saturation Data

There is no oxygen step-up at right atrial level unless sampling is in the immediate vicinity of the interatrial communication. There is always right to left shunting at atrial level with consequent desaturation of left atrial, left ventricular, and aortic blood. Saturations are variable in the left atrium, depending on whether sampling is in a stream from a pulmonary vein or near the interatrial communication. Saturations are usually similar in the left ventricle, aorta, and pulmonary artery and the degree of arterial desaturation is directly related to the severity of the pulmonic stenosis and/or the pulmonary vascular resistance.

Other Diagnostic and Therapeutic Procedures

If there is any suspicion that the interatrial communication is restrictive, the size of this communication should be estimated by a balloon measuring pullback from the left to the right atrium as described in Chapter 12. If the interatrial communication is determined to be significantly restrictive, a balloon atrial septostomy should be carried out as described in that chapter. A balloon atrial septostomy is likely to be effective

only in the neonatal period and in an older child, a blade atrial septostomy should be substituted (see Chapter 12).

Angiocardiography

Today, the basic intracardiac anatomy is defined by cross-sectional and Doppler echocardiographic study. Angiographically, the lack of direct communication between the right atrium and right ventricle can be demonstrated by a right atrial injection in either the anteroposterior or right anterior oblique projection. There is immediate passage of contrast media across an atrial septal defect or foramen ovale into the left atrium, but no early filling of the right ventricle. The coronary sinus may fill early and may resemble a hypoplastic right ventricle. However, the differentiation will be obvious in the complimentary lateral and left anterior oblique or four-chamber views since the coronary sinus lies posteriorly along the atrioventricular groove. The interatrial communication is best visualized angiographically in the four-chamber view and also can be well seen in the left anterior oblique projection. The hypoplastic right ventricle usually is visualized adequately by a left ventricular injection in the left anterior oblique or four-chamber view (Fig. 4). It fills via a ventricular septal defect, which may be either perimembranous or in the muscular septum. The right ventricle and possible sites of obstruction in the right ventricular outflow tract can be more clearly visualized with a direct injection into the right ventricle, approached by a retrograde arterial catheter passed across the aortic valve and through the ventricular septal defect (Fig. 3). The left ventricular angiogram also gives an indication of function of the left ventricle.

The ventriculoarterial connection can be assessed by either right or left ventricular angiography. Most commonly, the connection is concordant with the aorta filling from the left ventricle and the pulmonary artery from the right. Ventriculoarterial discord-

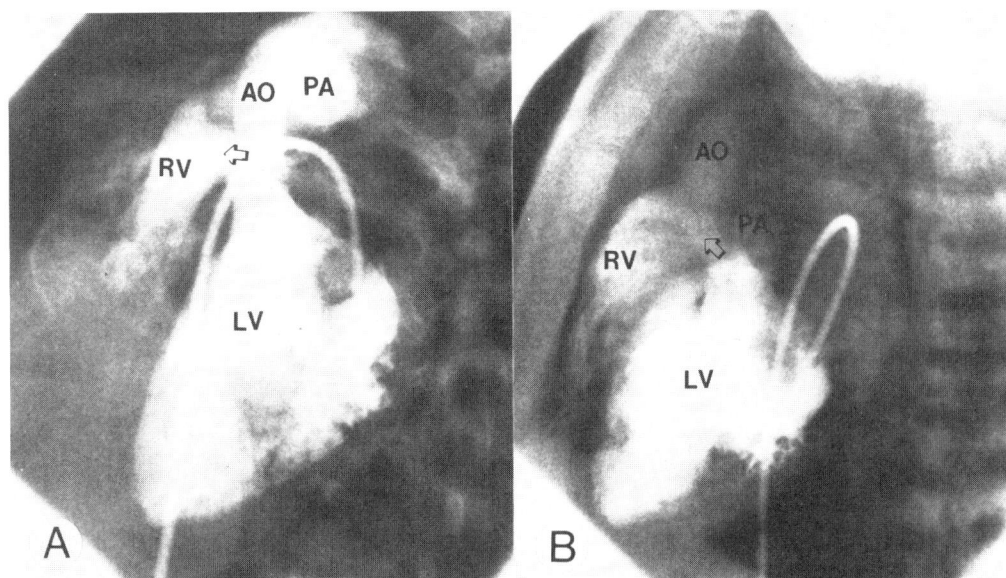

Figure 4. Selective left ventricular injections in tricuspid atresia. A: Left anterior oblique projection demonstrating a hypoplastic right ventricle filling via a ventricular septal defect (arrow). B: Lateral view demonstrating transposition of the great arteries with a hypoplastic right ventricle filling via a ventricular septal defect (arrow). AO = Aorta; LV = Left ventricle; PA = Pulmonary artery; RV = Right ventricle.

ance may also be seen, as well as the unusual situation where both great arteries connect to the right ventricular outflow tract. It is very difficult to be sure of this latter atrioventricular connection by injection into the left ventricle, but injection into the right ventricular outflow tract, approached with a retrograde arterial catheter, usually defines the anatomy quite clearly. This is best viewed in the left and right anterior oblique projections.

The most important aspect of the preoperative angiographic evaluation of a patient with right atrioventricular valve atresia is the morphology of the pulmonary arteries. It is crucial to recognize pulmonary artery stenosis or discontinuity between the right and left pulmonary arteries in a patient who is to undergo a Fontan operation. This is best accomplished by a pulmonary arteriogram or right ventricular angiogram, both sites usually being approached via a retrograde arterial catheterization in patients with con-

cordant ventriculoarterial connection (tricuspid atresia with normally connected great arteries). If there was a previous systemic to pulmonary shunt, this provides access to the pulmonary artery. If not, the right ventricle can be entered with the retrograde catheter across the ventricular septal defect as was described above. Quantitative assessment of pulmonary artery size is accomplished by calculating the pulmonary artery area index as was described in detail in Chapter 25. Ideally, the index should be above 200 mm^2/m^2.

Associated Lesions

Other cardiac anomalies may occur in patients with tricuspid atresia and may be three to four times more common in patients with ventriculoarterial discordance (transposition) as compared to those with ventriculoarterial concordance (normal great arteries) (63% vs. 18%, respectively) (Driscoll 1990). These include venous inflow anomalies such as a persistent left superior vena cava, and others such as juxtaposed atrial appendages and coarctation of the aorta. The possibility of an associated coarctation of the aorta should be suspected, especially in the setting of congestive heart failure and increased pulmonary blood flow.

Cautions and Precautions

The presence of juxtaposed atrial appendages makes entry to the left ventricle more difficult and if unrecognized, may enhance the possibility of perforation of the atrial appendage. In view of the common association of a persistent left superior cava either to the coronary sinus or to the left atrium, it is essential that this lesion be identified since it may preclude a successful Glenn or Fontan operation if unrecognized preoperatively.

Left Atrioventricular Valve (Mitral) Atresia

Anatomy

Left atrioventricular valve atresia associated with aortic atresia is included in Chapter 33; only the variety with a patent aortic orifice will be considered here. In all forms of this anomaly, the usual outlet from the left atrium is absent (Fig. 5). Pulmonary venous return exits the left atrium via an atrial septal defect or patent foramen ovale, or less commonly via a connection to the systemic venous system. This is usually in the form of an ascending vertical vein to the left innominate vein, but may rarely be a communication between the left atrium and the coronary sinus. The ventricular morphology and ventriculoarterial connection are variable (Mickell et al. 1983). In the most common type, both great arteries arise from the right ventricle and the left ventricular

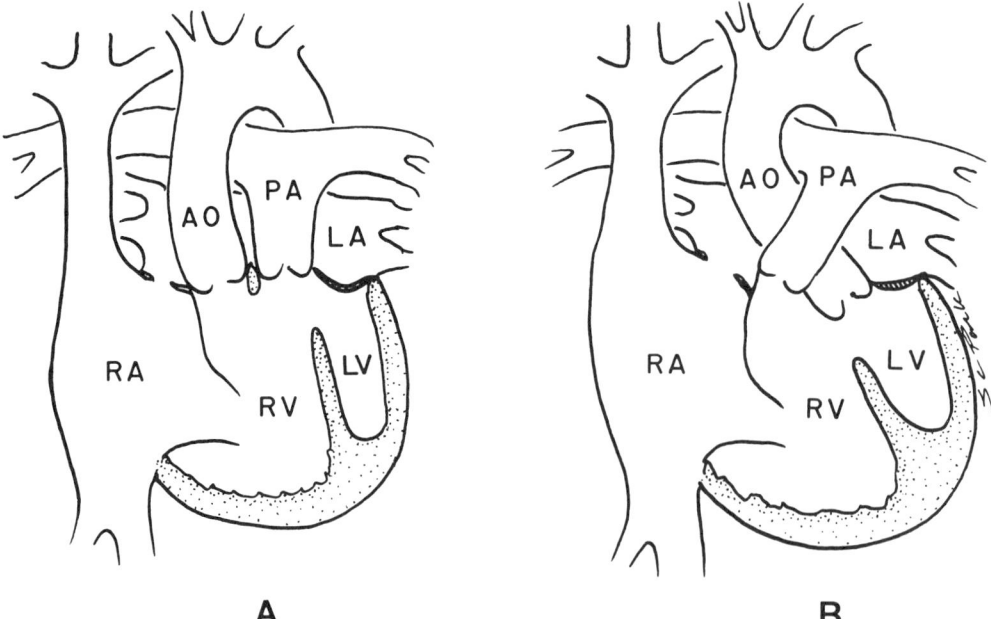

A   **B**

Figure 5. Diagrams of mitral atresia A: With double outlet right ventricle. B: With normal great artery arrangement (aorta arising from the left ventricle).

cavity is markedly hypoplastic or absent. In another common variety, there is a hypoplastic left ventricle which receives blood from the right ventricle through a ventricular septal defect. In this latter case there is usually ventriculoarterial concordance (aorta from left ventricle, pulmonary from right ventricle).

Hemodynamic Considerations

All patients with left atrioventricular valve atresia have arterial unsaturation, because there is mixing of systemic and pulmonary venous returns in the right atrium. Saturations are similar in the aorta and pulmonary artery and the degree of arterial desaturation is dependant upon pulmonary blood flow; high flow resulting in relatively mild desaturation. The exit from the left atrium is commonly restrictive. If the only outlet is a patent foramen ovale, the obstruction may be quite severe, leading to high pressure in the left atrium and pulmonary veins. In many infants, the interatrial communication may not appear to be restrictive in the first week of life while 3 to 4 weeks later, a considerable interatrial gradient is found (Mickell et al. 1980). This phenomenon may be explained by the high neonatal pulmonary vascular resistance preventing a markedly increased pulmonary blood flow in the early neonatal period. Then as pulmonary vascular resistance falls, pulmonary blood flow increases to a considerable degree resulting in increased pulmonary venous return and unmasking of the restriction to flow across the interatrial communication. Because associated pulmonic stenosis is relatively uncommon, pulmonary artery pressure is usually at or near systemic levels.

Indications for Cardiac Catheterization

As with right atrioventricular valve atresia, the diagnosis is established by cross-sectional and Doppler echocardiography. The common indications for cardiac catheterization include assessment prior to pulmonary banding if pulmonary blood flow is excessive, or to enlarge a restrictive interatrial communication. Unfortunately, balloon atrial septostomy is often less effective than in other anomalies. Nonetheless, it should be attempted if catheterization is done during the first month or two of life. In older infants and children a blade septostomy is more appropriate (Park et al. 1978).

Following palliation, postoperative cardiac catheterization is indicated to assess the adequacy of a pulmonary artery band or to size an atrial defect if it still seems restrictive clinically. If a patient is to be considered a candidate for a Fontan procedure in the future, it is essential to document a normal pulmonary artery pressure following initial palliation with a banding.

Catheterization Techniques

It is usually easy to cross the atrial septum in early infancy if the femoral approach is used. However, in older children, the interatrial opening is often distorted and may be oriented more superiorly and posteriorly than usual. This may make passage of the catheter across the atrial septum difficult. Once the catheter crosses the atrial septum, it then enters a pulmonary vein or the left atrial appendage, but not the left ventricle. Because the diagnosis is usually evident on echocardiography, repeated probing of the "mitral" area is clearly unnecessary. A withdrawal pressure tracing from left atrium to right atrium should be recorded to document adequacy of the interatrial communication. The right ventricle is entered in the usual fashion and if there is a double outlet right ventricle, both great arteries usually can be entered from this chamber. If there are two ventricles and little or no aortic override, it may be difficult to traverse the ventricular septal defect with a standard catheter, although the pass sometimes may be accomplished using a flow-directed balloon catheter. In this situation, however, it usually is necessary to use an arterial approach. A withdrawal pressure recording across the distal arch should be done to rule out coarctation of the aorta, which is relatively commonly associated with mitral atresia, especially if the aorta arises from the left ventricle.

Hemodynamic Evaluation

The hemodynamic abnormalities which lead directly or indirectly to cardiac catheterization in most patients with this anomaly are high pulmonary blood flow and pressure, and restriction at the interatrial communication. It is therefore very important to enter the pulmonary artery for pressure determination. Relative pulmonary and systemic blood flows are measured in the usual way, using blood samples obtained in the superior vena cava, pulmonary vein, aorta, and pulmonary artery. (Saturations in aorta and pulmonary artery are usually quite similar). The adequacy of the interatrial communication is evidenced by the gradient obtained on withdrawal pressure recording from the left to the right atrium. The opening also should be sized angiographically or with a balloon catheter.

In patients with two ventricles, the possibility of obstruction to systemic arterial blood flow must always be considered and ruled out. Such obstruction is most commonly in the form of coarctation of the aorta. Because it is usually difficult to enter the hypoplastic left ventricle and aorta prograde (unless there is a double outlet right ventricle), a retrograde arterial catheterization is required if there is clinical or echocardiographic evidence of coarctation. The diagnosis can be established by pressure measurement during withdrawal of the catheter across the distal aortic arch into the descending aorta. In patients with a normal ventriculoarterial relationship, a restrictive ventricular septal defect constitutes subaortic stenosis. This is a less common site of obstruction to systemic blood flow. Its presence is suggested by finding higher pressure in the right ventricle than in a peripheral artery, as determined by simultaneous pressure measurement or indirectly by comparing the right ventricular pressure with a simultaneous pressure measurement with a blood pressure cuff. If a discrepancy is found with the latter technique, it must be confirmed with a retrograde arterial study, with direct measurement of left and right ventricular pressures simultaneously or in rapid succession.

Other Diagnostic or Therapeutic Procedures

If the interatrial communication is restrictive and left atrial pressure is high, balloon or blade atrial septostomy should be considered. In our experience, a balloon

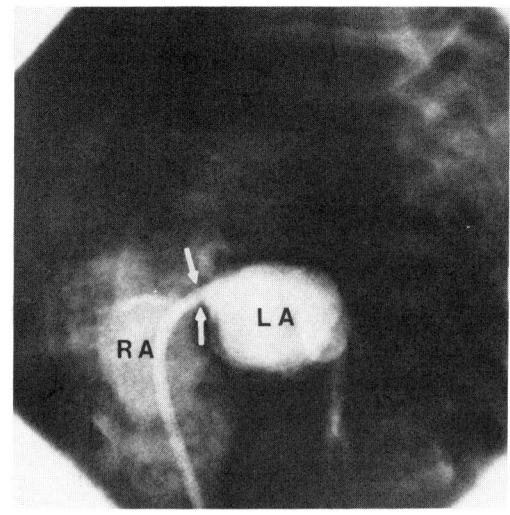

Figure 6. Selective left atrial injection in mitral atresia in the left anterior oblique projection demonstrating absence of the atrioventricular connection and a restrictive interatrial communication (arrows). LA = Left atrium; RA = Right atrium.

atrial septostomy usually is not often effective because even the flap of the foramen ovale tends to be thick and tough in this anomaly. Blade atrial septostomy is carried out as described in Chapter 12. One should be certain that the interatrial opening is in the fossa ovalis if this procedure is to be done; if the communication is a sinus venosus type atrial defect or via the coronary sinus, a blade septostomy is likely to be disastrous.

Angiocardiography

A left atrial angiogram is usually done early in the cardiac catheterization to determine the size of the interatrial communication. Contrast medium does not enter the left ventricle directly, but occasionally an imperforate mitral valve can be seen. This may be in the form of a "wind sock" extending into the left ventricle. In most cases there is an atrial septal defect or a patent foramen ovale and contrast passes from left atrium to right atrium directly (Fig. 6). In some infants, although the left atrium may be entered via a patent foramen ovale, exit is by way of an ascending vertical vein entering the left innominate vein. Rarely, blood may leave the left atrium via a communication with the coronary sinus, recognized by the unusually caudal site of left to right flow. In an unreported case from our institution, a long tortuous venous channel led from the posterior inferior wall of the left atrium to the posterior wall of the right atrium and constituted the only exit from the left atrium.

Ventricular morphology and ventriculoarterial connection are best defined by right ventricular angiography in anteroposterior and lateral views or in the left anterior oblique or four-chamber views (Fig. 7). In an occasional patient the ventricular septum is in an unusually transverse plane, and a small

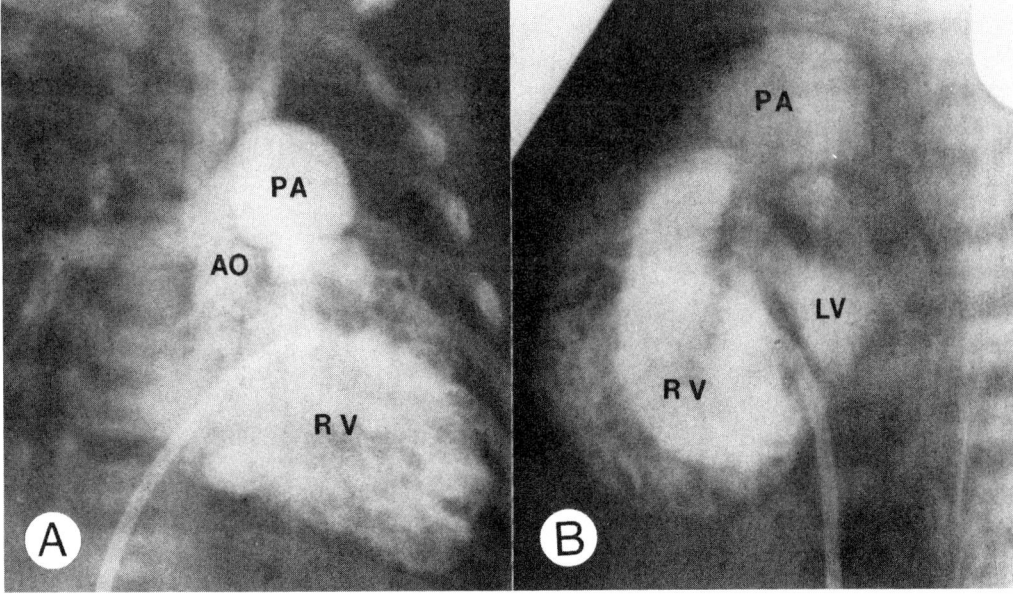

Figure 7. Selective right ventricular angiogram in mitral atresia demonstrating a double outlet right ventricle and small rudimentary left ventricle (LV). A = Anteroposterior view; B = Lateral view. AO = Aorta; LV = Left ventricle; PA = Pulmonary artery; RV = Right ventricle.

left ventricle can be missed unless the lateral view is recorded. If the distal aortic arch is not well defined an aortogram should be done in the left anterior oblique or the lateral view.

Associated Lesions

Left atrioventricular valve atresia is most commonly found in association with aortic atresia and this combination is considered in Chapter 33. Anomalies of venous return are common and the variety of anatomic patterns to decompress the left atrium have been described earlier in this chapter. Because there is usually no or mild pulmonary stenosis, increased pulmonary blood flow is the rule and a patent ductus arteriosus is often present as well. Coarctation of the aorta is a frequent additional problem and should always be considered in patients with this anomaly.

Cautions and Precautions

A restrictive interatrial communication almost always accompanies this lesion and the size of the defect therefore always must be evaluated. As was mentioned earlier, even if this communication was thought to be adequate initially, the possibility that the communication is restrictive should always be considered if any deterioration occurs.

References and Suggested Reading

Driscoll DJ. Tricuspid atresia. In: The Science and Practice of Pediatric Cardiology. Garson A, Bricker JT, McNamara DG (eds). Philadelphia, PA; Lea and Febiger, 1990:1118–1126.

Mickell JJ, Mathews RA, Park SC, et al. Left atrioventricular valve atresia: Clinical management. Circulation 1980;61:123–127.

Mickell JJ, Mathews RA, Anderson RH, et al. The anatomical heterogeneity of hearts lacking a patent communication between the left atrium and the ventricular mass ("mitral atresia") in presence of a patent aortic valve. Eur Heart J 1983;477–486.

Neches WH, Park SC, Lenox CC, et al. Tricuspid atresia with transposition of the great arteries and closing ventricular septal defect. J Thorac Cardiovasc Surg 1973;65:538–542.

Park SC, Neches WH, Zuberbuhler JR, et al. Clinical use of blade atrial septostomy. Circulation 1978;58:600–606.

Tynan MJ, Becker AE, Maccartney FJ, et al. Nomenclature and classification of congenital heart disease. Br Heart J 1979;41:544–553.

31

Double Inlet Ventricle

J.R. Zuberbuhler, M.D.

Anatomy

There has been much confusion and contention regarding the nomenclature of the anomaly dealt with in this chapter. It most often has been called "single ventricle" or "univentricular heart", but there are usually two ventricular chambers. One receives the atrial inflow, while the other is hypoplastic and without atrioventricular connection. It therefore seems preferable to call this anomaly a "double inlet ventricle", because this term describes an atrioventricular connection in which both atria empty into one ventricular cavity, either via two atrioventricular valves or a common valve. Double inlet ventricle is one variety of univentricular atrioventricular connection, the others being absent right and absent left atrioventricular connection (Anderson et al. 1983A). It should be noted that there is a distinction between "absent" and "imperforate" atrioventricular connection. If an imperforate valve abuts on the ventricular cavity that receives the inflow from the other atrioventricular valve, a double inlet ventricle is considered to be present. In such hearts the mode of connection is imperforate.

Once the diagnosis of double inlet ventricle has been made, details of ventricular morphology, the mode of atrioventricular connection, the ventriculoarterial connection and any associated anomalies can then be specified. Cross-sectional and Doppler echocardiography are essential tools for the elucidation of these features prior to performing cardiac catheterization.

Double Inlet Left Ventricle

The most common variety of double inlet ventricle consists of a left ventricle, which receives atrial inflow, and a rudimentary right ventricle, situated superior and anterior to the left ventricle and connected to it by a ventricular septal defect (Anderson et al. 1979) (Fig. 1). There is usually ventriculoarterial discordance, with the rudimentary right ventricle supporting the aorta and the left ventricle supporting the pulmonary artery (Fig 1A; Fig. 2). Less commonly, there is ventriculoarterial concordance, with reversal of the above described connections (Holmes heart) (Anderson et al. 1983B) (Fig. 1B; Fig. 3). Rarely, both aorta and pulmonary artery arise from the rudimentary right ventricle; in other words there is a double inlet left ventricle and a double outlet right ventricle (Fig. 4). Pulmonic stenosis is common and may be valvar, subvalvar, or at a restrictive ventricular septal defect if there is ventriculoarterial concordance. Aortic stenosis is rare but occurs if there is a restrictive ventricular septal defect in the setting of ventriculoarterial discordance. Straddling of one atrioventricular valve is not rare with double inlet ventricle. The connection is considered to be double inlet if more than 50% of the straddling orifice connects to the ventricle which receives the other atrioventricular valve. Also, in double inlet left ventricle one of the atrioventricular valves may be stenotic (Fig. 5). This has important hemodynamic consequences if the atrial septum is intact, or if an interatrial communication is restrictive.

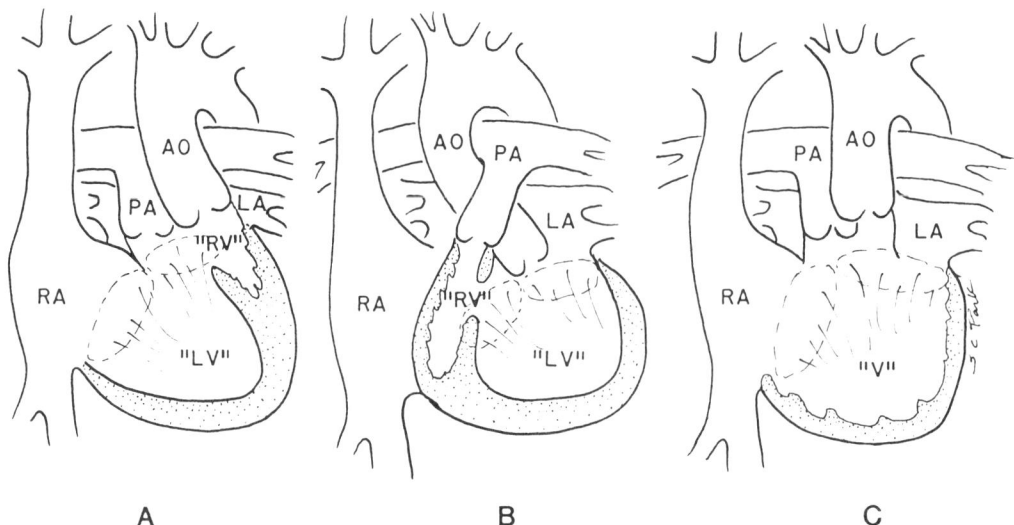

Figure 1. Diagrams of double inlet left ventricle. A: Common form—The pulmonary artery arises from the main ventricular chamber and the aorta from the rudimentary right ventricular outlet chamber (transposition). B: Holmes heart—The pulmonary artery arises from a small rudimentary right-sided right ventricle. The aorta arises from the main ventricular chamber. C: indeterminate form.

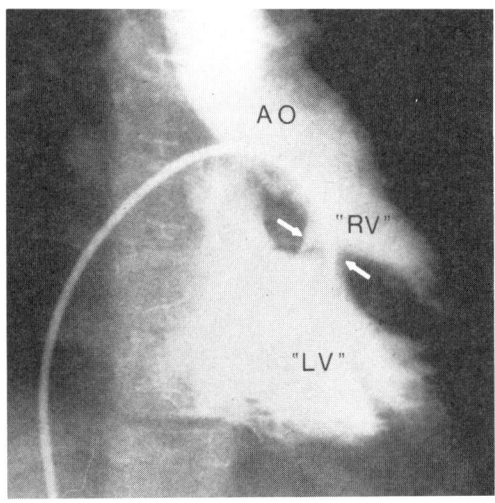

Figure 2. Cineangiogram of double inlet left ventricle with the aorta arising from a small outlet chamber. The ventricular septal defect is restrictive (arrows). AO = Aorta; LV = Left ventricle; RV = right ventricle; (outflow chamber).

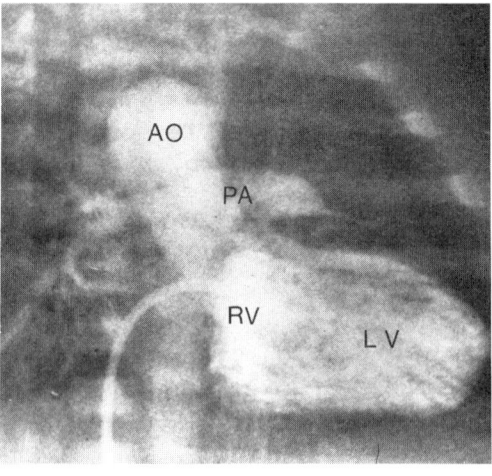

Figure 3. Cineangiogram of double inlet left ventricle with normally connected great arteries (Holmes heart). The aorta arises from the left ventricular chamber, the pulmonary artery from the outlet chamber. AO = Aorta; LV = Left ventricle; PA = Pulmonary artery; RV = right ventricle (outflow chamber).

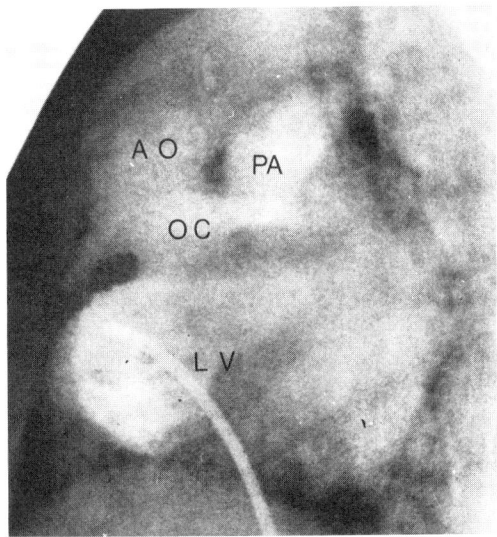

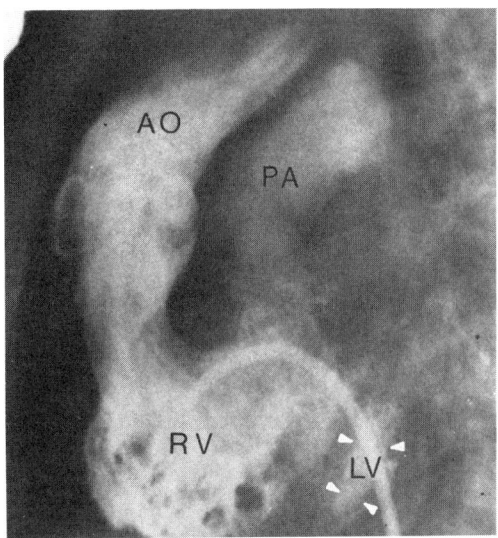

Figure 4. Cineangiogram of double inlet left ventricle with double outlet chamber in the lateral view. Both the aorta and pulmonary artery arise from the outlet chamber that is situated cephalad to the left ventricle. AO = aorta; LV = left ventricle; OC = outlet chamber; PA = pulmonary artery.

Figure 6. Right ventricular cineangiogram in double outlet right ventricle. The aorta is directly anterior to the pulmonary artery. There is a small left ventricular pouch situated posteriorly (arrows). AO = aorta; LV = Left ventricle; PA = pulmonary artery; RV = right ventricle.

Double Inlet Right Ventricle

In this anomaly, both atrioventricular valves (or a common atrioventricular valve) enter the right ventricle (Keeton et al. 1979). There may or may not be a rudimentary left ventricle, usually only the trabecular portion, situated posterior to the right ventricle (Fig. 6). Both aorta and pulmonary artery arise from the right ventricle.

Double Inlet Indeterminate Ventricle

The ventricle receiving inflow from the atria may have bizarre trabeculations and not be identifiable as a right or left ventricle (Fig. 1C; Fig. 7). In such hearts there is no rudimentary second ventricle (Anderson et al. 1979).

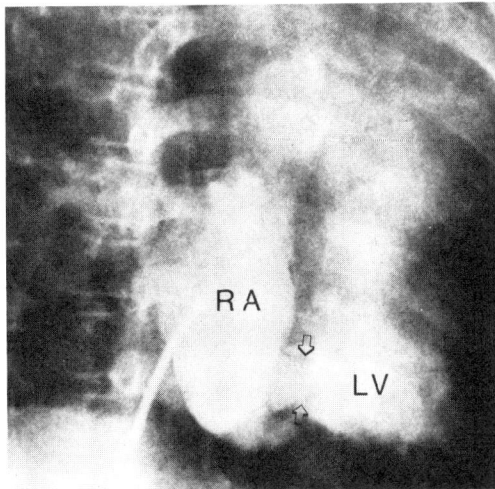

Figure 5. Right atrial injection in a patient with double inlet ventricle and a stenotic right-sided atrioventricular valve (arrows). LV = left ventricle; RA = right atrium.

Hemodynamic Considerations

As indicated above, hearts with double inlet ventricle have widely varying mor-

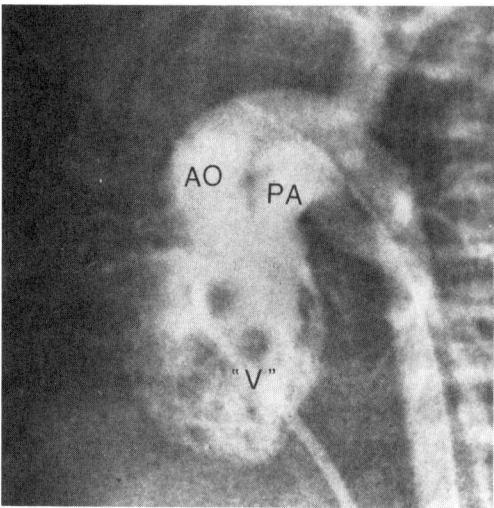

Figure 7. Cineangiogram of a double inlet indeterminate ventricle. The trabeculations are large and bizarre. AO = aorta; PA = pulmonary artery; V = ventricle.

phology. The only universal hemodynamic consequence of this connection is arterial unsaturation, which occurs because of mixing of systemic and pulmonary venous returns in the ventricle receiving the atrial inflow. The severity of unsaturation depends upon the relative magnitude of pulmonary and systemic flows, a large pulmonary flow resulting in relatively high arterial saturation. The magnitude of pulmonary blood flow is, in turn, related to the presence or absence of pulmonic stenosis and to the level of pulmonary vascular resistance. Although high pulmonary blood flow improves oxygen saturation, it is an important cause of congestive heart failure in patients with double inlet ventricle. Also, pulmonary vascular disease is an inevitable eventual consequence of high pulmonary artery pressure and flow.

In patients with double inlet ventricle, the systolic pressure in the pulmonary artery is at systemic level unless there is pulmonic stenosis. If there is an outlet chamber, a restrictive ventricular septal defect results in lower pressure in the outlet chamber and

in the great artery supported by it than in the main ventricular chamber. Such a restrictive ventricular septal defect constitutes subaortic stenosis or subpulmonary stenosis, depending upon the ventriculoarterial connection.

Atrioventricular valve regurgitation is relatively common in older children and adults with this anomaly and is another important cause of congestive heart failure. Stenosis of an atrioventricular valve has important hemodynamic consequences only if the atrial septum is intact or if an interatrial communication is restrictive.

To summarize some patients with double inlet ventricle may have pulmonary hypertension, with varying severity of pulmonary vascular disease. It is therefore important to measure pulmonary artery pressure and to estimate relative pulmonary and systemic blood flows. In other patients with double inlet ventricle there is outflow obstruction, and the degree of the obstruction should be assessed. Also, the obstruction should be localized to a semilunar valve, the infundibulum, or the ventricular septal defect. Atrioventricular valve function should be evaluated.

Indications for Cardiac Catheterization

Preoperative

The diagnosis of double inlet ventricle can be made echocardiographically, but cardiac catheterization is usually necessary prior to surgical intervention. In patients with double inlet ventricle, operation is most commonly undertaken to regulate pulmonary blood flow. If a systemic to pulmonary artery shunt is to be done in a child with severe pulmonic stenosis, an assessment of the morphology of the pulmonary arteries and the aortic arch and its branches is essential. In a patient being considered for pulmonary artery banding, preoperative measurement of pulmonary artery pressure and flow is required. If a Fontan procedure is planned, a very careful evaluation of pulmonary artery pressure and flow and pulmonary vascular resistance is even more vital. Rarely, surgery is undertaken because of atrioventricular valve malfunction and may consist of an atrial septectomy if the left-sided atrioventricular valve is stenotic, or valve replacement if there is severe valvar regurgitation. In either case, valve function should be evaluated by cardiac catheterization and angiography prior to surgical intervention.

Postoperative

Postoperative cardiac catheterization is indicated if there is a question of the adequacy of a pulmonary band or patency of a systemic-pulmonary artery shunt. In our laboratory postoperative cardiac catheterization is routinely recommended approximately 1 year following the Fontan operation.

Cardiac Catheterization Technique

Cardiac catheterization is usually done from the femoral approach unless there is iliofemoral venous thrombosis from a previous study. The main ventricle is usually accessible from the right atrium through the right atrioventricular valve, unless this valve is imperforate or severely stenotic. The distinction between an imperforate valve (rare) and a stenotic one (somewhat more common) is best made echocardiographically.

In double inlet left ventricle, the rudimentary right ventricle is usually located on the left anterior aspect of the ventricular mass. If the catheter is rotated clockwise and aimed toward the patient's left shoulder, it usually traverses the ventricular septal de-

fect and enters the outlet chamber. It can then be advanced into the great artery supported by this outlet chamber, usually the aorta (Fig. 1). Entering the artery supported by the main ventricle may be more difficult, especially if there is valvar or subvalvar obstruction. The orifice is usually more medial and posterior than the outlet chamber and a catheter with a more sharply curved tip may be helpful in the pass. If the artery cannot easily be entered, a flow-directed balloon catheter should be tried. If the aorta cannot be entered antegrade, the retrograde arterial approach may be utilized. If ventriculoarterial discordance is present, the rudimentary right ventricle usually can be entered from the aortic root.

An attempt should always be made to traverse the interatrial septum. A subsequent pass from the left atrium to a ventricular zone establishes patency of the left atrioventricular valve. In addition, a left atrial or pulmonary venous sample for oxygen saturation and a left atrial pressure can be obtained. If possible, pressure should always be measured in each atrium, in the main ventricle, in the rudimentary ventricle if one is present, and in the pulmonary artery and aorta.

Left atrioventricular valve stenosis is occasionally seen with double inlet ventricle, and in some of our patients was sufficiently severe to necessitate either blade atrial septostomy or surgical atrial septectomy. Therefore, if left atrial or pulmonary artery wedge pressure is high, pressure in the main ventricle should be recorded simultaneously, permitting measurement of the gradient across the left atrioventricular valve. Measuring pressures in both the ventricle and outlet chamber identifies a restrictive ventricular septal defect. It is very important that the pulmonary artery be entered in a patient with double inlet ventricle. If there is pulmonic stenosis it is necessary unequivocally to establish its presence and severity by measuring the ventricular-pulmonary artery gradient. Also, pulmonary vascular resistance can be calculated only if pulmonary artery pressure is known.

Hemodynamic Evaluation

Pressure Data

In the absence of pulmonic stenosis, systolic pressure is equal in the main ventricle and pulmonary artery. Pulmonary artery diastolic pressure is typically lower than aortic, however, if pulmonary vascular resistance is low and pulmonary flow high. If pulmonic stenosis is present it can be defined as valvar or subvalvar by a pullback from the pulmonary artery to the ventricle. High pressure in the pulmonary artery wedge position or in the left atrium is usually on the basis of high ventricular diastolic pressure. But if left ventricular diastolic pressure is not elevated, left atrioventricular valve stenosis is likely. Careful simultaneous recording of wedge or left atrial pressure and ventricular pressure is required to establish the presence of obstruction at the left atrioventricular valve. It should be noted that a large atrial septal communication precludes a gradient across even a very stenotic atrioventricular valve. The diagnosis must then be made echocardiographically or by angiocardiogram. Conversely, a difference in pressure in the right and left atria does not establish the presence of anatomic atrioventricular valve stenosis. If pulmonary blood flow is very large, a gradient will be on the basis of relative stenosis.

Oximetry Data

If there is an atrial septal defect there may be an oxygen step-up at atrial as well as ventricular level. Because of streaming, oxygen saturations are often quite variable in the main ventricular chamber. Also, because of streaming, saturation in the aorta and pulmonary artery may differ, and aortic saturation may be higher or lower than that in the pulmonary artery (Macartney et al. 1976). In many patients, however, saturations are similar in the outlet chamber and in the aorta and pulmonary artery. The pulmonary to systemic flow ratio is determined in the usual way, using saturations obtained in the superior vena cava, aorta, pulmonary artery and in either a pulmonary vein or a pulmonary artery wedge position. The lack of an oxygen step-up in the pulmonary artery does not, of course, rule out a patent ductus arteriosus, because oxygen saturation is similar in aorta and pulmonary artery.

Angiocardiography

Selective angiography most accurately defines ventricular morphology in double inlet ventricle. The structural characteristics of the ventricle can be defined; most importantly its trabecular pattern and the presence of a rudimentary ventricle. If the main ventricle is thought to be a morphological right ventricle, a trabecular pouch (Fig. 8) should be searched for. Because this structure is always posterior to the morphologic right ventricle, a lateral view of the ventricular injection is usually best. Occasionally, a steep left anterior oblique view better profiles the remnant of muscular septum and separates the ventricle and the pouch. With double inlet left ventricle, the position of the rudimentary right ventricle is more variable. It is always an anterior structure but may be to the right, left, or directly anterior to the left ventricle. An anteroposterior view often shows the outlet chamber well, but occasionally a right or left oblique view is better. Cranio-caudal angulation may better profile the ventricular septal defect and more clearly define the size of the rudimentary ventricle. If an outlet chamber is visualized after a main ventricular injection, it is usually wise to perform a selective injection into the rudimentary ventricle itself better to define its morphology and connections. For example, in a patient with corrected transposition and a ven-

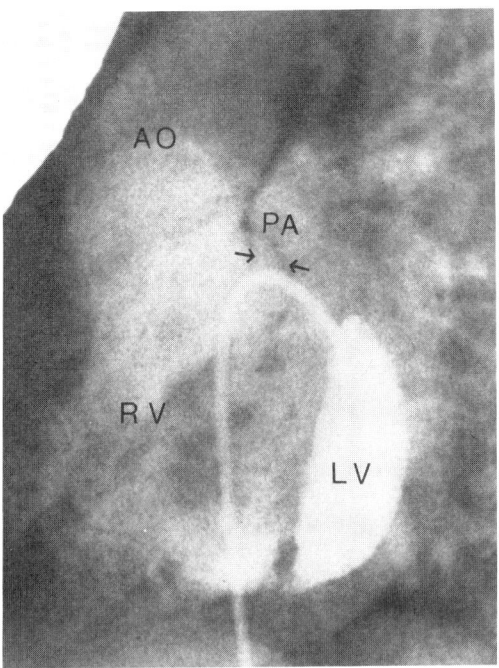

Figure 8. Steep left anterior oblique projection of a selective injection into a left ventricular pouch in a patient with double inlet right ventricle (arrows = pulmonary stenosis). AO = aorta; LV = left ventricular pouch; PA = pulmonary artery; RV = right ventricle.

tricular septal defect with severe pulmonic stenosis, a right-sided ventricular injection may show what appears to be a small left-sided rudimentary ventricle supporting the aorta. A selective injection into the supposed outlet chamber may, in this situation, show the left-sided cavity to be larger than expected. Also, inflow from the left atrium to the left-sided ventricle may be demonstrated, ruling out a double inlet ventricle. If there is doubt as to whether there is corrected transposition with a somewhat hypoplastic left-sided ventricle, or a double inlet left ventricle with a left-sided rudimentary right ventricle, an injection into the left atrium is mandatory. If there is a double inlet left ventricle, the left atrium will empty through the left-sided atrioventricular valve into the morphologically left ventricle. With corrected transposition, contrast medium

passes from the left atrium directly to the left-sided but morphologically right ventricle.

A main ventricular injection should show the size and location of the ventricular septal defect if a rudimentary ventricle is present. In some patients an injection into the rudimentary ventricle itself will define the defect, since contrast medium often briefly refluxes through it. Again, craniocaudal angulation may help to outline the ventricular septal defect. Pulmonic stenosis may be difficult to define angiographically and several ventricular injections in various projections, including standard oblique, angulated right anterior oblique and four chamber views may be necessary. Atrioventricular valvar regurgitation can also be identified and quantitated with a ventricular injection. The ventriculogram also serves as a rough measure of ventricular function. If semilunar valve regurgitation is suspected clinically, aortic root and pulmonary artery injections are desirable to identify aortic and pulmonic regurgitation, respectively. An aortic injection is often recommended to rule out a patent ductus arteriosus and/or aortic arch anomalies including coarctation of the aorta.

Associated Lesions

Because of the hemodynamic import of associated anomalies, they have been discussed above. To summarize, the most frequent associated anomaly is pulmonic stenosis. Pulmonary atresia is also seen and has profound clinical consequences. With double inlet left ventricle, a restrictive ventricular septal defect constitutes either subaortic or subpulmonic stenosis, depending on the ventriculoarterial connections. Abnormalities of the atrioventricular valves are the second most common group of associated malformations. Atresia of the right and left valves occur, as does stenosis of either valve. Stenosis of the left valve is more importantly hemodynamically. Atrioventricular valvar regurgitation is usually acquired and tends to be progressive.

Cautions or Precautions

Atrioventricular block can be induced during attempts to enter the pulmonary artery in a child with double inlet left ventricle and transposition, especially if the right ventricular outlet chamber is to the left (Becker et al. 1979). In this particular malformation the atrioventricular conduction axis traverses the subpulmonary outflow tract anteriorly and is therefore vulnerable to catheter manipulation in this area. Use of a flow-directed balloon catheter is likely to be less traumatic, but may be ineffective in the presence of pulmonic stenosis and restricted outflow from the dominant ventricle to the pulmonary artery.

The possibility of stenosis of the left atrioventricular valve should always be considered in a patient with double inlet left ventricle. Such stenosis may not be obvious clinically, but the consequences of constructing a systemic to pulmonary artery shunt or doing a Fontan operation in the presence of "mitral" stenosis can be very

serious. It is also mandatory to assess severity of atrioventricular valve regurgitation and dominant ventricular function in any child with double inlet ventricle being considered for a Fontan operation.

References and Suggested Reading

Anderson RH, Lenox CC, Zuberbuhler JR, et al. Double inlet left ventricle with rudimentary right ventricle and ventriculoarterial concordance. Am J Cardiol 1983B;52:573–577.

Anderson RH, Macartney FJ, Tynan M, et al. Univentricular atrioventricular connection: The single ventricle trap unsprung. Pediatr Cardiol 1983A;4:273–280.

Anderson RH, Tynan M, Freedom RM, et al. Ventricular morphology in the univentricular heart. Herz 1979;4:184–197.

Becker AE, Wilkinson JL, Anderson RH. Atrioventricular conduction tissues in univentricular hearts of left ventricular type. Herz 1979;4:166–175.

Keeton BR, Macartney FJ, Hunter S, et al. Univentricular heart of the right ventricular type with double or common inlet. Circulation 1979;59:403–411.

Macartney FJ, Partridge JB, Scott O, et al. Common or single ventricle. An angiocardiography and hemodynamic study of 42 patients. Circulation 1976;53:543–554.

32

Left Heart Inlet Obstruction

José A. Ettedgui, M.D.

Pulmonary vein stenosis, cor triatriatum and mitral stenosis will be considered together since each of these anomalies produces left heart inlet obstruction, although at different levels. Individual anomalies will be considered separately when there are significant differences in approach. Most patients with left heart inlet obstruction present with congestive heart failure, decreased exercise tolerance, dyspnea on exertion, or pulmonary hypertension. The diagnosis of cor triatriatum or pulmonary vein stenosis is never obvious clinically because there are no specific physical findings, only those of the resulting pulmonary hypertension. Clinical signs of mitral stenosis are more specific, and consist of an apical mid diastolic murmur with presystolic accentuation. If present, the signs of pulmonary hypertension also will be noted.

Anatomy

Pulmonary Vein Atresia

In this rare anomaly there is either no connection or a fibrous cord without a lumen between the confluence of the pulmonary veins and the left atrium or the systemic venous system. Life may be sustained for a few hours to a few days by flow through small accessary pulmonary veins which drain part of lung to a systemic vein. At times the atresia involves only one or two veins (Fig. 1F) and the clinical presentation is more subtle, and often masked by coexisting lesions (Beerman 1983).

Pulmonary Vein Stenosis

In pulmonary vein stenosis the obstruction is usually discrete and localized at the venoatrial junction. It may also be more tubular due to hypoplasia of the pulmonary vein and occasionally is located entirely within the pulmonary parenchyma. The obstruction may involve all veins, veins from only one lung, or even a single vein (Fig. 1D and 1E). The degree of obstruction is highly variable (Sade 1974).

Cor Triatriatum

In cor triatriatum the left atrium is partitioned into two chambers, a proximal one into which the pulmonary veins drain, and a distal one which includes the left atrial appendage and the mitral orifice (Fig. 1C). The size of the opening in the membrane between the two chambers is quite variable. It ranges from large and unrestrictive, and therefore of minimal clinical significance, to one or more small perforations located centrally or peripherally in the membrane and producing obstruction to left ventricular filling. There may be a patent foramen ovale or secundum atrial septal defect entering the distal chamber. Less commonly, an opening is present between the right atrium and the proximal chamber.

A supravalvar mitral ring is a membranous structure that produces inflow obstruction similar to cor triatriatum. However, this membrane is located distally just above the mitral valve.

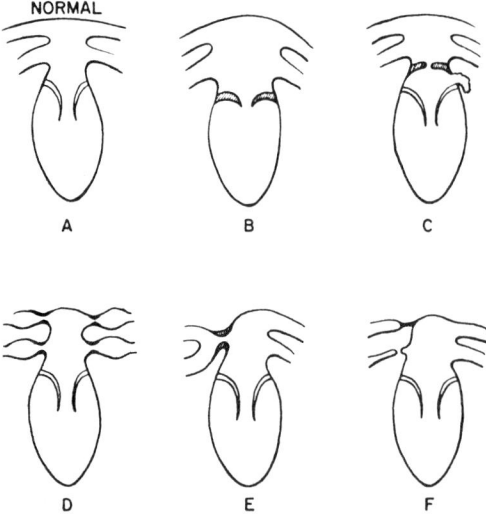

Figure 1. Diagram showing various levels of left heart inflow obstruction. A: Normal. B: Valvar mitral stenosis. C: Cor triatriatum. D: Stenosis of all pulmonary veins. E: Unilateral common pulmonary vein stenosis. F: Pulmonary vein atresia with fibrous cord or complete interruption.

Mitral Stenosis

Congenital mitral stenosis is a rare anomaly and differs in some morphologic features from acquired rheumatic mitral stenosis (Roberts 1983). The mitral valve is usually grossly abnormal with thickened leaflets, poorly defined commissures, and abnormal chordae and papillary muscles (Fig. 1B). In one variety of congenital mitral stenosis there is a single papillary muscle that receives all of the chordae from the mitral leaflets (parachute mitral valve).

Hemodynamic Considerations

If obstruction to left heart inflow is significant, it inevitably causes pulmonary venous hypertension and an elevation of the pulmonary artery wedge pressure. It is important to realize that the increased wedge pressure may be unilateral or may even be unilobar in isolated pulmonary vein stenosis where not all veins are obstructed. In this situation the diagnosis can be missed if wedge pressures are not obtained from several positions within the lung (Neches 1977). This is an especially important consideration in a patient with unexplained pulmonary hypertension. The pulmonary arterial hypertension associated with left heart inlet obstruction is partly "passive", a direct consequence of the increased pulmonary venous pressure. An "active" pulmonary arteriolar constrictive component may be present if the obstruction is severe. Cardiac output is usually normal, as is systemic arterial saturation. In rare cases of cor triatriatum or pulmonary vein stenosis, systemic arterial desaturation may be present, but is always higher than the saturation in the pulmonary artery. An oxygen step-up at the right atrial level may occur with either mitral stenosis, or cor triatriatum, if there is an accompanying interatrial communication (to the proximal chamber in cor triatriatum). In one reported case of cor triatriatum, a persistent left superior vena cava connected to the left atrium and provided a run-off from the high-pressure proximal chamber.

Indications for Cardiac Catheterization

The usual indication for cardiac catheterization in a patient suspected of having one of this group of anomalies is clinical evidence of pulmonary venous hypertension (Glancy 1976). Symptoms of increased pressure in the pulmonary veins ranges from dyspnea on exertion if the obstruction is mild, to orthopnea or paroxysmal nocturnal dyspnea if the obstruction is severe. Physical findings suggestive of pulmonary hypertension, such as a loud pulmonic closure sound or a right ventricular lift also indicate severe obstruction. Radiographic signs of pulmonary venous hypertension include an increase in pulmonary venous markings, especially in the hilar areas, and the presence of Kerley "B" lines at the lung bases.

Cross-sectional and Doppler echocardiography provide accurate, noninvasive diagnosis of this constellation of anomalies. However, the diagnosis of pulmonary vein stenosis and atresia using echocardiography is difficult. Color flow imaging greatly contributes to the noninvasive diagnosis of pulmonary venous obstruction but, unless sought for carefully, pulmonary vein stenosis or atresia can be missed easily. Echocardiography has replaced cardiac catheterization for the diagnosis of cor triatriatum. In this condition, preoperative catheterization is rarely indicated.

Cardiac Catheterization Technique

The importance of obtaining accurate pulmonary artery wedge pressures in patients with pulmonary hypertension cannot be overemphasized, because an elevation of pulmonary artery wedge pressure is the most prominent hemodynamic abnormality in this group of malformations. A single normal pulmonary artery wedge pressure recording, or even normal recordings from more than one area of lung, will eliminate left atrial hypertension due to mitral stenosis or cor triatriatum but should never be taken as firm evidence that pulmonary vein stenosis is absent. Wedge pressure recordings from multiple areas of both lungs must be obtained before pulmonary vein stenosis can be ruled out. An adequate wedge pressure usually can be obtained with an end-hole catheter, especially if pulmonary venous hypertension is present, but occasionally a balloon-tipped catheter must be utilized. If pulmonary venous hypertension is found, wedge pressures should be recorded simultaneously or in rapid succession with high gain left ventricular pressure. Cardiac output should always be measured since it

influences the level of pulmonary venous hypertension in a patient with a given amount of obstruction. Cardiac output will usually decrease in presence of severe obstruction.

Pulmonary Vein Stenosis

The adequate evaluation of a patient with pulmonary vein stenosis poses some special problems, particularly since this anomaly may occur in association with other congenital cardiac defects such as a ventricular septal defect. Unless an accurate pulmonary artery wedge pressure from more than one location is obtained, the presence of pulmonary vein stenosis may be missed (Park 1974). Pulmonary vein stenosis is a likely diagnosis in any patient with elevated pulmonary arterial wedge pressure and a normal left ventricular end diastolic pressure if mitral stenosis and cor triatriatum have been ruled out by cross-sectional echocardiography. However, the adequate visualization of pulmonary vein stenosis necessitates selective injection of contrast media into individual pulmonary veins (See Angiography later in this chapter). Entering the pulmonary veins is relatively easy if there is an interatrial communication and if the catheterization is done from the femoral approach. As the catheter is passed across the interatrial septum, it points to the patient's left and the left-sided pulmonary veins are usually entered readily. If any difficulty is encountered the catheter should be rotated slightly clockwise to make the tip point posteriorly toward the orifice of the left pulmonary veins. To enter right pulmonary veins the catheter is rotated clockwise with more torque until the tip points to the right. A sharply curved catheter is often helpful for entering the right pulmonary veins. In a patient with an intact atrial septum, entry into the pulmonary veins is more difficult. A transseptal catheterization is the recommended approach (see Chapter 14). Alternatively, an effort can be made to enter the pulmonary veins using a retrograde arterial catheter. The catheter is looped in the aortic root with the tip pointing to the patient's right (anteroposterior view). The catheter loop is advanced across the aortic valve into the left ventricle. It then may be possible to maneuver the catheter across the mitral valve and further advance the tip into a pulmonary vein (see also Chapter 5). This latter maneuver is difficult and should be attempted only when a transseptal approach is not feasible (e.g., bilateral iliac vein or inferior vena cava thrombosis, or an absent inferior vena cava with azygos continuation to the superior vena cava.)

Mitral Stenosis or Cor Triatriatum

The technique for entering the left atrium has just been described. In either of these anomalies a similar approach would be used. In mitral stenosis, however, a retrograde catheter pass may be difficult due to the anomalies of the valve. In cor triatriatum, it may be possible to pass the catheter retrogradely across the mitral valve, but it may be difficult to advance it further into the proximal, high-pressure chamber. In either situation, the appearance of a gradient between the pulmonary artery wedge position and the left ventricular end diastolic pressure will signify the presence of obstruction.

Hemodynamic Evaluation

An elevation of pulmonary artery wedge pressure is a universal finding in this group of anomalies. In addition, left ventricular end diastolic pressure is normal, indicating a gradient between the pulmonary arteriolar bed and the left ventricle. The magnitude of this gradient depends upon pulmonary blood flow and can be relatively modest if cardiac output is diminished, even in the presence of severe obstruction.

Pulmonary Vein Atresia

Hemodynamic findings in this rare anomaly include a low oxygen saturation throughout the heart, with no demonstrable step-up at any level. Severe pulmonary hypertension invariably is present and pulmonary artery wedge pressure is higher than left atrial pressure, effectively differentiating this anomaly from persistent fetal circulation (Ledbetter 1978).

Pulmonary Vein Stenosis

Left atrial pressure is normal in patients with pulmonary vein stenosis. The combination of elevated pulmonary arterial wedge pressure and a normal left atrial pressure is pathognomonic of pulmonary vein stenosis. The site of obstruction within the pulmonary vein can be demonstrated if the vein can be entered directly with an end-hole catheter. It should be noted that the gradient demonstrated with the catheter in the pulmonary vein is usually greater than the gradient calculated from simultaneous pulmonary artery wedge and either left atrial or left ventricular and diastolic pressure recordings. This occurs because the catheter lying across an area of stenosis in a pulmonary vein can add substantially to the degree of obstruction. Also, one must be sure when measuring pulmonary venous pressure that the catheter is not too far out into the pulmonary vein and is not actually measuring a pulmonary venous wedge pressure. The latter pressure, of course, is more indicative of pulmonary artery pressure than of pressure within the pulmonary vein. It may be necessary to check the position of the catheter tip with a small injection of contrast media.

In this anomaly there is usually no evidence of right to left or left to right shunting by oximetry. However, if there is severe pulmonary hypertension and right atrial pressures are sufficiently elevated, there may be right to left shunting through a patent foramen ovale. There is then desaturation in the left atrium, left ventricle and aorta. If obstruction is very severe, cardiac output may be reduced and mixed venous saturation is low.

Cor Triatriatum

As with the other anomalies in this group, an elevated pulmonary artery wedge pressure is a constant hemodynamic finding. It is easy to miss the diagnosis of cor triatriatum if another cardiac anomaly is present which can also cause an elevation in wedge pressure. Occasionally, there is an oxygen step-up at right atrial level secondary to shunting from the proximal left atrial chamber to the right atrium. If there is a communication between the right atrium and the distal chamber as well, there may be right to left shunting with resulting systemic arterial desaturation. The rare combination of a runoff from the proximal chamber and right to left shunting into the distal chamber should minimize the hemodynamic consequences of the cor triatriatum, because the combination of associated defects detours the pulmonary venous return around the obstructing membrane.

Mitral Stenosis

A diastolic gradient across the mitral valve is the hemodynamic hallmark of significant mitral stenosis. If obstruction is severe there will also be an elevation of pulmonary artery pressure. However, both the mitral valve gradient and the pulmonary hypertension have other determinates than the severity of the stenosis. The magnitude of flow across the mitral valve directly affects the gradient and in the presence of low cardiac output there may be only a modest gradient in spite of severe obstruction. Conversely, high cardiac output will cause a relatively high gradient in the presence of modest obstruction. Pulmonary artery pressure is influenced by the level of flow, and

by pulmonary arteriolar resistance as well as obstruction at the mitral valve. Both the level of pulmonary artery pressure and the transmitral gradient must be interpreted in the light of the other hemodynamic variables that influence them. Thus, to accurately assess the severity of mitral stenosis, both cardiac output and the mitral gradient must be measured. The latter is best accomplished by recording left ventricular and either left atrial or pulmonary artery wedge pressure simultaneously at a high gain. Because mitral flow occurs only in diastole the diastolic flow rate and diastolic gradient should be ascertained.

The mitral valve area can be calculated from these measurements by the following formulas:

$$MVF \ (mL/dfs) = \frac{CO \ (mL/min)}{DFP \ (sec/min)}$$

$$CO = Cardiac \ output$$

$$DFP = Diastolic \ filling \ period$$

$$dfs = Diastolic \ filling \ seconds$$

$$MVF = Mitral \ valve \ flow$$

where:

$$DFP \ (sec/min) = \frac{dfs}{beat} \times HR \ (beats/min)$$

$$HR = heart \ rate$$

then:

$$MVA \ (cm^2) = \frac{MVF \ (mL/dfs)}{38 \ \sqrt{MVG}}$$

MVA = mitral valve area
MVG = mean mitral valve gradient
MVF = Mitral valve flow
  38 = Gravity acceleration constant
        for the mitral valve

Cardiac output can be measured by any of a number of accepted methods (see Chapter 8). The diastolic filling period (DFP in seconds/minute) is demarcated by the

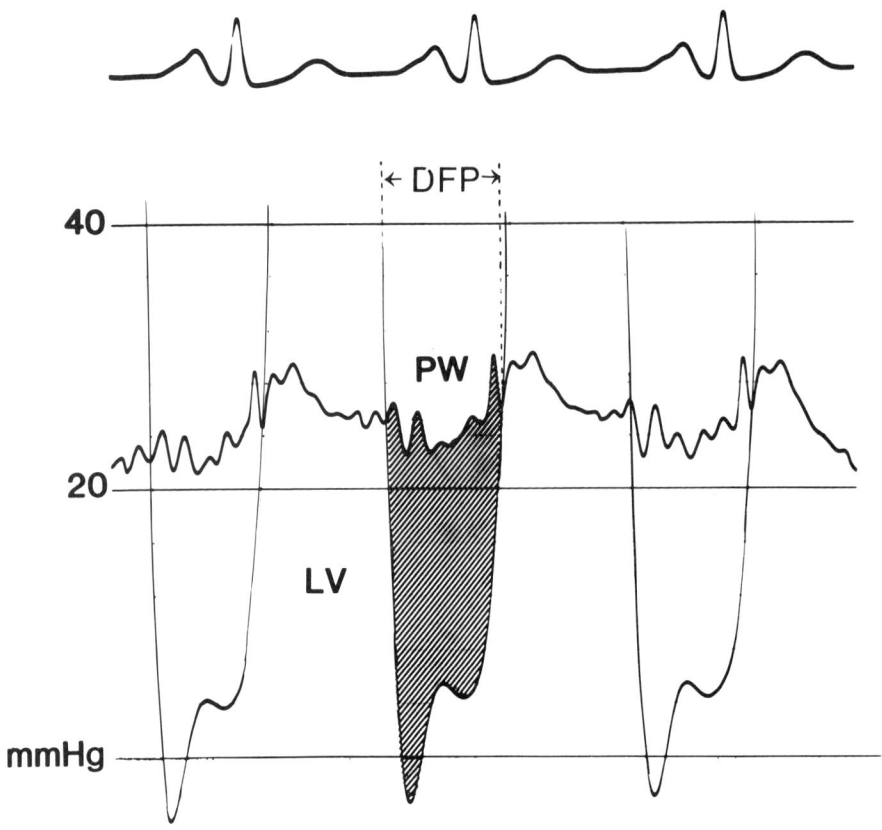

Figure 2. Simultaneous recording of the left ventricular end diastolic and pulmonary artery wedge pressures. The diastolic filling period is demarcated by the cross-hatched area.

crossovers of left ventricular and either pulmonary artery wedge or left atrial pressure tracings (Fig. 2). The mean diastolic gradient can be determined from the same tracing by averaging instantaneous gradients measured at fixed small time intervals throughout diastole. Alternatively, a computer can be utilized to calculate cardiac output and mitral valve area.

In adults, the normal mitral valve orifice is 4–6 cm². Generally, an orifice of less than 2 cm² results in elevation of left atrial and pulmonary artery wedge pressure. An orifice of less than 1 cm² constitutes severe mitral stenosis and a gradient of approximately 20 mm Hg (mean left atrial pressure 25 mm Hg) is required to maintain a normal cardiac output.

Other Diagnostic or Therapeutic Procedures

Balloon mitral valvotomy has been performed successfully in congenital mitral stenosis (Kveselis 1986). The double balloon technique is preferable due to the large area of the mitral valve. An "ideal" balloon:mitral valve ratio has not yet been identified, though most operators will use 1:1. The antegrade approach, usually by transseptal puncture, is recommended (See Chapter 14).

Balloon angioplasty of congenital pulmonary vein stenosis provides little, if any, relief of the obstruction, and is not recommended. Intravascular stents may be suitable for these lesions, however, this application is, at best, highly experimental and of unproven value.

Angiography

Pulmonary Vein Atresia

The premortem diagnosis of pulmonary vein atresia is a difficult one but the angiographic appearance is distinctive. Following a right ventricular or main pulmonary artery injection there is slow filling of the pulmonary arterial tree and the entire lung field "lights up". There may be faint visualization of the confluence of the pulmonary veins, but there is no visible return of contrast media to the vena cava or to the left atrium. A pulmonary artery wedge angiogram may be helpful and may result in better visualization of the confluence of the pulmonary veins. The differential diagnosis of pulmonary vein atresia includes total anomalous pulmonary venous return with severe obstruction, but in the latter entity there is almost always visualization of the pulmonary venous return beyond the confluence,

delayed and faint though it may be. If unilateral pulmonary vein atresia is present, contrast flows preferentially into the unaffected lung following injection into the main pulmonary artery. The branch pulmonary arteries to the affected lung will be hypoplastic and may not be visualized readily without a selective injection, or preferably a pulmonary artery wedge injection, on the affected site (Fig. 3).

Pulmonary Vein Stenosis

The diagnosis of pulmonary vein stenosis should be suspected if there is a discrepancy between pulmonary artery wedge pressure and left atrial pressure, but a definitive diagnosis is always angiographic. It is very difficult to be sure of pulmonary vein stenosis with a right heart injection of contrast media. Even a large bolus delivered rapidly into the pulmonary artery rarely results in adequate visualization of the obstruction. Therefore, contrast media must be injected into individual pulmonary veins if the diagnosis of pulmonary vein stenosis is to be established (Fig. 4). Pulmonary ar-

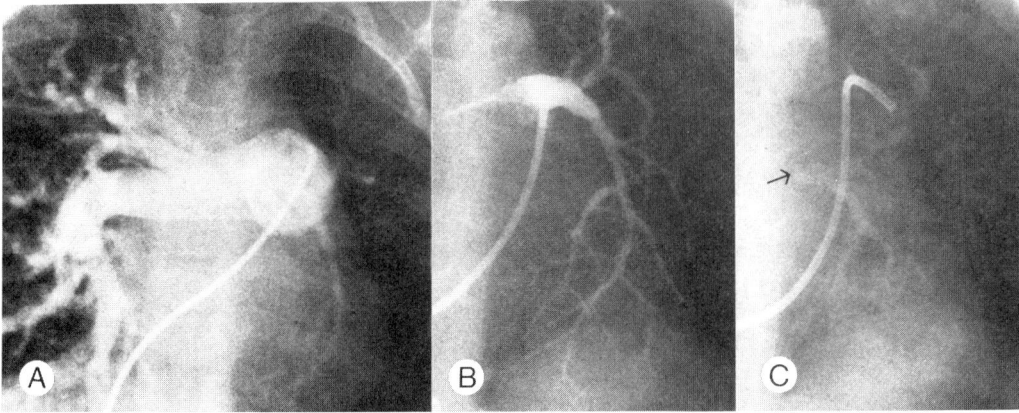

Figure 3. Pulmonary artery angiograms in unilateral pulmonary vein atresia. A: Main pulmonary artery angiogram demonstrating marked preferential flow to the right side. A small left pulmonary artery is barely seen. B: Selective angiogram in the left pulmonary artery demonstrating marked hypoplasia of the entire vessel. C: Late levophase following the angiogram in "B" demonstrating faint opacification of the blind ending atretic pulmonary vein (arrow).

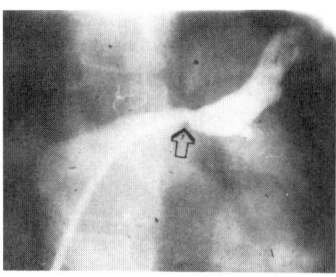

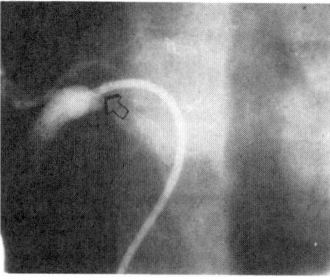

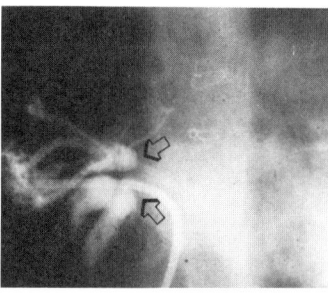

Figure 4. Selective angiograms in the pulmonary veins in a patient with multiple vessel stenoses (arrows). Top = Left upper pulmonary vein; Middle = Right upper pulmonary vein; Bottom = Right lower pulmonary vein.

tery wedge angiography may be helpful to visualize the pulmonary vein stenosis if a selective pulmonary vein injection is not possible (Bini 1984).

With unilateral pulmonary vein atresia or stenosis, the unaffected pulmonary artery fills promptly after a right heart injection of contrast media, and there is rapid visualization of the pulmonary veins on that side and of the left atrium. The pulmonary artery on the affected side is often small and fills slowly. The affected pulmonary veins are rarely seen, and must be visualized directly as discussed above.

Cor Triatriatum

The cineangiographic appearance of cor triatriatum is quite distinctive. The membrane appears as a thin radiolucent line extending obliquely across the left atrium from just medial to the left atrial appendage to the area of the right inferior wall of the left atrium. The membrane can be visualized on the levophase of a pulmonary artery injection and is usually best seen in the right anterior oblique projection (Fig. 5). If the membrane is not well visualized following a pulmonary arteriogram, a retrograde arterial catheter can be passed across the aortic and mitral valves and a direct left atrial injection made. Unless the catheter has traversed a perforation in the membrane, only the distal left atrial chamber and left atrial appendage are visualized.

It should be noted that the appearance of the left atrium in total anomalous pulmonary venous return may mimic a cor triatriatum. In the former malformation, the left atrium is small and in the right anterior oblique projection the right border may be straight or even slightly concave. Because the pulmonary veins are not visualized on left atrial injection the appearance is strikingly similar to that of a cor triatriatum. The site of pulmonary venous return is usually apparent, however, if the possibility of total anomalous pulmonary venous return is considered.

Mitral Stenosis

Following a pulmonary artery injection there is slow emptying of the left atrium in a patient with mitral stenosis (Fig. 6). The left atrial chamber is generally large but may be normal or even small in size, especially if there is severe endocardial fibroelastosis. A left ventricular angiogram may further define the mitral valve abnormality and it is especially useful in quantitating associated mitral regurgitation (Macartney 1976). Again, the right anterior oblique view is preferable.

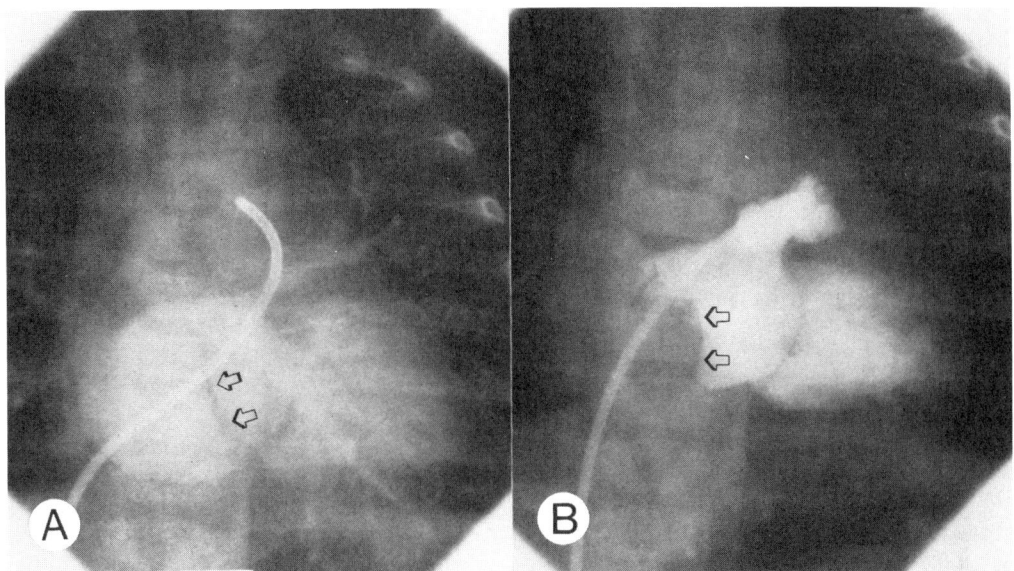

Figure 5. Angiography in cor triatriatum. A: Levophase following a selective pulmonary arteriogram in the anteroposterior view demonstrating the membrane (arrows). B: Selective injection in the distal left atrial compartment. Note that the left atrial appendage is connected to this area and there is no reflux of contrast into the pulmonary veins. Arrows indicate the site of the membrane.

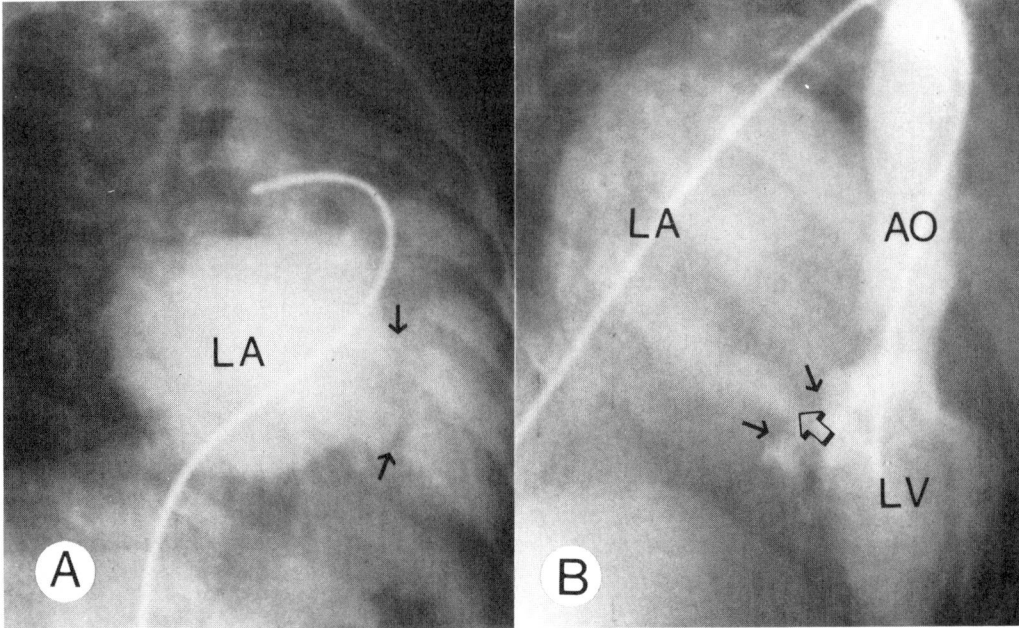

Figure 6. Angiography in mitral valve stenosis. A: Levophase following a selective pulmonary arteriogram in the right anterior oblique view demonstrating a thickened stenotic mitral valve (arrows). B: Selective left ventricular (LV) angiogram in the elongated right anterior oblique view demonstrating a jet of mitral regurgitation (open arrow) through a thickened, stenotic mitral valve (arrows). Ao = Aorta; LA = Left atrium.

Associated Lesions

Pulmonary vein stenosis, cor triatriatum or mitral stenosis may occur as isolated lesions or in combination with other types of congenital cardiac anomalies. Pulmonary vein stenosis and cor triatriatum have been seen in conjunction with left to right shunt lesions at atrial and/or ventricular level. Mitral stenosis may be found together with forms of left heart outflow obstruction such as aortic stenosis and/or coarctation of the aorta. We therefore recommend that pulmonary artery wedge pressure be measured routinely and if it is elevated it should be compared to the left ventricular end diastolic pressure. Bilateral pulmonary artery wedge pressure measurement is mandatory in all patients in whom pulmonary artery hypertension is present.

Cautions and Precautions

The pulmonary veins are delicate structures, therefore any catheter manipulation within a pulmonary vein must be gentle in order to avoid laceration or perforation of the vessel wall. When probing for the pulmonary veins within the left atrium, care must be taken not to perforate the atrial wall. The left margin of the atrium and the left lateral appendage are particularly vulnerable. Manipulation of a catheter in retrograde fashion across the mitral valve may produce extensive ventricular ectopy. The complications of transseptal catheterization are discussed in Chapter 14.

References and Suggested Reading

Beerman LB, Oh KS, Park SC, et al. Unilateral pulmonary vein atresia: Clinical and radiographic spectrum. Ped Cardiol 1983;4:105–112.

Bini RA, Cleveland DC, Ceballos R, et al. Congenital pulmonary vein stenosis. Am J Cardiol 1984;54:369–375.

Glancy DK, Roberts WC. Congenital obstructive lesions involving the major pulmonary veins, left atrium, or mitral valve. A clinical, laboratory and morphologic survey. Catheterization Cardiovasc Diagn 1976;2:215–252.

Kveselis DA, Rocchini AP, Beekman R, et al. Balloon angioplasty for congenital and rheumatic mitral stenosis. Am J Cardiol 1986;57:348–350.

Ledbetter MK, Wells DH, Connors DM. Common pulmonary vein atresia. Am Heart J 1978;96:580–586.

Macartney FJ, Bain HH, Ionescu MI, et al. Angiocardiographic/Pathologic correlations in congenital mitral valve anomalies. Eur J Cardiol 1976;4(2):191–211.

Neches WH, Park SC, Lenox CC, et al. Pulmonary artery wedge pressures in congenital heart disease. Catheterization Cardiovasc Diagn 1977;3:11–19.

Park SC, Neches WH, Lenox CC, et al. Diagnosis and surgical treatment of bilateral plmonary vein stenosis. J Thorac Cardiovasc Surg 1974;67:755–761.

Roberts WC. Morphologic features of the normal and abnormal mitral valve. Am J Cardiol 1983;51:1005–1028.

Sade RM, Freed MD, Matthews EC, et al. Stenosis of individual pulmonary veins. J Thorac Cardiovasc Surg 67:953–962.

33

Aortic Stenosis or Atresia

F. Jay Fricker, M.D.

This chapter will consider cardiac malformations that cause obstruction to the ejection of blood from the left ventricle to the aorta. These include valvar, subvalvar, and supravalvar aortic stenosis, as well as the aortic atresia complex (Fig. 1). Aortic arch anomalies that cause left ventricular outflow obstruction, such as coarctation of the aorta, will be considered in the following chapter. These defects can occur as isolated malformations, or in association with other lesions causing obstruction in the left heart. For example, there is an association between aortic valve disease and coarctation of the aorta (Tawes 1969). The clinical presentations are a spectrum ranging from the asymptomatic child to the neonate in severe congestive heart failure. The isolated defects of valvar, subvalvar, and supravalvar aortic stenosis will be considered together, while the problem of aortic atresia or hypoplastic left heart syndrome will be discussed toward the end of the chapter.

Aortic Stenosis

Anatomy

Valvar Aortic Stenosis

A congenitally abnormal aortic valve is usually either bicuspid or unicuspid. When fusion of the right and noncoronary leaflet occurs, a nonsuspended raphe divides this leaflet and the valve commissure has a right-left orientation with a coronary artery arising from each related sinus of valsalva. Fusion of the left and right leaflets occurs with similar frequency. The nonsuspended raphe bisects this anterior common leaflet, and the valve leaflets assume an anterior-posterior relationship. A unicuspid valve consists of an eccentrically placed commissure in any position. The other commissures are represented by ridges or raphe. The unicuspid valve is invariably stenotic but the bileaflet valve may be either stenotic or nonobstructive depending on the degree of commissural fusion (Roberts 1973) (Goor and Lillehei 1975). The aortic valve in the neonate with critical aortic valve stenosis is often unicuspid with poorly defined valve anatomy. It tends to be myxomatous and adequate valvotomy is difficult.

Subaortic Stenosis

The anatomical feature of discrete subaortic stenosis is a shelf of tissue positioned from just beneath, to several centimeters below, the aortic valve (Newfeld 1976). This shelf may be circumferential and attached to the anterior (aortic) leaflet of the mitral valve. Anderson (1983) noted that in some cases this subaortic tissue was a remnant of the spontaneous closure of a ventricular septal defect. Others have noted that subaortic stenosis is a spectrum of left ventricular outflow obstruction varying from a discrete membrane to fibromuscular tubular narrowing (Maron 1976).

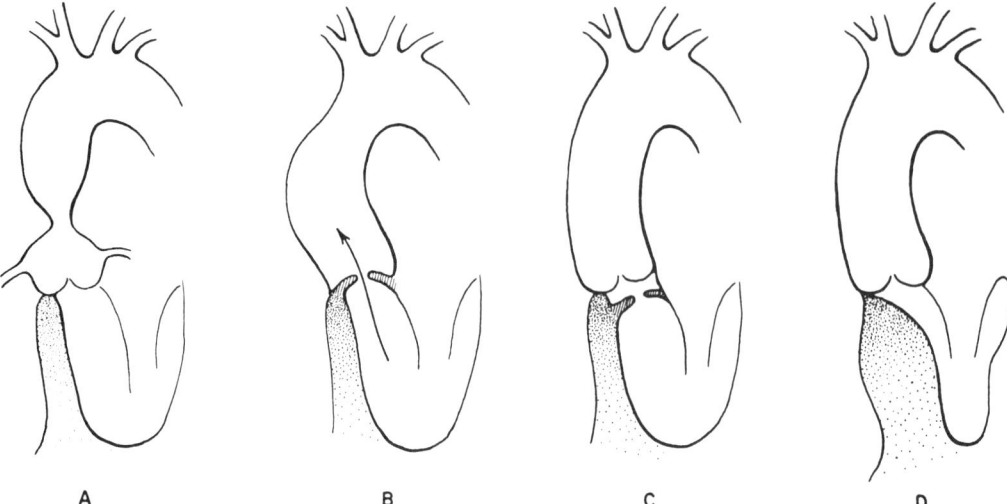

Figure 1. Diagrams illustrating various forms of aortic stenosis. A: Supravalvar. B: Valvar. C: Membranous subvalvar. D: Hypertrophic cardiomyopathy.

Supravalvar Aortic Stenosis

Supravalvar aortic stenosis occurs in varied anatomical forms, including an hourglass constricting annular ridge at the superior margin of the sinuses of valsalva, a fibromuscular diaphragm, and hypoplasia of the ascending aorta. Supravalvar aortic stenosis may be associated with Williams syndrome, or infantile hypercalcemia (Black 1963), with its typical "elfin facies".

Hemodynamic Considerations

Valvar Aortic Stenosis

Critical valvar aortic stenosis in the neonate is a different disease from aortic stenosis that presents in childhood (Edmunds 1980). Aortic stenosis in the neonate is recognized because of a harsh variably intense systolic murmur that is maximal at the high right sternal border. The most striking finding is that peripheral pulses are decreased. Symptoms are absent early, but our experience is that the natural history of this disease is early left ventricular dysfunction with congestive heart failure occurring in the first 2 months of life.

The older child with valvar aortic stenosis rarely has symptoms of angina or syncope even with severe obstruction. The character of the carotid upstroke and a thrill at the high right sternal border are the most reliable clinical signs in moderate to severe aortic valvar stenosis. However, once a murmur reaches grade IV/VI in intensity, it's character and length mean little in assessing severity of aortic valve obstruction (Zuberbuhler 1981). Left ventricular hypertrophy by voltage criteria on the electrocardiogram is not a sensitive index of severity but the presence of a strain pattern is good supporting evidence for significant obstruction (Hugenholz 1962). From retrospective reviews of serial hemodynamic studies in patients with congenital aortic valve stenosis, the degree of left ventricular outlet obstruction was found to progress irrespective of the age at time of diagnosis (Cohen 1972; Friedman 1971). Stress exercise testing also has a role in the assessment of aortic stenosis (Hossack, 1980). In the preadolescent with clinical evidence of moderate to severe aortic valve stenosis who has had a previous aortic valvulotomy, valve replacement usually is the only surgical option. Serial exercise studies measuring S-T segment changes on the electrocardiogram and systolic blood pressure responses, are valuable in timing repeat hemodynamic evaluation and subsequent surgery.

Subvalvar Stenosis

The infant or child presenting with clinical findings of subaortic stenosis is generally asymptomatic. A ventricular septal defect is the malformation most often confused with subvalvular stenosis (Fisher 1982). Attention to the character of the peripheral pulses, radiation of the murmur to the high right sternal border, and the presence of aortic regurgitation are important clues to the correct diagnosis. Cross-sectional and Doppler echocardiography have made the diagnosis of a subaortic membrane much easier but we would use caution in assessing severity from the echocardiographic observations alone. The attachment to the mitral valve is well visualized but the extent of impingement into the left ventricular outflow tract may be overestimated. The presence of a precordial thrill is clear indication for a hemodynamic assessment.

Discrete subaortic stenosis is a progressive lesion both in terms of severity of obstruction and degree of aortic valve damage (Wright 1983; Somerville 1980). Therefore, early surgical intervention is justified and a peak systolic pressure gradient of 40–50 mm Hg warrants repair. It should be remembered that left bundle branch block, complete heart block, mitral valve injury, and iatrogenic ventricular septal defect are complications related to surgery. Recurrence of obstruction may occur by proliferation of subaortic tissue (Newfeld 1976; Katz 1977).

Supravalvar Stenosis

The clinical findings of supravalvar stenosis can be distinguished from valvar aortic stenosis by the absence of an early systolic ejection sound and the disparity of systolic blood pressure in the upper extremities, because right arm systolic pressure may exceed the left arm by 25 mm Hg or more. This has been attributed to selective streaming of blood into the innominate artery (Coanda effect) (Goldstein 1970; French 1970).

Supravalvar aortic stenosis is the least remedial to surgical intervention among forms of congenital left ventricular outflow obstruction. Criteria for operation include a peak systolic gradient of greater than 50 mm Hg with an anatomically discrete obstruction (Weisz 1976). Coronary artery involvement may complicate the operative approach. Attempts to surgically manage diffuse hypoplasia of the ascending aorta generally have not been very successful.

Indications for Catheterization

In patients with all forms of aortic outflow obstruction, the assessment of the severity of obstruction and determination of left ventricular function are the primary reasons for a hemodynamic study. A decision regarding catheterization is based on the physical examination and on the noninvasive findings on the electrocardiogram and cross-sectional and Doppler echocardiogram. Serial echocardiographic measurements of left ventricular wall thickness and the assessment of the gradient by Doppler studies are helpful supporting evidence to proceed with hemodynamic evaluation and possibly balloon dilation valvotomy (See Chapter 13).

Cardiac Catheterization Technique

In the neonate, the standard femoral approach by percutaneous technique or saphenous vein cutdown has been used in the past. Invariably the foramen ovale is patent in this age group and left ventricular pressure easily can be measured. In patients less than 1 week of age, insertion of an umbilical artery catheter into the ascending aorta may be possible and is valuable for determining aortic pressure (and thus the peak systolic gradient across the valve) and for assessing aortic valve anatomy by angiography. Until the advent of balloon dilation valvotomy, it was rarely necessary to pass the retrograde arterial catheter across the aortic valve in this age group. Today, the diagnosis is established and an estimate of severity is provided readily by cross sectional and Doppler echocardiography. In view of the poor results with surgical management of the neonate with this lesion, many centers have begun to recommend balloon dilation valvotomy. The carotid arterial approach was originally reported from our center (Fischer 1985), and has proven to be extremely valuable in the neonate (see Chapter 13).

In older children, the femoral percutaneous approach is used and retrograde passage of the arterial catheter across the aortic valve into the left ventricle generally is successful. Initially an end-hole catheter (Lehman) is advanced around the aortic arch into the left ventricle. This allows a better definition of the site of stenosis and will delineate subvalvar and supravalvar aortic stenosis (see Chapter 7, Figure 5). When difficulty is encountered in crossing the valve, a pigtail angiographic catheter or a guide wire followed by a catheter have been successful (see Chapter 5). The other option available is the transseptal technique. However, this method involves the use of intravenous general anesthesia (Ketamine). The brachial artery approach has not been used in our recent experience and may offer some advantage in crossing the aortic valve if it is not possible from the femoral approach.

Hemodynamic Evaluation

Pressure Data

Valvar Stenosis

The transvalvular aortic gradient and the cardiac output are two important pieces of information in assessing the need for surgery. A peak systolic gradient across the aortic valve of greater than 60 mm Hg with a normal cardiac output is an indication for aortic valvotomy in our institution. With a peak systolic gradient of less than 60 mm Hg, other factors need to be considered. These include age of patient, previous aortic valve surgery, left ventricular wall thickness and function as well as the electrocardiogram and blood pressure response to exercise. The character of the central aortic pulse tracing also is helpful in the assessment in that it has a slow systolic rise, a prominent anacrotic notch and a late peak in significant aortic valve stenosis. The anacrotic notch is positioned lower on the upstroke with increasing stenosis. The left ventricular end diastolic pressure increases with hypertrophy and decreasing left ventricular compliance.

Although the calculated aortic valve area is an important concept in understanding aortic valve stenosis, the actual valve area obtained has not been a more useful index in making a decision for valvotomy than is the peak systolic gradient. Gorlin reported the hydraulic formula for calculation of aortic valve area in the early 1950s before anyone had ever measured left ventricular pressure (Gorlin 1951). The basic formula used:

Aortic Valve Area (cm^2)

$$= \frac{\text{Aortic valve flow}}{\text{Mean pressure difference across the orifice}}$$

Since the aortic valve flow occurs only in systole, this is determined as follows:

1. LVET (sec/beat) × HR (beats/min)

$$= SEP(sec/min)$$

HR = heart rate

LVET = Left ventricular ejection time

SEP = Systolic ejection period

2. Aortic Valve Flow (mL/min)

$$= \frac{Cardiac\ output\ (mL/sec)}{SEP\ (sec/min)}$$

3. Aortic Valve Area (cm²)

$$= \frac{Aortic\ valve\ flow\ (mL/sec)}{44.5\ \sqrt{P1\ -\ P2}}$$

Where: 44.5 is the acceleration constant
P1 − P2 = Mean pressure gradient across the aortic valve.

The mean systolic pressure gradient is calculated from the left ventricular and aortic pressure contours. Superimposing these two pressures, the area between them during systole can be planimetered and the mean gradient can be obtained (Fig. 2). There is some concern over the influence of the catheter across the aortic valve on the transvalvular gradient. Carbello et al (1979) noted a small increase in peripheral artery pressure (5–10 mm Hg) when the catheter was withdrawn from the left ventricle to aorta. All patients with this finding had calculated aortic valve areas of less than 0.7 cm². However, in general, a catheter crossing a stenotic valve would occupy less than 10% of the cross sectional area of even a severely stenotic aortic valve, and would have little influence on peak systolic gradient.

Another point of more practical concern is the influence of downstream resistance on transvalvar gradient. It has been shown experimentally that the gradient

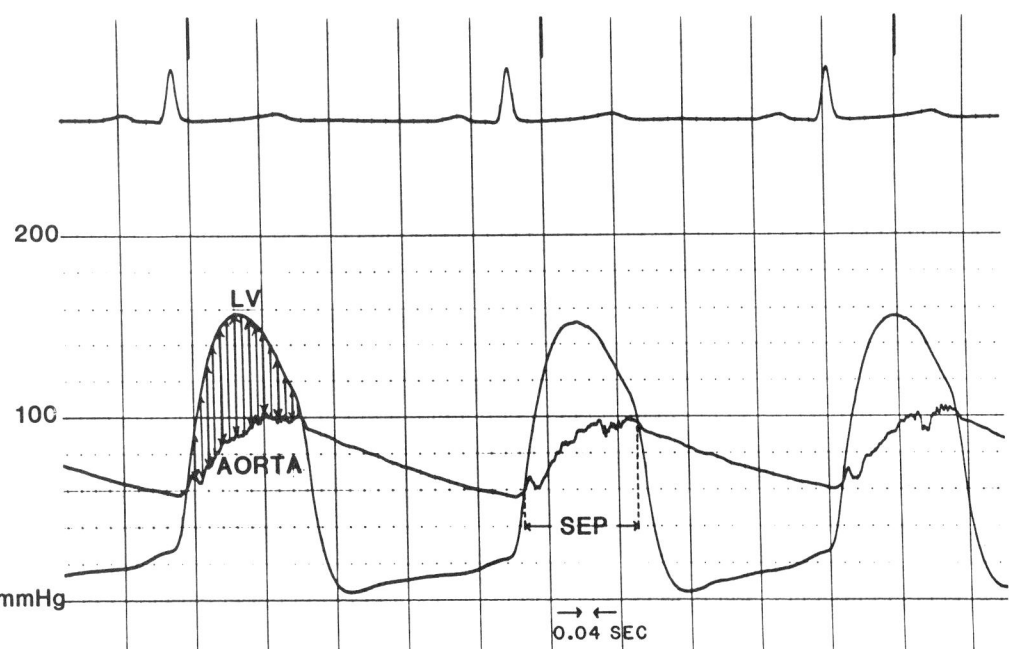

Figure 2. Calculation of mean pressure gradient by integration of the area between superimposed or simultaneously recorded left ventricular (LV) and aortic pressures. SEP = Systolic ejection period.

across a fixed stenosis is influenced and, in fact, can be abolished by downstream resistance (Silove 1968). Infusion of angiotension to increase systemic vascular resistance can also modify transvalvar aortic gradient (Perloff 1969). Thus, in the common clinical situation of aortic stenosis in the child with coarctation of the aorta, assessment of the degree of aortic valve disease can only be made at restudy following coarctation repair.

Subvalvar Stenosis

The catheterization approach to a patient with subaortic stenosis is similar to that in the patient with aortic valve stenosis. Retrograde catheterization of the left ventricle is begun with an end-hole, fluid-filled, catheter. The subaortic chamber may be small and this catheter optimizes the chance of documenting the level of obstruction. When the catheter is withdrawn from the left ventricular cavity to the aortic root, subvalvar, valvar and supravalvar stenosis can be distinguished one from the other (see Figure 5 in Chapter 7). The pulse contour is normal with discrete subaortic stenosis and can be differentiated from the delayed upstroke of aortic valve stenosis and the bifid pulse contour of hypertrophic cardiomyopathy (idiopathic hypertrophic subaortic stenosis). When catheter movement artifact makes accurate determination of the peak systolic gradient difficult, substitution of a Millar microtip catheter (Millar Corporation, Houston, Texas, USA) may well obviate the problem (this may require the use of a long sheath to enable passage of the microtip catheter around the aortic arch and into the left ventricle). Important hemodynamic variables that should be obtained include peak systolic gradient, left ventricular end diastolic pressure, and the degree of aortic regurgitation. A peak systolic gradient of 40 to 50 mm Hg in association with aortic regurgitation is an indication for surgical resection. The observation of progressive left

ventricular outflow obstruction and concern about future damage to the aortic valve are reasons for the less stringent criteria for operation as compared to those recommended in aortic valve stenosis. In fact Somerville (1980) has proposed operating on all patients with discrete subaortic stenosis regardless of the gradient. Right heart hemodynamics are generally normal in patients with discrete forms of subaortic stenosis.

Supravalvar Stenosis

Demonstration of the supravalvular aortic chamber by retrograde aortic catheterization confirms the diagnosis. The Coanda effect can be documented by pressure measurements in the innominate and left subclavian arteries. During right heart catheterization, pulmonary artery pressure gradients should be looked for because branch pulmonary artery stenosis is a commonly associated malformation.

The hemodynamics in the infant with critical aortic stenosis requires further comment. The aortic pulse pressure is usually low, often less than 20 mm Hg, and the transvalvar aortic gradient is highly variable and dependent on the degree of left ventricular failure (cardiac output). Right heart catheterization reflects left ventricular failure if there is elevated pulmonary artery wedge pressure and an intermediate degree of pulmonary hypertension.

Oxygen Saturation Data

In most patients with aortic outflow obstruction, there is no left to right shunt and therefore oximetry will be normal. The mixed venous saturation will of course, reflect the cardiac output status. In the neonate with critical aortic stenosis, the foramen ovale may be stretched and a significant left to right atrial shunt can occur, adding to the hemodynamic difficulties of the infant.

Angiocardiography

Both a left ventricular and aortic root angiogram provide valuable essential information in assessing valvar aortic stenosis. The angiographic anatomy of the aortic valve and annulus, the presence of associated subvalvar or supravalvar aortic stenosis and of aortic regurgitation, are demonstrated. Typical angiographic findings in aortic valve disease include a thickened and doming bileaflet aortic valve. A jet through the stenotic orifice can be seen impinging on the anterolateral aortic wall, accounting for the poststenotic dilation of the ascending aorta (Fig. 3). A left ventricular angiogram in the anteroposterior and lateral or axial four-chamber views, will show the level of left ventricular outflow obstruction, as well as left ventricular function, wall thickness, and cavity size. The aortic root injection is performed in anteroposterior and lateral, oblique or axial projections. In uncomplicated significant aortic valve stenosis, left ventricular size and function are normal, or the left ventricular contraction may be hyperkinetic with systolic cavity obliteration. In the infant, a right-sided angiogram should be done to look for the presence of a left to right shunt and associated mitral valve disease.

In patients with subaortic stenosis, a left ventricular angiogram in the anterior-posterior and axial left anterior oblique (four-chamber) view will usually demonstrate the subaortic chamber and membrane (Fig. 4). An aortic root injection is essential to estimate the degree of aortic regurgitation. If aortic regurgitation is present, con-

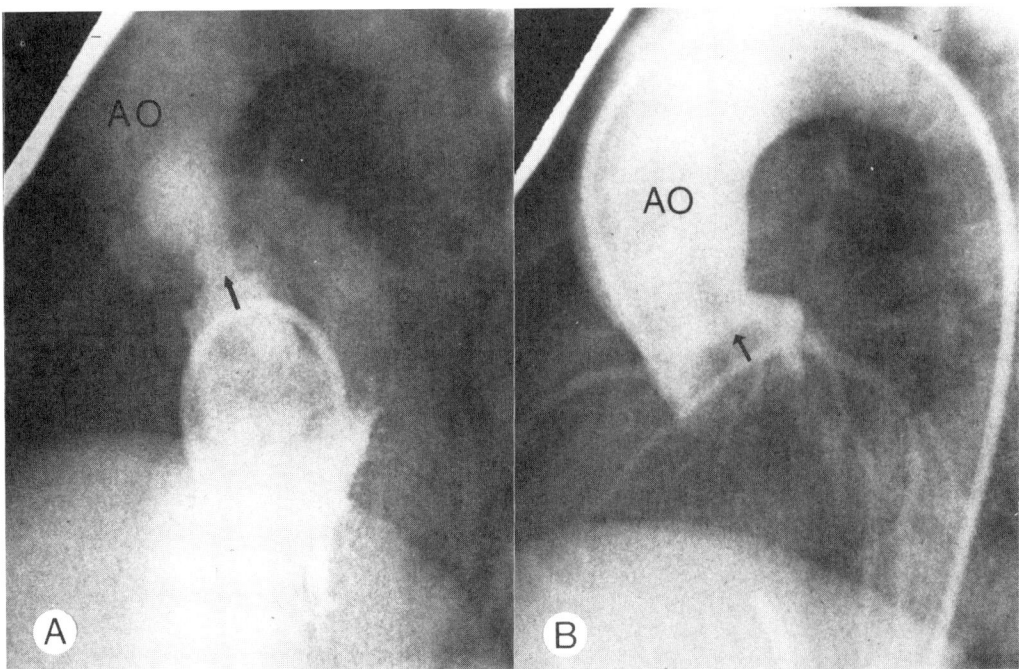

Figure 3. Angiocardiograms in valvar aortic stenosis. A: Left ventricular ejection in the four-chamber view demonstrating a thickened, doming aortic valve with a jet of contrast (arrows) through the stenotic orifice. B: Aortic root injection in the four-chamber view. A doming aortic valve and a negative jet of unopacified blood (arrows) through the stenotic orifice are seen. AO = Aorta.

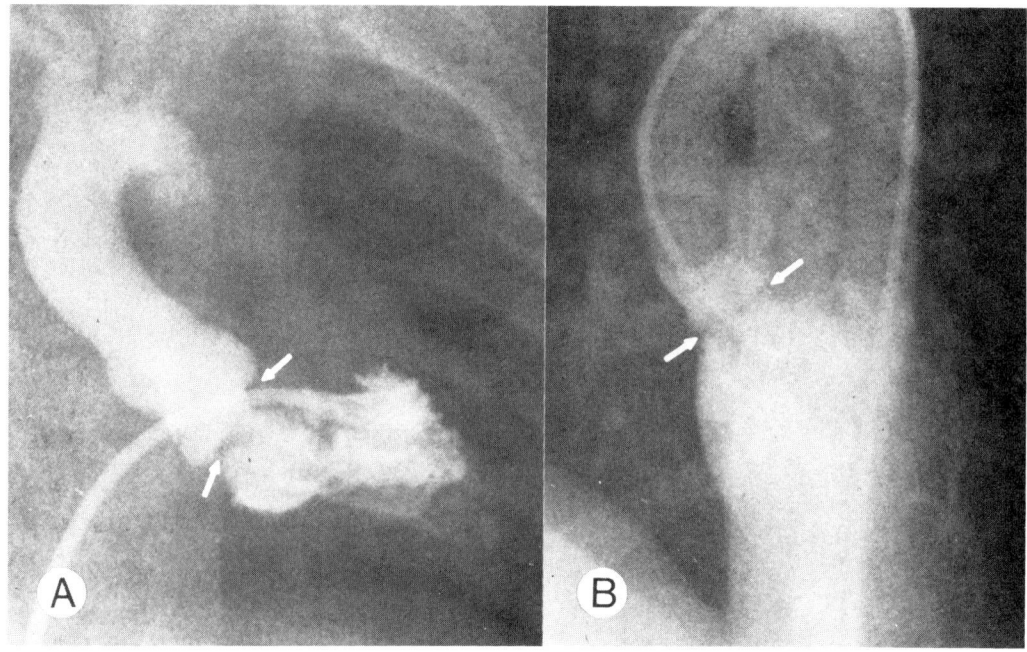

Figure 4. Left ventricular angiograms in subaortic stenosis demonstrating the subaortic membrane (arrows). A: Anteroposterior view. B: Four-chamber view.

trast from the root injection will fill the subaortic chamber and also help outline the subaortic membrane. In the tunnel form of subaortic stenosis, angiography demonstrates the long tubular narrowing in the four-chamber view. This narrowing is relatively fixed in that it changes little during the cardiac cycle (Maron 1976).

An aortic root or left ventricular angiogram in multiple views gives essential information about localization and severity of the supravalvar obstruction (Fig. 5). Coronary ostial stenosis may occur and selective coronary arteriography should be considered during the procedure. The coronary arteries tend to be dilated because they are subjected to the elevated left ventricular pressure. A pulmonary arteriogram should be performed to note the presence and severity of branch pulmonary artery stenosis.

Associated Lesions

Whenever an obstructive lesion to the left ventricle is found, other abnormalities of the left heart should be sought. Shone (1965) described infants with multiple levels of left heart inflow and outflow obstructive lesions consisting of parachute mitral valve, supravalvular mitral ring, subaortic stenosis, and coarctation of the aorta. The most common association seen with aortic valve disease is coarctation of the aorta, but mitral valve abnormalities are frequent as well. Finally, in the infant with critical aortic stenosis, a stretched foramen ovale or atrial septal defect may permit a significant left to right shunt.

Discrete and tunnel subaortic stenosis may complicate other congenital cardiac malformations. These include ventricular septal defect, atrioventricular septal defect and, especially, multiple left heart obstructive lesions. A variety of tunnel narrowing occurs in atrioventricular septal defects when there is marked deficiency of the inlet ventricular septum and the attachment of the left atrioventricular valve impinges on the outflow tract of the left ventricle. The discrete variety of subaortic stenosis is an

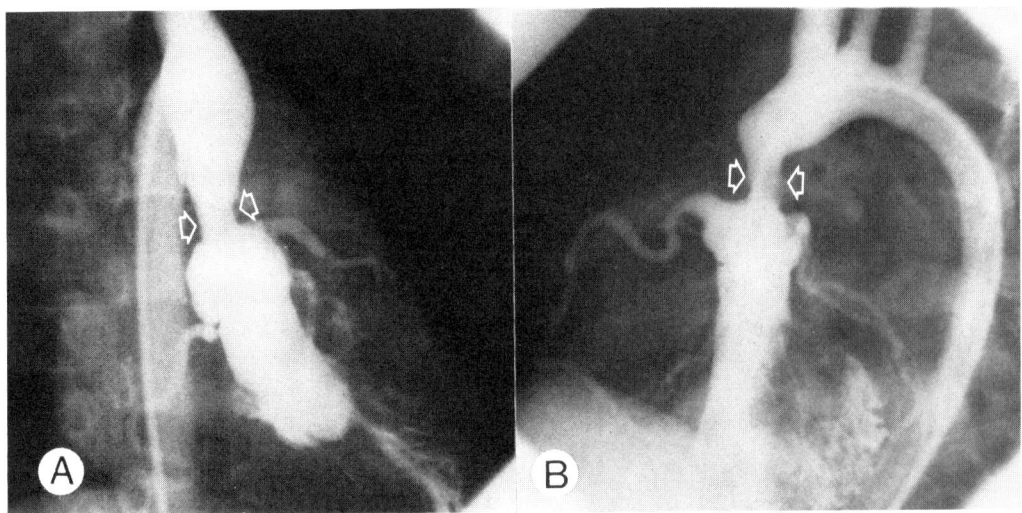

Figure 5. Left ventricular angiogram in supravalvar aortic stenosis (arrows). A: Right ventricular oblique view. B: Four-chamber view.

uncommon association with atrioventricular septal defects.

Aortic Atresia

Anatomy

The term hypoplastic left heart syndrome was first designated by Lev to describe the aortic atresia complex (Lev 1963). This section will consider the group of anomalies that have aortic atresia as the common denominator. Alteration of fetal hemodynamics, particularly premature closure of the foramen ovale, has been cited as a possible explanation for the occurrence of aortic atresia, but in fact the foramen ovale is open in most cases. Roberts proposed a classification of morphology based on the status of the ventricular septum (Roberts 1976). In most cases the ventricular septum is intact and the left ventricle is very hypoplastic or minute (Fig. 6). The mitral valve is atretic, or stenotic and hypoplastic, consistent with the size of left ventricle. In a minority of cases there is an associated ventricular septal defect and the left ventricular

cavity may be of nearly normal size. In these cases the mitral valve can be either atretic or well formed.

Indications for Catheterization

Cross-sectional and Doppler echocardiography provide the information previously obtained only by angiography. In fact, appropriate management decisions and recommendations, regarding treatment options are today based on echocardiographic findings alone and cardiac catheterization is not performed routinely. Specific echocardiographic information should include ascending aorta dimension, status of the aortic and mitral valves, size of the left ventricle and presence of an associated ventricular septal defect. Atypical findings on echocardiography, such as a normal sized aortic root, or larger than expected left ventricle, may lead to angiography if there is any doubt regarding the diagnosis, patency of the aortic valve, or whether the left ventricle is of adequate size to potentially support the systemic circulation. If increasing the size of the

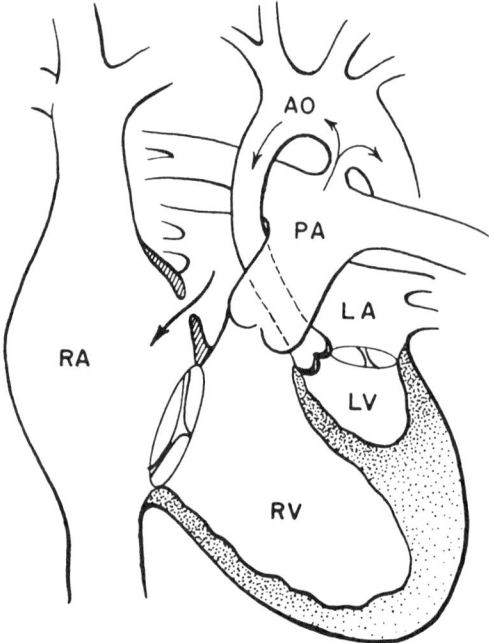

Figure 6. Diagram demonstrating the anatomy in aortic atresia. AO = aorta; LA = Left atrium; LV = Left ventricle; PA = Pulmonary artery; RA = Right atrium; RV = Right ventricle.

atrial septal communication is required for management, then cardiac catheterization clearly would be required to perform balloon or blade septostomy.

Hemodynamic Considerations

The major hemodynamic abnormality is ductus arteriosus dependent systemic blood flow. Because there is increased pulmonary blood flow, pulmonary artery saturation therefore is high and systemic oxygenation is not a problem. In fact, as the patent ductus arteriosus constricts thereby further diminishing systemic blood flow, pulmonary flow increases and systemic oxygen saturation remains high even in the face of an increasingly severe metabolic acidosis. The real problem is the decreased systemic blood flow and the consequent de-

crease in oxygen transport to the peripheral tissues.

Cardiac Catheterization Technique

An infant with aortic atresia/hypoplastic left heart syndrome is often critically ill with metabolic disturbances related to decreased systemic blood flow (i.e., hypoglycemia and metabolic acidosis). If a cardiac catheterization is required, an attempt should be made to correct these disturbances prior to catheterization with bicarbonate, glucose and prostaglandin E_1 infusion. The catheterization is from the femoral approach by percutaneous or cutdown technique, or via umbilical artery and vein. The umbilical artery catheter is particularly helpful in this situation because the aortic injection shows the presence of aortic atresia by retrograde filling of the ascending aorta and coronary arteries. Specific information that should be obtained at catheterization includes: presence of mitral and/or aortic atresia or degree of stenosis, size and function of the left ventricle, presence of a ventricular septal defect, size of the left atrium and the interatrial communication, presence of tricuspid regurgitation, and adequacy of right ventricular function.

Hemodynamic Evaluation

Pressure Data

Right and left atrial pressures are increased, and left atrial pressure is markedly elevated if there is a restrictive interatrial communication. In a recent review of our patients with this anomaly we found that the interatrial communication may be restrictive even in the absence of a gradient between the two atria. This may be due to elevated right atrial pressure caused by severe congestive heart failure and/or to tricuspid valve regurgitation. There is right ventricular and pulmonary artery hypertension. If the patent ductus is restrictive, pressure in the pulmonary artery will exceed descending aorta pressure.

Oxygen Saturation Data

Mixed venous oxygen saturation is low and a large oxygen step-up occurs in the right atrium from the obligatory atrial left to right shunt. In fact, oxygen saturation samples are similar in right atrium, right ventricle, pulmonary artery, and descending aorta. Calculated pulmonary blood flow is increased.

Angiocardiography

The diagnosis of aortic atresia is confirmed by a selective injection into the descending aorta at the level of the patent ductus. The umbilical artery catheter can be positioned there without difficulty, but if umbilical artery is unavailable, the venous catheter is passed from the pulmonary artery through the patent ductus to its junction with the descending aorta. Injection of contrast in this position demonstrates the typical angiographic findings of aortic atresia. A tiny ascending aorta with a diameter slightly larger than the coronary arteries fills retrogradely (Fig. 7). The aortic arch and brachiocephalic arteries are usually normal in caliber. An associated coarctation is often demonstrated. A right ventricular angiogram shows the large right ventricular chamber with filling of the descending aorta from the main pulmonary artery via the patent ductus. A small or minute left ventricle can only be demonstrated by selective injection. A selective left atrial injection in the left anterior oblique view will demonstrate the atrial communication, which often is restrictive.

Cautions and Precautions

Patients with severe aortic stenosis, particularly the neonate or young infant may

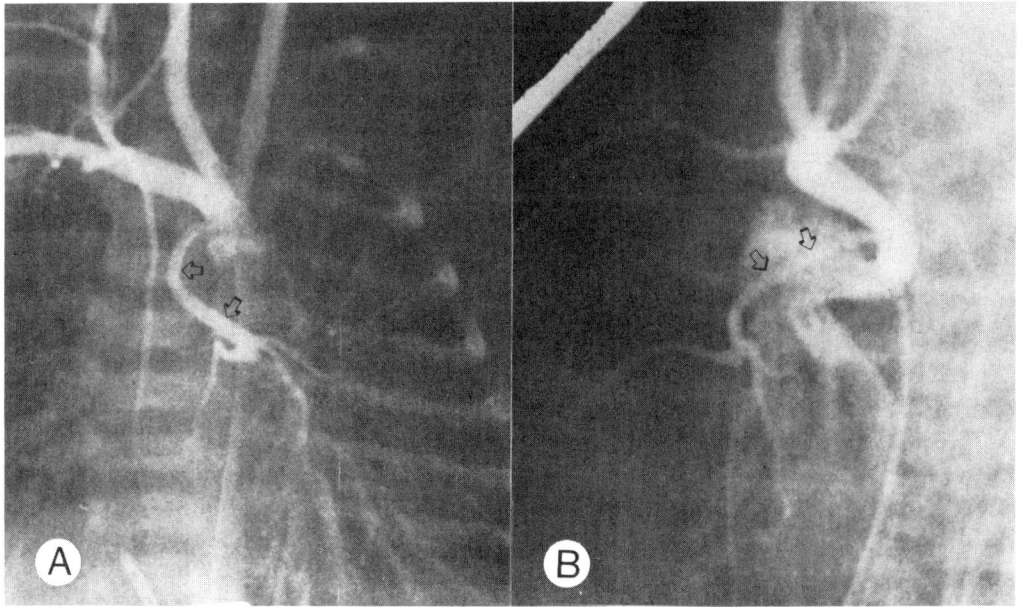

Figure 7. Selective injection in the transverse aortic arch demonstrating a very small ascending aorta (arrows) with filling of the coronary arteries. A: Anteroposterior view. B: Lateral view.

have decreased cardiac output and have borderline hemodynamic compensation. These patients are quite sensitive to excessive volume load with fluid and/or contrast material. Considerable caution should be used to avoid excessive volume infusion in these patients. Also, if hemodynamic compromise and low cardiac output exist, these patients are at greater risk for arterial thrombosis due to stasis. The use of heparin is therefore recommended for arterial catheterization in these patients.

It must be remembered that the hemodynamic data regarding outflow gradients are affected by the cardiac output. It is thus important to measure cardiac output directly either by oxygen consumption and oximetry data, thermodilution, or indocyanine green dye techniques. If the cardiac output is not measured and is actually below normal, the measured gradient will not reflect the severity of the stenosis accurately. Also, the presence of downstream obstruction may mask or minimize the proximal gradient as is seen often in patients with aortic stenosis and an associated coarctation of the aorta.

Left heart outflow obstruction often can be present at multiple levels. It is important to remember to consider the possibility of mitral valve, subaortic, supravalvar, and distal aortic obstruction in patients who have valvar aortic stenosis. In patients with supravalvar stenosis and suspected Williams syndrome, a pulmonary arteriogram should be performed to evaluate for pulmonary artery stenosis that is found frequently with this lesion.

References and Suggested Reading

Anderson RH, Lenox CC, Zuberbuhler JR. Morphology of ventricular septal defect associated with coarctation of the aorta. Br Heart J 1983;50:176–181.

Becker AE, Becker MJ, Edwards JE. Anomalies associated with coarctation of the aorta: Par-

ticular reference to infancy. Circulation 1970;41:1067–1075.

Black JA, Bonham-Carter RE. Association between aortic stenosis and facies of severe infantile hypercalcemia. Lancet 1963;2:745.

Carabello BA, Barry WH, Grossman W. Changes in arterial pressure during left heart pullback in patients with aortic stenosis. A sign of severe aortic stenosis. Am J Cardiol 1979; 44:424–427.

Cohen LS, Friedman WF, Braunwald E. Natural history of mild congenital aortic stenosis elucidated by serial hemodynamic studies. Am J Cardiol 1972;30:1–5.

Fischer DR, Park SC, Neches WH, et al. Successful dilatation of a stenotic Blalock-Taussig anastomosis by percutaneous transluminal balloon angioplasty. Am J Cardiol 1985;56:861–862.

Fisher DJ, Snider AR, Silverman NH, et al. Ventricular septal defect with silent discrete subaortic stenosis. Pediatr Cardiol 1982;2:265–269.

French JW, Guntheroth WG. An explanation of asymmetric upper extremity blood pressure in supravalvular aortic stenosis—The Coanda effect. Circulation 1970;42:31–36.

Friedman WF, Modinger J, Morgan JR. Serial hemodynamic observation in asymptomatic children with valvar aortic stenosis. Circulation 1971;43:91–97.

Goldstein RE, Ebstein SE. Mechanism of elevated innominate artery pressures in supravalvular aortic stenosis. Circulation 1970;42:23–29.

Gorr DA, Lillehei CW. Malformations of the aortic pathway. In: Congenital Malformations of the Heart. New York, NY; Grune & Stratton, 1975.

Gorlin R, Gorlin SG. Hydraulic formula for calculation of area of the stenotic mitral valve, other cardiac valves and central circulation shunts. Am Heart J 1951;41:1–29.

Hossack KF, Neutze JM, Lowe JB, et al. Congenital valvular aortic stenosis. Natural history and assessment for operation. Br Heart J 1980;43:561–573.

Hugenholtz PG, Lees MM, Nadas AS. The scalar electrocardiogram, vectorcardiogram and exercise electrocardiogram in the assessment of congenital aortic stenosis. Circulation 1962;26:79–91.

Katz NM, Buckley MJ, Liberthson RR. Discrete membranous subaortic stenosis. A report of 31 patients, review of the literature, and delineation of management. Circulation 1977;56:1034–1038.

Lev M, Arcilla R, Rimoldi HJ, et al. Premature narrowing or closure of the foramen ovale. Am Heart J 1963;65:638–647.

Maron BJ, Redwood DR, Roberts WC, et al. Tunnel subaortic stenosis. Left ventricular outflow obstruction produced by fibromuscular tubular narrowing. Circulation 1976;54:404–414.

Newfeld EA, Muster AJ, Paul MH, et al. Discrete subvalvular aortic stenosis in childhood. Am J Cardiol 1976;38:53–61.

Perloff JD, Binnion P, Caulfield WH, et al. The use of angiotension in the assessment of left ventricular function in fixed orifice aortic stenosis. Circulation 1967;35:347–357.

Roberts WC. Valvular, subvalvular and supravalvular aoartic stenosis: Morphologic features. Cardiovasc Clin. 1973;5:97–126.

Roberts WC, Perry LW, Chandra RS, et al. Aortic valve atresia: A new classification based on necropsy study of 73 cases. Am J Cardiol 1976;37:753–756.

Shone JD, Sellers RD, Anderson RC, et al. The developmental complex of "Parachute Mitral Valve", supravalvular ring of the left atrium, subaortic stenosis and coarctation of aorta. Am J Cardiol 1963;11:714–725.

Silove ED, Vogel JHK, Grover RF. The pressure gradient in ventricular outflow obstruction: Influence of peripheral resistance. Cardiovasc Res 1968;2:234–242.

Somerville J, Stone S, Ross D. Fate of patients with fixed subaortic stenosis after surgical removal. Br Heart J 1980;43:629–647.

Tawes RL, Aberdeen E, Waterston DJ, et al. Coarctation of the aorta in infants and children. Circulation 1969;39(Suppl I):173–184.

Weisz D, Hartmann AF, Weldon CS. Results of surgery for congenital supravalvular aortic stenosis. Am J Cardiol 1976;37:73–77.

Wright GB, Keane JF, Nadas AS, et al. Fixed subaortic stenosis in the young: Medical and surgical course in 83 patients. Am J Cardiol 1983;52:830–835.

Zuberbuhler JR. Aortic stenosis. In: Clinical Diagnosis in Pediatric Cardiology. Edinburgh. Churchill-Livingstone. 1981:75–82.

34

Coarctation of the Aorta or Interruption of the Aortic Arch

F. Jay Fricker, M.D.

Anatomy

The classification of aortic obstruction proposed by Rudolph (1974) into juxtaductal coarctation, aortic isthmus narrowing, and interruption is a useful concept. Juxtaductal coarctation occurs as an isolated defect, or may be associated with aortic valve disease or with a ventricular septal defect. Infants with aortic isthmus hypoplasia or interruption usually have more complicated associated malformations. In juxtaductal coarctation, a shelf-like process extends into the lumen from the posterolateral wall of the aorta opposite the insertion of the ductus arteriosus. This region has been studied histologically by Yen Ho and Anderson (1979) and they have shown that ductal tissue surrounds the aortic lumen and makes up a large portion of the obstructive lesion. In neonates there are varying degrees of isthmus hypoplasia associated with coarctation while older infants and children usually have an isthmus of normal caliber (Fig. 1). A bicuspid aortic valve is seen in up to 80% of patients with coarctation. Mitral valve abnormalities are common (Wood 1975; Rosenquist 1974). If a ventricular septal defect is present it is often moderate or small in size and perimembranous in location. Spontaneous closure of the defect is common in this group of patients.

Infants with isthmal hypoplasia of the aortic arch usually have, in addition, the same shelf of tissue causing discrete obstruction in the descending aorta. These patients usually have major intracardiac malformations as well. A large perimembranous or subarterial ventricular septal defect is common and other associated defects include double outlet right ventricle (Taussig Bing variety), atrioventricular septal defect and tricuspid atresia with transposition of the great arteries (Becker 1970).

A more distal origin of the subclavian artery is frequently associated with the aortic coarctation. Rarely, anomalous origin of the right subclavian artery may be present with its origin below the coarctation. If these occur concurrently, they will result in diminished pulses in both upper extremities. Interruption of the aorta deserves special comment. The types of interruption of aortic arch were classified by Celoria and Patton (1959) (Fig. 2). Interruption most often occurs between the left subclavian and left common carotid artery (type B) but it can occur in the aortic isthmus (type A) or rarely between the innominate and left common carotid arteries (Roberts 1962; Moller 1965; Van Praagh 1971). Variation in take-off of the right and left subclavian arteries or their connections with a right-sided patent ductus arteriosus occurs with some frequency (Roberts 1962). Interruption of the aortic arch is usually associated with a ventricular septal defect and a patent ductus. Rarely has it been reported as a solitary lesion (Dische 1975). The ventricular septal defect is large and subarterial in location. There is usually

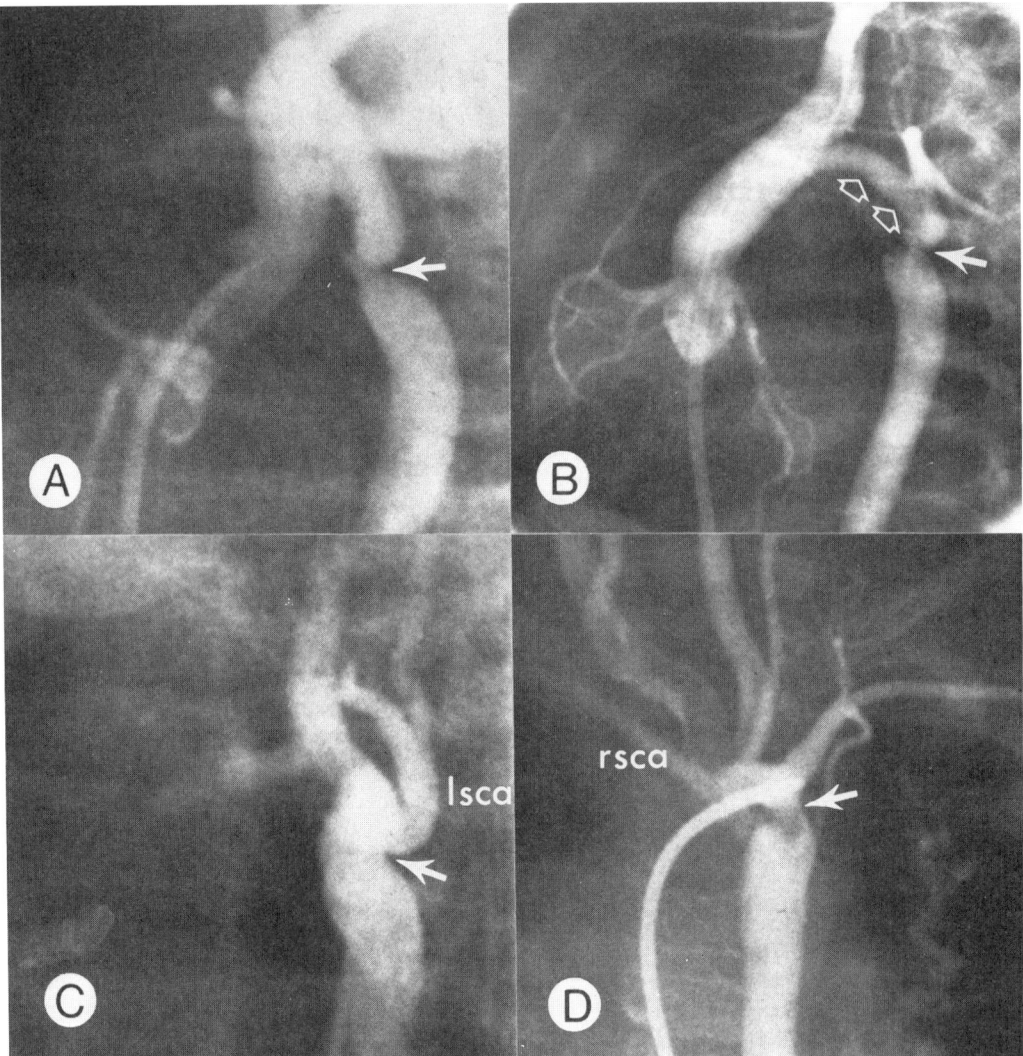

Figure 1. Selective aortograms in the lateral view demonstrating variations of coarctation of aorta (arrows) A: Usual form. B: Hypoplasia of the Isthmus (open arrows) common in early infancy. C: Distal take-off of the left subclavian artery (lsca). D: Anteroposterior view demonstrating anomalous origin of the right subclavian artery (rsca) distal to the coarctation.

malalignment of the outlet ventricular septum with deviation into the left ventricular outflow tract creating subaortic stenosis. The subaortic stenosis is an important cause of operative and postoperative mortality. Truncus arteriosus is rarely associated with interruption of the aortic arch.

Hemodynamic Considerations

Coarctation of the aorta may influence both right and left heart dynamics and selective blood flow to specific organs. Iso-

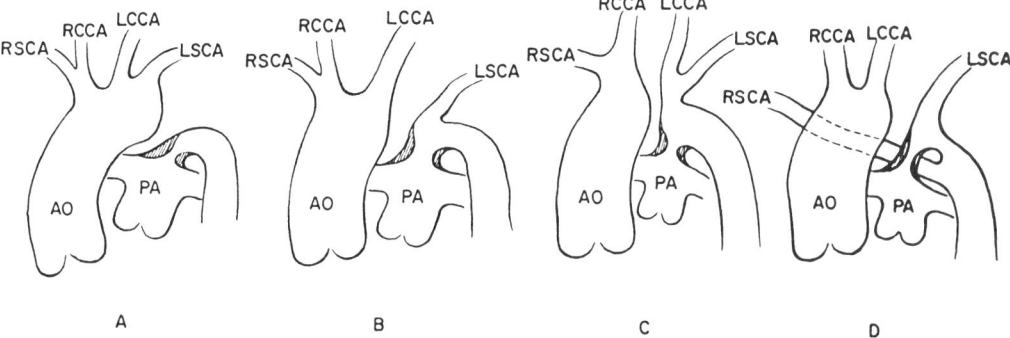

Figure 2. Variations in arch anatomy with interruption. A: Distal to the left subclavian artery (LSCA). B: Between the left subclavian and left common carotid (LCCA) arteries. C: Between the left and right common carotid (RCCA) arteries. D: Between the left subclavian and left common carotid arteries with distal origin of the right subclavian artery (RSCA). AO = aortic; PA = Pulmonary artery.

lated coarctation causes a spectrum of hemodynamic abnormalities that vary from systemic hypertension with increased left ventricular afterload that is well tolerated, to severe compromise of systemic blood flow producing renal failure and metabolic acidosis. When there is an associated intracardiac defect the increased afterload produced by the coarctation accentuates the left to right shunt. For example, in the neonate or young infant with coarctation of the aorta, the left ventricular overload and decreased compliance results in increased left atrial pressure and an atrial left to right shunt through a stretched foramen ovale. The increased pulmonary blood flow results in pulmonary artery and left atrial hypertension with subsequent obstructive large and small airway disease (Motoyama 1977). In the common situation of a coarctation of the aorta and ventricular septal defect, the increased afterload of the coarctation overcomes the neonatal pulmonary vascular resistance and congestive heart failure is commonly seen in the first week or so of life. This is in contrast to the patient with an isolated ventricular septal defect without coarctation of the aorta where congestive heart failure is uncommon before the third week of life. Coarctation of the aorta occurs

with other obstructive abnormalities of the left ventricular outflow particularly, valvar aortic stenosis. Because coarctation can mask significant aortic stenosis and this association occurs with some frequency, the presence of an aortic valve anomaly must be excluded during the catheterization of patients with coarctation of the aorta.

Indications for Cardiac Catheterization

Preoperative

Any infant who presents with congestive heart failure, especially in the first month of life, should have careful and detailed echocardiographic study of the aortic arch to exclude coarctation or interruption. Because associated intracardiac defects are usually identified by cross-sectional and Doppler echocardiography, cardiac catheterization is indicated if there is any question regarding the diagnosis or to define the anatomy further when required.

Congestive heart failure in infants without intracardiac defects is related to left ventricular dysfunction. If congestive heart failure or systemic hypertension is present in infancy, hemodynamic study and early operation are indicated. If the infant is asymptomatic, normotensive and has good left ventricular function by echocardiography, close observation is recommended. We have evaluated several infants with isthmus hypoplasia and large arm/leg systolic blood pressure differences whose mild hypertension and clinical findings of coarctation resolved during the first year of life.

The necessity of heart catheterization in the older child with clinical findings of coarctation has been debated. We have elected to perform magnetic resonance imaging or a preoperative catheterization to identify variations in arch anatomy, including length of coarcted segment, distal origin of subclavian arteries and rare variations in position of coarctation (i.e., abdominal coarctation).

The use of balloon dilation angioplasty for native, nonoperated coarctation of the aorta remains controversial but is being evaluated prospectively in a number of centers.

Postoperative

Some patients exhibit persistent systolic hypertension, particularly with exercise, and mild arm/leg blood pressure difference following operation. Diminution of the femoral pulses with or without brachial/femoral artery pulse delay is of particular concern. Hypertension with an arm/leg peak systolic pressure gradient of over 20 mm Hg indicates significant residual obstruction. This hypertension is thought to be related to abnormal aortic compliance. Balloon dilation angioplasty should be considered in patients with clinical evidence of significant residual coarctation and, of course, another indication for re-study. This procedure is discussed in Chapter 13.

Catheterization Technique

In the neonate, the umbilical vessels often may be used for catheterization. A #5

French feeding tube is passed from the umbilical artery in the usual fashion up to the aortic isthmus. Depending on arch anatomy, this catheter may pass anteriorly through the patent ductus into main pulmonary artery, directly into the left subclavian artery, or through the aortic isthmus into the transverse aortic arch. Because the foramen ovale is generally patent in this age group, a venous approach can be used to perform selective left ventricular angiography. In the infant with an associated ventricular septal defect, an attempt should be made to enter the ascending aorta through the defect. This is difficult or even impossible, if the defect is in the muscular septum. When the above approaches are unsuccessful, a right axillary cutdown can be performed. This makes both ascending and descending aorta approachable for selective angiography. Repair of the arteriotomy is done following catheter removal but if establishment of a patent axillary artery is not attained, viability of the arm is not threatened (see Chapter 4).

In the older child with isolated coarctation, the retrograde femoral arterial catheterization approach is still preferred. Difficulty in passing the catheter across the coarcted segment is occasionally encountered but usually can be accomplished with a guidewire and an end-hole catheter (Chapter 5). In the older patient with severe juxtaductal coarctation, a right brachial arterial approach percutaneously, or by cutdown, is an acceptable option. In the uncomplicated coarctation this may not be warranted, because arch anatomy may be seen well enough on levophase of a pulmonary arteriogram, by digital subtraction angiography, or by magnetic resonance imaging techniques.

Hemodynamic Evaluation

Pressure Data

In infants with isolated coarctation of the aorta, pulmonary artery pressure may be increased to more than nearly half of systemic arterial pressure. If congestive heart failure is present, right atrial pressure is raised and left ventricular end diastolic and left atrial pressures are significantly increased, reflecting increased intravascular volume and afterload. Left ventricular and aortic peak systolic pressures vary depending on cardiac output and whether associated aortic stenosis is present. Descending aortic pressure reflects the degree of obstruction and is characterized by a narrow pulse pressure (Fig. 3). In situations where the ductus arteriosus is open, the right to left ductal shunt masks the pressure gradient between the left ventricle and the descending aorta. Reduction of the peak systolic pressure gradient across the coarctation can also be caused by a large aortic ampulla (aortic end of the ductus insertion), which enlarges the effective cross-sectional area of the aorta at the level of the of coarctation.

In the older child, right heart hemodynamics are usually normal. Peak left ventricular pressure and the systolic gradient across the coarctation reflect cardiac output and the magnitude of collateral circulation. The infant with a large associated ventricular septal defect always has pulmonary artery and right ventricular hypertension. Congestive heart failure is more common, and right and left ventricular end diastolic and right and left atrial pressures are increased.

Oxygen Saturation Data

Oxygen saturation data reflect left to right shunts at atrial or ventricular level. In interrupted aortic arch and occasionally in coarctation, oxygen saturation is lower in the descending than in the ascending aorta because the patent ductus arteriosus supplies all or part of blood flow to the descending aorta. However, this difference is usually small because an associated left to right ven-

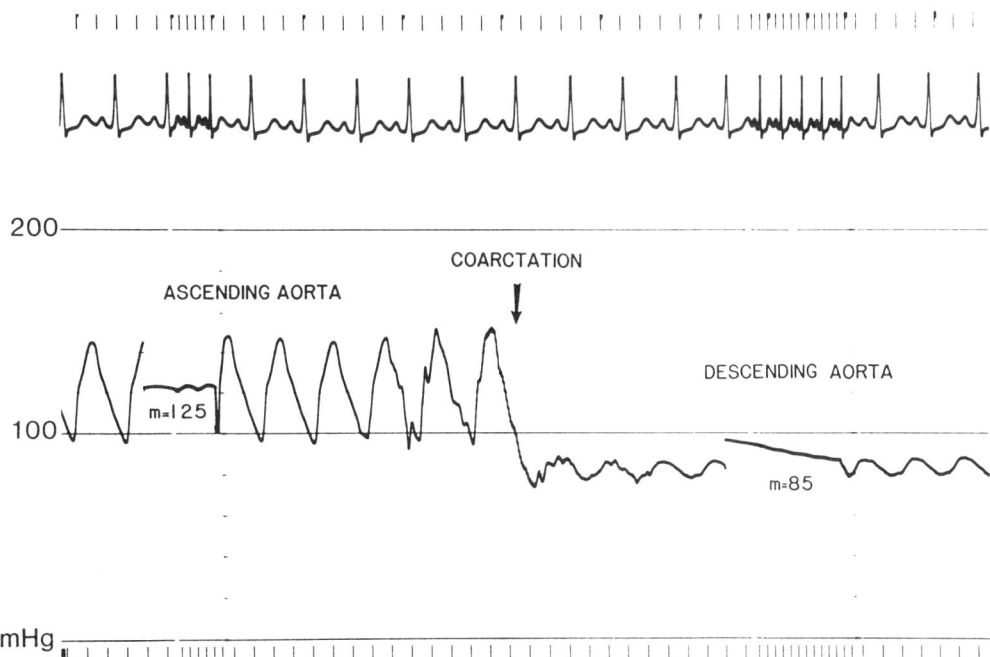

Figure 3. Withdrawal pressure tracing from the ascending aorta to descending aorta demonstrating a marked pressure difference across the area of coarctation.

tricular shunt increases pulmonary arterial saturation.

Angiocardiography

In the neonate with an isolated discrete coarctation, a left ventricular angiogram in the anteroposterior and lateral projection will usually delineate aortic arch anatomy. Selective injection through an umbilical artery catheter into the aorta near the coarctation is an alternative. If there is an associated ventricular septal defect, a left ventricular injection in the anteroposterior (or right anterior oblique) and four-chamber views is performed to evaluate the ventricular septum and aortic arch. The curtain lesion is recognized as an indentation in the lateral wall of the aorta opposite the ductus insertion. There is hypoplasia of the isthmus and the descending aorta is usually dilated (Fig. 4). The left subclavian artery often arises at or near the level of the coarctation. Rarely, the right subclavian also comes from the descending aorta (anomalous retroeso-

phageal right subclavian artery) (Fig. 1D). Collateral circulation is not well developed in infants.

In the infant with interruption of the aortic arch, the ascending aorta is visualized coursing straight toward the neck on the left ventricular angiogram and the site of interruption is usually evident (Fig. 5). The descending aorta fills following the right ventricular angiogram. Identifying the site of interruption requires selective injection into the ascending aorta. Visualization of the associated ventricular septal defect is best in the lateral or axial left oblique view of a right or left ventricular angiogram.

In the older patient with coarctation, there is concentric narrowing of the descending aorta, poststenotic dilatation, and a large pulsating ascending aorta and brachiocephalic arteries. The collateral circulation is usually well developed. Left ventricular and aortic root angiograms are done to assess aortic valve anomalies. Again, there should be specific attention paid to the origin of the right and left subclavian arteries since abnormal position of these vessels can alter the surgical approach. A descending aortogram has also been done routinely in our institution to exclude an associated renal vascular anomaly.

Associated Lesions

Coarctation of the aorta is found in association with a number of other lesions. As was already mentioned, left to right shunt lesions such as a patent ductus arteriosus or ventricular septal defect are particularly common associations (Neches 1977; Rosenquist 1974). Coarctation is also often seen as part of complex intracardiac malformations, particularly: mitral atresia, the Taussig-Bing anomaly and aortic atresia (hypoplastic left heart syndrome). Less commonly, it is also found in association with transposition of the great arteries, tricuspid atresia and single ventricle. Interestingly, coarctation of the aorta is rarely seen

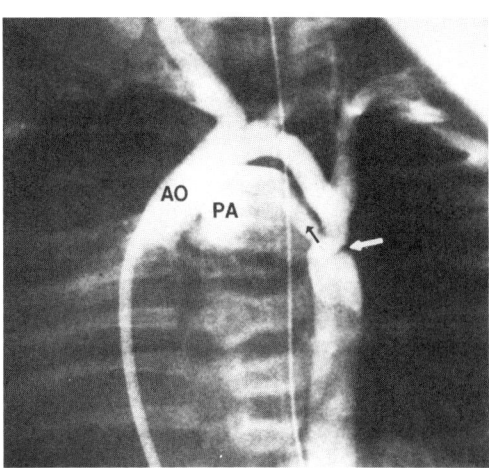

Figure 4. Aortogram in a neonate with juxtaductal coarctation of the aorta (arrow). There is hypoplasia of the transverse arch. There is flow into the pulmonary artery via a patent ductus arteriosus (black arrow). AO = aortic; PA = Pulmonary artery.

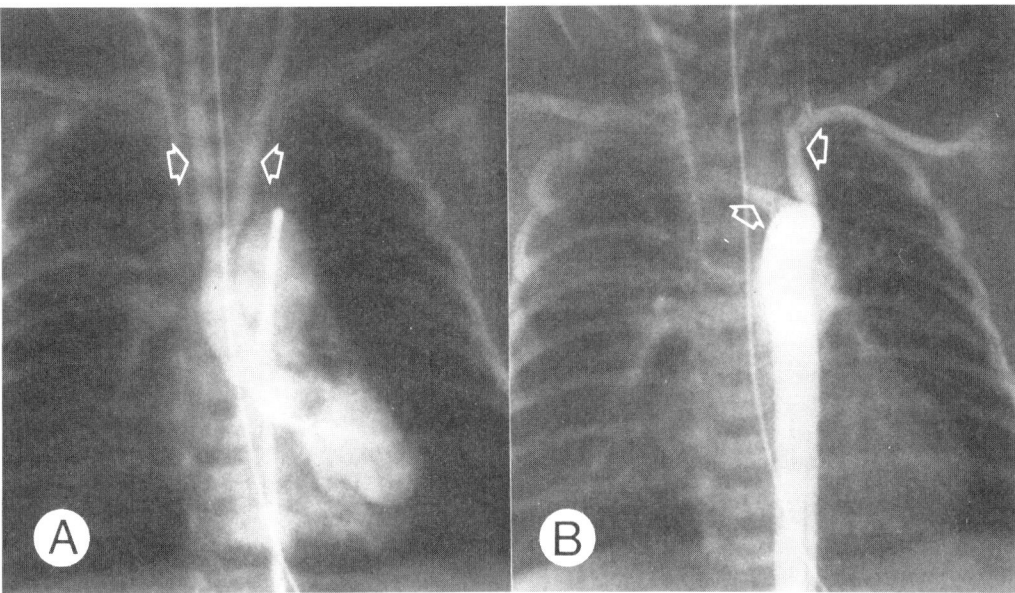

Figure 5. Angiograms in an interrupted aortic arch. A: Left ventricular angiogram in the anteroposterior view demonstrating filling of only both carotid arteries (arrows). The catheter pass is as follows: Descending aorta-patent ductus-pulmonary artery-right ventricle-left ventricle through a ventricular defect. B: Selective injection in the descending aorta at the level of the ductus arteriosus demonstrating filling of the pulmonary arteries as well as the left and an anomalous right subclavian arteries (arrows).

in association with tetralogy of Fallot and the reason for this lack of occurrence may be due to the increased flow through the aortic arch as a result of the pulmonary stenosis or atresia.

Pseudocoarctation

Pseudocoarctation (congenital kinking of the aorta) can be recognized by a typical angiographic appearance (Fig. 6) and lack of significant gradient on catheter withdrawal from ascending to descending aorta. Late aortic aneurysm formation is the only known sequelae (Hoeffel 1975).

Unusual Sites of Aortic Coarctation

Unusual sites for coarctation are the transverse arch, thoracic and abdominal aorta (Fig. 7). With the latter, there often is

associated stenosis of renal and/or mesenteric arteries.

Cautions and Precautions

The neonate with severe coarctation of the aorta tends to have metabolic acidosis due to decreased peripheral perfusion. Prostaglandin E_1 should be started to maintain patency of the ductus arteriosus and thereby improve flow to the distal aorta. Because these infants usually have congestive heart failure, the amount of contrast material should be kept to a minimum and nonionic contrast should be used.

In the infant with coarctation, the hemodynamic and angiographic features may be masked by the presence of a large patent ductus arteriosus. Thus, whenever an infant in the first month of life with a ventricular septal defect and/or patent ductus arterio-

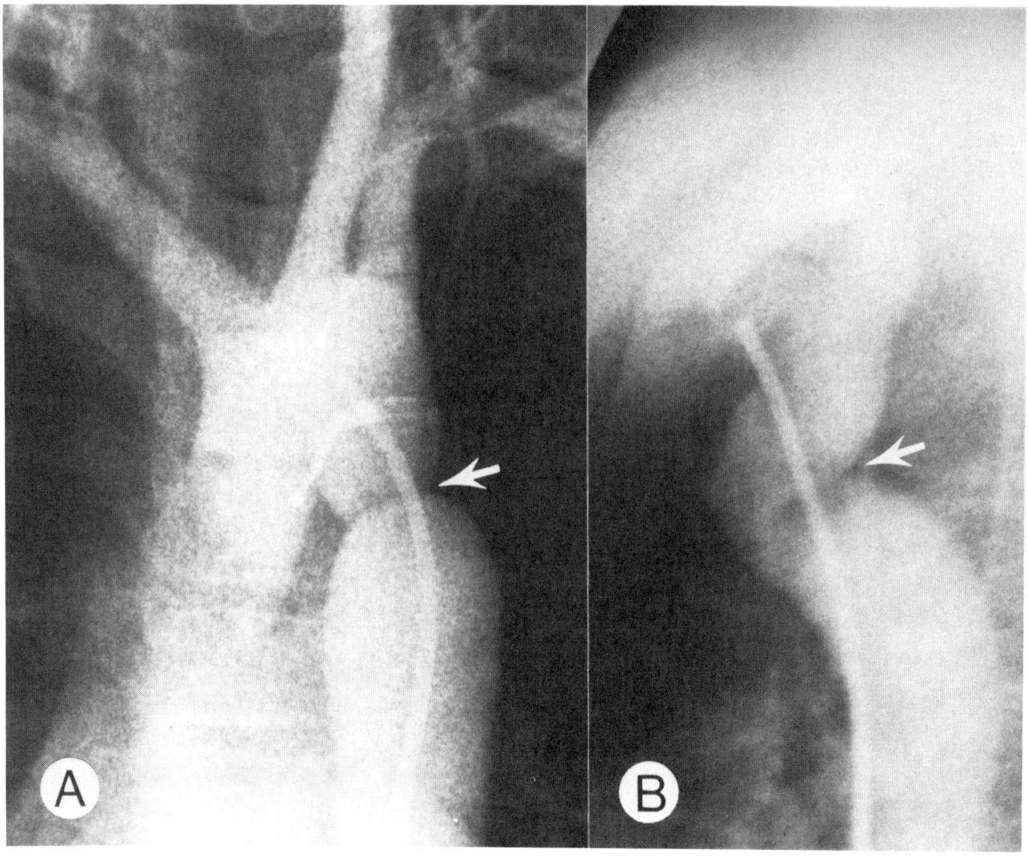

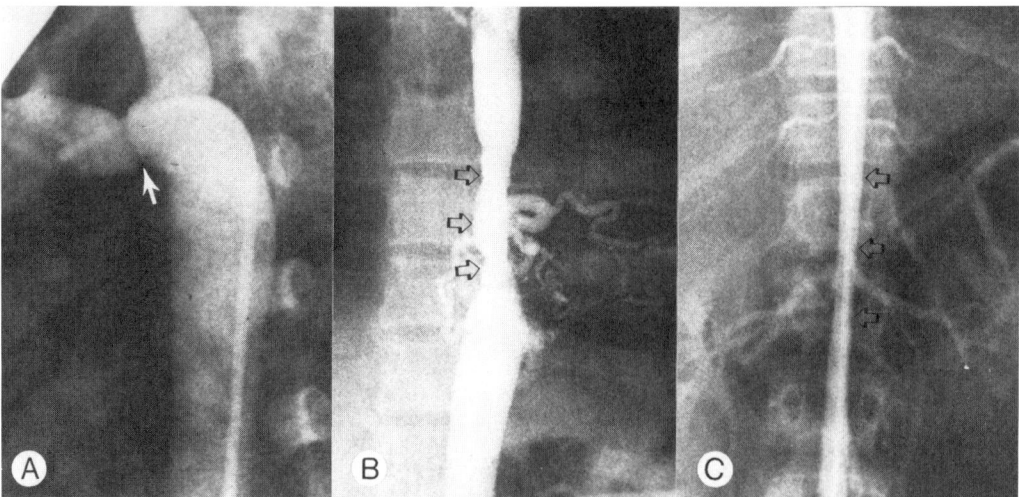

Figure 6. Selective aortogram demonstrating a pseudocoarctation of the aorta (arrows). A: Anteroposterior view. B: Lateral view.

Figure 7. Selective aortograms demonstrating unusual sites of aortic coarctation (arrows). A: Left anterior oblique view of a coarctation in the transverse aortic arch. B: Anteroposterior view of a coarctation in the lower thoracic aorta. C: Anteroposterior view of diffuse hypoplasia of the abdominal aorta.

sus presents with congestive heart failure, the possibility of an associated coarctation must be considered and carefully looked for by echocardiography and angiography.

References and Suggested Reading

Becker AE, Becker MJ, Edwards JT. Anomalies associated with coarctation of the aorta: Particular reference to infancy. Circulation 1970;41:1967–1075.

Celoria GC, Patton RB. Congenital absence of the aortic arch. Am Heart J 1959;58:407–413.

Dische R, Rsai M, Baltaxe HA. Solitary interruption of the arch of the aorta. Am J Cardiol 1975;35:271–277.

Hoeffel JC, Henry M, Mentre B, et al. Psdueo-coarctation or congenital kinking of the aorta, radiologic considerations. Am Heart J 1975;89:428–436.

Moller JH, Edwards JE. Interruption of aortic arch: Anatomic patterns and associated cardiac malformations. Am J Roentgenol 1965;95:557–572.

Motoyama EK. Pulmonary mechanics during early postnatal years. Pediatr Res 1977;11:220–223.

Neches WH, Park SC, Lenox CC, et al. Coarctation of the aorta with ventricular septal defect. Circulation 1977;55:189–194.

Roberts WC, Morrow AG, Braunwald E. Complete interruption of the aortic arch. Circulation 1962;26:39–59.

Rosenquist GC. Congenital mitral valve disease associated with coarctation of the aorta. Circulation 1974;49:985–993.

Rudolph AM. Congenital Diseases of the Heart. Yearbook Medical Publishers, 1974.

Van Praagh R, Bernhard WF, Rosenthal A, et al. Interrupted aortic arch: Surgical treatment. Am J Cardiol 1971;27:200–211.

Wood WC, Wood JC, Lower RR, et al. Associated coarctation of the aorta and mitral valve disease. J Pediatr 1975;87:217–220.

Yen Ho S, Anderson RH. Coarctation, tubular hypoplasia and the ductus arteriosus—Histological study of 35 specimens. Br Heart J 1979;41:268–274.

35

Anomalous Pulmonary Venous Return

Cora C. Lenox, M.D.

Anomalous pulmonary venous connection exists if one or more pulmonary veins connect to a systemic vein or directly to the right atrium. Anomalous connection may be partial or total, depending upon the number of pulmonary veins involved.

Total Anomalous Pulmonary Venous Connection

Anatomy

With total anomalous pulmonary venous connection there is no direct connection between the confluence of the pulmonary veins and the left atrium. In this anomaly, the confluence is usually normally placed immediately behind the left atrium, but it remains distinct from the left atrium rather than having been incorporated into its posterior wall during embryologic development. In addition, one or more primitive connections between the pulmonary veins and the systemic veins persist, allowing pulmonary venous blood to drain directly or indirectly to the right atrium (Delisle et al. 1960). This persistence of connections to the systemic venous system distinguishes total anomalous pulmonary venous connection from atresia of the common pulmonary vein that later develops embryologically after these connections have been lost (Lucas 1983) (see Chapter 32). Anomalous pulmonary venous connection

may be conveniently classified as supracardiac, cardiac, or infracardiac based upon the site of connection to the systemic venous system (Table 1) (Fig. 1). The supracardiac variety results from persistence of a connection between the pulmonary veins and a derivative of the anterior cardinal system. The connection may be to a left-sided systemic vein, either a persistent left superior vena cava or a left vertical vein, which drains into the innominate vein and then into the right superior vena cava. The connection is less commonly to the right superior vena cava, usually at or above the level of the azygos vein. Connection is occasionally to the azygos or hemiazygos veins that are derivatives of the posterior cardinal veins but the connection is still "supracardiac". Connection at the cardiac level may be to veins that enter the right atrium directly (usually just below the orifice of the superior vena cava), into the portion of the right atrium derived from the sinus venosus, or to the coronary sinus, also a derivative of the sinus venous. Infracardiac connection is to the inferior vena cava or to a derivative of the umbilico-vitelline system; either the portal vein or the ductus venosus. Occasionally there is mixed connection, in which there may be no common pulmonary vein or confluence behind the left atrium.

Hemodynamic Considerations

In total anomalous pulmonary venous return, all pulmonary venous return even-

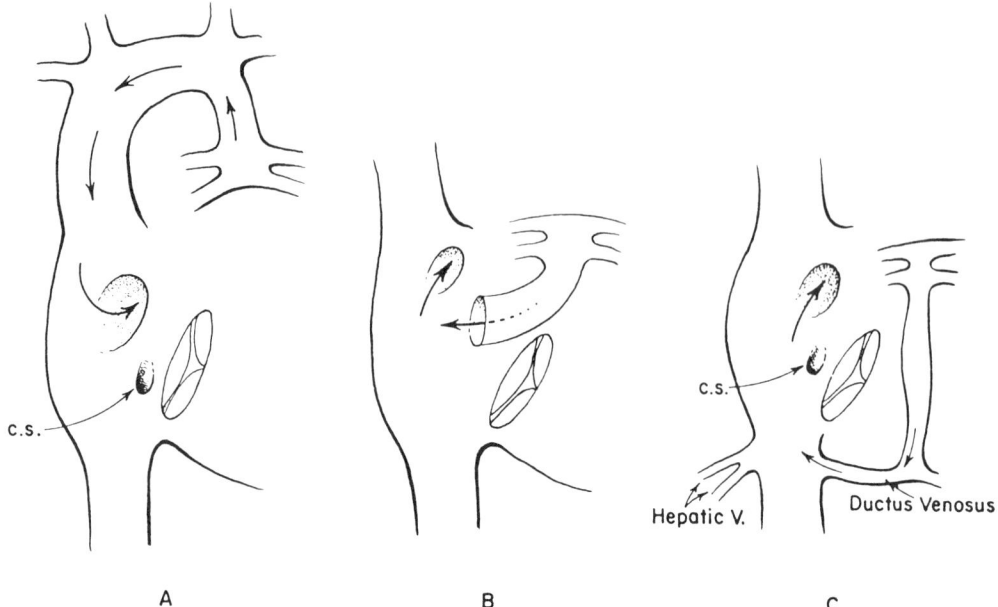

Figure 1. Diagrams of various forms of total anomalous pulmonary venous return. A: Supracardiac to a left vertical vein (left superior vena cava). B: Cardiac to coronary sinus (c.s.). C: Infracardiac (infradiaphragmatic) to the portal vein.

tually enters the right atrium and mixes there with systemic venous return. Pulmonary blood flow is by the usual route, but all systemic blood flow must cross the atrial septum into the left atrium before entering the left ventricle and aorta. The magnitude of pulmonary blood flow depends upon the impedance to diastolic filling of the right ventricle, and is therefore related to hypertrophy and function of this chamber. This in turn is also influenced by the pulmonary vascular resistance. In patients with severe obstruction within the anomalous channel, there is high pulmonary venous pressure, high pulmonary artery pressure, and resistance that result in low pulmonary blood flow. This is most commonly seen in the newborn infant with total anomalous pulmonary venous return below the diaphragm. The consequences of this hemodynamic derangement are marked arterial oxygen unsaturation and signs and symptoms of congestive heart failure. Tachypnea, respiratory distress, and frank pulmonary edema

occur if pulmonary venous pressure is sufficiently elevated. Hepatomegaly is the consequence of the right ventricular failure induced by right ventricular pressure overload.

If pulmonary venous obstruction is not present, the right ventricular hypertrophy and increased pulmonary vascular resistance normally present in the newborn may protect against very high pulmonary blood flow. With regression of this resistance and the right ventricular hypertrophy, the impedance to right ventricular filling decreases, pulmonary flow increases and congestive heart failure may then occur. In contrast to connection below the diaphragm that usually presents in the newborn, patients with connections above the diaphragm may present in the first few months of life or even much later. Cyanosis then is often mild or even inapparent because the pulmonary blood flow is relatively high.

Mixing of systemic and pulmonary venous returns usually is completely at atrial

Table 1

Anomalous Pulmonary Venous
Connection

I. Total
  A. Supracardiac
    1. Left superior vena cava
    2. Right superior vena cava
    3. Azygos or hemiazygos vein
  B. Cardiac-Right atrium
    1. Direct connection
    2. Coronary sinus
  C. Infracardiac
    1. Inferior vena cava
    2. Portal vein or its tributary
    3. Ductus venosus
  D. Mixed
    1. Pulmonary veins of one lung drain-
       ing to one systemic vein and veins
       of other lung draining to another
       systemic vein.
    2. One pulmonary vein draining to
       one systemic vein and all the others
       to another.
II. Partial
  A. Right pulmonary vein
    1. Right upper and lower pulmonary
       veins to right superior vena cava or
       right atrium. Usually atrial septal
       defect coexists.
    2. Right middle and lower lobe vein to
       inferior vena cava ("Scimitar")
      a. With or without a sequestered
         pulmonary lobe
      b. With or without arterial supply
         from the aorta
  B. Left-sided pulmonary veins
    1. Left upper lobe vein to left superior
       vena cava
      a. With associated cor triatriatum
      b. With associated mitral atresia
  C. Mixed
  D. Miscellaneous, (e.g., crossover from
    one side to systemic vein on contra-
    lateral side).

level but this does not always occur. Inferior vena caval return may be shunted preferentially across the foramen ovale, as seen in fetal life. If this occurs and the site of return is cardiac or supracardiac, the relatively unsaturated inferior vena caval blood will cross the foramen ovale and consequently the left ventricular and aortic blood will be less saturated than right ventricular and pulmonary arterial blood. One might also expect relatively high left ventricular and aortic saturation in a patient with infracardiac return, but because venous obstruction is almost universal in such patients, pulmonary blood flow is not large and there is usually no difference between aortic and pulmonary artery saturation.

Indications for Cardiac Catheterization

Preoperative

The most common indication for cardiac catheterization is to define further the nature of the anomalous connections when this lesion has been suspected or diagnosed by echocardiography. Cross-sectional echocardiography alone has not been completely reliable in defining the site of entry of pulmonary veins because it may appear that pulmonary veins are entering the left atrium when, in fact, anomalous return is present. The proximity of the confluence of the pulmonary veins to the left atrium in this anomaly may explain this illusion. However, with the advent of Doppler color flow mapping, the ability to diagnose this lesion has been greatly enhanced and the diagnosis is almost always made echocardiographically.

In some newborns and in older infants and children, cardiac catheterization and angiography are performed prior to surgical repair to assess adequacy of the left ventricle, to measure pulmonary vascular resistance, and to document the site of pulmonary venous return. The site is not necessarily important from the surgical standpoint but the occasional case with mixed return and/or a small, unusually positioned, or absent confluence makes an angiographic evaluation highly desirable.

Postoperative

Prior to the days of echocardiography, we recommended routinely performing cardiac catheterization a year or so after surgical repair of total anomalous pulmonary venous return. The major justification for this practice was the possibility that obstruction might be present at the anastomosis between the confluence and the left atrium and yet not be clinically apparent. At least one of our patients died suddenly and at autopsy was found to have severe obstruction at this site. Currently, cross-sectional and Doppler echocardiographic techniques enable visualization of the pulmonary venous connection and usually it is possible to rule out postoperative obstruction. Certainly, any evidence of pulmonary venous obstruction such as the typical radiographic findings, tachypnea, clinical evidence of pulmonary hypertension, or abnormal flow patterns echocardiographically, makes postoperative cardiac catheterization mandatory.

Catheterization Technique

Cardiac catheterization is usually not technically difficult in patients with this anomaly. The right ventricle and pulmonary artery are easily entered by the usual techniques, and from the femoral approach the catheter readily passes from the right to the left atrium. Entry into the left ventricle from the left atrium is easier than usual because the catheter never inadvertently enters a pulmonary vein. As long as the catheter tip is kept low in the left atrium, entry into the appendage is not a problem and the catheter often passes easily into the left ventricle. The aorta can be entered antegrade from the left ventricle with the use of a flow-directed balloon catheter, especially if the tip is sharply curved. However, in the newborn or young infant with a small left ventricle, this latter catheter pass may be extremely difficult.

If possible, the confluence of the pulmonary veins should also be entered, both to record pressure and for contrast injection. If return is to the left innominate vein

it may be difficult to turn the catheter caudally from the innominate vein unless a sharply curved guidewire is used. With return to the coronary sinus, entry into the confluence is easy; the difficulty is in being sure that the catheter is there and not in the right or left atrium. The distinction is cineangiographic.

Hemodynamic Evaluation

Pressure Data

Pressures in the right ventricle and pulmonary artery are largely dependent upon the presence or absence of obstruction within the course of the anomalous pulmonary venous connection. If there is significant obstruction, pulmonary hypertension is invariable; if there is no obstruction, pulmonary artery pressure usually is increased only mildly and even may be normal. Therefore, if pulmonary hypertension is found to be present, pulmonary artery wedge pressure should be measured and a site of obstruction should always be sought. When the anomalous connection is supracardiac, obstruction is uncommon but may occur where the anomalous channel courses between the pulmonary artery and the bronchus on its way to the right or left superior vena cava. If connection is directly to the right atrium or to the right superior vena cava, there may be obstruction at the venoatrial or venocaval junction. A connection to the coronary sinus is rarely associated with obstruction. Severe obstruction always accompanies connections below the diaphragm, because the portal venous blood must pass through the sinusoids of the liver after the ductus venosus closes soon after birth.

A pressure gradient is sometimes present along the course of the anomalous channel, due to increased flow even though there may be no angiographically or morphologically evident obstruction. With anomalous pulmonary venous connection to the left innominate, for instance, there may be a gradual drop of 10–15 mm Hg between the confluence and the superior vena cava-right atrial junction (Fig. 2). This pressure drop may be associated with a continuous "hum", audible externally and recordable internally with a phonocatheter. The hum is always loudest internally at or immediately down stream from the site of obstruction (or pressure drop if there is no actual anatomic narrowing of the channel).

A withdrawal or pullback pressure recording from the left atrium to the right atrium is important. Right atrial pressure is usually higher than the left atrial pressure, particularly when the interatrial opening is small.

Calculated total pulmonary resistance includes resistance in the anomalous venous channel and should not be misinterpreted as evidence of severe pulmonary vascular disease in the patient with severe obstruction within the channel.

Oxygen Saturation Data

At cardiac catheterization, right and left heart oximetry are important and should in-clude samples from the innominate vein and the superior and inferior vena cavae. Oxygen saturation is highest in an anomalous pulmonary vein and at the site where this anomalous vein joins a systemic vein. Because all pulmonary venous blood eventually enters the right atrium, oxygen saturation there is high and is maintained in the right ventricle and pulmonary artery. There is right to left shunting across an interatrial communication and a true atrial septal defect or a foramen ovale. If the anomalous pulmonary venous connection is supracardiac or to the right atrium, saturation in the left atrium, left ventricle, and aorta may be somewhat lower than in the right-sided chambers because relatively unsaturated inferior vena caval return is shunted preferentially across the atrial communication. If pulmonary venous pressure is very high, as in the newborn infant with anomalous pulmonary venous connection below the diaphragm, oxygen exchange may be impaired, leading to pulmonary venous unsaturation.

Relative pulmonary and systemic blood flows are calculated in the usual fashion, although obtaining a true mixed systemic ve-

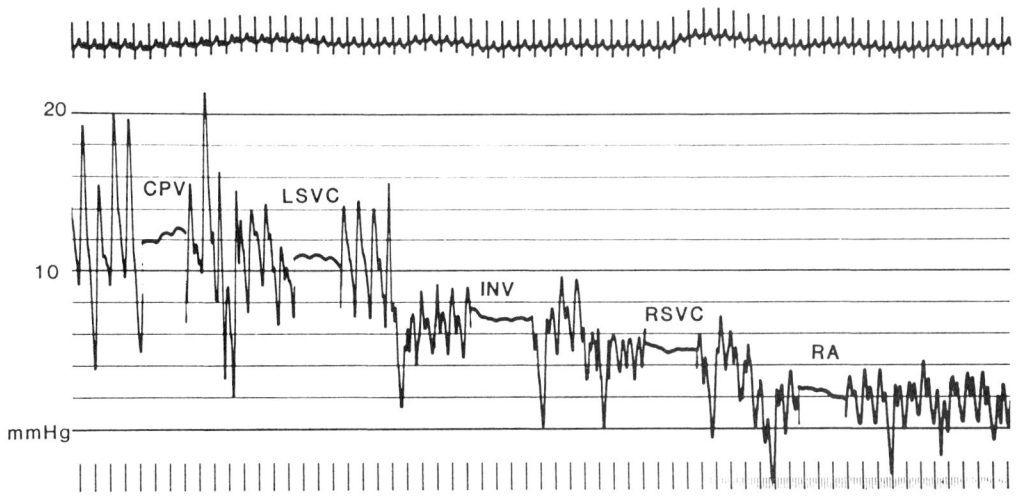

Figure 2. Withdrawal pressure tracing from the confluence of the pulmonary veins to the right atrium demonstrating pressure gradients at a number of sites despite the absence of anatomic obstruction. CPV = Common pulmonary vein; INV = Innominate vein; LSVC = Left superior vena cava; RA = Right atrium; RSVC = Right superior vena cava.

nous saturation may be difficult, especially if return is supracardiac. If return is to the left innominate vein, a sample drawn in the high right superior vena cava is probably most representative of systemic venous return, although there may be a problem with streaming from jugular and subclavian veins. If return is to the right superior vena cava an innominate sample is preferable.

Other Diagnostic or Therapeutic Procedures

Most patients with total anomalous pulmonary venous return now undergo surgical repair during the newborn period or early infancy as soon as diagnosis is established and in such patients balloon atrial septostomy may not be needed. However, in pa-

tients with a restrictive interatrial communication, low cardiac output, and severe pulmonary hypertension, balloon atrial septostomy is beneficial even if surgery is contemplated within a short time. In the occasional patient in whom surgery is deferred (e.g., mixed anomalous venous return without a confluence of the pulmonary veins), a balloon septostomy should be performed to insure unobstructed right to left atrial shunting (Ward 1986).

Angiocardiography

Although an injection of contrast media into the main pulmonary artery usually visualizes the anomalous channel, if possible the catheter should also be passed into the channel as far as the confluence of the pulmonary veins and an injection of contrast

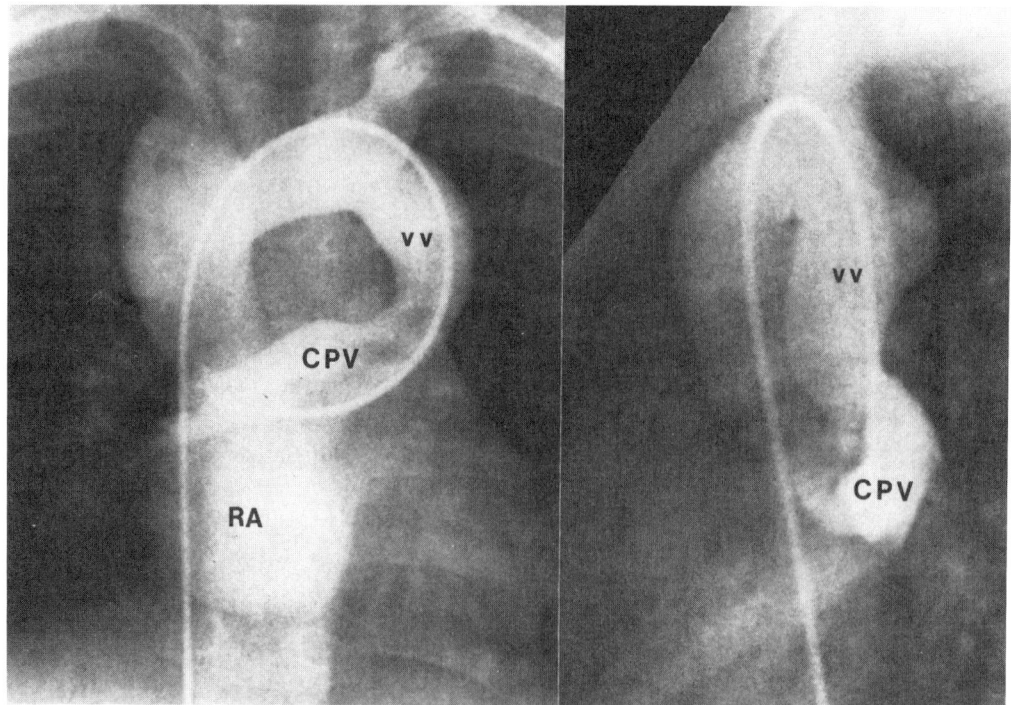

Figure 3. Selective angiogram in the pulmonary venous confluence in supracardiac total anomalous pulmonary venous return in the anteroposterior (left) and lateral (right) views. CPV = Common pulmonary vein; RA = Right atrium; VV = Vertical vein.

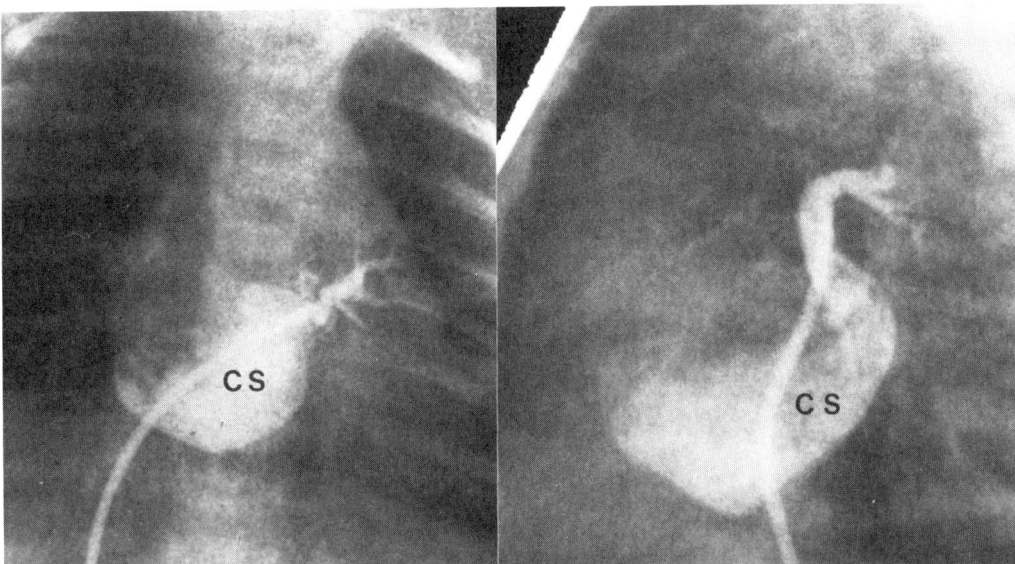

Figure 4. Selective angiogram in the left upper pulmonary vein in a total anomalous pulmonary venous return to the coronary sinus in the anteroposterior (left) and lateral (right) views. CS = Coronary sinus.

media made there (Figs. 3 and 4). In a newborn, if the anomalous connection is infracardiac, an injection of contrast media into the ductus venosus by way of an umbilical vein catheter may show the connection. If there is any question of a mixed connection, contrast media should be injected selectively into both right and left pulmonary arteries.

The anomalous venous channel is most difficult to visualize angiographically if there is severe obstruction within it. Under these circumstances it is usually impossible to enter the channel directly and one must rely on the pulmonary artery injection. It may be necessary to use up to 1.5 mL of contrast media/kg of body weight and since the transit time through the lungs is considerably longer than usual, a prolonged cine run may be necessary to visualize the delayed return. *In a symptomatic newborn suspected of having total anomalous pulmonary venous connection with obstruction, the field should always include the subdiaphragmatic area.* With return to the portal system, the confluence is usually faintly visualized and gives rise to a narrow venous channel which courses caudally parallel to the spine and then enters the portal system. It is usually difficult or impossible to see the contrast media returning through the hepatic veins to the right atrium. A selective injection of contrast material into the pulmonary artery wedge position is an effective way to visualize the pulmonary venous pattern, particularly when pulmonary venous obstruction is severe with slow flow (Figs. 5 and 6).

Associated Lesions

Total anomalous pulmonary venous connection is commonly found as part of the complex congenital heart disease in patients with the atrial isomerism syndromes. In right atrial isomerism (asplenia syndrome), there is usually a primitive-type heart with an undifferentiated type of ventricle, single ventricle, or complete atrioventricular septal defect. Severe pulmonary stenosis or

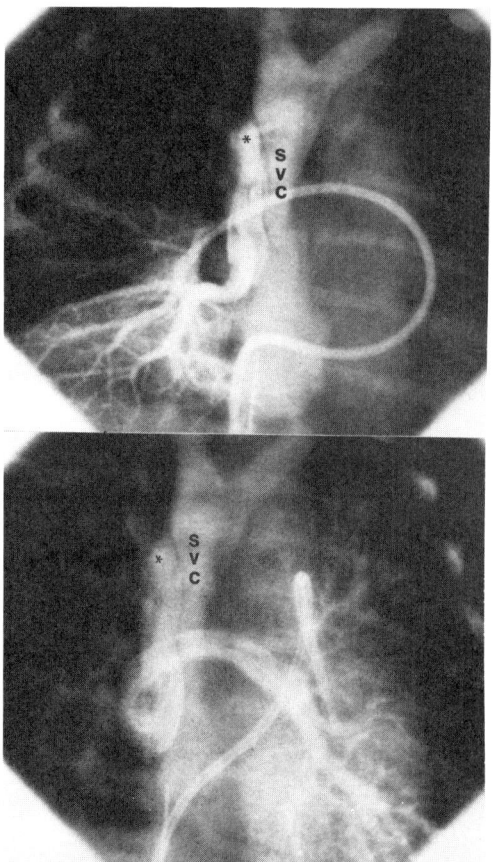

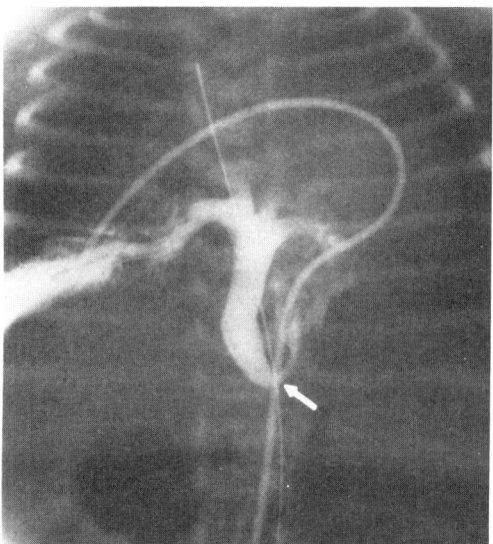

Figure 6. Selective pulmonary artery wedge injection demonstrating severe obstruction (arrow) at the site of entry into the portal vein in total anomalous pulmonary venous return below the diaphragm.

Figure 5. Selective right (top) and left (bottom) pulmonary artery wedge angiograms demonstrating total anomalous pulmonary venous return to the right superior vena cava (SVC). Asterisk indicates the point of entry of the anomalous vein.

atresia is almost always also present and this may mask the presentation of total anomalous pulmonary venous return due to the reduced pulmonary blood flow. This is also true in other situations where anomalous pulmonary venous return is found in conjunction with reduced pulmonary blood flow. Other cardiac lesions that have been seen in conjunction with total anomalous pulmonary venous return include transposition of the great arteries, single ventricle, and ductus arteriosus.

Cautions and Precautions

Newborns with total anomalous pulmonary venous connection often are quite ill and have pulmonary edema. If cardiac catheterization is indicated, an attempt must be made to stabilize the infant and correct acidosis as rapidly as possible prior to the procedure. Endotracheal intubation and mechanical ventilation with a fairly high level of positive end expiratory pressure is warranted to lessen the pulmonary edema caused by the pulmonary venous obstruction. Information should be obtained during the procedure as rapidly as possible.

Partial Anomalous Pulmonary Connection

Anatomy

Partial anomalous pulmonary venous connection may be isolated but is more commonly found associated with another anomaly. For example, a right upper lobe vein connected to the superior vena cava or high right atrium is usually associated with an atrial septal defect of the sinus venous type. A left upper lobe vein connection to the innominate vein is sometimes associated with obstructive lesions in the left heart such as mitral atresia or cor triatriatum. Right, mid, and lower lobe vein connection to the inferior vena cava may accompany a lung anomaly and either hypoplasia or absence of the right pulmonary artery. In this situation there may also be a sequestered lobe supplied by an anomalous artery from the descending aorta. The anomalous vein in this complex can often be seen on chest roentgenogram and has been described as resembling a curved sword, hence the "scimitar" syndrome (Neill et al. 1960).

Hemodynamic Considerations

The hemodynamic consequence of partial anomalous pulmonary venous return is an increase in pulmonary blood flow. Pulmonary artery pressure is usually normal, as it is with left to right shunting through a simple atrial septal defect. Pulmonary artery pressure may be elevated, however, if most pulmonary veins drain anomalously. There is no arterial unsaturation, even in patients with only one normally draining pulmonary vein. The presence of other significant cardiac or vascular anomalies profoundly may influence hemodynamics.

Indications for Cardiac Catheterization

Partial anomalous pulmonary venous return usually accompanies other congenital cardiac defects, and the indications for invasive study are usually those of the as-sociated anomaly. When partial return is found in association with an atrial septal defect, the usual indication is clinical evidence of a large left to right shunt and suspicion of the venous anomaly. At times, isolated partial anomalous pulmonary venous return can clinically manifest a significant right ventricular volume overload plus high pulmonary blood flow and warrant further investigation.

Catheterization Technique

Anomalous draining veins can be entered with the catheter. When anomalous right-sided pulmonary veins accompany a sinus venosus atrial defect the veins are entered from the lateral wall of the high right atrium or the superior vena cava. The catheter pass across this variety of atrial septal defect is unusually high. The pass into the left ventricle from the left atrium may be difficult and often requires aid of an curved guidewire. Left-sided pulmonary veins draining into the left innominate vein are easily entered from the innominate. With this particular anomaly there may be another channel (persistent left superior vena cava) leading from the left pulmonary veins to the coronary sinus and resulting in an oxygen step-up there. This channel can sometimes be entered from the coronary sinus.

Hemodynamic Evaluation

Right heart and pulmonary artery oxygen saturations and pressures should be recorded. Because individual pulmonary veins may be partially obstructed, pressure should be recorded in each, or if this is not possible, in the corresponding pulmonary arterial wedge position. Relative pulmonary and systemic blood flow can be calculated in the usual fashion, although the volume of flows through an individual pulmonary vein cannot be measured accurately by methods available in the usual catheterization laboratory. If more than one vein drains anomalously, the pulmonary to systemic flow ratio can be greater than 2:1. Pulmonary artery pressure is usually normal, but may be elevated with very high pulmonary blood flow. Pulmonary vascular resistance is usually normal unless there are associated anomalies. Systemic arterial saturation is normal as long as there is only partial anomalous venous return.

Angiocardiography

Partial anomalous pulmonary venous connection is usually well visualized following a pulmonary arteriogram in the posteroanterior projection. A selective right or left pulmonary arteriogram may then be done to define the connection further (Figs. 7 and 8). In the presence of an atrial septal defect it can be very difficult to differentiate whether a pulmonary vein joins the right atrium directly or if the connection is really to the left atrium and there is then flow of contrast media into the right atrium. The distinction can usually be made by an injection of con-

trast media into the vein in question in the four-chamber position (Fig. 9). This view best outlines the interatrial septum and the site of the connection is usually evident.

If a scimitar syndrome is present, an anomalous arterial supply to the right lower lobe should always be sought. The anomalous artery originates from the descending aorta, usually just below the diaphragm, and can be seen on a left ventriculogram or, preferably, on an aortogram in the anteroposterior projection (see Chapter 17).

Associated Lesions

Partial anomalous pulmonary venous return can be found in association with many forms of congenital heart disease and should be considered in any patient who is found to have a left to right shunt at atrial level. As was mentioned earlier, it is particularly common in association with atrial septal defects, especially those of the sinus venosus type. In patients with left atrial isomerism (polysplenia syndrome), the left-sided pulmonary veins drain appropriately to the left side of the atrium while the right-sided veins drain to the right-sided atrium.

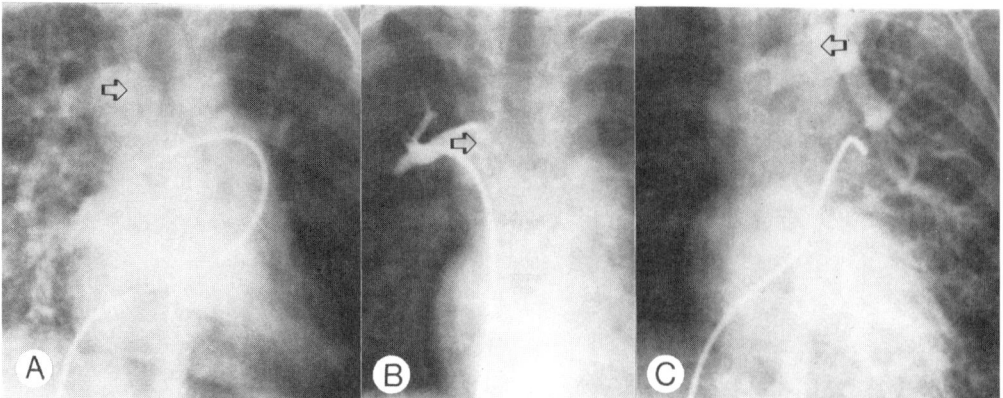

Figure 7. Selective angiogram in the pulmonary artery branches demonstrating partial anomalous pulmonary venous return. A: Right upper pulmonary vein to the superior vena cava (arrow). B: Selective injection in the anomalous right upper pulmonary vein in the same patient as in (A) demonstrating direct connection to the superior vena cava (arrow). C: Left upper pulmonary vein to the left innominate vein (arrow).

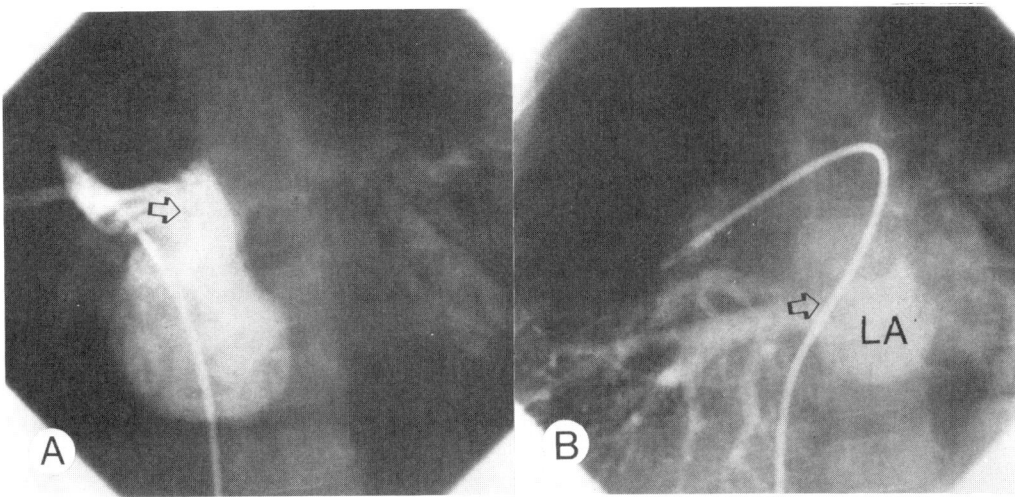

Figure 8. Angiograms demonstrating partial anomalous pulmonary venous return. A: Selective injection in the right upper pulmonary vein demonstrating drainage to the superior vena cava-right atrial junction (arrow). B: Selective injection in the right lower pulmonary artery demonstrating normal drainage of the right lower pulmonary vein (arrow) into the left atrium (LA).

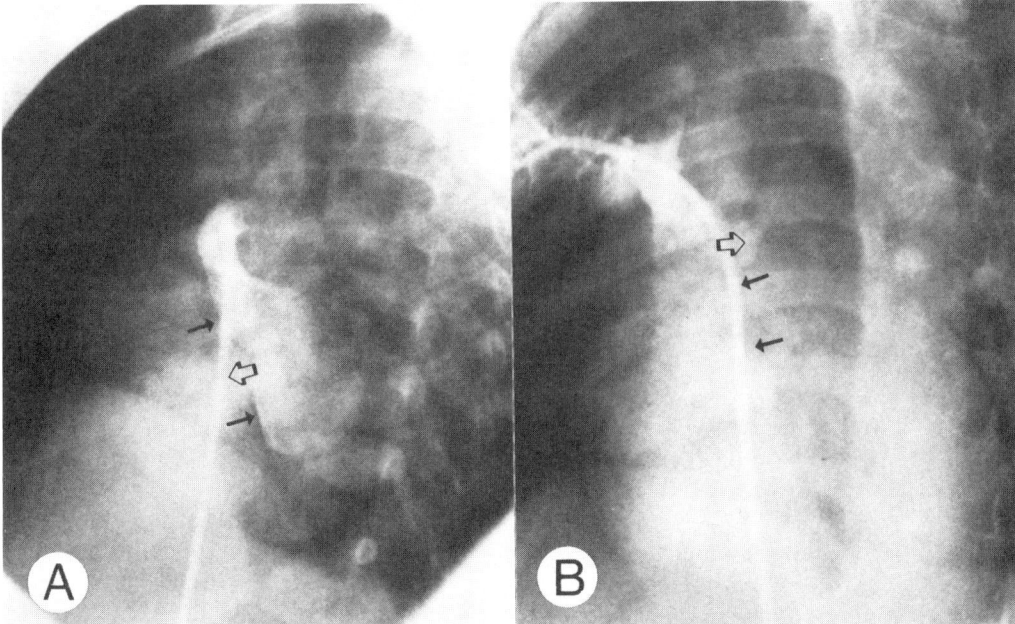

Figure 9. Selective angiograms in the right upper pulmonary vein in the four-chamber view. A: Normal pulmonary venous drainage on the left side of the atrial septum (arrows). There is shunting across the atrial defect (open arrow). B: Abnormal pulmonary venous drainage to the superior vena cava-right atrial junction is on the right side of the atrial septum (arrows). There is shunting across the atrial defects (open arrow).

Since this right-sided atrium is also morphologically a left atrium, one could argue about whether or not this belongs in the category of partial anomalous pulmonary venous return.

Cautions and Precautions

In any attempt to catheterize the pulmonary veins selectively, it must be remembered that these are relatively thin structures. Gentle manipulation in these vessels is essential to avoid the possibility of perforation.

References and Suggested Reading

DeLisle G, Ando M, Calder AL, et al. Total anomalous pulmonary venous connection: Report of 93 autopsied cases with emphasis on diagnostic and surgical considertion. Am Heart J 1976;91:99–122.

Lucas RV, Jr. In: Heart Disease in Infants, Children and Adolescents. Third ed. Baltimore, MD; Williams & Wilkins. 1983:459–475.

Neill CA, Ferencz C, Sabiston DC, et al. The familial occurrence of hypoplastic right lung with systemic arterial supply and venous drainage: "Scimitar syndrome". Bull Johns Hopkins Hosp 1960;107:1–15.

Ward KE, Mullins CE, Huhta JC, et al. Restrictive interatrial communication in total anomalous pulmonary venous connection. Am J Cardiol 1986;57:1131–1136.

36

Systemic Venous Anomalies

J.R. Zuberbuhler, M.D.

Systemic veins are more plastic structures than are arteries. For example, occlusion of a peripheral vein rarely leads to any permanent vascular embarrassment, rather, collateral veins enlarge and adequate venous drainage ensues. This is in striking contrast to the ischemic change that may follow occlusion of a peripheral artery. Veins are also more congenitally variable than arteries. The clinically important congenital venous anomalies involve the vena cavae. Certain anomalies, such as drainage of the left superior vena cava to the left atrium, have clinical consequences. Other anomalies are important only because they present technical problems during cardiac catheterization or cardiac surgery.

Congenital caval anomalies are most easily understood against the background of embryologic development. Systemic venous drainage of the developing embryo is by way of the cardinal venous system. On each side of the body, anterior and posterior cardinal veins drain the upper and lower portions of the body, respectively, and then combine to form the common cardinal veins. The right and left common cardinals, in turn, drain to the right and left horns of the sinus venous, the most proximal portion of the cardiac tube (Fig. 1A and 1B). The right horn of the sinus venous forms part of the developing right atrium, while the left horn becomes the coronary sinus (Fig. 1C).

Portions of the cardinal veins are incorporated into the developing vena caval system; the right common cardinal into the right superior vena cava, the left common cardinal into the left superior vena cava and the coronary sinus. Following development of the innominate vein as a connecting link between the right and left superior vena cavae, the portion of the left superior cava between the left innominate and the coronary sinus involutes, or may persist in part as the oblique vein of Marshal on the posterior surface of the heart (Fig. 1D). The right and left posterior cardinal veins contribute to the azygos and hemiazygos veins, respectively. Most congenital vena caval anomalies represent aberrations in the transition from the cardinal to the vena caval system.

Anomalies of the Superior Vena Cava

For the most part, anomalies of the superior vena cava consist of abnormal sites of entry into the atria.

Left Superior Vena Cava to the Coronary Sinus

By far the most common caval anomaly is drainage of a persistent left superior vena cava to the coronary sinus (persistence of the left common cardinal vein). This anomaly has been reported to occur in 0.3% of autopsies (Geissler and Albert 1956) and in 2.0% to 4.4% of patients with congenital heart disease (Campbell and Deuchar 1954; Frascr ct al. 1961; Cha and Khoury 1972). The incidence in patients undergoing cardiac catheterization in our laboratory is 2.0%.

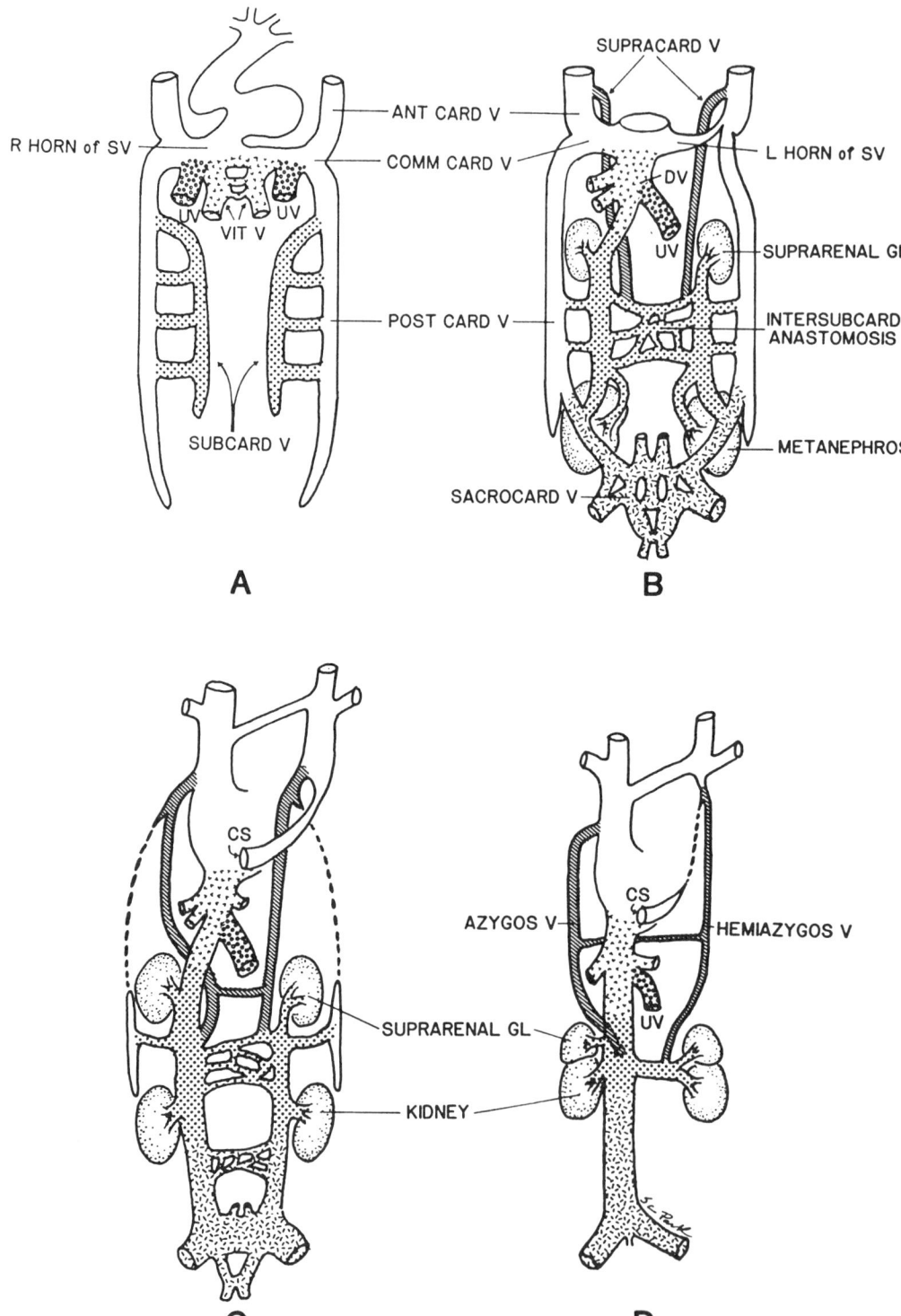

Figure 1. Diagrams of the embryogenesis of systemic venous system from early fetal life (A) to birth (D). Ant = Anterior; Card = Cardinal; Comm = Common; DV = Ductus venous; GL = Gland; L = Left; Post = Posterior; R = Right; SV = Sinus venosus; UV = umbilical vein; Vem Vit V = Viteline vein. (From Fischer, 1987).

The coronary sinus is abnormally large when the left superior vena cava empties into it, and a persistent left cava should be suspected when the coronary sinus is entered inadvertently during right heart catheterization. It is usually possible to advance the catheter from the large coronary sinus to the left superior vena cava itself, the catheter clearing the cardiac shadow as it is advanced cephalad. This anomaly has no intrinsic hemodynamic importance but may pose a problem during cardiopulmonary bypass. In this regard, it is important to know whether or not a left innominate vein is present in any patient with a left superior vena cava to coronary sinus connection who is a candidate for cardiopulmonary bypass. Winter (1954) reported that a connecting innominate vein is present in 60% of individuals with a left superior cava draining to the coronary sinus. The presence of a left innominate vein can be ascertained by probing from the right superior vena cava or by an injection of contrast media into the per-

sistent left superior vena cava at the expected level of an innominate vein (Fig. 2). If there is a well developed left innominate vein, the superior vena cava can be occluded at the time of operation without important consequence. Even without an innominate vein, there may be sufficient collaterals within the head and neck to prevent a serious rise in left superior vena caval pressure with occlusion. In some patients, however, the pressure may rise to dangerous levels. Some surgeons are comfortable with observing the effects of left superior vena cava occlusion during the surgical procedure; others prefer to have the effects of temporary occlusion tested in the catheterization laboratory. This can be done by passing an end-hole balloon catheter into the left superior vena cava via the coronary sinus and then occluding the cava by inflating the balloon. During the occlusion, the caval pressure above the balloon is monitored via the end hole in the catheter. One must be careful to have the balloon caudal to the left

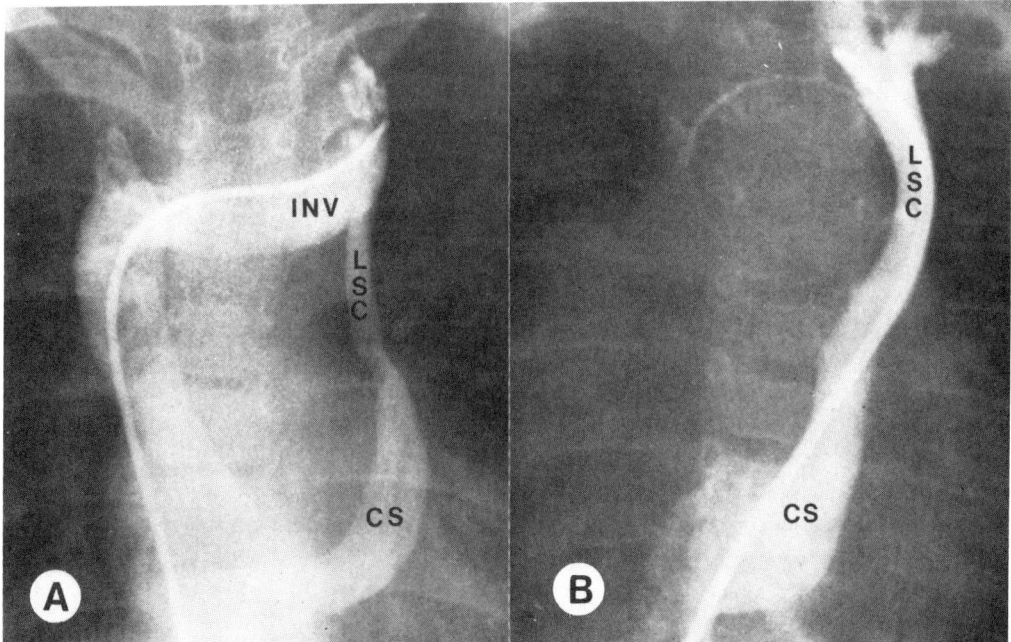

Figure 2. Persistent left superior vena cava (LSC) draining into coronary sinus (CS). A: With innominate vein connection (INV). B: Without innominate vein connection.

innominate vein if one is present. A rise in caval pressure to a level greater than 20 mm Hg is worrisome and should probably lead to a plan to cannulate the left superior vena cava separately during cardiopulmonary bypass.

Left Superior Vena Cava to the Left Atrium

Although a persistent left superior vena cava usually drains to the coronary sinus, it occasionally empties into the left atrium just medial to the left atrial appendage. This anomaly can best be explained by postulat-

ing resorption of the common wall between a persistent left superior vena cava and coronary sinus and the left atrium ("unroofing" of the coronary sinus). In the absence of this common wall, the left superior vena cava enters the left atrium, not the coronary sinus. Additionally, there is always an interatrial communication at the site of the entry of coronary sinus into the right atrium (see Chapter 17). In our laboratory, a left superior cava-left atrial connection has been noted in 0.4% of cardiac catheterizations, or in 18% of children having a persistent left superior vena cava. This is substantially higher than the 8% reported by Lucas and Schmidt (1977). There was atrial isomerism in 12%

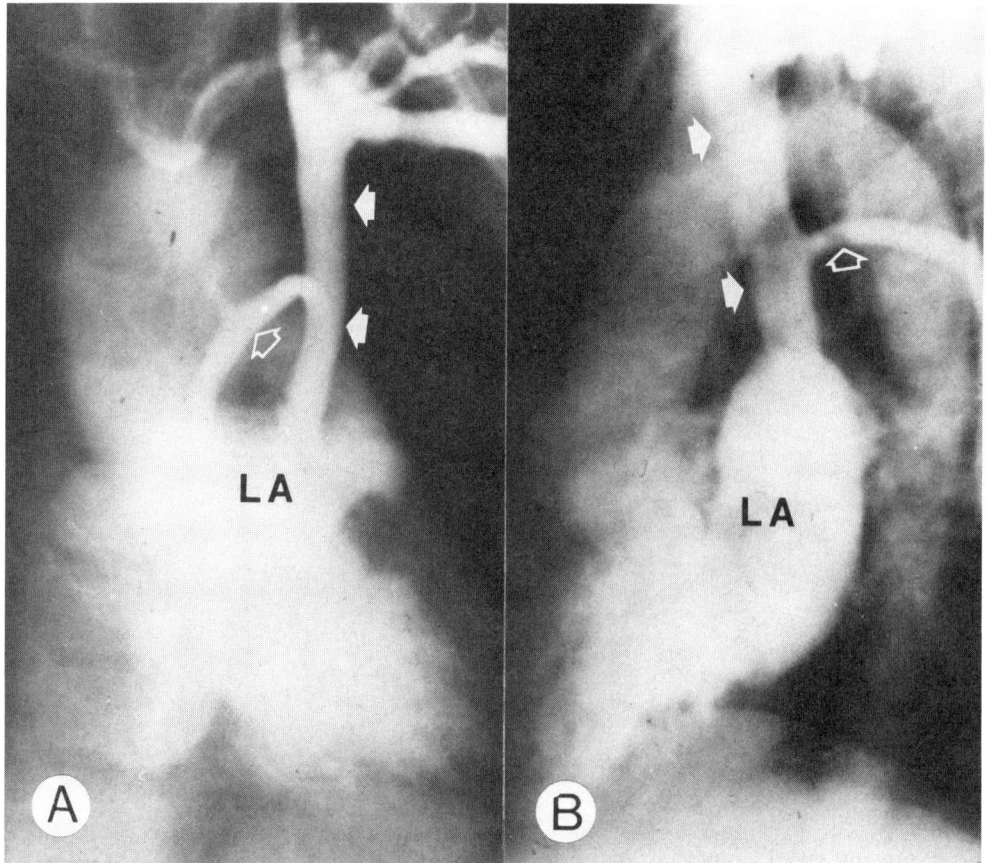

Figure 3. Injection of contrast into a left antecubital vein demonstrating a left superior vena cava (white arrows) draining into the left atrium (LA). There is also reflux seen into the hemiazygos system (open arrows).

of our 30 cases of left superior cava to the left atrium, with equal numbers of the left and right atrial varieties. Drainage of a left superior vena cava to the left atrium has important hemodynamic consequences, because unoxygenated systemic venous blood enters the left atrium. If flow is sufficiently great, cyanosis will be clinically evident. In patients with left superior vena caval drainage to the left atrium, the cava can be entered by probing the left superior portion of the left atrium, the left atrium having been entered via the coronary sinus type interatrial septal defect, or via a patent foramen ovale if one is present.

The drainage may be further defined with an injection of contrast medium into the left cava (Fig. 3). Usually, anteroposterior and lateral projections are adequate. Occasionally, contrast medium streams down into what appears to be an enlarged coronary sinus, and it may be difficult to distinguish direct entry of the cava into the left atrium from drainage to the coronary sinus with "unroofing" of the sinus (see below). It is obviously important to identify drainage of the left cava to the left atrium since the anomaly should be treated surgically at the time of repair of other defects. The status of the left innominate vein should be ascertained carefully, because the simplest surgical repair consists of ligation of the left superior vena cava below the innominate vein. If no innominate is present it is necessary to construct an intra-atrial baffle to direct left superior vena caval blood into the right atrium.

Bilateral Superior Vena Cavae

The incidence of bilateral superior vena cavae draining directly to an atrial chamber is highest in the presence of visceral situs ambiguous and atrial isomerism (44%) (Macartney et al. 1980). This anomaly is diagnosed by injection of contrast medium into both superior vena cavae.

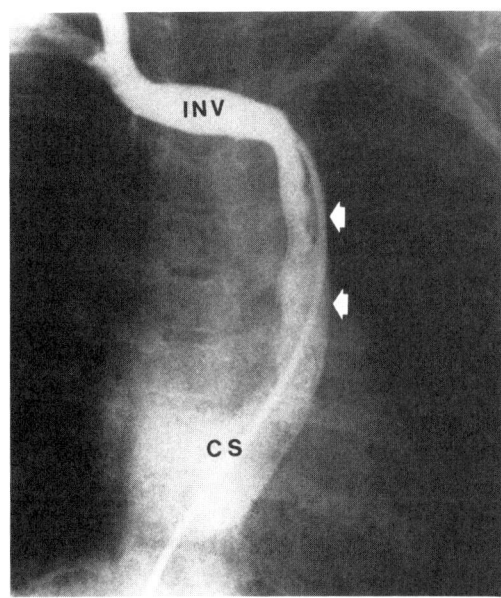

Figure 4. Injection of contrast into the innominate vein (INV) demonstrating absence of the right superior vena cava. The venous drainage is into a left superior vena cava (arrows) that drains to the coronary sinus (CS) and right atrium (RA).

Absent Right Superior Vena Cava

Absence of the right superior vena cava is a rare anomaly, occurring in only 0.1% of our cardiac catheterizations. Interestingly, 4 of our 7 cases have been in patients with discrete subaortic stenosis (Lenox et al. 1980). In this anomaly, the proximal right superior vena cava is absent and drainage of blood from the right arm and head is by way of the innominate vein to a persistent left superior vena cava and there to the coronary sinus (Fig. 4).

Anomalies of the Inferior Vena Cava

Absent Intrahepatic Portion

Azygos Continuation

The most common important anomaly of the inferior vena cava is absence of its intrahepatic portion. Systemic venous drainage of the lower body is by way of the azygos system to the superior vena cava. This malformation is most often part of the complex associated with left atrial isomerism, and occurs in 82% of such patients (Sharma et al. 1987). An azygos or hemiazygos continuation of an interrupted inferior vena cava was present in 0.7% of catheterizations done in our laboratory (Fig. 5A). This anomaly is not hemodynamically important, because drainage is ultimately to the right atrium. It does impose technical difficulty during right heart catheterization from the leg because it is necessary to turn the catheter 180° in passing from the azygos vein to the superior vena cava. Such a passage can usually be accomplished with a standard catheter in an older child but a flow directed balloon catheter is usually preferable in an infant. Completion of the right heart catheterization is also more difficult, because another nearly 180° turn is required to pass from the right atrium to the right ventricle and then into the pulmonary artery.

In an occasional patient there may be dual drainage of the inferior vena cava, both through its normal channel to the right atrium and through an unusually well developed azygos system. These cases are recognized when the venous catheter is passed from the inferior vena cava both into the right atrium directly and into the azygos system.

Hemiazygos Continuation

Rarely, in a patient with absence of the intrahepatic portion of the inferior vena cava, drainage of the lower body is by way of vein derived from the left, not the right

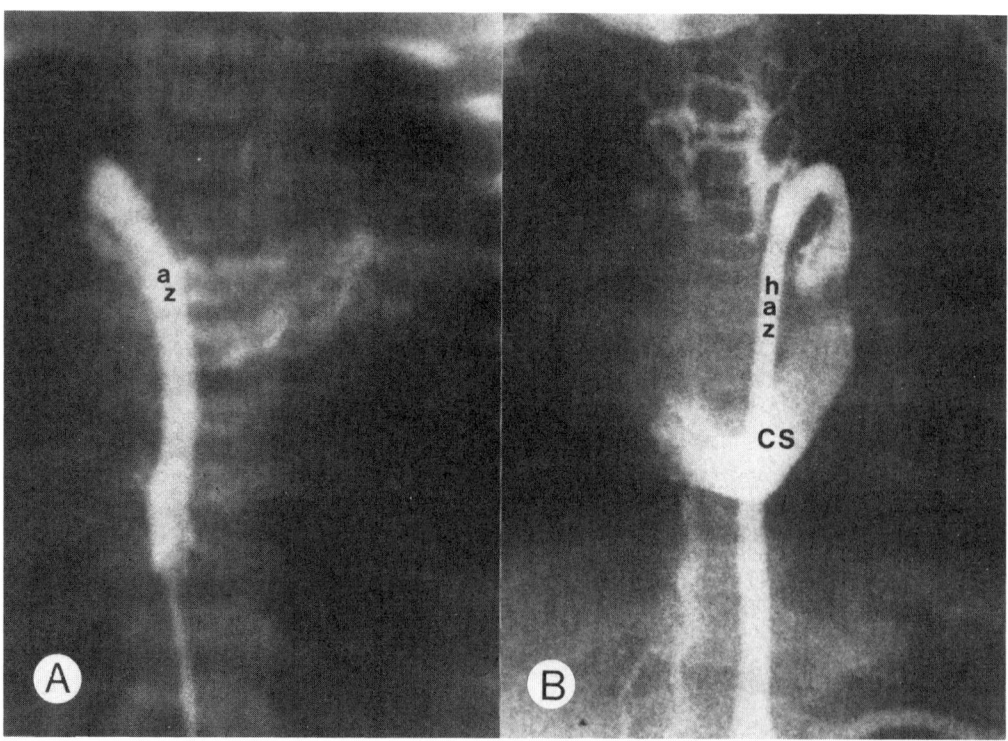

Figure 5. Absence of hepatic segment of the inferior vena cava. A: Draining via the azygos vein (AZ). B: Draining via the hemiazygos vein (HAZ). CS = coronary sinus.

cardinal system (Fig. 5B). The left-sided equivalent of the azygos vein is the hemiazygos, and this vein may serve as the main drainage channel for the lower body, emptying into a persistent left superior vena cava or into a left innominate vein and from there to the right superior vena cava. Drainage may be through a system derived from both right and left cardinal systems; a left-sided hemiazygos crossing the midline at about the level of the diaphragm as the accessory hemiazygos and then emptying into the right superior vena cava.

Inferior Vena Cava to Left Atrium

Inferior vena caval drainage into the left atrium is a rare malformation (Fig. 6). It is usually accompanied by a defect in the in-

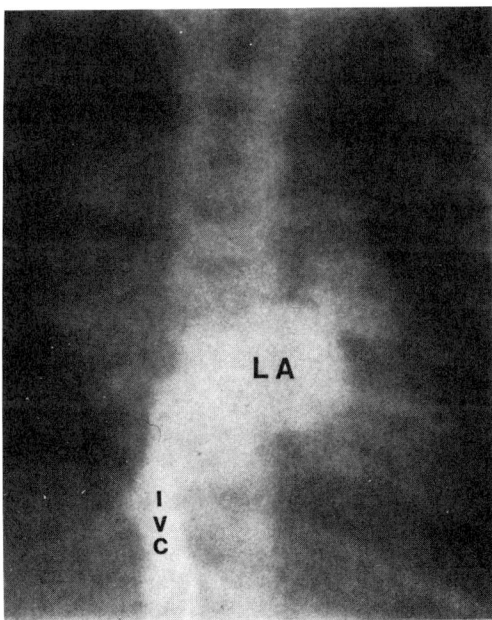

Figure 6. Drainage of the inferior vena cava (IVC) to the left atrium (LA).

teratrial septum immediately adjacent to the entry of the inferior vena cava (inferior sinus venosus defect). Also, there is usually partial anomalous pulmonary venous connection.

References and Suggested Reading

Campbell M, Deuchar DC. The left sided superior vena cava. Br Heart J 1954;16:423–439.

Cha EM, Khoury GH. Persistent left superior vena cava. Radiology 1972;103:375–381.

Fischer DR, Zuberbuhler JR. Anomalous systemic venous return In: Paediataric Cardiology. Anderson RH, Macartney FJ, Shinebourne EA, et al., eds. Edinburgh, Churchill Livingstone. 1987:497–508.

Fraser RS, Dvorkin J, Rossall RE, et al. Left superior vena cava; A review of associated congenital heart lesions, catheterization data and roentgenologic findings. Am J Med 1961;31:711–716.

Geissler W, Albert M. Persistierende linke obere Hohlvene und mitral stenose. Zeitshrift fur die Gesamte inhere Medizin und ihre. Grenzgebiete 1956;11:865–874.

Lenox CC, Zuberbuhler JR, Park SC. Absent right superior vena cava with persistent left superior vena cava: Implications and management. Am J Cardiol 1980;45:117–122.

Lucas RV, Schmidt RE. Anomalous venous connections, pulmonary and systemic. In: Heart Disease in Infants, Children, and Adolescents. Moss AJ, Adams FH, Emmanoulides GC (eds). Second ed. Baltimore, MD. Williams & Wilkins. pp. 437–470.

Macartney FJ, Zuberbuhler JR, Anderson RH. Morphological considerations pertaining to recognition of atrial isomerism. Consequences for sequential chamber localisation. Br Heart J 1980;44:657–667.

Sharma S, Devine W, Anderson RH, et al. Identification and analysis of left atrial isomerism. Am J Cardiol 1987;60:1157–1160.

Winter FS. Persistent left superior vena cava; survey of world literature and report of thirty additional cases. Angiology 5:90–132.

37

Vascular Ring and Pulmonary Sling

Sang C. Park, M.D.

Although the term "vascular ring" properly refers to a complete encirclement of the trachea and esophagus by connected vascular structures, it is often used to describe vascular anomalies that cause compression of the trachea or esophagus, but that do not always form a completely interconnected "ring". The majority of the many vascular anomalies that can occur do not cause significant encroachment on the trachea or the esophagus; only a few varieties lead to clinically significant airway obstruction and even fewer to esophageal obstruction. This chapter will describe the investigation of the patient suspected of having airway obstruction by a vascular structure.

Anatomy and Embryologic Considerations

To understand the genesis of the various aortic arch anomalies, it is important to review the embryologic development of the aortic arch (Stewart et al. 1964; Shuford and Sybers 1974; Park & Zuberbuhler 1987). The aortic arch begins as paired ventral and dorsal aortae (Fig. 1A). The proximal portions of the ventral aortae fuse to form an aortic sac while the distal dorsal aortae fuse to form the descending aorta (Fig. 1B). Six paired brachial arches develop between the ventral and dorsal aortae. Most of the first arch, as well as the second and fifth arches regress (the shaded area in the diagram). The third arch and the dorsal aorta cephalad to the fourth arch become the in-

ternal carotid artery, while the ventral aorta becomes the external carotid artery (Fig. 1C). The fourth arch forms the aortic arch proper and the sixth arch becomes the ductus arteriosus. The seventh dorsal intersegmental arteries migrate in the cephalad direction and become the subclavian arteries (Fig. 1D). Edwards (1953) suggested that there was a primitive double aortic arch, bilateral ductus, and independent common carotid and subclavian arteries on each side in the early embryonic stage. Using this assumption, it then follows that the aortic arch anomalies occur as a result of either regression of a part that normally persists, or patency of a part that normally regresses during embryonic development.

Figure 2 illustrates the possible aortic arch anomalies that occur as a result of regression or interruption at the various sites in the aortic arch. To simplify the sites of the aortic arch that may be involved, the segments are designated numerically as follows; 1 = distal to the ductus; 2 = between the subclavian artery and the ductus; 3 = between the carotid and subclavian arteries; and 4 = proximal to the carotid arteries. The normal left aortic arch is produced by an interruption at position 1 on the right arch indicated as "R-1". When the interruption is on the left side (L-1), a right-sided aortic arch with mirror image branching of the brachiocephalic vessels results. An interruption at position 2 "R-2 or L-2" results in a rather tight vascular ring due to a ductus arteriosus arising from the diverticulum-like remnant from the descending aorta (diverticulum of Kommerell). Only a few cases of

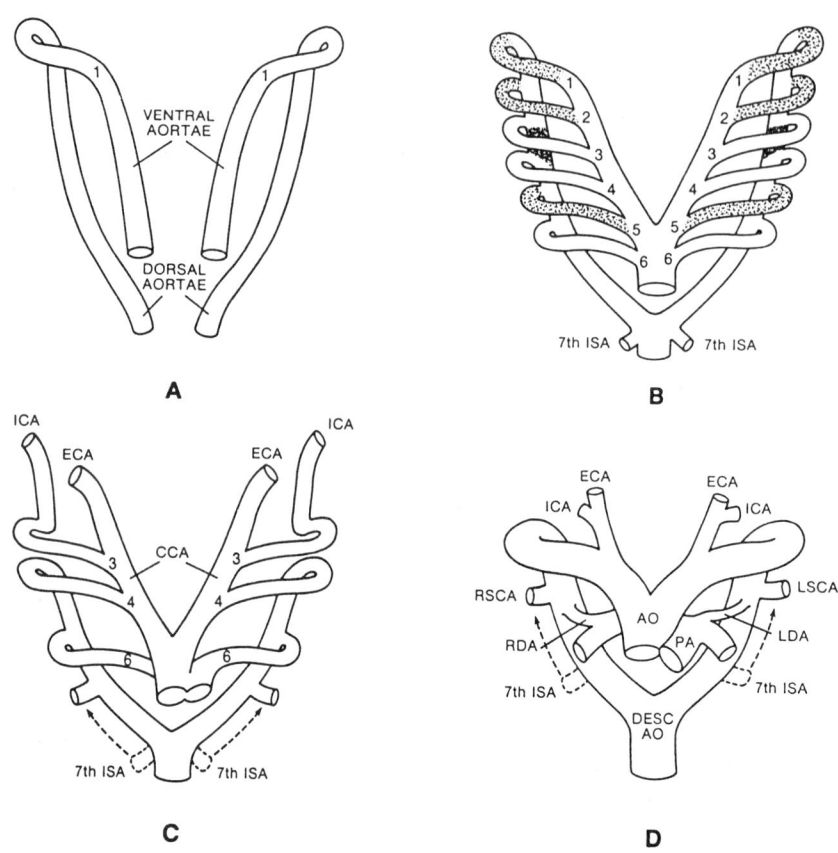

Figure 1. Schematic diagram of the embryonic development of the aortic arch. CCA = Common carotid arteries; ECA = External carotid arteries; ICA = Internal carotid arteries; ISA = Intersegmental arteries; LDA = Left ductus arteriosus; LSCA = Left subclavian arteries; RDA = right ductus arteriosus; RSCA = right subclavian arteries. The shaded area indicates a regression during development. (From Park, 1987).

such involvement in a left arch have been reported previously. Interruption between the subclavian artery and the common carotid artery (position 3), is rather common and results in a right or left aortic arch with anomalous origin of the contralateral subclavian artery (eg left arch and anomalous or distal origin of the right subclavian artery). Generally, this anomaly (L-3a or L-3b) produces no significant airway compromise because it does not result in a ring of contiguous vascular structures. However, when the ductus originates from the diverticulum of Kommerell (as seen in L-3C, R-3B, or R-3C), a complete ring with tighter arrangement of the vessels may result in airway compromise. Finally, interruption of the

arch in the area proximal to common carotid artery (position 4), results in an anomalous retroesophageal innominate artery. Airway compromise is unusual with this anomaly. When there is no interruption of the arch, a double aortic arch is formed (Fig. 2).

Diagnostic Considerations and Indications for Cardiac Catheterization

Although there are many other causes of chronic airway obstruction in infants and children, the possibility of a vascular anomaly should be considered in any patient with

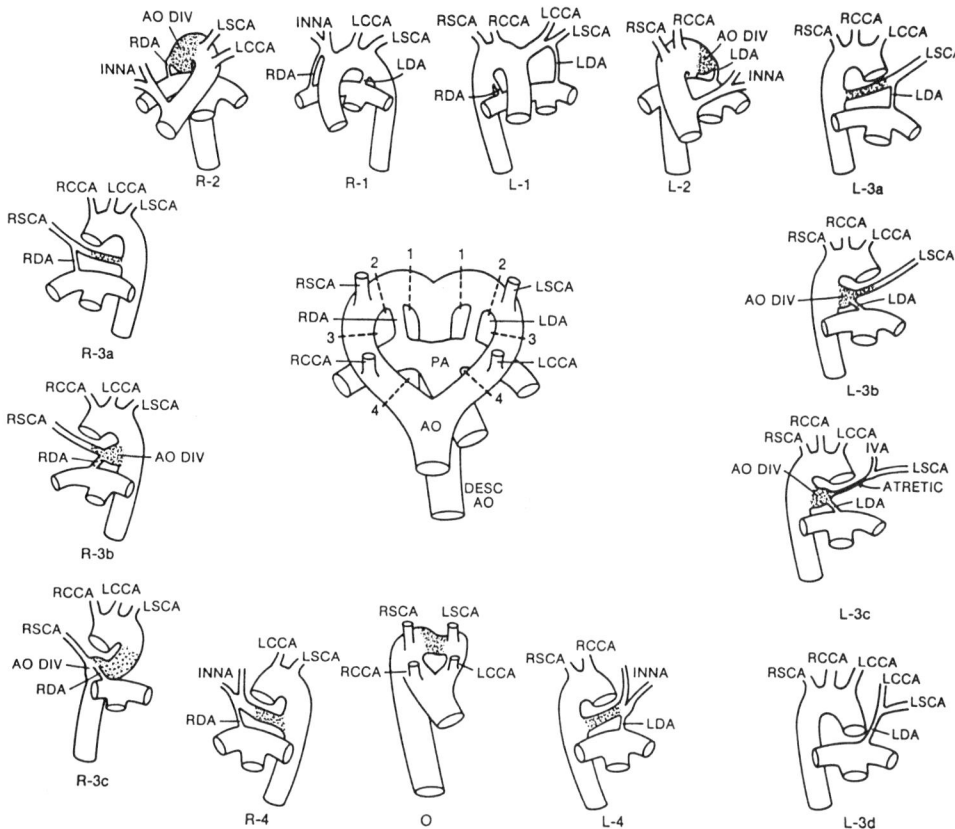

Figure 2. Diagrams of possible aortic arch anomalies depending upon the site of interruption (dotted lines) in the primitive double arch seen in the center. The code under each figure indicates the side of the aortic arch (L = left, R = right) and the site of the interruption. The shaded area indicates the retroesophageal component (see text). AO = aorta; Desc = descending; Div = diverticulum; INNA = innominate artery; LCCA = left common carotid artery; LDA = left ductus arteriosus; LSCA = left subclavian artery; RCCA = right common carotid artery; RDA = right ductus arteriosus; RSCA = right subclavian artery; VA = vetebral artery. (From Park, 1987).

symptoms or signs of airway compromise. On review of the causes of airway obstruction in the pediatric age group, vascular origin was found in approximately 5% (Kahn et al. 1977). It is quite important to consider a vascular abnormality in the differential diagnosis of airway disease, because a potentially correctable condition might otherwise be overlooked. It is not unusual for a patient with a vascular ring to be misdiagnosed initially as having an allergic problem or chronic respiratory tract infection.

The most valuable noninvasive study is a four-view cardiac series with barium in the esophagus (barium esophagram). It provides information as to the size of the aortic arch and to the presence of retroesophageal vascular components. A barium swallow with fluoroscopy may provide additional information in certain cases, such as tracheoesophageal fistula, particularly when dysphagia or aspiration coexist with evidence of airway obstruction. As shown in Table 1, the barium filled esophagus and tracheal air shadow on various views of chest roentgenogram often provide valuable clues to the presence of various vascular abnormalities. Bronchoscopy also may contribute useful

Table 1

Possible Vascular Abnormality Based on the Barium Esophagram

Vascular anomalies	Compression or indentation	
	Esophagus	Trachea
Pulmonary (vascular)sling—(distal origin of the left pulmonary artery) Ductus arteriosus sling (Anomalous duct between the right pulmonary artery and the left descending aorta)	Anterior	Posterior

Double aortic arch
  Both arches patent
  One arch atretic
 Right aortic arch with left ductus arteriosus
	Posterior	Anterior

Aberrant subclavian artery with ipsilateral ductus arteriosus Aberrant innominate artery Left aortic arch with right descending aorta	Posterior	None
Trachea compression by innominate artery or brachiocephalic trunk	None	Anterior

information, although it should be recognized that bronchoscopic findings in a child with a suspected vascular ring may be equivocal or even misleading. Differentiating normal vascular pulsation from the pulsation of an anomalous artery is not always easy and a decision for surgical intervention cannot be always made reliably on bronchoscopic findings alone. It should be noted that a vascular ring can be an incidental finding without clinical symptoms. Therefore, invasive diagnostic studies in patients with asymptomatic vascular anomalies are not warranted.

In recent years, with increased experience with cross-sectional echocardiography, the status of the aortic arch and brachiocephalic vessels can be investigated by the suprasternal approach. In fact, some patients with double aortic arch were diagnosed by echocardiography alone and corrective surgery has been performed without further angiographic confirmation. Similarly, magnetic resonance imaging techniques also can be used for the evaluation of aortic arch abnormalities. However, this

noninvasive diagnostic method has some limitations in defining complex vascular abnormalities. Cardiac catheterization with aortography and selective angiography of the brachiocephalic arteries remains the best way precisely to define the anatomy of the aorta and its branches. A pulmonary arteriogram is essential to diagnose a pulmonary vascular sling (distal origin of the left pulmonary artery) (Lenox et al. 1979).

Another cause of symptomatic airway compromise in the pediatric age group is related to anterior tracheal compression by an innominate artery which abnormally originates somewhat distally and posteriorly from the aortic arch as shown in Figure 3. Although skepticism as to the existence of this condition persists, we have seen dramatic improvement in respiratory symptoms following innominate artery suspension surgery in a number of patients as has been reported by others (Fearon 1963; Ardito 1980). This lesion is demonstrated on the lateral view of the chest roentgenogram by an anterior indentation of the trachea.

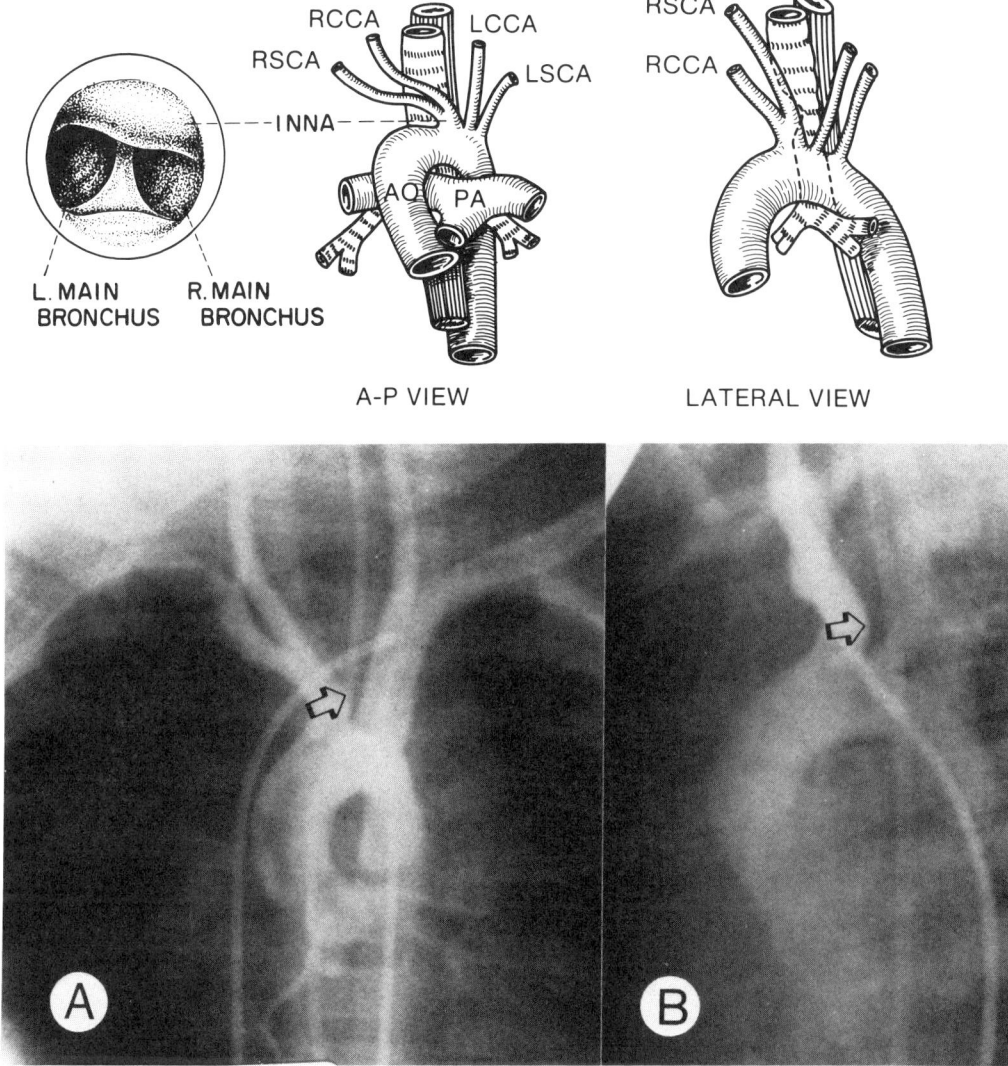

Figure 3. Innominate artery compression of the trachea Top: Diagram illustrating the anomaly in the anteroposterior (AP) and lateral views (see Figure 2 for abbreviations). In the circle, the bronchoscopic finding of an oblique pulsatile compression is evident anteriorly. Bottom: (A) Anterior-posterior view of an aortogram demonstrating distal origin of the innominate artery just past the midline (arrow). (B) Selective angiogram in the innominate artery in the left anterior oblique view demonstrating posterior bowing (arrow) that causes compression of the trachea. (Modified from Park, 1987).

The barium esophagram is usually normal without an abnormal indentation. Angiography is helpful at times to delineate the distal takeoff of the innominate artery which arises to the left of the mid line. However, this finding alone does not confirm this di-

agnosis since normal individuals also may have such distal origins of the vessel from the midline. Bronchoscopy is the ideal diagnostic tool for this condition and demonstrates an oblique anterior pulsatile compression of the trachea, extending from lcft inferior to right superior, about 1 to 2 cm above the carina (Fig. 3). Angiographic study usually is recommended only when associated lesions are suspected.

Cardiac Catheterization Technique

Premedication is carried out in the usual manner for cardiac catheterization. However, in patients with significant airway compromise a smaller dose of morphine or meperidine is recommended to minimize the chance of respiratory depression. Prior to cardiac catheterization, a small radiopaque tube, such as a premature infant feeding tube, can be inserted through the nostril, down the esophagus and into the stomach to mark the location of the esophagus. Although most vascular anomalies involve the aorta and its branches, the femoral vein approach is usually used initially, since left ventricular angiography can be performed through an interatrial communication in some infants. Older children and infants with an intact atrial septum usually require retrograde arterial catheterization for selective aortography.

Measurement of pressures and oxygen saturations from various sites of the cardiovascular system are usually performed to rule out associated intracardiac anomalies. Arterial PO_2 and PCO_2 should be determined if the ventilatory status of the patient is in question.

The course of the catheter in the right heart is not unusual except in the presence of a pulmonary vascular sling. With this anomaly, it is not possible to pass the catheter into the left pulmonary artery from the main pulmonary artery. The presence of a right aortic arch is obvious during a retrograde study. If the barium swallow is suggestive of a double aortic arch, an attempt should be made to enter both right and left distal arches individually by angling the catheter both to the right and the left as it is advanced from the descending aorta. If the catheter passes around the arch first to one side of the trachea and then to the other, the presence of a double aortic arch can be established.

Pressure Data

Pressure data in patients with a vascular anomaly are normal unless there is an associated cardiac lesion or unless there is severe airway obstruction.

Patients with severe obstruction may have a mild to moderate degree of pulmonary hypertension secondary to hypoxia, and show marked respiratory variation in both systemic and pulmonary pressure, with a pronounced negative dip during the inspiratory phase. This phenomenon is usually more pronounced in the right side of the heart than the left side, and it can be minimized by hyperextension of the neck, which may reduce airway compromise.

Oxygen Saturation Data

Systemic oxygen saturation is generally within normal limits despite an obstructive airway component. However, if there is an associated pulmonary disorder such as aspiration pneumonia or intracardiac right to left shunting, desaturation in systemic arterial blood may be observed.

Angiocardiography

Selective aortography or left ventriculography are the preferred initial angiographic studies. If aortography is done, the injection of the contrast material should be in the aortic root so that the entire aortic arch system can be visualized. The sequence of origin of the brachiocephalic vessels are obviously of considerable importance. Generally, simultaneous anteroposterior and lateral views are obtained first, followed, if necessary, by oblique or cranio-caudal (sitting-up) views. When a double aortic arch is suspected, adequate visualization of each arch must be attempted. At times, a selective angiogram in each arch may be required to determine the size and patency of each arch accurately (Fig. 4). According to a review of several series of double arch cases (Klinkhamer et al. 1969), the right arch was dominant in 73% while a dominant left arch was found in 18%. However, in 9% of the cases, both arches were of equal size. A selective injection of contrast using an end-hole catheter is important to confirm the presence of an atretic segment (Fig. 5). Atresia of one arch occurs in 17% of patients with double aortic arch; 77% occurring distal to the left subclavian and 23% between the left subclavian and the left carotid arteries (Klinkhamer 1969). Occasionally there is severe stenosis rather than atresia (Fig. 6). Rarely, one arch only may be probe patent (Fig. 7). An atretic arch consists of a fibrous cord and is not visualized angiographically. However, it can be contiguous with other surrounding vessels resulting in a clinically significant vascular ring.

Patients with a small retroesophageal

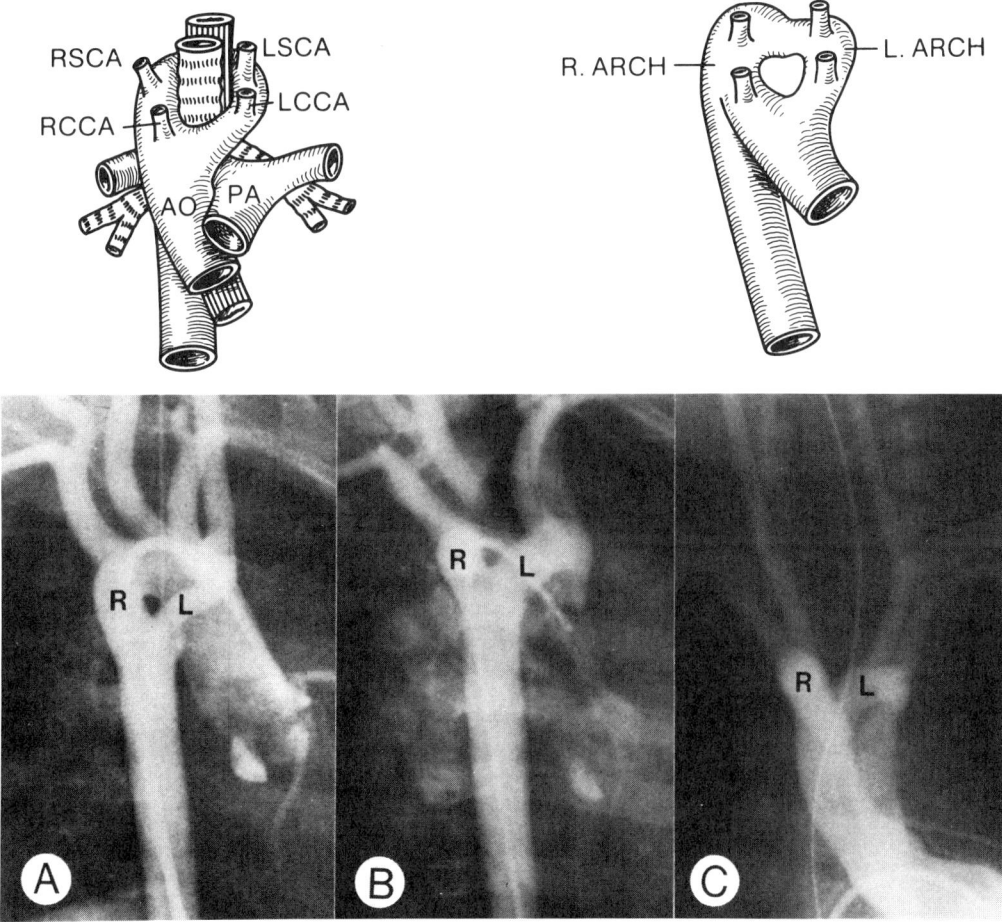

Figure 4. Double aortic arch. Top: Diagram illustrating the anomaly (see Figures 1 and 2 for abbreviations). (A) Dominant right arch. (B) Dominant left arch. (C) Equal size arches. (Modifed from Park, 1987).

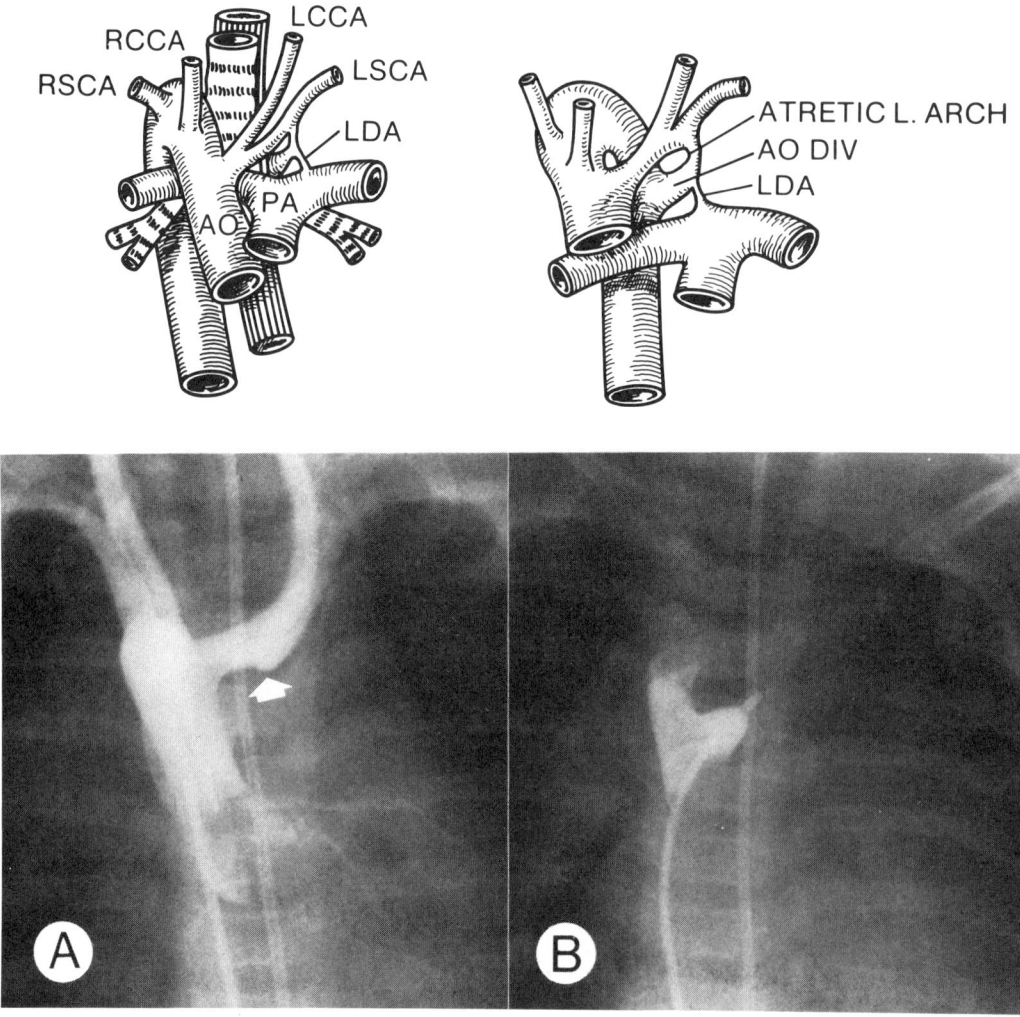

Figure 5. Double aortic arch with one arch atretic. Top: Diagram illustrating the anatomy (see Figures 1 and 2 for abbreviations). Bottom: (A) Aortogram in anteroposterior view shows an apparently usual right aortic arch. However, there is tenting of the proximal portion of the left subclavian artery (arrow) suggesting the presence of an atretic left arch. (B) Selective injection of contrast in the descending aorta demonstrating a blind pouch. (Modified from Park, 1987).

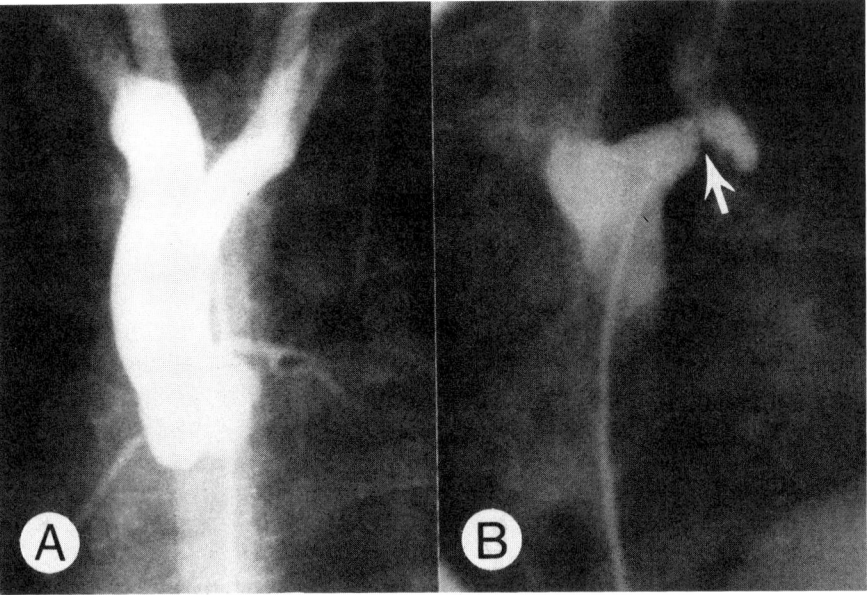

Figure 6. Double aortic arch with one arch stenotic. A: Aortogram in the anteroposterior view demonstrating what appears to be a double aortic arch with both arches equally patent. B: Selective injection in the left arch in the left anterior oblique view demonstrating severe stenosis (arrow).

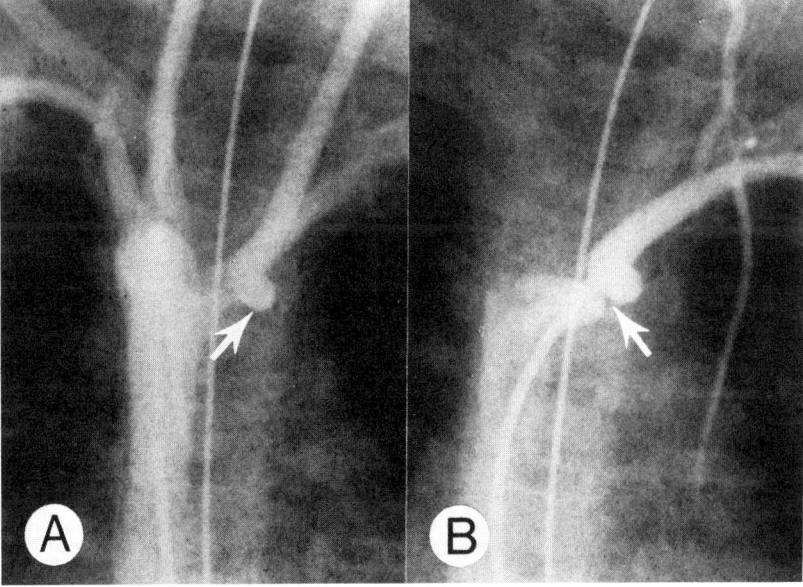

Figure 7. Double aortic arch with a probe patent left segment. A: Aortogram demonstrating what appears to be a double arch with an atretic left segment(arrow) as seen in Figure 5. B: Selective injection in the left arch segment demonstrating that it is probe patent(arrow) but not atretic.

indentation on barium esophagram usually have an aberrant subclavian artery. This occurs with either a left or right aortic arch. An aberrant right subclavian artery may occur as an isolated anomaly or in association with other congenital heart disease such as coarctation of the aorta or interrupted arch. Aberrant left subclavian artery, which is found with a right aortic arch, often is associated with more complex congenital heart disease such as tetralogy of Fallot, truncus arteriosus and transposition of the great arteries (Fig. 8). However, some patients may have a large indentation of the esophagus in association with an aberrant subclavian artery. This usually is due to the presence of a remnant of the distal arch (diverticulum of Kommerell) seen in Figure 9. A vascular ring caused by a ductus arterious or ligamentous cord arising from the diverticulum should always be considered, particularly when there are airway symptoms.

Other patients with a large retroesophageal indentation on barium esophagram

require careful arch study with special spatial orientation. In addition to the already described double aortic arch, a few arch anomalies produce such a large indentation. A left aortic arch with a right descending aorta, or a right aortic arch with a left descending aorta, causes a large retroesophageal indentation (Fig. 10). However, these anomalies usually do not result in airway compromise since they to not form a contiguous vascular ring. On the other hand, when an aberrant subclavian artery also is associated, significant right bronchial compression may result due to a tight ligamentous duct originating from the diverticular structure (Kommerell) of the right descending aorta (Park et al. 1976) (Fig. 11). Lastly, an aberrant innominate artery also causes a large retroesophageal indentation but airway compromise is unusual with this condition because it does not form a vascular ring (Fig. 12).

If an anterior indentation of the esophagus is present on a barium swallow, the

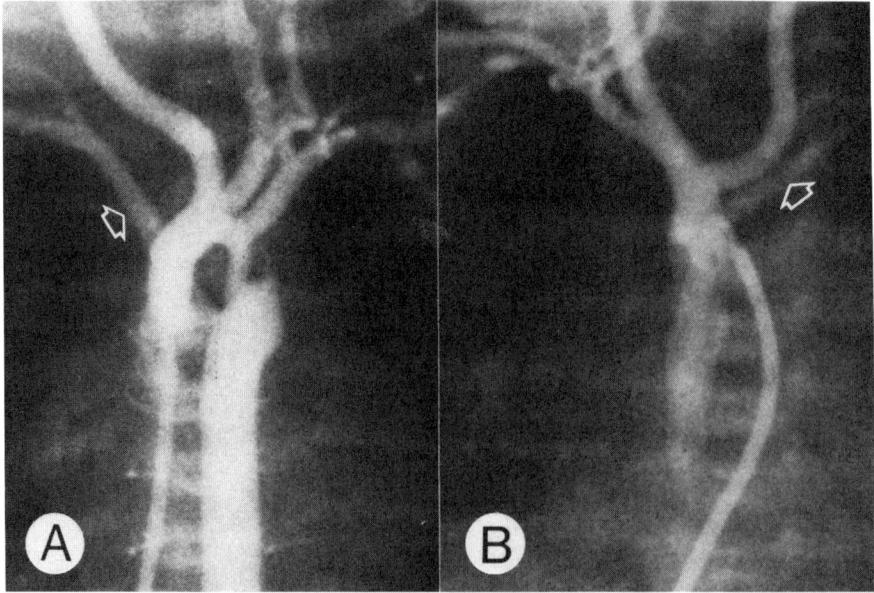

Figure 8. Angiographic findings of aberrant subclavian artery in the anteroposterior view. A: Aberrant right subclavian artery (arrow) in association with coarctation of the aorta. B: Aberrant left subclavian artery (arrow) in association with right aortic arch and ventricular septal defect.

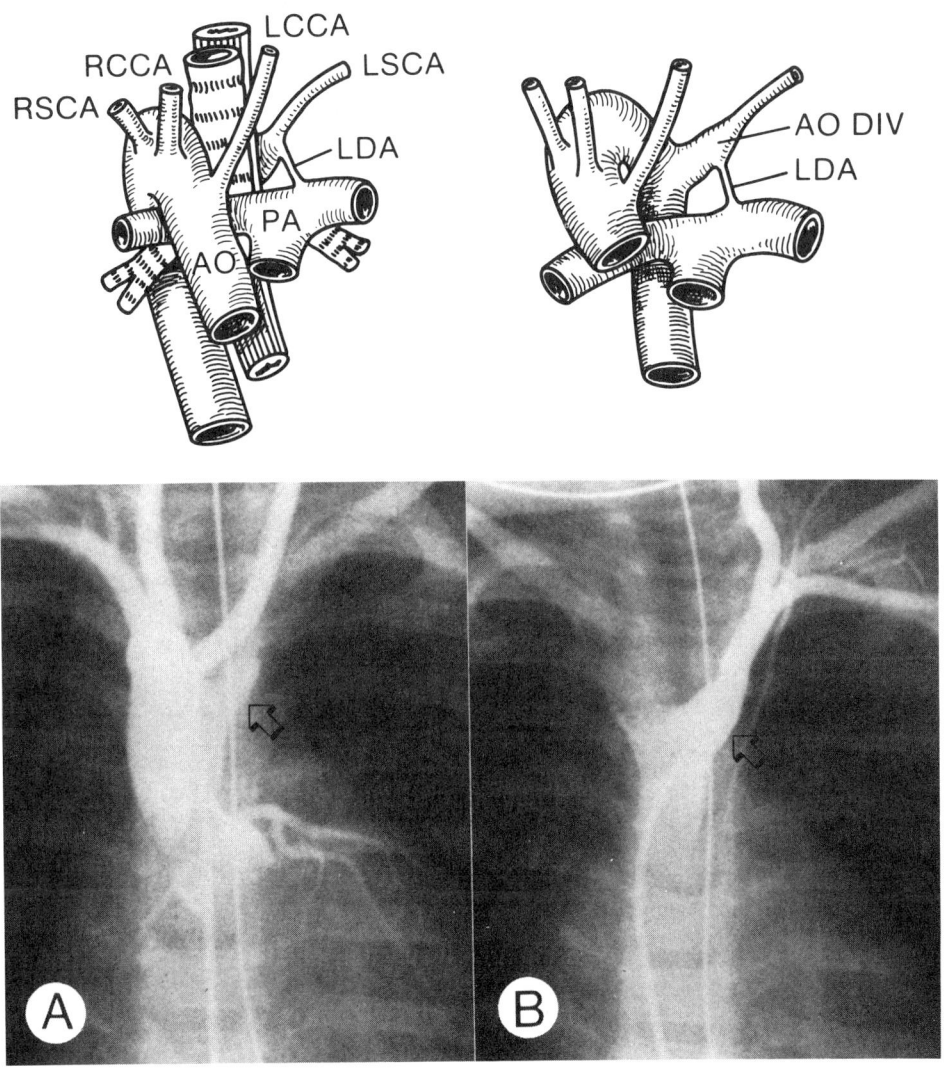

Figure 9. Right aortic arch with an aberrant left subclavian artery originating from a diverticular structure (diverticulum of Kommerell) (arrow). A: Diagramatic illustration (see Figures 1 and 2 for abbreviations). B: Angiographic view. (From Park, 1987).

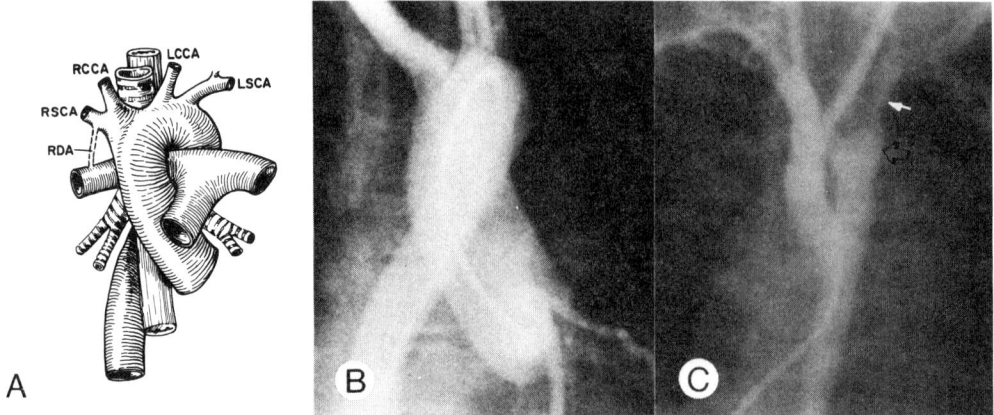

Figure 10. Ascending aorta with a contralateral descending aorta. A: Diagram of a left aortic arch with a right descending aorta. B: Angiograms of a left aortic arch with a right descending aorta. C: Angiogram of a right aortic arch with a left descending aorta. The left subclavian anatomy (white arrow) arises from a diverticulum of Kommerell (open arrow). (From Park, 1987).

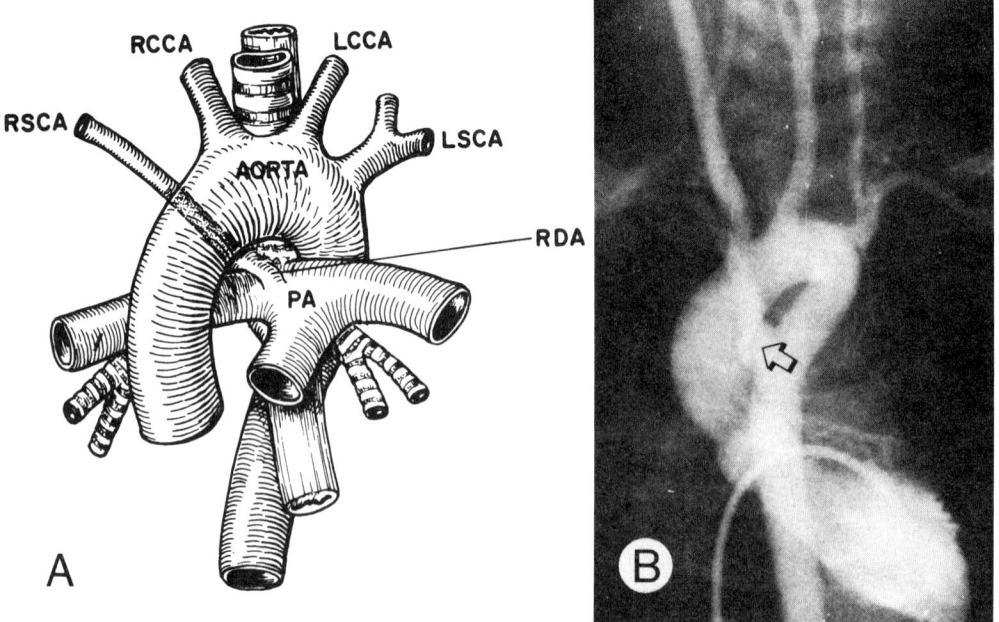

Figure 11. Left aortic arch with an aberrant right subclavian artery originating from the diverticulum of Kommerell on descending aorta. A: Diagrammatic illustration (see Figures 1 and 2 for abbreviations). B: Selection left ventriculogram demonstrating the lesion and diverticular structure (arrow) from the descending aorta. (From Park, 1987).

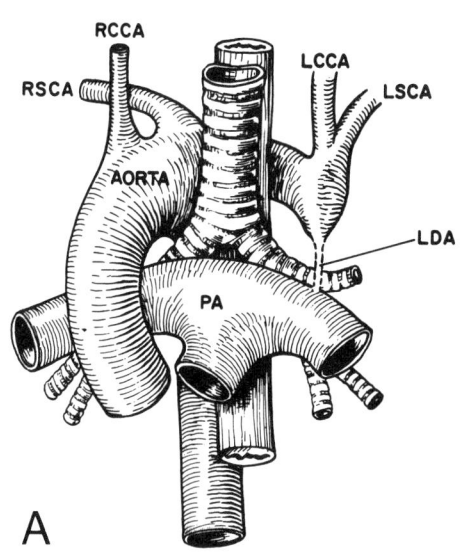

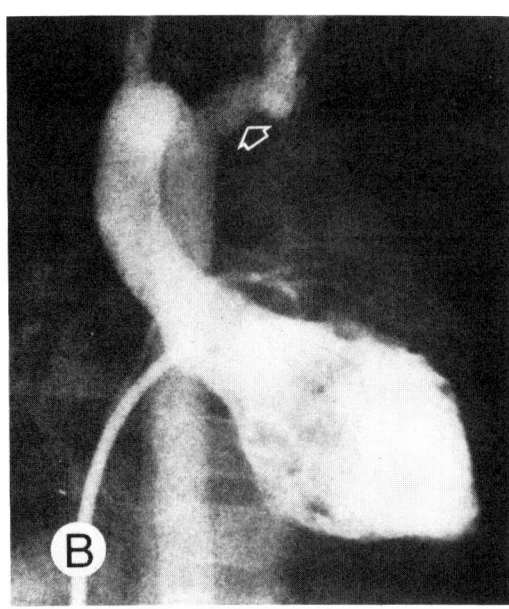

Figure 12. Aberrant innominate artery. A: Diagramatic illustration of the anomaly (see Figures 1 and 2 for abbreviations). B: Selective left ventriculogram in the anteroposterior view demonstrating the aberrant innominate artery (arrow). (From Park, 1987).

possibility of a pulmonary vascular sling (distal origin of the left pulmonary artery) or a rare condition, a ductus arteriosus sling, should be considered. In this latter situation, an anomalous duct between the right pulmonary artery and the left descending aorta causes tracheobronchial compression (Binet et al. 1978). An anteroposterior view with maximum cranio-caudal angulation (sitting-up view) is best to demonstrate the origin of the right and left pulmonary arteries. With a pulmonary vascular sling, the left pulmonary artery originates from the right pulmonary artery to the right of the trachea, then turns sharply posteriorly and to the left to enter the left to enter the left hilus (Fig. 13). Patients with evidence of unilateral pulmonary abnormalities such as hyperinflation or atelectasis should have a pulmonary arteriogram to rule out this vascular abnormality.

The following important information should be observed during review of angiographic studies:

1. The side of the ascending aorta and descending aorta. For example, right aortic arch, left aortic arch with right descending aorta, etc. The side of the ascending aorta is contralateral to the side of the first carotid artery branch from the aortic root. Thus, if the first carotid artery is on the left (left-sided innominate artery or a left carotid with distal origin of a retroesophageal right subclavian artery), the aortic arch is on the right. The exception to this is a double aortic arch or when there is an aberrant innominate artery (distal origin of the innominate from the descending aorta). The side of the descending aorta is based upon its relationship to the midline of the spinal column.

2. Single versus double aortic arch. If a double arch is present, the dominant arch should be identi-

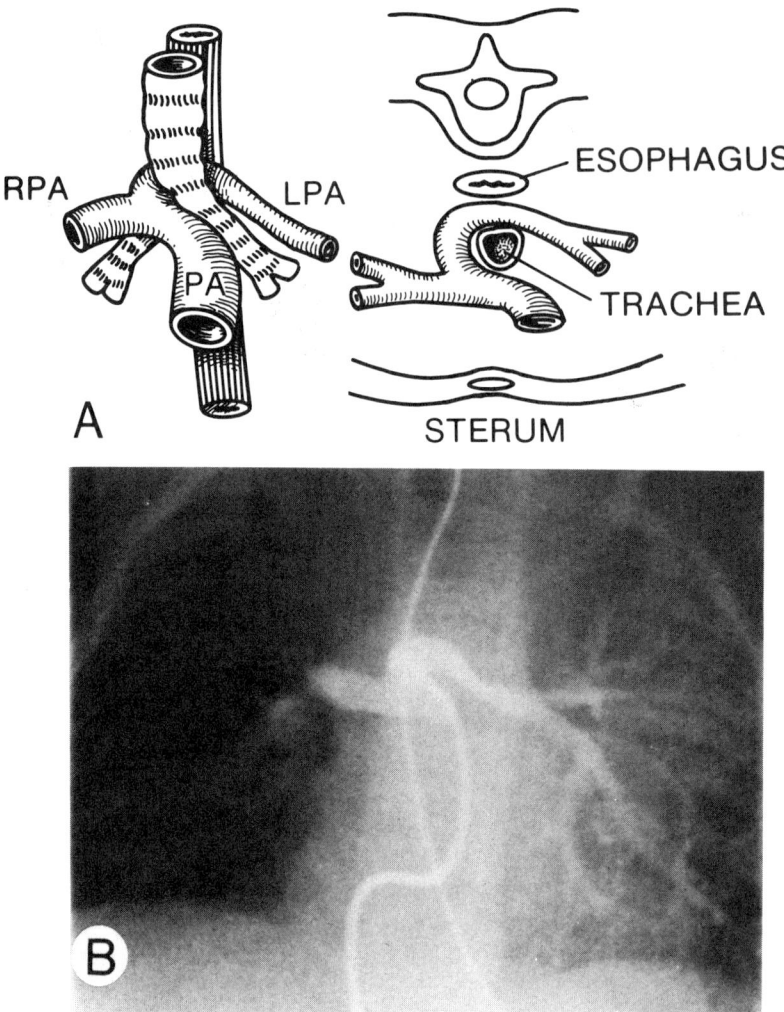

Figure 13. Pulmonary vascular sling (distal origin of the left pulmonary artery). A: Diagramatic illustrations of the anomaly demonstrating the left pulmonary artery (LPA) originating from the right pulmonary artery (RPA). It courses between the trachea and esophagus. B: Selective pulmonary angiogram in the sitting up view demonstrating the anomaly. (From Park, 1987).

fied. The possibility of unilateral arch atresia should be considered when double arch features are present without bilateral patency.

3. Common origin of the innominate arteries and the left common carotic artery may be present. Also, a separate origin of the vertebral artery directly from the aortic arch may coexist. Thus, the origin of each brachiocephalic vessel should be visualized sufficiently in the cephalad direction to determine the anatomic arrangement.

4. The sequence of the origin of the brachiocephalic arteries from the aortic root. Normally, the innominate, carotid and subclavian arteries originate in order. An abnormal sequence should be carefully observed.

5. Unusual angulation of the innominate or subclavian arteries should be observed. Tenting of an artery may indicate the site of an atretic vessel, or a ligamentous duct which may be part of a vascular ring (Fig. 14).

6. When a subclavian artery is not visualized in the early phase of an aortogram, the possibility of a subclavian steal syndrome should be suspected (Fig. 2, L-3C). The late phase of the angiogram should be observed carefully to document retrograde filling of the vessel via the vertebral artery (Fig. 15).

7. Unusual dilation of the proximal portion of a retroesophageal subclavian artery may indicate the presence of diverticulum of Kommerell. When the diverticulum alone is seen, the proximal portion of the subclavian artery may be atretic as is seen in Figure 2 (L-3C).

8. The spatial relationship between airway (trachea or bronchus) and the surrounding blood vessels should be carefully studied.

Cautions and Precautions

The angiographic findings are usually diagnostic for most vascular abnormalities. However, a ligamentous duct or an atretic segment of an aortic arch is not demonstrable angiographically. If a ring is suspected but cannot be visualized directly, a careful search for distortion, such as the abovementioned tenting of the innominate or subclavian artery, should be undertaken. If found, the presence of an atretic cord should be considered. Careful correlation between angiography and clinical findings is always very important. Despite severe airway compromise in association with various vascular abnormalities, the patient may have minimal respiratory symptoms during rest, particularly when asleep. Thus, the severity of the airway obstruction should not be underes-

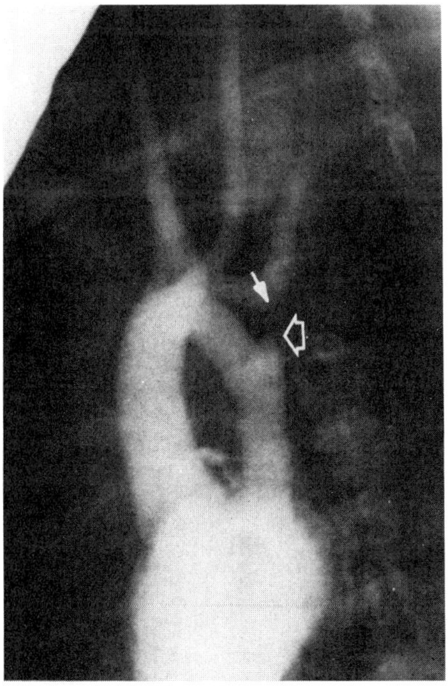

Figure 14. Left ventricular angiogram in the left anterior oblique view in a patient with a double aortic arch and an atretic left arch. Note the tenting of the subclavian artery (arrow) and of the diverticulum (open arrow) indicating the presence of an atretic segment connecting the two structures.

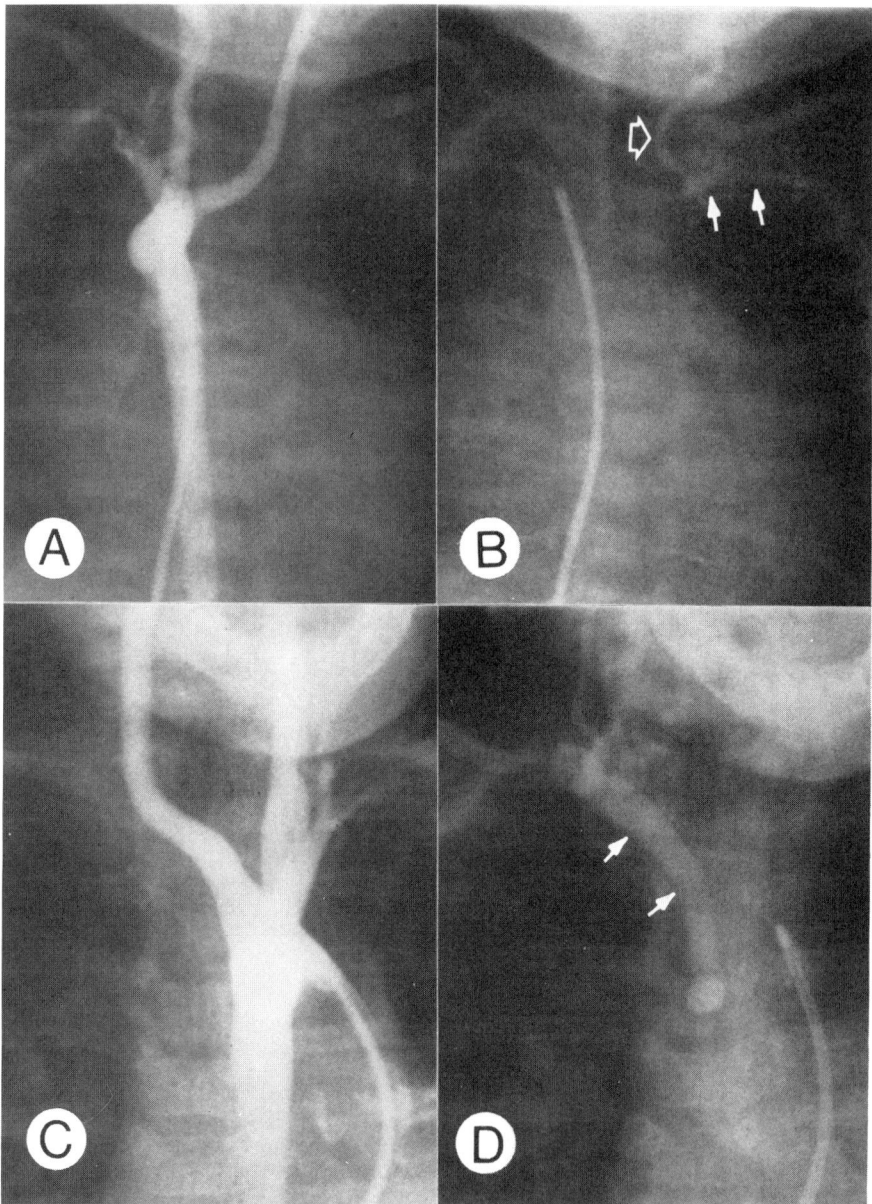

Figure 15. Subclavian steal syndrome. Top: Selective aortogram in a patient with a right aortic arch (anteroposterior views). A: The left subclavian artery is not visualized. B: Late phase demonstrating the left subclavian artery (solid arrows) filling by retrograde flow from the left vertebral artery (open arrow). Bottom: Selective aortogram in a patient with a left aortic arch and transposition of the great arteries (anteroposterior view). C: The right subclavian artery is not visualized. D: Late phase demonstrating filling of the right subclavian artery by retrograde flow from the vertebral artery and other collateral vessels. Note a large right-sided patent ductus arteriosus (arrows) arising from the right subclavian artery.

timated by such temporary observation. The best observer is the mother.

References and Suggested Reading

Ardito JM, Ossoff RH, Tucker GF, et al. Innominate artery compression of the trachea in infants with reflex apnea. Ann Otology, Rhino Laryngol 1980;89:401–405.

Binet JP, Conso JF, Losay J, et al. Ductus arteriosus sling: Report of a newly recognised anomaly and its surgical correction. Thorax 1978;33:72–75.

Edwards JE. Malformations of the aortic arch system manifested as 'vascular rings'. Lab Invest 1953;2:56–75.

Fearon B, Shortreed R. Tracheobronchial compression by congenital cardiovascular anomalies in children: Syndrome of apnea. Ann Otology, Rhino, Laryngol 1963;72:949–969.

Kahn A, Baron D, Spehl M, et al. Congenital Stridor in infancy. Clinical lesions derived from a survey of 31 instances. Clin Pediatr 1977;16:19–26.

Klinkhamer AC. Esopghagography in Anomalies of the Aortic Arch System. Baltimore, MD. Williams & Wilkins. 1969:16–30, 64–65.

Lenox CC, Crisler C, Zuberbuhler JR, et al. Anomalous left pulmonary artery. J Thorac Cardiovasc Surg 1979;77:748–752.

Park SC, Siewers RD, Neches WH. Left aortic arch with right descending aorta and right ligamentum arteriosum. J Thorac Cardiovasc Surg 1976;71:779–784.

Park SC, Zuberbuhler JR. Vascular ring and pulmonary sling. In: Paediatric Cardiology. Anderson RH, Macartney FJ, Shinebourne EA, et al., eds. Chapter 46, Edinburgh. Churchill Livingstone. 1987:1123–1136.

Shuford WH, Sybers RG. The Aortic Arch and its Malformations. Springfield, MA. Charles C. Thomas. 1974:4–9, 51.

Stewart JR, Kincaid OW, Edwards JE. An Atlas of Vascular Rings and Related Malformations of the Aortic Arch System. Springfield., MA. Charles C. Thomas, 1964:8–13, 124, 219.

Index

Absent pulmonary valve syndrome, 293–294
Acid-base equilibrium in newborn, 7
Acidosis, metabolic
  coarctation of aorta and, 395
  transposition of great arteries and, 313
Adolescent, cardiac catheterization and, 3–4
Adriamycin toxicity, 176
Airway, vascular obstruction of. *See* Vascular
  obstruction of airway
Alcohol in endomyocardial biopsy, 178
Allagille syndrome, 274
Amplifier in electrophysiology, 124
Anesthesia
  cutdown technique and, 37, 40
  percutaneous technique and, 27, 33–34
Aneurysm, ventricular septal defect and,
  234–235, 237
Angiocardiography, 101–119. *See also*
  Angiography
  of aberrant subclavian artery, 428, 429, 430,
  431
  in anomalous pulmonary venous return,
  404–405, 408
  in aortic arch anomaly, 425, 426, 427
  in aortic valve atresia, 385
  in aortic valve stenosis, 381–382
  in aortopulmonary window, 258–259
  in atrial septal defect, 223–225
  in atrioventricular septal defect, 245–248
  in coarctation of aorta, 166, 394, 397
  complications of, 115–119
  contrast media and, 102
  in double inlet ventricle, 362–363
  in double outlet right ventricle, 305–306
  in Ebstein's anomaly, 339–341
  in mitral atresia, 355–356
  in patent ductus arteriosus, 253–255
  power injectors and, 103
  projections for, 104–115. *See also* Projections
  in pulmonary valve stenosis, 271–272
  radiographic equipment in, 101–102
  selection of catheters for, 20–22, 103, 166

in tetralogy of Fallot with pulmonary atresia,
  295–298
in transposition of great arteries, 319–324
in tricuspid atresia, 350–351
in truncus arteriosus, 263–265
in vascular obstruction of airway, 424–433
in ventricular septal defect, 232–235
Angiography. *See also* Angiocardiography
  biplane equipment for, 11
  catheter for, 103
  in coarctation of aorta, 166
  in corrected transposition of great arteries,
  330–332
  in cor triatriatum, 372
  in mitral valve stenosis, 372–373
  in pulmonary valve atresia with intact
  ventricular septum, 280–283
  pulmonary vein, in atrioventricular septal
  defect, 246, 248
  in pulmonary vein atresia, 371
  in pulmonary vein stenosis, 371–372
  in tetralogy of Fallot, 288–293
  transseptal catheterization and, 172
  in ventricular septal defect, 229, 234
Angioplasty, balloon. *See* Balloon angioplasty
Anomalous pulmonary venous return, 399–410
  anatomy of, 399, 406–407
  angiocardiography in, 404–405, 408
  associated lesions in, 405–406, 408–410
  catheterization indications in, 401–402, 407
  catheterization technique for, 402, 407
  cautions for, 406, 410
  hemodynamic considerations in, 399–401,
  407
  hemodynamic evaluation of, 402–404,
  407–408
Anomaly
  aortic arch. *See* Aortic arch anomaly
  Ebstein's. *See* Ebstein's anomaly
  systemic venous. *See* Systemic venous
  anomaly
  Taussig-Bing. *See* Taussig-Bing anomaly

Antecubital fossa cutdown, 41
Anterior oblique views, 106
Anteroposterior view, 106, 107–108
Aorta
  coarctation of. See Coarctation of aorta
  congenital kinking of, 395, 396
  origin of single pulmonary artery from. See
    Truncus arteriosus
  patent ductus arteriosus and pressure tracing
    of, 254
  transcatheter coil embolization and, 198
  transposition of great arteries and, 309
  vascular obstruction of airway and, 431
Aortic arch
  anomaly of. See Aortic arch anomaly
  double outlet right ventricle and interrupted,
    306
  patent ductus arteriosus and, 251
  vascular obstruction of airway and, 431–432
Aortic arch anomaly
  angiocardiography in, 425, 426, 427
  double, 425, 426, 427
  tetralogy of Fallot and, 293
  truncus arteriosus and, 265
  vascular obstruction of airway and, 419, 420,
    421, 422
Aortic arch interruption. See Coarctation of
  aorta
Aortic isthmus hypoplasia, 389
Aorticopulmonary window, 263
Aortic outflow
  double outlet right ventricle and, 302
  obstruction of, 87
Aortic pulse pressure
  coarctation of aorta and, 393
  patent ductus arteriosus and, 253
Aortic valve area, 378
Aortic valve atresia, 383–386
  anatomy of, 383
  angiocardiography in, 385
  catheterization indications in, 383–384
  catheterization technique for, 384
  cautions for, 385–386
  coarctation of aorta and, 394
  hemodynamic considerations in, 384
  hemodynamic evaluation of, 384–385
Aortic valve herniation, 234, 236
Aortic valve stenosis, 375–383
  anatomy of, 375–376
  angiocardiography in, 381–382
  associated lesions in, 382–383
  balloon angioplasty in, 163–165
  catheterization indications in, 377
  catheterization procedure for, 163–165
  catheterization technique for, 377–378
  complications of, 165
  double inlet ventricle and, 357
  double outlet right ventricle and, 306

hemodynamic considerations in, 376–377
hemodynamic evaluation of, 378–380
in newborn, 164, 165–166
Aortogram in ventricular septal defect,
  232–234, 235
Aortopulmonary fenestration. See
  Aortopulmonary window
Aortopulmonary septal defect. See
  Aortopulmonary window
Aortopulmonary window, 257–260
  anatomy of, 257
  angiocardiography in, 258–259
  aortic root injection of contrast media in,
    258–259
  catheterization indications in, 257–258
  catheterization technique for, 258
  cautions for, 259–260
  hemodynamic considerations in, 257
  hemodynamic evaluation of, 258
Approach
  femoral. See Femoral approach
  retrograde, 103, 164
  subxiphoid, 178–180
  venous, for patent ductus arteriosus,
    252–253
Arrhythmia
  atrial. See Atrial arrhythmia
  preexcitation phenomenon with, 122
  supraventricular. See Supraventricular
    tachycardia
  ventricular. See Ventricular arrhythmia
Arterial spasm, 204–205
Arterial switch in transposition of great
  arteries, 318
Arterial transposition. See Transposition of
  great arteries
Arterial trunk, common. See Truncus arteriosus
Arteriography. See also Angiocardiography;
  Angiography
  transseptal catheterization and, 172
  ventricular septal defect and pulmonary, 234
Arteriotomy, 44–47
Asplenia syndrome, 404–405
Atrial arrhythmia
  atrial flutter in, 135
  catheterization and, 208–209
  ectopic tachycardia in, 135
Atrial deflection, 135
Atrial ectopic tachycardia, 135
Atrial extrastimulus technique, 132, 133
Atrial flutter, 135
Atrial isomerism
  anomalous pulmonary venous return and,
    404–405, 408
  atrioventricular septal defect and, 249
  superior vena caval anomaly and, 414–415
Atrial muscle function assessment, 131
Atrial obstructive lesion, 84

Atrial pacing, 128–132
    rapid, 131
Atrial pressure, 84, 85
    coarctation of aorta and, 393
    tracing of, 89
Atrial septal defect, 217–226
    anatomy of, 217
    angiocardiography in, 223–225
    anomalous pulmonary venous return and,
        407
    associated lesions in, 225–226
    atrioventricular septal defect and, 241
    balloon catheter in, 222–223
    catheterization indications for, 218–219
    catheterization technique for, 219–220
    cautions for, 226
    hemodynamic considerations in, 217–218
    hemodynamic evaluation of, 220–222
    indicator dye dilution and, 222, 223
    tetralogy of Fallot and, 293
    transseptal catheterization and, 175
    truncus arteriosus and, 265
Atrial septostomy, 147–155
    balloon, 8, 23, 147–150, 404
    blade, 23–24, 150–154, 354–355
Atrial septum. *See also* Atrial septal defect;
        Atrial septostomy
    atrioventricular septal defect and, 241
    double inlet ventricle and, 361
    transseptal catheterization and puncture of,
        173–175
Atrial wall perforation, 153
Atrioventricular block
    corrected transposition of great arteries and,
        329
    electrophysiology and, 121–122
Atrioventricular canal defect. *See*
        Atrioventricular septal defect
Atrioventricular conduction electrophysiology,
        130
Atrioventricular dissociation
    pressure measurements in, 86
    supraventricular arrhythmias and, 135
Atrioventricular node assessment, 131–132
Atrioventricular septal defect, 241–250
    anatomy of, 241–243
    angiocardiography in, 245–248
    arterial blood in, 245
    associated lesions in, 249
    cardiac anomalies and, 249
    catheterization indications in, 243–244
    catheterization technique for, 244
    cautions for, 249
    hemodynamic considerations in, 243
    hemodynamic evaluation of, 244–245
    patent ductus arteriosus and, 251
    pulmonary vein angiography in, 246, 248
    valve orifice and, 241

    in ventricular septal defect classification, 227
Atrioventricular septum in ventricular septal
        defect, 235, 237
Atrioventricular valve atresia, 345–356
    left, 352–356. *See also* Mitral atresia
    right, 345–352. *See also* Tricuspid valve
        atresia
Atrioventricular valve regurgitation, 328–329.
        See also Tricuspid valve regurgitation
Atrioventricular valve stenosis, 361
Atrium
    anomalous pulmonary venous return and,
        399
    atrial septal defect and pressure in, 220
    electrophysiology and, 126–127
    inferior vena caval anomaly and, 417
    superior vena caval anomaly and, 414–415
Atropine
    before cardiac catheterization, 5
    supraventricular arrhythmias and, 135
Audiovisual materials, 3
Axial oblique view, 112–115
Axial view, long, 106
    ventricular septal defect and, 232, 234
Axilla in cutdown technique, 39–41
Axillary vein catheterization, 41
Azygos continuation, 415–416
    catheter manipulation and, 55

Balloon in balloon angioplasty, 158, 160
    malfunction of, 210
Balloon angioplasty, 157–170
    in aortic stenosis in newborn, 165–166
    in aortic valve stenosis, 163–165
    balloon for, 158, 160
    balloon malfunction in, 210
    in coarctation of aorta, 166, 167
    delivery of catheter in, 159
    development of, 24, 157
    in left heart inlet obstruction, 370–371
    in mitral valve stenosis, 169
    in newborn, 8, 162–166
    principles of, 157
    procedures of, 157–159
    in pulmonary artery stenosis, 166–169
    in pulmonary valve stenosis, 160–162,
        270–271
    in pulmonary valve stenosis in newborn,
        162–163
    size of catheter for, 160
    in tetralogy of Fallot, 288
Balloon atrial septostomy, 23, 147–150. *See
        also* Balloon angioplasty
    in anomalous pulmonary venous return, 404
    catheter for, 147, 148
    sequence of, 149
    in transposition of great arteries, 313–314

Balloon catheter, 22–23. *See also* Balloon angioplasty; Balloon atrial septostomy
in atrial septal defect, 222–223
in ductus arteriosus and ventricular septal defect occlusion, 232
manipulation of flow-directed, 66–69
Balloon dilation. *See* Balloon angioplasty; Balloon atrial septostomy
Balloon embolization, 198–201
catheter insertion in, 199
Balloon-tipped catheter, 22–23
angiography and, 22, 103
Balloon valvotomy. *See* Balloon angioplasty
Barium esophagram, 421–423
Basket snare for foreign body retrieval, 182, 183
Berman catheter, 19, 67
Betadine. *See* Povidone-iodine
Biopsy, endomyocardial, 176–180
Bioptome, 176, 177, 178
Blade atrial septostomy, 150–154
catheter for, 151
development of, 23–24
in mitral atresia, 354–355
Block, complete, 86, 89, 121–122
Blood flow
anomalous pulmonary venous return and, 403–404
calculation of, 93–94, 95
indicator dilution method for, 95
pulmonary. *See* Pulmonary blood flow
transposition of great arteries and, 311
Blood gas analysis, 12
shunt determination and, 74–75
Blood loss
balloon atrial septostomy and, 150
blade atrial septostomy and, 151
catheterization in transposition of great arteries and, 313
Booklets for teaching, 3
Brachiocephalic artery, 432, 433
Bradycardia
catheterization and, 209
in corrected transposition of great arteries, 329
pacing for, 137
Bridging leaflet, 243
Brockenbrough transseptal needle, 171, 173
Bronchoscopy, 421–424
Bypass, cardiopulmonary, 413

Cabinets for storage, 10
Cardiac catheter. *See* Catheter
Cardiac catheterization. *See* Catheterization
Cardiac malposition, 334
Cardiac output, 93–100
direct Fick method for, 93–95

indicator dilution method for. *See* Indicator dilution method
transposition of great arteries and, 316
Cardiac perforation in catheterization, 175, 207
Cardiac surgery, conduction disturbances after, 123–124
Cardiac tamponade, 86
Cardiac transplantation, 176
Cardiogreen. *See* Indocyanine green
Cardiomyopathy, congestive, 176
Cardiopulmonary bypass, 413
Cardiovascular aide, 12, 15
Cardiovascular injury, 175, 204, 207–209
Cardiovascular technician, 12, 15
Cardioverter/defibrillator, 12
C-arm equipment, 11, 101
in angiocardiography, 115, 117
projection and, 104, 105
Carotid artery in coarctation of aorta, 391
Catheter
balloon. *See* Balloon catheter
Berman, 19, 67
Cournand, 17, 19
double-lumen, 103
double-lumen thermodilution, 98
electrode, 22, 24, 124
end-hole, 17–18, 161, 164
endomyocardial biopsy, 178
flow-directed, 22–23, 66–69. *See also* Balloon catheter
flow-velocity, 24
fluid-filled, 20, 81
Fogarty, 23, 147, 148
fracture of, 210
Gensini, 19
Goodale-Lubin, 18, 19
immobilization of, 210–211
introduction of. *See* Catheter introduction
kinking of, 209–210
knotting of, 210
Lehman, 17, 19, 21
manipulation of. *See* Catheter manipulation
micromanometer-tipped, 23
Mullins transseptal, 154, 172, 173
NIH, 19, 21
pigtail, 21–22
positioning of fluoroscopic, 127, 128
preformed, 19
problems of, 204, 209–211
Rashkind. *See* Rashkind patent ductus arteriosus occluder
Schwartz, 67
storage racks for, 10
Swan-Ganz, 17, 19, 67
Teflon, 178
thermal-dilution, 24
umbilical, 313
Catheter deflector system, 183

Catheter delivery system, 186–187
Catheter embolization, 181–182, 198–201
Catheter insertion
    in balloon embolization, 199
    in endomyocardial biopsy, 179–180
    percutaneous, 28–32
Catheter introduction, 25–49
    arteriotomy in, 44–47
    cutdown technique of, 36–44. *See also*
        Cutdown
    general considerations in, 25–26
    percutaneous technique of, 25, 26–36. *See*
        also Percutaneous technique
    in transseptal catheterization, 173
    venotomy in, 48
Catheterization, 17–24
    angiocardiography and, 20–22
    balloon angioplasty/valvotomy and, 24. *See*
        also Balloon angioplasty
    balloon atrial septostomy and, 23. *See also*
        Balloon atrial septostomy
    blade atrial septostomy and, 23–24
    electrode catheters and, 24
    fiberoptic oximetry and, 24
    flow-directed catheters and, 22–23. *See also*
        Balloon angioplasty
    flow-velocity catheter and, 24, 66–69
    hemodynamic measurements and, 17–20
    introduction of catheter in. *See* Catheter
        introduction
    micromanometer-tipped catheters and, 23
    systemic complications of, 204, 211–213
    therapeutic maneuvers in, 8, 181–182,
        186–187, 198–201
    thermal-dilution catheters and, 24
    transseptal puncture and, 24, 154, 172, 173
Catheterization complications, 203–214
    arterial, 204–206
    atrial arrhythmias and, 208–209
    cardiovascular injury and, 204, 207–209
    catheter problems and, 204, 209–211
    local, 204, 211
    mortality and, 203–204
    systemic, 204, 211–213
    vascular system and, 204–207
    wall dissection and, 205
Catheterization indications, 1–2
    in anomalous pulmonary venous return,
        401–402, 407
    in aortic valve atresia, 383–384, 384
    in aortic valve stenosis, 377–378
    in aortopulmonary window, 257–258
    in atrial septal defect, 218–219
    in atrioventricular septal defect, 243–244
    in coarctation of aorta, 391–392
    in corrected transposition of great arteries,
        328–329
    in double inlet ventricle, 360–361

    in double outlet right ventricle, 303
    in Ebstein's anomaly, 338
    in left heart inlet obstruction, 366–367
    in mitral atresia, 353
    in patent ductus arteriosus, 252
    in pulmonary valve atresia, 278
    in pulmonary valve stenosis, 268–269
    in tetralogy of Fallot, 286
    in transposition of great arteries, 312
    in tricuspid atresia, 346–347
    in truncus arteriosus, 262–263
    in vascular obstruction of airway, 420–424
    in ventricular septal defect, 228–229
Catheterization laboratory, 9–15
    equipment in, 10–12
    personnel for, 12–15
    room design and layout in, 9–10
Catheterization technique
    for aortopulmonary window, 258
    for atrial septal defect, 219–220
    for atrioventricular septal defect, 244
    for coarctation of aorta, 392
    for double inlet ventricle, 361–362
    for double outlet right ventricle, 303–304
    for Ebstein's anomaly, 338–339
    for left heart inlet obstruction, 367–368
    for mitral atresia, 353–354
    for patent ductus arteriosus, 252–253
    for pulmonary atresia, 278–279
    for pulmonary valve stenosis, 269
    for tetralogy of Fallot, 286–287
    for transposition of great arteries, 313–318
    for tricuspid atresia, 347–349
    for truncus arteriosus, 263
    for vascular obstruction of airway, 424
    for ventricular septal defect, 229–230
Catheter loading
    balloon embolization and, 199
    ductus arteriosus catheter occlusion and,
        188–180
Catheter loop
    in jugular vein, 56
    removal of, 65, 66
Catheter manipulation, 55–69
    aorta to left ventricle, 63–64
    atrium to right ventricle, 56–58
    catheter loop removal and, 65
    flow-directed balloon, 66–69
    left atrium to left ventricle, 62–63
    left atrium to pulmonary veins, 61–62
    pulmonary artery branches, 59–60
    in retrograde passage across atrioventricular
        valve, 64–65
    right atrium to left atrium, 60–61
    right atrium to superior vena cava, 56
    right ventricle to pulmonary artery, 58–59
    in venous system, 55–56
Cava-Shultz bioptome, 176, 177

Cherry pit hypoplasia, 277, 280–281
Chlorpromazine
    catheterization and, 4, 172
    in electrophysiology, 125
Chromosomal damage, 212
Cineangiography, 20–21, 101–102
    equipment for, 11
Clamps
    arteriotomy and, 44
    endomyocardial biopsy and, 178
Coarctation of aorta, 389–397
    anatomy and, 389–390
    angiocardiography in, 166, 394, 397
    associated lesions in, 394–395, 396
    atrial septal defect and, 226
    atrioventricular septal defect and, 249
    balloon angioplasty in, 166, 167
    catheterization indications in, 391–392
    catheterization technique for, 392
    cautions for, 395–397
    double outlet right ventricle and, 306
    hemodynamic considerations in, 390–391
    hemodynamic evaluation of, 392–394
    juxtaductal, 389
Coils, Gianturco, 194–198
Complete heart block
    electrophysiology and, 121–122
    pressure measurements in, 86, 89
Conduction disturbances after cardiac surgery,
        123–124
Conduction interval
    baseline, 127–128
    electrophysiology and, 130
    sinoatrial, 130
Congestive heart failure
    aortopulmonary window and, 257
    atrioventricular septal defect and, 243
    coarctation of aorta and, 391–392, 393
    double outlet right ventricle and, 303
    patent ductus arteriosus and, 251
    transposition of great arteries and, 313
    truncus arteriosus and, 262
Conotruncal abnormality, 107
Conray contrast media, 102
Contrast media
    angiocardiography and, 102
    angiography and, 104
    anomalous pulmonary venous return and,
        404–405
    aortopulmonary window and, 258–259
    complications from, 116–117, 211–212
    patent ductus arteriosus and, 253–255
    pulmonary atresia and, 280
Cordis disposable bioptome, 176, 177
Coronary artery
    tetralogy of Fallot and, 291–293
    truncus arteriosus and, 266
Coronary sinus

multiple intracardiac catheters and, 128
    superior vena caval anomaly and, 411–414
Corrected transposition of great arteries,
        327–335
    anatomy in, 327–328
    angiography in, 107, 330–332
    associated lesions in, 332–335
    catheterization indications in, 328–329
    catheterization technique for, 329–330
    cautions for, 335
    Ebstein's anomaly and, 343
    hemodynamic considerations in, 328
    hemodynamic evaluation of, 330
Cor triatriatum
    anatomy of, 365–366
    angiography in, 372
    catheterization technique for, 368
    hemodynamic evaluation of, 369
Cournand catheter, 17, 19
Cranio-caudal view, 106, 115, 116, 117, 118
Cutdown, 36–44
    antecubital fossa and, 41
    axilla and, 39–41
    femoral vessels and, 37–39
    umbilical vessels and, 41–44
    use of, 25–26
Cut film changer, 101
Cyanosis
    anomalous pulmonary venous return and,
        400
    newborn catheterization and, 5–8
    pulmonary atresia and, 277
    tetralogy of Fallot with pulmonary atresia
        and, 294
    transposition of great arteries and, 312
    truncus arteriosus and, 262

Damped pressure tracing, 84
Deflector system, 183
Demerol. See Meperidine
Diastolic pressure, 84
    aortopulmonary window and, 258
    patent ductus arteriosus and pulmonary, 253
DiGeorge's syndrome, 266
Dilation, balloon. See Balloon angioplasty
Dilator
    arteriotomy and, 46
    percutaneous technique and, 30, 32, 33, 34
Double aortic arch, angiocardiography in, 425,
        426, 427
Double chamber right ventricle, 267
Double inlet ventricle, 357–364
    anatomy of, 357–359
    angiocardiography in, 362–363
    angiography in, 362–363
    associated lesions in, 363–364
    catheterization indications in, 360–361
    catheterization technique for, 361–362

Double inlet ventricle (*cont.*)
  cautions for, 364
  cineangiogram of, 358, 359
  corrected transposition of great arteries and,
      334
  diagram of, 358
  hemodynamic considerations in, 359–360
  hemodynamic evaluation of, 362
  ventriculoarterial concordance and, 357
Double-lumen catheter
  angiography and, 103
  in cardiac output measurement, 98
Double outlet right ventricle, 301–307
  anatomy of, 301–302
  angiocardiography in, 305–306
  angiography and, 107
  associated lesions in, 306–307
  catheterization indications in, 303
  catheterization technique for, 303–304
  cautions for, 307
  hemodynamic considerations in, 302–303
  hemodynamic evaluation of, 304–305
Ductus arteriosus, patent, 251–256
  anatomy of, 251
  angiocardiography in, 253–255
  aortopulmonary window and, 257
  atrial septal defect and, 226
  atrioventricular septal defect and, 249
  balloon occlusion of, 232
  catheterization indications in, 252
  catheterization technique for, 252–253
  cautions for, 255–256
  coarctation of aorta and, 393
  hemodynamic considerations in, 251–252
  hemodynamic evaluation of, 253
  prostaglandin E$_1$ and, 7
  pulmonary stenosis in newborn and, 163
  venous approach for, 252–253
Ductus arteriosus catheter occlusion, 185–194
  polyurethane foam plug and, 185–186
  Rashkind occluder and, 186–194. *See also*
      Rashkind patent ductus arteriosus
      occluder
Ductus venosus, 278
Dye for indicator dilution method. *See*
    Indicator dilution method

Ebstein's anomaly, 337–343
  anatomy of, 337–338
  angiocardiography in, 339–341
  associated lesions in, 341–343
  catheterization indications in, 338
  catheterization technique for, 338–339
  cautions for, 343
  corrected transposition of great arteries and,
      327, 332–334
  diagram of, 337
  hemodynamic considerations in, 338

  hemodynamic evaluation of, 339
  imperforate, 341
  pulmonary atresia and, 283
  pulmonary valve stenosis and, 273
Echocardiography
  in pericardial effusion, 177–178
  in vascular obstruction of airway, 422
Electrical hazards, 213
Electrical stimulator, 124–125
Electrocardiography in catheterization
    complications, 204, 208–209. *See also*
    Electrophysiology
Electrode catheter, 22, 24, 124
Electrophysiology, 121–139
  atrial pacing and, 128–132
  complications of, 139
  corrected transposition of great arteries and,
      329
  equipment for, 124–125
  indications for, 121–124
  normal values in, 130
  recording sites in, 125–127
  refractory periods in, 130, 133
  stimulator in, 124–125
  supraventricular arrhythmias and, 134–137
  switch box and, 124
  techniques of, 125–128
  tetralogy of Fallot and, 287–288
  therapeutic pacing and, 137–139
  transposition of great arteries and, 317
  ventricular arrhythmias and, 137
  ventricular pacing and, 132–134
Embolism, pulmonary, 207
Embolization
  balloon, 198–201
  of catheter fragment, 181–182
  ductus arteriosus catheter occlusion and,
      193–194
  particulate, 201
  Rashkind patent ductus arteriosus occluder
      and, 193
End-hole catheter, 17–18, 124
  in aortic valve stenosis, 164
  in pulmonary valve stenosis, 161
Endocardial cushion defect. *See*
    Atrioventricular septal defect
Endomyocardial biopsy, 176–177
  catheter for, 178
  catheter insertion for, 179–180
Equipment
  in catheterization laboratory, 10–12
  for electrophysiology, 124–125
Esophagram, barium, 421–423

Fallot
  pentalogy of, 293
  tetralogy of. *See* Tetralogy of Fallot

Femoral approach, 18
  for aortic valve stenosis, 378
  in atrial septal defect, 219–220
  corrected transposition of great arteries and,
    329–330
  cutdown technique and, 37–39
  in double outlet right ventricle, 303–304
  in Ebstein's anomaly, 338–339
  in electrophysiology, 125
  in endomyocardial biopsy, 176
  percutaneous technique and, 26, 27–33
  in pulmonary valve stenosis, 269
  in ventricular septal defect, 229–230
Femoral artery
  cutdown technique and, 37–39
  endomyocardial biopsy and, 176
  percutaneous technique and, 26, 27–33
Femoral triangle, 27, 28, 37, 38
Fenestration, aortopulmonary. See
    Aortopulmonary window
Fibrillation, ventricular, 137
Fick method for cardiac output, 93–95
Fick principle, 72
Film changer, 101
First heart sound, 141
Flow-directed catheter, 22–23, 24. See also
    Balloon catheter
  manipulation of, 66–69
Flow ratio
  pulmonary-to-systemic, 74
  shunt detection and, 74
Flow-velocity catheter, 24
Fluid-filled pressure curve, 83
Fogarty septostomy catheter, 23
  balloon atrial septostomy and, 147, 148
Forceps in foreign body retrieval, 182
Foreign body retrieval, 181–183
Fore 'n Aft Triangle method, 95, 97
Four-chamber view, 106, 110–112

Gas analyzer, 12
Gensini catheter, 19
Gianturco coils, 194–198
Goodale-Lubin catheter, 18, 19
Goose-neck deformity, 245, 247
Gould-Statham P-23-ID transducer, 81
Gown pack, 15
Gradients, pressure. See Pressure gradient
Graham-Steele murmur, 143–144
Great arteries
  catheterization perforation of, 207
  transposition of. See Transposition of great
    arteries
Grounding system, 10
Group teaching sessions, 2
Guidewire, 51–55
  in aortic valve stenosis, 164

  in ductus arteriosus catheter occlusion, 188,
    190
  in percutaneous technique, 29–32, 33
  in pulmonary valve stenosis, 161
  in pulmonary valve stenosis in newborn, 163

Hazards, electrical, 213
Heart
  malposition of, 334
  perforation of, 175, 207
Heart block, complete, 86, 89, 121–122
Heart failure, congestive. See Congestive heart
    failure
Heart sounds, 141–142
Hemaquet, 151
Hemiazygos continuation, 416–417
Hemitruncus. See Truncus arteriosus
Hemodynamic complications of catheterization,
    211
Hemodynamic evaluation. See also
    Hemodynamics
  of anomalous pulmonary venous return,
    402–404, 407–408
  of aortic valve atresia, 384–385
  of aortic valve stenosis, 378–380
  of aortopulmonary window, 258
  of atrial septal defect, 220–222
  of atrioventricular septal defect, 244–245
  of coarctation of aorta, 392–394
  of corrected transposition of great arteries,
    330
  of double inlet ventricle, 362
  of double outlet right ventricle, 304–305
  of Ebstein's anomaly, 339
  of left heart inlet obstruction, 368–370
  of mitral atresia, 354
  of patent ductus arteriosus, 253
  of pulmonary atresia, 279–280
  of pulmonary valve stenosis, 269–270
  of tetralogy of Fallot, 287
  of transposition of great arteries, 318–319
  of tricuspid atresia, 349–350
  of truncus arteriosus, 263
  of ventricular septal defect, 230–231
Hemodynamics. See also Hemodynamic
    evaluation
  in anomalous pulmonary venous return,
    399–401, 407
  in aortic valve atresia, 384
  in aortic valve stenosis, 377–377
  in aortopulmonary window, 257
  in atrial septal defect, 217–218
  in atrioventricular septal defect, 243
  cardiac catheterization and, 17–20, 211
  in coarctation of aorta, 390–391
  in corrected transposition of great arteries,
    328
  in double inlet ventricle, 359–360

Hemodynamics (*cont.*)
  in double outlet right ventricle, 302–303
  in Ebstein's anomaly, 338
  in left heart inlet obstruction, 366
  in mitral atresia, 353
  in patent ductus arteriosus, 251–252
  in pulmonary atresia, 277–278
  in pulmonary valve stenosis, 267–268
  in tetralogy of Fallot, 285–286
  in tetralogy of Fallot with pulmonary atresia, 295
  in transposition of great arteries, 310–312
  in tricuspid atresia, 345–346
  in truncus arteriosus, 262
  in ventricular septal defect, 227–228
Hemostat
  arteriotomy and, 46
  percutaneous technique and, 29, 32
Heparin
  aortic valve stenosis and, 163
  arteriotomy and, 45–46
  balloon dilation and, 158
  coarctation of aorta and, 166
  percutaneous technique and, 36
Hepatoclavicular view, 110–112
Hepatomegaly, 400
Herniation of aortic valve, 234, 236
Hexabrix, 102
His bundle electrophysiology, 27, 121, 123, 125, 126
Holmes heart, 357, 358
Hypaque contrast medium, 102
Hypertension
  coarctation of aorta and, 392
  pulmonary. *See* Pulmonary hypertension
  ventricular, in pulmonary valve stenosis, 268
Hypertrophy, ventricular, 400
Hypoplasia
  aortic isthmus, 389, 390
  in hypoplastic left heart syndrome. *See* Aortic valve atresia
  pulmonary atresia and, 280, 281
Hypothermia, 313
Hypovolemia, 313
Hypoxemia
  in pulmonary valve stenosis, 268
  in tetralogy of Fallot, 286–287, 294
  in transposition of great arteries, 310–311, 313

Image intensifier, 101
Immobilization, 5, 6, 7
Immunosuppressive therapy, 176
Incision
  skin, 29, 32, 40–41
Incision in arteriotomy, 44. *See also* Femoral approachIncisura, pulmonary artery, 141–142

Indicator dilution method, 95–99
  appearance time in, 75
  atrial septal defect and, 222, 223
  calibration factor in, 96–97
  shunt determination and, 75–79
Indocyanine green, 75, 95–98
Infarction, 209
Inferior vena cava
  absent intrahepatic portion of, 415–417
  azygous or hemiazygos continuation of, 415–416
  catheter manipulation in, 55–56
  to left atrium, 417
Infundibula, bilateral, 305–306
Injector, power, 103
Inlet obstruction of left heart. *See* Left heart inlet obstruction
Innominate artery, 422–424, 432, 433
Innominate vein, 415
Instruments
  in cardiac catheterization, 13, 14–15
  cutdown, 14, 15
  percutaneous, 13, 15
Interatrial communication in pulmonary stenosis, 272–273
Interatrial septum in double inlet ventricle, 361
Iodine
  in contrast media, 102
  in endomyocardial biopsy, 178
Ischemia
  during catheterization, 209
  tricuspid atresia and, 346
Isoproterenol, 135
Isovue 370, 102

Jugular vein, 33–36
Junction box, 124
Juxtaductal coarctation, 389

Ketalar. *See* Ketamine
Ketamine
  balloon dilation and, 159
  ductus arteriosus catheter occlusion and, 190
  in electrophysiology, 125
  laryngeal spasm and airway compromise and, 5

Laboratory, catheterization. *See* Catheterization laboratory
Laboratory table, 11
Lateral view, 106, 107–108
Left heart inlet obstruction, 365–374
  anatomy of, 365–366
  angiography and, 371–373
  associated lesions in, 374
  balloon angioplasty in, 370–371
  catheterization indications in, 366–367
  catheterization technique for, 367–368

Left heart inlet obstruction (*cont.*)
  cautions for, 374
  diagram of, 366
  hemodynamic considerations in, 366
  hemodynamic evaluation of, 368–370
Lehman catheter, 17, 19, 21
Lidocaine
  balloon dilation and, 158
  cutdown technique and, 37
  endomyocardial biopsy and, 178
  percutaneous technique and, 27
  pulmonary valve stenosis and, 161
Linen pack, 15
Literature for teaching, 3
Lobe vein connection, 407
Long axial view, 106
  ventricular septal defect and, 232, 234
Loop snare in foreign body retrieval, 182

Medicut cannula in percutaneous technique, 32
Membranous defect, 227
Meperidine
  catheterization and, 4, 172
  in electrophysiology, 125
Metabolic acidosis
  coarctation of aorta and, 395
  transposition of great arteries and, 313
Metabolism of newborn, 6–7
Micromanometer
  catheter and, 23
  phonocardiography and, 141
  pressure curve of, 83
Mitral atresia, 352–356
  anatomy of, 352–353
  angiocardiography in, 355–356
  associated lesions in, 356
  catheterization indications in, 353
  catheterization technique for, 353–354
  cautions for, 356
  coarctation of aorta and, 394
  diagram of, 352
  hemodynamic considerations in, 353
  hemodynamic evaluation of, 354
Mitral regurgitation, 245. *See also* Tricuspid
    valve regurgitation
Mitral valve stenosis
  anatomy of, 366
  angiography in, 372–373
  balloon angioplasty in, 169
  catheterization technique for, 368
  hemodynamic evaluation of, 369–370
Mixed venous oxygen saturation, 72
Morphine sulfate
  cardiac catheterization premedication and, 4
  tetralogy of Fallot and, 294
Mortality, 203–204
Mullins transseptal catheter, 154, 172, 173
Multichannel recorder, 11–12
Murmurs

evaluation of, 142–145
  Graham-Steele, 143–144
Muscular defect, 227
Myocardial infarction, 209
Myocardial injury, 208
Myocardial ischemia
  during catheterization, 209
  tricuspid atresia and, 346
Myocardial sinusoids, 277
Myocarditis, inflammatory, 176
Myocardium
  catheter perforation of, 208
  transcatheter coil embolization and, 198

Neck in percutaneous technique, 33–34, 35
Needle
  Brockenbrough transseptal, 171, 173
  endomyocardial biopsy, 178
  percutaneous insertion of, 28–29
Neurologic complications, 213
Newborn
  aortic stenosis in, 164, 165–166
  catheterization and, 5–8
  Ebstein's anomaly in, 340–341
  pulmonary stenosis in, 162–163, 268,
    277–278
  transposition of great arteries in, 313–315,
    318
NIH catheter, 19, 21
Noonan syndrome, 271
Nurse in cardiac catheterization laboratory, 13

Oblique view, 108–110
  anterior, 106
  elongated right anterior, 106, 114, 115
  long axial, 110–112, 112–115
Oblique views, anterior, 106
Occluder delivery system, 189–190
Occlusion
  ductus arteriosus catheter, 185–194
  Rashkind patent ductus arteriosus. *See*
    Rashkind patent ductus arteriosus
    occluder
  superior vena caval anomaly and, 413–414
  transcatheter vascular. *See* Transcatheter
    vascular occlusion
Omnipaque 350, 102
Osmolality, contrast media and, 102
Ostium primum and ostium secundum defects,
    217
Outflow obstruction
  aortic, 87
  ventricular, 88, 269
Overdamped pressure tracing, 84
Oximetry, 12
  double inlet ventricle and, 362
  fiberoptic, 24
  pulmonary atresia and, 279–280
  shunt detection and, 71–75
  truncus arteriosus and, 263

Oxygen. *See also* Oxygen saturation
  aortopulmonary window and, 258
  in arterial blood, 94
  atrioventricular septal defect and, 245
  for cyanotic newborn, 7
  measurement of arterial, 94
  patent ductus arteriosus and, 253
  shunt determination with, 74–75
  ventricular septal defect and, 231–232
Oxygen saturation. *See also* Oxygen
  anomalous pulmonary venous return and,
    403, 407–408
  aortic valve atresia and, 385
  aortic valve stenosis and, 380
  aortopulmonary window and, 258
  atrial septal defect and, 220–222
  atrioventricular septal defect and, 245
  coarctation of aorta and, 393–394
  double inlet ventricle and, 360
  double outlet right ventricle and, 305
  Ebstein's anomaly and, 339
  patent ductus arteriosus and, 253
  pulmonary valve stenosis and, 269–270
  shunt detection and, 71–72
  tetralogy of Fallot and, 287
  tetralogy of Fallot with pulmonary atresia
    and, 295
  transposition of great arteries and, 311
  tricuspid atresia and, 350
  vascular obstruction of airway and, 424
  ventricular septal defect and, 230–231

Pacing, 124, 137–139
  atrial, 128–132
  rapid atrial, 131
  ventricular, 132–134
Packs, detailed listing of, 15
Paley stopcock bank, 15
Parent groups, 2
Parent's role, 4
Patent ductus arteriosus. *See* Ductus
  arteriosus, patent
Patient, 1–8
  cardiac catheterization indications for, 1–2
  immobilization of, 5, 6, 7
  newborn as, 5–8
  premedication in, 4–5
  psychological concerns for, 2–4
Patient table, 11
Pentalogy of Fallot, 293
Percutaneous balloon dilation. *See* Balloon
  angioplasty
Percutaneous technique, 25, 26–36
  in aortic valve stenosis, 377–378
  aperture drape in, 27
  catheter insertion in, 28–32
  femoral vein and artery in, 27–33. *See also*
    Femoral approach

  heparinization in, 36
  internal jugular vein in, 33–36
  introducing unit in, 30, 32–33
  postcatheterization care and, 36
  site preparation for, 26–27
  in transposition of great arteries, 313
Pericardial drainage, indwelling, 180
Pericardial effusion, 177–178
Pericardiocentesis, 177–181
  catheter insertion and, 179–180
  complications of, 181
  emergency, 181
  indwelling pericardial drainage and, 180
  pericardial effusion and, 177–178
  preparation for, 178
  procedure for, 178–179
  set for, 179, 180
Peripheral arterial pulse, 36
Phenergan. *See* Promethazine
Phonocardiography, 141–145
  heart sounds and, 141–142
  murmur evaluation and, 142–145
Picker-Amplatz film changer, 101
Pigtail catheter, 21–22
Plastic cannula in percutaneous technique, 32
Play therapy, 3
Polysplenia syndrome, 408
Polyurethane foam plug, 185–186
Postcatheterization care, 36
Postoperative catheterization in transposition
  of great arteries, 315–317, 318
Povidone-iodine
  in endomyocardial biopsy, 178
  percutaneous technique and, 26–27
Power injector, 103
Preexcitation phenomenon, 122, 135
Premature ventricular contractions, 208
Premedication, 4–5
  reaction to, 212
  for transseptal catheterization, 172
Pressure curve, micromanometer versus fluid-
  filled, 83
Pressure data. *See also* Pressure measurement
  in anomalous pulmonary venous return, 402,
    407–408
  in aortic valve atresia, 384–385
  in aortic valve stenosis, 378–380
  in aortopulmonary window, 258
  in atrioventricular septal defect, 244–245
  in coarctation of aorta, 392–393
  in double inlet ventricle, 362
  in double outlet right ventricle, 304
  in Ebstein's anomaly, 339
  in patent ductus arteriosus, 253
  in pulmonary atresia, 279
  in pulmonary valve stenosis, 269
  in tetralogy of Fallot, 285–286, 287, 290–291

Pressure data (*cont.*)
  in tetralogy of Fallot with pulmonary atresia, 295
  in transposition of great arteries, 311
  in tricuspid atresia, 349–350
  in vascular obstruction of airway, 424
Pressure drop, angiography catheters and, 103
Pressure gradient, 20
  in anomalous pulmonary venous return, 402–403
  in atrial septal defect, 220
  in double outlet right ventricle, 302
Pressure measurement, 81–86. *See also*
      Pressure data; Pressure tracing
  in atrial septal defect, 220
  instrumentation in, 81–82
  resistance calculation in, 86–91
  in ventricular septal defect, 230
Pressure tracing, 84, 85
  atrial, 89
  damped, 84
  overdamped, 84
  in patent ductus arteriosus, 254
Pressure volume chart, 20, 21
Priscoline. *See* Tolazoline
Programmed stimulation, 134, 137
Projections, 104–115
  anteroposterior and lateral view, 106, 107–108
  axial four-chamber view, 110–112
  elongated right anterior oblique view, 115
  hepatoclavicular view, 110–112
  long axial oblique view, 112–115
  oblique view, 108–110
  sitting up view, 106, 115, 116, 117, 118
Promethazine
  in catheterization premedication, 4, 172
  in electrophysiology, 125
Propranolol, 294
Prostaglandin D_1, 161
Prostaglandin E_1, 5, 7
  in coarctation of aorta, 395
  in pulmonary atresia, 278, 283–284
  in pulmonary valve stenosis, 163, 274
  in transposition of great arteries, 312
Prosthesis, catheter occlusion and, 186–187, 188–189, 190, 191
Pseudocoarctation, 395, 396
Psychological concerns, 2–4
Pullback pressure, 84, 86
  anomalous pulmonary venous return and, 403
Pullback tracing, 20
Pulmonary arteriogram, 234
Pulmonary artery
  cardiac catheterization and, 18, 208
  dissection of, 208
  patent ductus arteriosus and disease of, 251

pressure in. *See* Pulmonary artery pressure
Pulmonary artery incisura, 141–142
Pulmonary artery pressure. *See also* Pulmonary
      artery stenosis; Pulmonary artery wedge
      pressure
  in aortopulmonary window, 257, 258
  in atrioventricular septal defect, 244–245
  in coarctation of aorta, 392–393
  in corrected transposition of great arteries, 328
  in patent ductus arteriosus, 253, 254
  in pulmonary stenosis in newborn, 163
Pulmonary artery stenosis
  atrioventricular septal defect and, 249
  balloon angioplasty in, 166–169
  corrected transposition of great arteries and, 330, 332
  double outlet right ventricle and, 304, 306
  Ebstein's anomaly and, 341
  isolated muscular, 267
  isolated subvalvar, 267
  patent ductus arteriosus and, 251
  truncus arteriosus and, 262
Pulmonary artery stenosis in newborn, 162–163, 268
  with pulmonary atresia, 277–278
Pulmonary artery wedge pressure, 86. *See also*
      Pulmonary artery pressure
  atrial septal defect and, 220, 221
Pulmonary blood flow
  atrioventricular septal defect and, 243
  Fick method for calculation of, 93–94
  patent ductus arteriosus and, 253
  pulmonary atresia and, 277
  shunt detection, 72–73
  transposition of great arteries and, 311
Pulmonary embolism, 207
Pulmonary hypertension
  in anomalous pulmonary venous return, 402
  in aortopulmonary window, 258
  in atrioventricular septal defect, 243
  in double outlet right ventricle, 304
  in patent ductus arteriosus, 251, 253
  shunt determination and, 74
  in tetralogy of Fallot with pulmonary atresia, 295
Pulmonary outflow in double outlet right ventricle, 302
Pulmonary sling. *See* Vascular obstruction of airway
Pulmonary-to-systemic flow ratio, 74
Pulmonary valve
  double outlet right ventricle and, 301–302
  syndrome of absent, 293–294
Pulmonary valve annulus, 160
Pulmonary valve atresia with anomalous pulmonary venous return, 405–406

Pulmonary valve atresia with intact ventricular
    septum, 277–284
  anatomy of, 277
  angiocardiography in, 280–283
  angiography in, 280–283
  associated lesions in, 283
  catheterization indications in, 278
  catheterization technique for, 278–279
  cautions for, 283–284
  Ebstein's anomaly and, 342–343
  hemodynamic considerations in, 277–278
  hemodynamic evaluation of, 279–280
  systemic pressure in, 279
Pulmonary valve atresia with tetralogy of
    Fallot, 294–298, 324. See also Tetralogy of
    Fallot
Pulmonary valve regurgitation, 143–144
Pulmonary valve stenosis, 267–275
  anatomy of, 267
  angiocardiography in, 271–272
  anomalous pulmonary venous return and,
    405–406
  associated lesions in, 272–274
  atrial septal defect and, 225
  balloon angioplasty in, 160–163
  catheterization indications in, 268–269
  catheterization procedure for, 160–161, 269
  cautions for, 274–275
  complications of, 161–162
  double inlet ventricle and, 357
  hemodynamic considerations in, 20, 267–268
  hemodynamic evaluation of, 269–270
  suprasystemic pressure and, 268
  valvar obstruction in, 272
Pulmonary vascular resistance, 90
  anomalous pulmonary venous return and,
    400
  atrial septal defect and, 220
Pulmonary vein
  angiography of, 371–372
  anomalous pulmonary venous return and.
    See Anomalous pulmonary venous return
  atresia of. See Pulmonary vein atresia
  atrial septal defect and, 225
  atrioventricular septal defect and, 246, 248
  mitral atresia and, 352
  stenosis of. See Pulmonary vein stenosis
Pulmonary vein atresia
  anatomy of, 365
  angiography of, 371
  hemodynamic evaluation of, 368
Pulmonary vein stenosis
  anatomy of, 365
  angiography of, 371–372
  catheterization technique for, 367–368
  hemodynamic evaluation of, 368–369
Pulmonary venous return

anomalous. See Anomalous pulmonary
    venous return
  atrial septal defect and, 225
  mitral atresia and, 352
Pulse pressure, aortic, 253
Puppet therapy, 3

Radiation hazards, 212–213
Radiographic unit, 10–11
  angiocardiography and, 101–102
  biplane, 104, 105
Radiography
  angulation in, 104
  rotation in, 104
Rashkind atrial septostomy 23, 147–150
Rashkind patent ductus arteriosus occluder,
    186–194
  complications of, 193–194
  loading of, 188–189
  occlusion technique and, 189–193
  system design and, 186–188
Recorder, multichannel, 11–12
Recurrent supraventricular tachycardia, 122
Recurrent ventricular tachycardia, 122
Refractory periods in electrophysiology, 130,
    133
Regurgitation
  atrioventricular valve. See Tricuspid valve
    regurgitation
  mitral, 245
  pulmonic, 143–144
  tricuspid. See Tricuspid valve regurgitation
Renografin contrast medium, 102
Resistance
  anomalous pulmonary venous return and,
    400
  atrial septal defect and, 220
  pulmonary vascular, 90, 400
  systemic, 90
Respiratory insufficiency in transposition of
    great arteries, 313
Retroesophageal indentation, 425–431
Retrograde approach
  angiography and, 103
  aortic valve stenosis and, 164
Rhythm disturbance mechanism, 134–135
Roll film changer, 101
Ross transseptal needle, 171, 173
Rubella syndrome
  patent ductus arteriosus and, 251
  pulmonary valve stenosis and, 274

Sanchez-Perez film changer, 101
Sandbags in restraint, 5, 6
Sapheno-femoral junction, 37–39
Saphenous bulb, 37–39
Saphenous vein cutdown, 37–39
  for aortic valve stenosis, 377–378

Saturation, oxygen. *See* Oxygen saturation
Schoenader film changer, 101
Schwartz catheter, 67
Scimitar syndrome, 408
Second heart sound, 141–142
Sepsis, 211
Septal defect
  angiography and, 107
  aortopulmonary. *See* Aortopulmonary
    window
  atrial. *See* Atrial septal defect
  atrioventricular. *See* Atrioventricular septal
    defect
  ventricular. *See* Ventricular septal defect
Septostomy, atrial. *See* Atrial septostomy
Septum
  atrial. *See* Atrial septum
  ventricular. *See* Ventricular septum
Sheath
  aortic valve stenosis and, 164, 165–166
  blade atrial septostomy and, 153
  ductus arteriosus catheter occlusion and,
    189–190
  Mullins transseptal long, 154, 172, 173
  percutaneous technique and, 33, 34
  transseptal catheterization and, 154, 172, 173
Shielding in catheterization laboratory, 10
Shunt
  aortopulmonary window and, 257
  atrial septal defect and, 217
  atrioventricular septal defect and, 243
  corrected transposition of great arteries and,
    332
  detection of, 71–79
  left-to-right, 73–74, 77, 78, 217, 227–228,
    230–231, 243, 257
  left ventricular-right atrial, 144–145
  oxygen saturation and, 230–231
  quantitation of, 77–79
  right-to-left, 73, 77–79, 332
  transposition of great arteries and, 311–312
  ventricular septal defect and, 227–228
  ventricular septal defect and left ventricle-
    right atrial, 235–238, 239
Shunt detection, 71–79
  flow ratio and, 74
  indicator dilution method in, 75–79
  oximetry and, 71–75
Sinoatrial conduction time, 130
Sinoatrial node reentry, 135
Sinus node function, atrial pacing and, 129–131
Sinus node recovery time, 129–130, 131
Sinus rhythm, atrial pressure tracing and, 89
Sinus venosus defect, 217
Sitting up view, 106, 115, 116, 117, 118
Skin closure, 48
Skin incision

cutdown technique, 40–41
percutaneous technique, 29, 32
Snare in foreign body retrieval, 182
SNRT. *See* Sinus node recovery time
Sodium, contrast media and, 102
Stenosis
  aortic valve. *See* Aortic valve stenosis
  mitral valve. *See* Mitral valve stenosis
  pulmonary artery. *See* Pulmonary artery
    stenosis
  pulmonary valve. *See* Pulmonary valve
    stenosis
  pulmonary vein. *See* Pulmonary vein stenosis
  subvalvar, 377, 380
  supravalvar, 377, 380
Stewart-Hamilton logarithmic extrapolation
  method, 95–97
Stimulation, programmed, 134, 137
Stimulator in electrophysiology, 124–125
Storage cabinets, 10
Subaortic stenosis, 375–376
  coarctation of aorta and, 390
Subaortic ventricular septal defect, 303
Subclavian artery
  angiocardiography of, 428, 429, 430, 431
  coarctation of aorta and, 389, 390, 391
Subclavian steal syndrome, 433, 434
Subvalvar stenosis, 377, 380
Subxiphoid approach for pericardiocentesis,
  178–180
Superior vena cava
  anomalies of, 411–415
  bilateral vena cavae and, 415
  left, to left atrium, 414–415
  transposition of great arteries and, 311
  transseptal catheterization via, 175
Supracristal defect, 227
Supravalvar stenosis, 377, 380
Supraventricular tachycardia
  electrophysiology in, 127, 134–137
  pacing for, 137–139
  recurrent, 122
Suture, arteriotomy and, 47
Swan-Ganz catheter, 17, 19, 67
Switch box, 124
Syncope
  corrected transposition of great arteries and,
    329
  of uncertain etiology, 122–123
Syndromes
  Allagille, 274
  DiGeorge, 266
  Noonan, 271
  scimitar, 408
  Williams, 274
  Wolff-Parkinson-White. *See* Wolff-Parkinson-
    White syndrome

Systemic blood flow
  Fick method for calculation of, 94
  shunt detection and, 72–73
  transposition of great arteries and, 311
Systemic vascular resistance, 90
Systemic venous anomaly, 411–417
  of inferior vena cava, 415–417
  of superior vena cava, 411–415
Systemic venous system embryogenesis, 411,
    412
Systolic pressure, 84
  aortopulmonary window and, 258
  double inlet ventricle and, 360
  patent ductus arteriosus and, 253

Tachycardia
  ectopic, 135
  reentrant, 135
  supraventricular. See Supraventricular
    tachycardia
  ventricular. See Ventricular tachycardia
  wide QRS, 122
Tamponade, 86
Taussig-Bing anomaly
  coarctation of aorta and, 394
  double outlet right ventricle and, 302, 304,
    305, 306, 307
  transposition of great arteries and, 324–325
Teflon catheter, 178
Tetralogy of Fallot, 285–294
  anatomy of, 285
  angiocardiography in, 288–293
  angiography in, 107, 288–293
  arterial pressure in, 285–286
  associated lesions in, 293–294, 298
  catheterization indications in, 286
  catheterization technique for, 286–287
  cautions for, 294
  diagram of, 286
  electrophysiology in, 287–288
  flow-directed balloon catheter manipulation
    in, 66
  hemodynamic considerations in, 18–20,
    285–286
  hemodynamic evaluation of, 287, 295
  interventional catheterization in, 288
  with pulmonary atresia, 294–298, 295–298
  pulmonary valve stenosis and, 274
Tetralogy of Fallot with pulmonary atresia,
    angiocardiography in, 294–298
Thermal-dilution catheter, 24
Thermal environment for newborn, 5–6, 8
Thermodilution method, 98–99. See also
    Indicator dilution method
  catheter for, 24
Thorazine. See Chlorpromazine
Thromboembolism, 204, 206–207
Thrombosis, 204, 206–207

arterial, 204–205
  balloon embolization and, 199
  transseptal catheterization and, 175
  venous, 206
Tissue adhesive, 201
Tolazoline
  shunt determination with oxygen
    administration and, 74
  ventricular septal defect and, 232
Toxicity of adriamycin, 176
Tracheal compression, 422–424
Transcatheter vascular occlusion, 185–202
  balloon embolization in, 198–201
  ductus arteriosus and, 185–194. See also
    Ductus arteriosus catheter occlusion
  Gianturco coils and, 194–198
  particulate embolization and, 201
  tissue adhesive and, 201
Transducer, 81–82
  Gould-Statham P-23-ID, 81
  strain gauge, 81
Transducer pack, 15
Transplantation, cardiac, 176
Transposition of great arteries, 309–326
  anatomy of, 309–310
  angiocardiography in, 310, 319–324
  angiography in, 107
  associated anomalies in, 324–326
  balloon atrial septostomy in, 147
  catheterization indications in, 312
  catheterization technique for, 313–318
  cautions for, 326
  corrected. See Corrected transposition of
    great arteries
  diagram of, 309
  flow-directed balloon catheter manipulation
    in, 66
  hemodynamic considerations in, 310–312
  hemodynamic evaluation of, 318–319
  pulmonary valve stenosis and, 274
Transseptal catheterization, 171–176
  blade atrial septostomy and, 153
  catheter introduction in, 173
  complications of, 175–176
  development of, 24
  equipment for, 171–172
  indications for, 171
  interatrial septum puncture in, 173–175
  intramyocardial infiltration in, 175
  long-sheath technique in, 175
  Mullins catheter in, 154, 172, 173
  preparation for, 172–173
  via superior vena cava, 175
Transseptal needle of Ross and Brockenbrough,
    171, 173
Tricuspid valve
  Ebstein's anomaly of. See Ebstein's anomaly
  pulmonary atresia and, 277

Tricuspid valve atresia, 345–352
  anatomy of, 345
  angiocardiography in, 350–351
  associated lesions in, 351–352
  catheterization indications in, 346–347
  catheterization technique for, 347–349
  cautions for, 352
  diagram of, 346
  hemodynamic considerations in, 345–346
  hemodynamic evaluation of, 349–350
  ventriculoarterial discordance and, 346
Tricuspid valve regurgitation
  atrioventricular septal defect and, 245
  Ebstein's anomaly and, 338
  phonocardiography and, 143
  pulmonary atresia and, 277, 282
  pulmonary valve stenosis and, 273
  transposition of great arteries and, 328–329
Tricuspid valve rupture, 150
Tricuspid valve stenosis, 338
Truncus arteriosus, 261–266
  anatomy of, 261–262
  angiocardiography in, 263–265
  angiography and, 107
  aortopulmonary window and, 259
  associated anomalies in, 265–266
  catheterization indications in, 262–263
  catheterization technique for, 263
  cautions for, 266
  hemodynamic considerations in, 262
  hemodynamic evaluation of, 263
  valve in, 263–265

Umbilical catheter, 313
Umbilical vessels in cutdown, 41–44
Underdamped pressure tracing, 84

Valve
  aortic. See Aortic valve entries
  atrioventricular. See Atrioventricular valve
    atresia
  pulmonary. See Pulmonary valve; Pulmonary
    valve entries
  tricuspid. See Tricuspid valve entries
Valvotomy, balloon. See Balloon angioplasty
Vascular complications of catheterization,
  204–207
Vascular obstruction of airway, 419–435
  anatomy in, 419–420, 421, 422
  angiocardiography in, 424–433
  catheterization indications in, 420–424
  catheterization technique for, 424
  cautions for, 433–435
Vascular occlusion, transcatheter. See
  Transcatheter vascular occlusion
Vascular resistance. See Resistance
Vascular ring. See Vascular obstruction of
  airway

Vein tearing in catheterization, 206
Vena cava
  absent intrahepatic portion of inferior,
    55–56, 415–417
  superior. See Superior vena cava
Venotomy, 48
Venous oxygen saturation, 72
  patent ductus arteriosus and, 253
Venous spasm, 206
Venous system
  catheterization complications of, 204, 206
  embryogenesis of, 411, 412
  systemic anomaly of, 411–417
Ventricle
  double inlet. See Double inlet ventricle
  double outlet right. See Double outlet right
    ventricle
Ventricular angiogram, 109
Ventricular arrhythmia
  electrophysiology of, 137
  tetralogy of Fallot and, 288
Ventricular dysfunction, Ebstein's anomaly and,
  338
Ventricular end-diastolic pressure
  atrial septal defect and, 220
  left, 84, 85, 86
Ventricular fibrillation, 137
Ventricular filling in atrial septal defect, 217
Ventricular hypertension, 268
Ventricular hypertrophy, 400
Ventricular inflow obstruction in atrial septal
  defect, 217
Ventricular outflow obstruction, 88
  in pulmonary valve stenosis, 269
Ventricular outflow tract
  atrioventricular septal defect and, 245
  blade atrial septostomy perforation of, 153
  pulmonary valve stenosis and, 274
Ventricular pacing, 132–134
Ventricular pressure, 84, 85
  atrial septal defect and, 217
  coarctation of aorta and, 393
  pulmonary valve atresia and, 279
  pulmonary valve stenosis and, 269
  tetralogy of Fallot and, 285–286, 290–291
Ventricular septal defect, 227–240
  anatomy of, 227
  angiocardiography in, 232–235
  angiography in, 229
  in aortopulmonary window, 257
  associated lesions in, 235–238, 239
  atrial septal defect and, 225
  balloon occlusion of ductus arteriosus in,
    232
  catheterization indications in, 228–229
  catheterization technique for, 229–230
  cautions for, 238
  classification of, 227

Ventricular septal defect (*cont.*)
  in coarctation of aorta, 393, 394
  corrected transposition of great arteries and, 330, 332
  in double outlet right ventricle, 301, 302–303, 303
  in Ebstein's anomaly, 341–342
  flow-directed balloon catheter manipulation in, 67
  hemodynamic considerations in, 227–228
  hemodynamic evaluation of, 230–231
  in patent ductus arteriosus, 251
  pharmacology and, 231–232
  subaortic, 303
  in transposition of great arteries, 309
  in truncus arteriosus, 265
Ventricular septum
  angiography of, 245, 246
  atrioventricular septal defect and, 241, 245, 246
  pulmonary atresia with intact. *See* Pulmonary valve atresia with intact ventricular septum
  pulmonary stenosis with. *See* Pulmonary valve stenosis
Ventricular tachycardia
  programmed stimulation and, 137

recurrent, 122
sustained, 138
Ventricular volume overload, 407
Ventriculoarterial concordance, in double inlet ventricle, 357
Ventriculoarterial discordance, in tricuspid atresia, 346
Ventriculoatrial interval, 135
Ventriculography
  Lehman catheter for, 21
  right, 108
  transseptal catheterization and, 172
  ventricular septal defect and, 232, 233
Venturi effect, 269

Warming mattress, 6, 8
Whetstone bridge, 81
Williams syndrome, 274
Withdrawal pressure in anomalous pulmonary venous return, 403
Wolff-Parkinson-White syndrome
  corrected transposition of great arteries and, 329
  electrophysiology in, 127
  supraventricular arrhythmias in, 135, 136

Xylocaine. *See* Lidocaine